Hydrotherapy:
Principles and Practice

Long have the praises of water been sung. It has cleansed cult and creed, cured pysche and soma.
Christa and Jost Benedum

To accomplish great things, we must not only act but also dream, not only plan but also believe.

Anon.

Hydrotherapy:
Principles and Practice

Edited by

Margaret Reid Campion

Grad. Dip Physiotherapy (UK) MCSP
Consultant in Hydrotherapy
Formerly, Lecturer, School of Physiotherapy,
Curtin University of Technology,
and Hydrotherapy Consultant,
Lifecare Rehabilitation Centre,
Perth, Western Australia

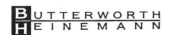
BUTTERWORTH
HEINEMANN

Butterworth-Heinemann
Linacre House, Jordan Hill, Oxford OX2 8DP
A division of Reed Educational & Professional Publishing Ltd

 A member of the Reed Elsevier plc group

OXFORD   BOSTON   JOHANNESBURG
MELBOURNE   NEW DELHI   SINGAPORE

First published 1997

© Margaret Reid Campion

British Library Cataloguing in Publication Data
Hydrotherapy: principles and practice
  1. Hydrotherapy
  I. Reid Campion, Margaret
  615.8'53
  ISBN 0 7506 2261 X

Campion, Margaret Reid.
  Hydrotherapy: principles and practice/Margaret Reid Campion.   p. cm.
  Includes bibliographical references and index.
  ISBN 0 7506 2261 X
  1 Hydrotherapy. I.   Title.
  [DNLM: 1   Hydrotherapy.   2   Health Promotion.   WB 520 C196hc]
  RM811.C35.
  615.8'53—dc20

                                                              96–7479
                                                                  CIP

Typeset by Interactive Sciences Ltd, Gloucester
Printed and bound in Great Britain by Martins the Printers, Berwick upon Tweed

Contents

This book is dedicated in gratitude to

'Mac'

the late James McMillan MBE
who devised the Halliwick Method providing
ideas and techniques for water activity to
physiotherapists worldwide.

Preface

There is a place for therapy and recreation for all who suffer a disability, providing physical, psychological and social benefits. The guiding light in preparing this book has been the belief of my colleagues and myself in hydrotherapy. It is our wish to advance activity in water as a means of rehabilitation in its own right. Our aim is to provide a definitive but practical account of both paediatric and adult hydrotherapy, including aspects such as pool design and the pool environment.

Water is a wonderful medium for exercise, offering exciting opportunities for movement not available within traditional land-based exercise programmes. Different forces apply in water. Buoyancy, metacentre and the rotational effects provide scope for specialized techniques. Turbulence in water can be appreciated in a manner not possible in air and the weight of water means that it can be leant against and used as a force against which an individual can work.

Early treatment in a weight relieving situation is possible and the warmth and support of the water provide beneficial effects. A greater perception of rotation with the need to control this demands considerable balance and coordination as well as precise muscle work.

The contributors to the adult section have provided a practical guide to hydrotherapy for a variety of conditions. Recent developments in spinal mobilization in water form part of the text and newer ideas such as 'Watsu' are indicated. The chapters are linked by an awareness of the Halliwick Method's ideas and techniques. Even when applying the 'conventional' method or Bad Ragaz patterns, there is an underlying perception of using water very specifically based on the critical nature of water, shape and density and an awareness of the effects of these on the human being immersed in water and on the ways to handle the disabled in water – all themes and techniques advocated in the teaching and application of 'Halliwick'.

The paediatric section provides detailed information on the Halliwick Method but throughout the text the reader is advised to appreciate its application to the treatment of adults.

It is hoped that all this will provoke both undergraduate and postgraduate physiotherapists to give careful consideration to hydrotherapy and to how the effective conduct of treatment programmes in water can be enhanced. Through a wider knowledge of water, its potential, the techniques and skills, improved assessment and recording, the advantages and benefits of hydrotherapy as a valuable treatment modality may be recognized by doctors and physiotherapists as part of the total rehabilitation programme for innumerable conditions.

Acknowledgements

In the second edition of *Hydrotherapy in Paediatrics*, the inspiration provided by Neil, who had a marked visual defect and severe hypotonia delaying his development, who when launching himself from a 'sitting' position on the poolside, submerged completely and surfaced laughing uproariously, was truly superb.

Life is made up of such inspirational moments. It is not only children who bring joys of that kind. Many adults have achieved unknown potential in the water and gladdened the hearts and minds of all. The disabled who provide such inspiration teach us all a great deal and make every effort worthwhile. To all our 'swimmers', young and old alike, our thanks are extended – our gratitude recorded for accepting our ministrations, for teaching and helping us so much.

My personal thanks are extended to each of the authors for their acceptance of the challenge and their efforts in contributing to this book. Their personal acknowledgements and thanks follow their chapters.

To Caroline Makepeace, Tim Brown and Catherine Zank-McKelvey and to all at Butterworth-Heineman – my grateful thanks for their support and encouragement without which I would have faltered. A number of my colleagues among them Alison Skinner, Ann Thomson and 'Jega' Jegasothy have sustained me in ways which are perhaps only apparent to me and I am more than grateful.

Last but by no means least I would like to record my thanks to all the partners and families of the co-authors who supported and accepted the necessary deprivations of the writers as they met the demands of putting pen to paper to meet the deadlines thus contributing to this publication.

Margaret Reid Campion
Editor and Author

Contributors

Aliçon Bennie, GradDip Physiotherapy

Aliçon has worked in three Spinal Injuries units over the last 13 years including nearly six years as Superintendent Physiotherapist of the Hydrotherapy Pool at Stoke Mandeville Hospital. She also coached the Great Britain Disabled Swimming Team for 10 years, including three Paralympic Games. She has been involved in the Hydrotherapy Association of Chartered Physiotherapists and worked on the production of *Hydrotherapy Standards of Good Practice* published by the Chartered Society of Physiotherapy.

Margaret Reid Campion, GradDip Physiotherapy (UK), MCSP

After qualification Margaret undertook general work in a number of fields. Specializing in paediatrics and hydrotherapy she worked in Special Schools and was later appointed Deputy Superintendent at the Hospital for Sick Children, Great Ormond Street, London before leaving England and working in Western Australia. In 1978 she joined the teaching staff of the School of Physiotherapy as a lecturer. Travelling and teaching in Australia and many countries world-wide – in addition to teaching under- and postgraduate students – are all part of Margaret's life. After retiring from the University she spent four years as Hydrotherapy Consultant but continued travelling. She returned to England on a visit and decided to stay and be with her family and in her 'milieu'. The working pattern continues and the air miles are still clocking up. Author of *Hydrotherapy in Paediatrics*, author/editor of *Adult Hydrotherapy – A Practical Approach* she has contributed to Duffield's *Exercise in Water* and written extensively. Although hydrotherapy and related topics are of especial interest to Margaret she says she has other loves, such as all forms of movement, women's health, paediatrics and neurology.

Georgina Evans, MCSP

Georgina, who worked in rehabilitation before specializing in obstetrics and gynaecology, is currently physiotherapy manager at the Acland Hospital in Oxford. Since 1990 she has been on the executive committee and the education subcommittee of the Association of Chartered Physiotherapists in Women's Health; she edited the Association's journal from 1990 to 1993 and was responsible for its new *Aquanatal Guidelines* in 1995. She and a midwife colleague have led aquanatal classes in Oxford since 1991; together they have run various training courses for aquanatal instructors, including an ENB-approved course for midwives. She has three children of her own.

David Fitzgerald, GradDip Manip Ther, MCSP

Having a background in mechanical engineering David graduated from Cardiff School of Physiotherapy in 1988 and completed a postgraduate diploma in Manipulative Therapy from Curtin University, Western Australia in 1991. As a member of the International Association for the Study of Pain, David has a particular interest in the treatment of chronic pain by physiotherapy intervention. His clinical practice involves a cross-section of people from casual to elite athletes, chronic dysfunction and work-related upper limb disorders. A common theme in the treatment of these conditions is the use of therapeutic exercise either on land or in water.

Sue Gray, MSc, MCSP, SRP, HT

Sue has worked in her present post for six years. Her work has been in paediatric and adult neurological physiotherapy for a large part of her 18-year career. She is particularly interested in the intuitive approach to therapeutic treatment and the idea that movement is an experience rather than a technique. She is nearing the end of an MSc in Rehabilitation Counselling which she pursued because of her interest in the psychological effects of neurological disability.

Jan Hill, BAppSC (physio), DipPty

Jan has been involved with Hydrotherapy since the early 1970s while working in the UK, and finally undertook the Bath Hydrotherapy

Course in 1975/6. Since then she has been involved in developing courses and lecturing for the Australian Physiotherapy Association (Victoria branch) Certificate Hydrotherapy Course since its inception in 1988, as well as for Vic Levin. Jan also manages a physiotherapy and hydrotherapy department at Caulfield General Medical Centre, has her own hydrotherapy private practice and consults on hydrotherapy issues and pool design. For the last two years she has been Chairperson of the Hydrotherapy Special Interest Group of the Australian Physiotherapy Association (Victoria branch). Aside from developing Hydrotherapy Jan has other interests, in neurology movement awareness and manual handling.

G. 'Jega' Jegsothy, Associateship Physiotherapy, MAPA

'Jega' qualified in 1972 and for four years worked as a physiotherapist in the University Hospital, Kuala Lumpur, Malaysia. Since returning to Western Australia, where she trained, Jega has worked in the Neurosurgical Unit at Royal Perth Rehabilitation Hospital and has been Senior Physiotherapist to the 28-bed ward for eight years. Her hydrotherapy programmes have some very innovative features.

Christine Lee, BAppSc (Physio)

Christine has been involved in hydrotherapy since 1987 when she joined the staff at Fremantle Hospital. In 1988 she attended the hydrotherapy course in Melbourne. While travelling in 1993 and 1994 she attended the Bath hydrotherapy course in England. She is now working in private practice at Southcare Physiotherapy and Como Physiotherapy, Perth, Western Australia.

Anne M. Levin, Bsc PT, HT, MCPA

Anne practises at the Baycrest Centre for Geriatric Care in Toronto, Canada. She is the co-ordinator for the Arthritis Education/Exercise Programme, and has a strong interest in health promotion. Anne is involved in clinical work, programme development, research, consultation and education. She teaches hydrotherapy across Canada. Anne holds a lecturer status appointment in the Department of Physical Therapy, Faculty of Medicine, University of Toronto. In 1993, Anne was awarded a fellowship from the World Health Organization which enabled her to obtain her certification in hydrotherapy in Bath, England.

Rosalie Mori, BAppSc (Physio), MAPA

After qualifying in 1981 Rosalie worked at Albany Regional Hospital treating orthopaedic out-patients and in-patients, both adults and children. A two-year spell at a Special School in Perth followed. Here she treated the physically handicapped pupils at the school as well as children with MCD from the surrounding community. In March 1984, Rosalie returned to Albany as the Paediatric Physiotherapist. She works in the hospital, in homes, schools and the community in general which means her case load is very diverse.

Lynette Tinsley, DipPty (WA), MAPA

Lyn is currently involved with treatment and patient education of rheumatic diseased patients as well as teaching undergraduate and postgraduate physiotherapists, and other health professionals. She has worked in varied posts in Western Australia and is presently Senior Physiotherapist to the Rheumatic Diseases Unit at Royal Perth Rehabilitation Hospital. Her overseas experience was gained in London, Norway and Denmark. In 1981 she was awarded a Churchill Fellowship and travelled in the UK and Scandinavia. Ankylosing Spondylosis is an area of special interest to Lyn.

Introduction to hydrotherapy

Margaret Reid Campion

Hydrotherapy as a modality for rehabilitation has a long history and is as important today as it was in the past. With the current upsurge in the popularity of hydrotherapy, physiotherapists are encouraged to use water, making the most of its unique properties. Hydrotherapeutic techniques must be learnt and new ideas explored and developed.

Water is fun! The majority of people enjoy water and it is an integral part of life. Water allows us all to achieve marvellous feats of movement which can be performed on land only with difficulty if at all.

The word hydrotherapy is derived from the Greek words *hydor* (water) and *therapeia* (healing) (Duffield, 1976, p. 1). Hydrotherapy is as old as the history of mankind (Finnerty and Corbitt, 1960, p. 1), and information on activity in water for both therapeutic and recreational purposes has been documented despite the fact that the popularity of this modality has fluctuated through the ages. One authority (Behrend, 1960) believes that the use of hydrotherapy antedates that of all other modalities employed in physical medicine. The past shows us that many forms of treatment once greeted with enthusiasm have long since been abandoned, while hydrotherapy has continued even though the rationale is largely empirical. But this picture is changing. New knowledge regarding the physiology of hydrotherapy and new techniques using patterns of movement adapted to water and more water-specific exercises are ensuring that hydrotherapy is becoming increasingly accepted as a medium for rehabilitation in its own right. That it should be considered thus is, in the author's opinion, correct. To go into water – one of only two environments available to the human – is a unique experience. Here the body is simultaneously acted upon by two forces – gravity (or downthrust) and buoyancy (or upthrust) – providing us with the possibility of three-dimensional exercise not available in the medium of air, and allowing movement and non-weight-bearing activities to occur before they are possible on land.

With greater understanding of the advantages of activity in water, increasing numbers of facilities are being provided, and physiotherapists are becoming both interested and skilled in the application of techniques and more aware of the benefits of swimming as an adjunct to fitness and performance generally.

HISTORICAL BACKGROUND

By necessity this is a brief review of the use of water for therapeutic purposes throughout the ages. The study of the historical background of both the curative and recreational aspects of water is fascinating. It has been dealt with by a number of authors (Wyman, 1944; Krizek, 1963; Price, 1981) and the interested reader is referred to their work.

The history of hydrotherapy as a modality used in physical medicine goes back many thousands of years. At which moment in time hydrotherapy was first used therapeutically is not known, but records dating back to 2400 BC suggest that Proto-Indian culture made hygienic installations and that the early Egyptians, Assyrians and Mohammedans used mineral waters for curative purposes. The Hindus in 1500 BC used water to combat fevers.

Most peoples in ancient times respected or worshipped running water, especially springs of pure water. Japanese medical men, the Chinese as well as the Greeks and Romans used baths long before the coming of Christ. Homer suggested the use of warm baths for reducing fatigue, for promoting the healing of wounds and for combating dejection and low spirits.

The Greeks were among the first to appreciate the relationship between physical and mental well-being. They developed centres near springs and rivers using them for bathing and recreation. By 500 BC the transition from mysticism and cult to a logical use of water for physical treatment had occurred. The Romans, with their skills in construction, developed and expanded upon the Greek system of athletics followed by a cold plunge; they produced a series of baths ranging from the caldarium through the tepidarium to the frigidarium. The baths were centres where intellectual, recreational activities, health and hygiene were pursued.

Around AD 339 some of these baths were used solely for healing purposes and treatment was indicated first of all for symptoms of rheumatic disease, paralysis and the after effects of injuries. Burns were treated in prolonged baths. There was a decrease in the use of the baths as the Roman Empire declined. The standards of hygiene and morals were lowered. Thus, the early Christians banned the use of the public baths, and the church in the Middle Ages condemned the use of physical forces, such as water, as being associated with paganism. The suppression of hydrotherapy in the West was sustained more or less through medieval times but by the fifteenth, sixteenth and seventeenth centuries the use of water for healing purposes acquired some recognition from a few European physicians.

Early pioneers of hydrotherapy were Sir John Floyer who wrote a treatise in 1697 'An enquiry into the right use and abuse of hot, cold and temperate baths'; John Wesley, the founder of Methodism, who published a book on hydrotherapy in 1747, called it 'An easy and natural way of curing most diseases'; and Dr Wright who in 1779 published a work on the use of cold in small pox. In the main, however, the academic clinicians at this time were busy diagnosing diseases and working on wards and

in the dissecting rooms. Natural therapy hardly concerned them at all. A Silesian peasant, Vincent Pressnitz, had plenty of time and plenty of water. He set up outdoor baths in a woodland setting and placed his clients on treatment programmes that included cold douches, massage and chopping wood. The medical profession viewed his success with concern and tried to put a stop to the craze. During this period a Bavarian priest, Sebastian Kniepp, became well known for his water cures. In America, Dr Joel Shaw developed a more systematic water cure at his hydropathic establishment in New York. Professor Winterwitz of Vienna dedicated his life to the scientific study of the practice of hydratics and gave an accurate foundation to modern hydrotherapy.

Advances in the use of water continued in Europe but America lagged behind during the nineteenth century. However, the warm bath gradually gained popularity and was used in decubiti and other surgical, neuralgic and psychiatric conditions (Kamenetz, 1963). Dr Simon Baruch who worked with Professor Winterwitz furthered the use of hydrotherapy through his work which revolved round the fact that heat or cold was conveyed to the central nervous system by the cutaneous nerves and thus became reflected in the motor pathways. Hydrogymnastics or underwater exercise in warm water was advised in the late nineteenth century. However, it was not until the first Hubbard tank was made in the 1920s that therapeutic pool exercises really began to be developed systematically.

The two world wars, especially the second, highlighted the need for the use of water for exercise and the maintenance of fitness and acted as precursors for the current resurgence of the use of the hydrotherapy pool using total immersion as a means of rehabilitation for a wide range of conditions (Harris, 1963).

Today, the ever increasing popularity and value of hydrotherapy appears to be highlighted by an upsurge in research into many different aspects of water, the physiology of exercise in water and so on. Recognition of the ways in which the characteristics and properties of water may be used to create techniques that enhance activity in the water as an integral part of the total physical and psychological care of many and varied conditions will ensure the place of hydrotherapy in their total rehabilitation.

REFERENCES

Behrend H.J. (1960). Foreword. In *Hydrotherapy* (F.G. Finnerty and T. Corbitt, eds), London: Ungar.

Duffield M.H. (1979). *Exercise in Water*, London: Baillière Tindall and Cassell.

Finnerty F.G. and Corbitt T. (1960). *Hydrotherapy*, London: Ungar.

Harris R. (1963). Therapeutic pools. In *Medical Hydrology* (S. Licht, ed.), New Haven: Elizabeth Licht Publisher.

Kamenetz H.L. (1963). History of American spas and hydrotherapy. In *Medical Hydrology* (S. Licht, ed.), New Haven: Elizabeth Licht Publisher.

Krizek V. (1963). History of balenotherapy. In *Medical Hydrology* (S. Licht, ed.), New Haven: Elizabeth Licht Publisher.

Price R. (1981). Hydrotherapy in England 1840–70, *Medical History*, 25: 269–80.

Wyman J. (1944). *Hydrotherapy in Medical Physics, 1* (O. Glazer, ed.), Chicago: Year Book Publishers, pp. 619–22.

Principles

INTRODUCTION

This section of the book reviews hydrotherapy in general and sets the scene, as it were, for the ensuing sections and chapters. In discussing the physiological, therapeutic and psychological effects and benefits of activity in water the author has endeavoured to show the scope water has for therapy and recreation.

The ideas on pool design, equipment and maintenance are based on experiences gained from working in a vast range of hydrotherapy and recreational pools throughout the world. In offering these an attempt has been made to avoid many pitfalls. Since numerous authors have produced works on hydrodynamic laws and the mechanics of fluids, only those principles particularly relevant to hydrotherapy and to the Halliwick Method are discussed in this text. Additionally, ideas for the introduction of people to water in order to enhance their treatment and/or their recreation are presented, and, both the importance of assessment and recording, and a method of achieving these are explored.

1

The physiological, therapeutic and psychological effects of activity in water

Margaret Reid Campion

To go into water is a unique experience (p. i) affording everyone opportunities of widening their knowledge and skills physically, mentally and psychologically.

The uniqueness of water lies mainly in its buoyancy, which relieves stress on weight-bearing joints and permits movement to take place with reduced gravitational forces, thus non-weight-bearing activities can be commenced before they are possible on land.

The physiological effects of exercise combined with those brought about by the warmth of the water are one of the advantages of activity in this medium. The outcome of immersion in warm water is similar in adults and children and is related to body temperature, circulation and the severity of exercise, with variations allowing for size.

The body possesses mechanisms for regulating its heat, and the maintenance of balance between the production of heat and heat loss requires fine adjustment (Chaffee and Lytle, 1980). A distinction has to be made between the core temperature of the body and that of the periphery (Janig, 1978), but under standard conditions body temperature in man remains remarkably constant. Fine diurnal changes in body temperature do occur throughout the day and vary for different parts of the body. Factors such as exercise, emotional disturbance and extremes of environmental temperatures may affect it, as well as age and sex (Downey, 1971). It is suggested by several authorities that the temperature of the skin is 33.3°C (92°F), though this may decrease in the most distal parts of the extremities (Finnerty and Corbitt, 1960; Bierman, 1963) (p. 7).

The therapeutic effects of exercise in water relate to:

(a) the relief of pain and muscle spasm,
(b) the maintenance or increase in range of motion of joints,
(c) the strengthening of weak muscles and an increase in their tolerance to exercise,
(d) the re-education of paralysed muscles,
(e) the improvement of the circulation,
(f) the encouragement of functional activities,
(g) the maintenance and improvement of balance, co-ordination and posture.

In addition, water provides the potential for exercise in three dimensions which cannot be achieved on land. There is also the possibility of considerable perceptual stimulation:

(a) visually,
(b) aurally,
(c) via the skin proprioceptors,
(d) by heat.

The eyes have to accommodate to the constantly changing levels of the water due to movement of the liquid in relation to the poolside above the surface. When the ears are submerged there is greater pressure on them than there is in air. The skin reacts to different temperatures as well as appreciating the all-embracing effect of water on the body when immersed. Turbulent effects are initially felt by the skin, and when a limb is moving through the water the greatest appreciation of turbulence will be in the distal part.

Also, from a psychological standpoint there is much to recommend activity in water. Most of the information regarding the use of water i* the treatment of mental illness throughout the ages came from disciplines such as sociology and anthropology. In more recent times the sedative effect of warm water and the value of swimming programmes for those persons affected by mental illness have been recognized (Wilson and Kasch, 1963; Kraus, 1973). From a humanistic point of view, the social and psychological significance that may be attached to the ability to swim is undoubtedly considerable.

The person who can swim and participate in other aquatic activities has gained a social asset. This ability places them on an equal footing with other members of the family and with friends, whether able-bodied or disabled. They can compete at a similar level. The ability to be independent in water, to achieve skills that may be difficult or impossible on land, can only have favourable and lasting psychological effects which boost confidence and morale, and these may well be carried over into life on land.

TRAINING FOR HYDROTHERAPY

The training of physiotherapists of hydrotherapy skills should reflect the upsurge in interest in and use of the modality in many conditions.

A wide disparity exists in the amount of undergraduate training in hydrotherapy between the schools of physiotherapy worldwide. Minimum hours covering theory and practical work are recommended in some countries, and placement of the student with physiotherapists who have expertise in hydrotherapy is also advocated.

The limitations of undergraduate hydrotherapy training have implications for postgraduate study and qualification. The specific knowledge and skills should cover the subjects related to:

- the mechanics of fluids and hydrodynamical laws
- the critical nature of water
- the application and effects of the above on the human being in water
- the physiological effects of immersion
- the therapeutic effects of hydrotherapy
- the theory and application of techniques
- methods of promoting movement and acquiring independence in water
- assessment and recording procedures

- safety and emergency procedures
- care and maintenance of the water and pool areas.

Without adequate knowledge and skills and an ability to control their own bodies in water against any disturbing factors physiotherapists will not provide effective treatments and may produce tension, anxiety and adverse reactions in their patients.

CLINICAL STANDARDS FOR HYDROTHERAPY

Some countries and Physiotherapy Associations have developed clinical standards for hydrotherapy providing guidelines for a minimum standard.

Such standards cover client/staff safety; safety in relation to the facilities; the physiotherapist's knowledge and skills; professional conduct and quality assurance. The subdivisions of these standards are comprehensive and include all aspects of hydrotherapy and such a document should be readily available in all relevant schools, departments and centres providing hydrotherapy.

REFERENCES

Bierman W. (1963). Physiologic changes produced by heat. In *Medical Hydrology* (S. Licht, ed.), New Haven: Elizabeth Licht, pp. 78–116.

Chaffee E.E. and Lytle I.M. (1980). *Basic Physiology and Anatomy*, 4th edn, Philadelphia: J.B. Lippincott.

Downey J. (1971). Physiology of temperature regulation in man. In *Physiological Bases of Rehabilitation Medicine* (J. Downey and R. Darling, eds), London: W.B. Saunders, pp. 137–148.

Finnerty F.G. and Corbitt T. (1960). *Hydrotherapy*, London: Ungar.

Janig W. (1978). The autonomic nervous system, Section 8.5: The hypothalamus, osmolarity of the extracellular space, and the endocrine glands. In *Fundamentals of Neurophysiology*, 2nd edn (R.F. Schmidt, ed.), New York: Springer-Verlag, pp. 250–260.

Kraus R. (1973). *Therapeutic Recreation Services – Principles and Practices*. Philadelphia: W.B. Saunders.

Wilson I.H. and Kasch F.W. (1963). Medical aspects of swimming. In *Medical Hydrology* (S. Licht, ed.), New Haven: Elizabeth Licht, pp. 229–238.

2

Key features of pool design and caring for the pool

Margaret Reid Campion

The environment in which water activity takes place has a considerable bearing on all pool users.

However, practical considerations are vital when planning and designing a pool and its facilities and must take precedence over excessive aesthetic ideas for design. The simpler the design and construction the more useful the pool becomes for both specific therapy and more general recreational activity.

Assessing the need takes into account the disabilities of those who will use the pool and those of other groups who may also wish to avail themselves of it, such as water exercise programmes, disabled swimming groups, ante- and post-natal groups and other rehabilitation centres desirous of providing hydrotherapy.

In practice an uncluttered rectangular below-ground-level pool is the most advantageous; its dimensions will be determined by the size of the site and the finance available.

There is little or no need for a specifically designed pool when taking children into water. Facilities that are available may be used; the advantages of deeper water usually outweighing those of a shallower depth (p. 6).

The following discussion is intended to provide general information and to outline major points about pool design which have evolved from the experience of working in a wide variety of pools throughout the world.

The main factors for consideration are:

- pool design and dimensions
- type, size, shape, depth, floor and entry
- temperatures and ventilation
- equipment
- lighting
- facilities
- surfaces
- noise factors
- staffing
- care and maintenance
- safety and emergency equipment
- costs and costing.

POOL DESIGN AND DIMENSIONS

Having assessed the need, the type of pool requires consideration. The main options are below ground, below-ground deck-level, semi-raised or raised. From experience the desired option would be below ground with or without deck-level construction.

Should a below-ground pool without a deck level be chosen the height of the bathside from the surface of the water must be kept to a minimum. This means a distance of no more than 15.24 cm (6 inches) and preferably 7.62 cm (3 inches). Too great a height decreases the ease of entry and exit over the side and increases the difficulties of handling in an emergency. While a deck-level assembly has obvious advantages – easy exiting, a decrease in turbulence and no scum line – unless the surrounds of the pool are correctly constructed the concourse can be awash compromising safety and leading to unclean water being washed back into the pool. In an extreme situation a 15.24 cm (6 inch) brick wall had to be erected on the concourse side of the deck-level grill to prevent an excess of water from the pool flowing over the walkways making them unsafe and to prevent unclean water returning to the pool. The small wall seriously hindered entry to and exit from the water.

The use of a sunken pool means that the physiotherapist must be in the pool while carrying out treatments. This certainly provides the optimum situation for treatment and is considered by this author to be incumbent on the physiotherapist who provides hydrotherapy treatment. It is inappropriate to ask people to go into the water with all the potential risks and not enter with them to offer assurance and to help with any difficulties with balance and control the person may experience.

Some sunken pools are constructed with a well on one side designed for use by the staff but the physiotherapist should not be lured by this as once again safety is compromised. It is also not unknown for pool users to fall into the pit.

The *dimensions* of the pool cover size, shape and depth. The pool should be large enough for the users to carry out a full rehabilitation programme from total support on a plinth through ambulation to swimming and other recreational activities (Skinner and Thomson, 1983).

The dimensions are frequently governed by the size of the site and the finance available as well as the proposed usage. It is suggested by Whitelock and Barefoot (1993) among others that the minimum space for each person is 2.50 m by 2.25 m. In practice pools no smaller than 9.24 m (30 feet) by 4.57 m (15 feet) provide a good working size for approximately eight people and can be used for most activities including swimming; when possible a pool of larger dimensions should be constructed.

The *shape* of the pool should be simple. The most common shape is that of a rectangle and is strongly advocated. A square pool leaves one with 'nowhere to go' and generally causes adverse comment from the users. Pools that are designed with curves, for example a kidney shape, are impractical for treatment and for swimming; above all they produce increased turbulence which can be most disturbing and compromises balance. All movement in water produces turbulence but any item such as curves, off which the water 'bounces', makes the situation worse.

When considering the *depth* of water the vertical balance of the user is important. At two-thirds a person's height, that is at the lower end of the sternum, vertical balance becomes critical. At this buoyancy neutral point it is possible to stabilize the body. For an optimum working depth a further 15.24 cm (6 inches) of water, bringing the level to shoulder height, is adequate. It is suggested that a depth that varies between 0.84 m and 1.42 m is ideal. The shallower depth may be useful where children are concerned when walking forms part of the child's rehabilitation programme, but the advantages of deeper water usually outweigh those of the shallower depth. If a base is required for the child the physiotherapist can provide this by using the stable 'sitting' position, the child using the physiotherapist's thighs as a platform.

A variety of pool floors are available; they may be level throughout, stepped or sloping. The latter provides the most satisfactory situation and gradients vary between 1 in 15 (Skinner and Thomson, 1983) through 1 in 20 (Reid Campion, 1991) to 1 in 30 (Davis and Harrison, 1988).

The advantage of a stepped floor is that it offers several depths, but the edge of each step must be clearly marked. The limitations are that however visible the markings there are risks of inadvertently stepping or slipping into deeper water with resultant anxiety for all, especially where a person's vision is deficient. When carrying out Bad Ragaz techniques, steps prove disconcerting as the physiotherapist, who has to move around the pool actively, finds the steps cramp that mobility and may bring about a loss of control.

The level overall type of floor allows freedom of movement over the whole pool area but it does not permit the use of different levels of water for exercise and can make non and partial weight-bearing exercise difficult or impossible. Skinner and Thomson (1983) suggest that a 1.1 m depth of water provides sufficient buoyancy but in some instances taller people are disadvantaged.

Some authorities advocate bays which provide space for individual exercise in a shallower depth. However, this author's experience of pools with bays is that they interrupt the working area of the pool, increase turbulence and that, among square, rectangular, circular and horseshoe shaped bays, none has proved satisfactory.

Entry to the pool can be by several methods. They are:

- steps
- ramps
- hoists
- over the side.

Steps leading into the pool should be situated at the shallow end and recessed so that the working area of the pool is kept clear. Skinner and Thomson (1983) advocate that the steps have 150 mm risers, be 300 mm in depth and the width of the steps should be 600 mm so that the rails on either side can be grasped. The front edges of the steps must be clearly defined preferably by different coloured tiles. Where a raised type of pool is in use it is advisable to have a platform at the top of the steps and another flight of steps down into the concourse.

Ramps take up considerable space and also tend to break up the water, increasing turbulence. They can, however, ease entry to the pool for wheelchair users. The gradient should be very shallow and the surface of the ramp must be non-slip.

The main types of hoists are:

- mechanical
- hydraulic
- electric

and can be fitted with a stretcher, a seat or both. Ideally they should be designed to be operated by one person.

Mechanical hoists are not so commonly used today but they can be of value in small pool areas or where finance is limited. Hydraulically operated hoists may be slow in lowering and raising and this can present a difficulty in an emergency when it is vital to remove the person from the water quickly.

Whatever type of hoist is used it must be sited at the shallower end of the pool and have a clear space surrounding it to allow for an uninterrupted 360° turn.

Entries over the side of the pool are described in the paediatric section; although all the entries shown there are applicable to adults and the aim should be for such entries to be undertaken by the person independently.

The pool surrounds need to be sufficiently wide to accommodate wheelchairs and stretchers which require a 2 m turning circle. This should be provided on at least two sides of the pool and such areas must be free of any hazards. Suitable grading of the non-slip surface will ensure that water drains away from the pool edge.

TEMPERATURE AND VENTILATION

Temperature of Water for Activity

When considering water temperature, the things to bear in mind are the type and severity of the exercise in addition to the duration of the activity. Whenever exercise is undertaken certain physiological effects occur. In water the physiological effects of exercise are combined with those brought about by the warmth of the water. In addition, the results of buoyancy and hydrostatic pressure must be considered when the whole body is immersed (Franchimont *et al.*, 1983).

The thermoregulatory system of the body needs to be efficient to cope with exercise in warm water. The hypothalamus responds to the stimulation of the cutaneous thermoreceptors or to the temperature of the blood passing through it. When immersed in water the natural mechanisms for losing heat, such as evaporation, are rendered largely ineffective, since only those parts of the body not under water can lose heat by sweating. As the patient exercises there is increased heating to compound further the problem of losing heat.

The body has elaborate mechanisms for the maintenance of thermal homeostasis. Heat dissipation is balanced against the heat gained from the body's metabolic activities and from the environment. The temperature of the human being is not uniform and varies with the body's ability to transfer heat from the area to which it is applied. Under normal circumstances the heat regulating mechanisms maintain the body temperature within narrow limits. In comfortable surroundings the skin temperature of the head and torso is 33.3°C (92°F) which according to Finnerty and Corbitt (1960) is the point of thermal indifference of the skin for water. On exposure to a hot environment subcutaneous temperatures rise most rapidly in the peripheral parts of the body so that the difference in temperature between the torso and the extremities is obliterated. In warm water, heat loss is limited so a systemic rise in temperature occurs.

Throughout the literature on hydrotherapy there is wide variation as to the temperature a which water should be kept in the hydrotherapy pool. Skinner and Thomson (1983) advocate an average temperature between 35.5°C and 36.6°C (96 and 98°F). While accepting that pool temperatures will vary with the different conditions treated in the hydrotherapy department and according to local environmental factors, Bolton and Goodwin (1974) suggest that the water temperature should be between 34.4°C (94°F) and 37.8°C (100°F).

Davis and Harrison (1988) recommend a range between 35°C and 37°C (95 and 98.6°F) although as they point out the temperature should be set so that it is suitable for the majority of people using the pool – both patients and physiotherapists. Maintaining the temperature at a required level between 33 and 37°C (92 and 98°F) is advised by Golland (1981) although this author also proposes varying temperature ranges for different age groups and conditions. For instance, patients in a younger age bracket with orthopaedic problems could be treated at a lower temperature while the older person and those with rheumatic conditions are considered to require a temperature as high as 37°C (98°F).

Huddleston (1961) believed a pool temperature of 30.5 to 33.3°C (87 to 92°F) was ideal for therapeutic exercise and general physical programmes providing both sedative and stimulating effects. Palmer (1978, p. 111) argues that 'the thermal effects of hydrotherapy depend on the exact temperature of the pool' and advocates variations in the temperature of the water from summer to winter of 32 to 33°C (89.3 to 91.2°F) in the former and 34°C (92.6°F) in the latter. This was possibly taking into account the environmental factors pertaining to Queensland, Australia, but nevertheless shows that in cooler ranges it is possible to treat patients satisfactorily.

The work of Finnerty and Corbitt (1960) shows that 33.3°C (92°F) is neutral and has a sedative effect. Temperatures just above this are warm yet still produce sedation, but when the heat rises above 35.5°C (96°F) and upwards the effects are stimulating and temperature is into the hot range. These authors propose that 28.8°C (84°F) is tepid and that below 26.6°C (80°F) produces stimulating effects.

When working with ante- and postnatal women in water exercise programmes Vleminckx (1988) advocates a temperature range between 30 and 32°C (86 and 89.6°F). The advantage of this range especially at the highest point is that it allows for relaxation and permits activities to take place at a more leisurely pace. When the water is cooler it is important that exercise is carried out at a faster rate. The information cited above provides sufficient evidence of the variations and requirements of temperature thought necessary by a number of authors. The advocates of higher temperature ranges express concern for the patient and physiotherapist alike and propose shorter treatment sessions in the water, packing following treatment and other measures.

The work of Franchimont *et al.* (1983) stresses that temperatures above 35°C (95°C) are disadvantageous as the beneficial effects of treatment in warm water are dissipated due to alterations in the cardiovascular system which may produce untoward consequences. Higher temperatures do produce relaxation but when patients are subjected to more than 15–20 min in water heated to 35°C (95°F) or above they become ennervated, tired and frequently sleep for up to three hours following treatment. Koga (1985) found that a neutral water temperature for light exercise was 31°C (87.4°F) and that light exercise in temperatures of 27°C (80.3°F), 31°C (87.4°F) and 35°C (95°F) showed no discrepancies as far as the thermal response of the body was concerned.

All the desired effects of hydrotherapy for the neurological patient, such as relaxation of muscles, decrease of pain which is a result of muscle spasm, the improvement in the circulation and the removal of waste metabolic products from hypertonic muscle groups are considered by Palmer (1978) to be achieved in water temperatures ranging from 32°C (89.3°F) to 34°C (92.6°F). Furthermore, Palmer suggests that to work with neurological conditions in water where the temperature is above 34°C (92.6°F) will produce debilitating consequences for the patient as well as the physiotherapist.

Tenseness may be brought about in the neurological patient by work in water that is too cool, that is below 32°C (89.3°F) (Palmer, 1978). According to Vleminckx (1988) when water is too cold the response of the skin thermoreceptors is reduced and an increase in tone may occur due to stimulation of the motor neurons. There are those physiotherapists who would argue that the geographical location may have an influence in deciding at what temperature the water should be kept. Since most hydrotherapy pools are enclosed this argument would appear to have little weight. Where an outdoor pool is used it may well be that a variation in temperature between summer and winter would be considered. In tropical and sub-tropical climates the pool temperature might range between 34–35°C (92.6–98.6°F) in winter and 31–33°C (87.4–92°F) in summer.

It is impractical to change the temperature of the water, and in hydrotherapy pools where a variety of conditions and age groups are treated it is impossible to vary it to suit everyone. Golland (1981) recommends a water temperature range between 35 and 35°C (95 and 97°F) to cover all contingencies. Whitelock and Barefoot (1993) advocate a thermo-neutral water temperature of 35°C and a temperature range of 32 to 37°C.

However, in this author's experience the pool water should be heated to a range between 32°C (89.6°F) and 34°C (93.2°F) or 35°C (95°C) but no higher. This caters for all conditions and avoids any debilitating or untoward effects provided that all contra-indications to hydrotherapy have been considered. In the past, and in many pools even today, the trend of keeping the water temperature in the higher ranges goes against research findings, ignores the thermal indifference of the skin temperature and puts patients and physiotherapists at risk.

Ventilation

Air temperature should be slightly lower than that of the water to allow gentle cooling. The rate of cooling of a body in a given time is proportional to the difference in temperature between the body and its surroundings. The greater the difference in temperature, the greater will be the rate of cooling – this is Newton's law of cooling. The air temperature of the pool area is usually kept at 25°C and the changing rooms 4°C lower.

Ventilation should ensure that excessive condensation does not build up and that humidity is maintained at approximately 50 per cent. Air conditioning of the dehumidifying type offers the best solution for ventilation and controlling condensation which, if excessive, affects the body, increasing its difficulty in losing heat as well as affecting the walls, ceilings and equipment, unless these have been constructed from materials unaffected by humidity.

EQUIPMENT

Equipment involves both in-pool – fixed and movable – and external equipment items.

Handrails are fixed in-pool items and should be made of stainless steel and have a diameter of 40 mm. Handrails are provided on either side of the steps and should be continuous with the rail around the sides of the pool. Breaks in the handrail for whatever reason reduce safety. It may not be necessary or desirable to provide a handrail on all sides of the pool but there should be one on three sides. One side without a rail allows easy entry and exit over the side and makes it easier for the physiotherapist to assist.

Care must be taken as to the installation of the handrail; it should be sited at water level and the distance from the wall should not be too great so that the protruding rail impedes access over the side, nor too small so that arms may become trapped.

Underwater jets are installed in some pools to provide a massaging effect and for impedance to movement and swimming, thus improving strength and endurance. The positioning of these jets needs to be carefully considered as the turbulence they create will compromise the balance of those using the pool. It is important that if installed the jets can be easily controlled from inside and outside the pool. The inlet for the water to the pool needs to be sited at the deep end and the flow should be slow and gentle, causing as little turbulence as possible. Some pools have been built where the circulation of the water was so poor that a 'stagnant' situation occurred. To counteract this jets were installed to move the water on but were so powerful that the turbulence sucked the user under and swept them to the deep end. Nor does a line of small jets placed centrally the full length of the pool prove satisfactory, however slowly the water entry may be. They produce turbulence inappropriately when working across the pool altering balance and there is increased difficulty with underwater visibility due to the 'bubbling' effects.

Other equipment items, such as parallel bars stools of varying heights, seats and plinths should be movable, not permanently fixed

Floats, of all types, are usually made of rubber, plastic or polystyrene; rings, toys, kickboards, balls, bats and flippers can be moved from the bathside at the end of the day and hosed down and stored on hooks or wooden slatted shelves. On the poolside during treatment sessions, these items can be stored in meshed plastic baskets or, in the case of rings, neck and ankle floats, placed over traffic cones thus keeping the area safe and tidy.

Around the sides of the pool chairs should be provided and either hooks or an 'umbrella stand' in which to place walking sticks and crutches so that these items do not present a hazard while the users are in the water.

LIGHTING

The pool area needs to be well lit. Whether natural or artificial lighting is used the fact that refraction and reflection take place must be taken into account because, at all times, visibility throughout the whole pool area and to the full depth of water is vital in the interests of treatment and safety. Windows should be sited so as to avoid reflections on the water. Setting these well back from the pool edge invariably achieves this, although in one instance the setting sun produced a black area in the deep end of the pool totally reducing visibility. Overhead skylights produce bands of light across the water again destroying visibility in those patches. Windows set high up in the walls may provide the solution.

Suitably placed artificial lighting that produces indirect and even distribution is advocated. If this lighting is directly over the pool access for maintenance purposes must be available from above the ceiling.

FACILITIES

Facilities in the hydrotherapy unit comprise:

- changing areas
- showers
- resting space
- toilets

or both patients and staff. Additional facilities clude an office area for staff, rooms for drying n and clothing, plant room and storage e for equipment and chemicals.

The number of changing rooms and showers is determined by the needs of the users and the total number of people passing through the unit. The location of these in the overall layout of the unit depends on the needs of the users. Sufficient space must be provided for changing and resting and at least one facility constructed for wheelchair bound persons. Bench-type seats and chairs should be provided and for the severely disabled a couch should be available.

Curtained partitions for cubicles prove more adaptable than fixed ones; showers and toilets should be located in separate areas from the changing rooms but within easy reach and should be sufficiently large to take wheelchairs. Throughout the changing areas items such as handrails, mirrors, lockers, and clothes hooks should be provided. Separate changing and resting areas, showers, toilets and lockers are required for staff usage.

Handrails installed in changing and shower areas may be placed vertically, horizontally or sloping. Showers need to be adjustable and/or hand held, taps accessible for all and thermostatically controlled with a set temperature no higher than 43°C (Whitelock and Barefoot, 1993).

The drying room should provide facilities for the washing and drying of swimwear and towels and consideration may need to be given to space for containers for sterilizing items such as caps and bathside footwear. Additional storage space for linen may be required.

The plant room houses the plant required for heating, filtering, sterilizing and circulating the water. It should be sufficiently large for the storage of dangerous chemicals in accordance with the rules and regulations pertaining locally, nationally or internationally.

Further storage space is required for the pool equipment such as floats, rings, kickboards and toys. These items should be hosed down after use to remove the chemicals, maintain cleanliness and lengthen their life. Wooden slatted shelving provides an easy and effective means of storage for such equipment.

SURFACES

Surfaces, both those in the pool, those around the pool and in the facilities need to be non-slip, non-abrasive and easily cleaned.

In the pool specially manufactured tiles with non-slip surfaces should be used on the floor. When selecting the tiles it is well worth testing them underwater for their non-slip qualities as the makes and designs vary in this regard. When the tiles are laid the grouting needs to be precise and level with the surface of the tiles to ensure the non-slip nature of the pool floor. It also avoids sharp edges which can contribute to cuts and abrasions especially in conditions where the skin and circulation are affected such as in paraplegia and spina bifida.

Some authorities advocate that the junction between the pool floor and the walls should be rounded for ease of cleaning and to reduce turbulence. Others would argue that a right angle, which is not difficult to clean but, not being rounded, does not produce any turbulence, is best. A further argument for the right angle is that it makes it easier for staff to position themselves closer to the wall and more appropriately for assisting entry to and exit from the water, since the distribution of their weight is correct for lifting. A curve means that the forward foot and leg cannot be placed flat and the body weight is thrown on to the back leg stressing the body and making lifting unsafe. If a curve is constructed the radius should be kept to an *absolute minimum*.

The surfaces of the pool surrounds should have the same qualities – non-slip, non-abrasive and easy to clean. They should also be appropriately graded so that when cleaned dirty waste water does not flow back into the pool. Again good grouting is vital. Whitelock and Barefoot (1993) advocate the addition of poly-resin to the grouting to withstand vigorous cleaning.

The surfaces in the changing rooms and showers need careful attention. There will be wet and dry areas and it is essential that these are kept separate. The floors must be non-slip and non-abrasive – the safety of the users being of particular importance. Ease of cleaning also needs to be considered. Wheelchair access must be provided in the changing areas, showers and toilets.

NOISE FACTORS

Pools tend to be noisy places where much activity, laughter, shouting and splashing inevitably occur. When designing and constructing a pool acoustic materials should be used for the walls and the ceiling of the pool area. This will help to avoid excessive noise which can produce anxiety and tension in children and adults alike and makes the work of the physiotherapist easier especially when conducting group sessions.

STAFFING/CARE AND MAINTENANCE

The staffing of the hydrotherapy department over and above the physiotherapists who are treating patients should include a bathside assistant(s), cleaning and maintenance staff. Some hydrotherapy departments appoint a physiotherapist to have an overall management role and it is essential that this person should be familiar with all aspects of care and maintenance.

SAFETY AND EMERGENCY PROCEDURES

Safety in the water is paramount. Therefore certain procedures should be followed. In the interests and safety of the patients the bathside assistant(s) must be in dry clothing so that the dressing and other needs of the patients can be catered for. Also in the event of an emergency they can readily give assistance.

An emergency routine must be in place and all staff must be fully aware of it and competent in the use of resuscitation equipment and CPR skills.

Maintenance staff are concerned with the general care of the department and specifically of the water and the plant. However, all physiotherapists should be familiar with the plant and its operation and be able to test the water for residual chlorine content and pH value (or with other chemicals such as bromine). A full bacteriological analysis of the water should be carried out every two to four weeks; this is usually the task of the hospital or local authority scientific laboratory.

Emergency equipment includes a test kit for testing the chemical levels of the water, an alarm system which can be operated from within the pool and throughout the poolside area, an air oxygen, oxy viva or air viva system and a telephone that can access an emergency call system.

COSTS

The costs of constructing, equipping, maintaining and running a hydrotherapy pool are high. However, the real advantages of this modality for rehabilitation are so great the provision of a pool is to be encouraged. Through careful and practical design, by the efficient and effective use by highly trained staff and by permitting its hiring and use by outside groups its potential can be maximized and its disadvantages minimized.

The initial expenditure covers the overall building, the pool, the plant, facilities and equipment. Apart from the staff, running costs are concerned with heating, lighting, chemicals, the volume of water, frequency of emptying, the number of patients treated, laundry and replacing equipment. Running costs will vary from department to department due to different design, size, patient numbers and so on.

THE PHYSIOTHERAPIST AND THE HYDROTHERAPY POOL

For the physiotherapist, high temperatures reduce the ability to carry out effective treatments and decrease the time that can be spent in the water. Generally speaking two or three hours in the pool in any one day is sufficient, particularly if the physiotherapist is working in the hydrotherapy department for several weeks or months at a time. It is advisable to divide the time spent in the water into sessions. If working three hours a day, then two $1\frac{1}{2}$ hour sessions with reasonable breaks between each is acceptable. Skinner and Thomson (1983) suggest 20 to 30 minutes is adequate time to recover after $1\frac{1}{2}$ hours in the water. A longer period for recovery is preferable. Davis and Harrison (1988) believe that two hours in the water is possible and should not be exceeded if the physiotherapist is working an extended tour of duty in the pool.

In this author's experience, especially when the warmth of the water is in the higher ranges, it is advantageous for the physiotherapist to emerge from the pool to bring in each patient. Not only is there time for some cooling to take place, but it provides an opportunity to observe the patient and to note asymmetry of shape. Analysis of the rotational effects likely to occur means that the person can be informed about these and instructed in the actions to take to counteract the rotations on entering the water. Thus the person becomes more adjusted to water activity and such mental adjustment is extended as the programme progresses.

If it is not possible to have these short times out of the water when conducting classes, the physiotherapist needs to adjust gradually by initially taking shorter sessions. Individually, physiotherapists vary in their reaction to the water and the temperature, but no one person should undertake longer periods in the water than those advocated earlier. When the water temperature is high, that is above 35°C (95°F), and if the physiotherapist spends two or more hours twice a day in the water, there is a build-up of fatigue and tiredness that at the end of two weeks may result in extreme reactions such as sleeping for as long as 24 hours.

Table 2.1 Pools' design and equipment – summary chart

Pool		
Type	Below ground with or without deck level	
Shape	Rectangular	
Size	The larger the pool the greater the use Consider funding and proposed usage Dimension 4–6 m accommodates 8 persons Minimum space per person 2.50 m × 2.25 m	
Floor	Sloping, gradient 1:20 to 1:30 Non-slip, grouting to height of tiles	
Depth	For adults and children 830 mm to 1270 mm For adults 1000 mm to 1350 mm (McMillan, 1977)	
Entry	Steps –	at shallow end, recessed to keep work area clear maximum riser height 150 mm minimum tread depth 300 mm minimum step width 600 mm (Skinner and Thomson, 1983)

Ramps – gradient no steeper
than 1:15
non-slip surface;
recessed where possible

Hoists – mechanical
– hydraulic
– electric
stretcher and seat
combination
placed at shallow end
and 360° turning area

Temperature and ventilation

Temperature   Water: thermo-neutral 35°C with
a range of 32°C to 36°C
Pool area: 25°C
Changing areas: 21°C

Ventilation   Maintain humidity at
approximately 50%
Dehumidifying air conditioning
Ceilings, walls constructed of
materials unaffected by humidity

Equipment

In pool   All large equipment – plinths,
parallel bars be movable
Handrails – stainless steel,
diameter 40 mm
Wall fixing – 50 mm from wall, at
or 75 mm below water surface
Underwater jets – cautious
approach, disadvantages may
outweigh advantages
Equipment for treatment – stools,
chairs, floats, rings, toys,
kickboards, balls, bats, flippers,
etc.

Ex pool   Alarm system
Telephone with access to
emergency call system
Air/oxygen system; air viva or oxy
viva
Test kit for chemical testing of
water

Lighting

Pool must be well lit
Natural or artificial
Absolute maximum visibility at all
times throughout whole pool area
and at every depth
Easy access for maintenance
essential

Facilities

Changing areas, showers, resting
space, toilets
Staff changing rooms, showers,

toilets and office
Laundry area
Plant room
Storage space for equipment,
chemicals
Handrails, mirrors, lockers,
clothes hooks

Surfaces

In pool, around pool and in the
facilities – non-slip, non-abrasive,
easily cleaned

Noise factors

Acoustic material for construction
of walls and ceiling

Staffing

Other than physiotherapists,
bathside assistant(s), cleaners,
maintenance staff

REFERENCES

Bolton E. and Goodwin D. (1974). *An Introduction to Pool Exercises*, Edinburgh: Churchill Livingstone.

Davis B.C. and Harrison R.A. (1988). *Hydrotherapy in Practice*, Edinburgh: Churchill Livingstone.

Franchimont P., Juchmes J. and Lecomte J. (1983). Hydrotherapy mechanisms and indications. *Pharmac. Ther.*, **20**: 79–93.

Finnerty F.G. and Corbitt T. (1960). *Hydrotherapy*, London: Ungar.

Golland A. (1981). Basic hydrotherapy, *Physiotherapy*, **67(9)**: 258–62.

Huddleston O.L. (1961). *Hydrotherapy in Therapeutic Exercises*, Philadelphia: F.A. Davis.

Koga S. (1985). The regional difference of thermal response to immersion during rest and exercise. *Annals Physiol. Anthrop.*, **4(2)**: 191–2.

Palmer R.P. (1978). *Guidelines to Neurological Rehabilitation*, 2nd edn, Queensland: Multiple Sclerosis Society.

Reid Campion M. (1991). Hydrotherapy in Paediatrics, 2nd edn, Oxford: Butterworth-Heinemann.

Skinner A.T. and Thomson A.M., eds (1983). *Duffield's Exercises in Water*, 3rd edn, London: Baillière Tindall.

Vleminckx M. (1988). Pregnancy and recovery: the aquatic approach in obstetrics and gynaecology. In *Obstetrics and Gynaecology* (McKenna J., ed.), Edinburgh: Churchill Livingstone.

Whitelock H. and Barefoot J. (1993). *Hydrotherapy pools: Considerations in Planning and Design*. Hydrotherapy Association of Chartered Physiotherapists.

3

Basic physics: shape and density

Margaret Reid Campion

HYDRODYNAMIC PRINCIPLES

When undertaking hydrotherapy the physiotherapist should have knowledge of the properties and characteristics of water (Table 3.1). The physical properties include mass, weight, density, specific gravity, buoyancy, hydrostatic pressure, surface tension, refraction and viscosity (Reid Campion, 1985).

The principles have been described in the literature and the majority of physiotherapists will be familiar with them (Macdonald, 1973; Massey, 1979; Skinner and Thomson, 1983; Davis and Harrison, 1988). It is not the author's intention to describe them further except where the laws of hydrodynamics have especial relevance to the following chapters where specific techniques and exercises are advocated in the text. The hydrodynamic principles which are of particular importance are those related to relative density, turbulence, metacentre, friction and hydrostatic pressure.

Relative Density ✓

Archimedes' principle states that when a body is immersed in a fluid it experiences a buoyant force equal to the weight of the fluid which the body has displaced. The relative density of water is taken as a ratio of one. Any object with a density of less than one will therefore float.

The relative density of the human body varies with age, the young child having a total relative density of approximately 0.86. In adolescence and early adulthood, the relative density of the body increases to approximately 0.97. Later in life the body tends to acquire more adipose tissue (Smith and Bierman,

Table 3.1 Laws of hydrodynamics

Author	Principle
Archimedes (c. 287–212 BC)	Relative density
Bougier (1690–1758)	Metacentre
Bernoulli (1700–82)	Turbulence
Reynolds (1849–1912)	Flow
Prandtl (1875–1953)	Boundary layer
Froude (1810–79) and	Friction
Zahm (1862–1945)	
Pascal (1623–62)	Pressure

1973) and the relative density tends to return towards 0.86. It can be seen therefore that at certain times in a human being's life it is easier and at others harder to float in water.

Each individual part and tissue of the body has its own relative density. The upper limbs are usually less dense than the lower limbs thus the arms float more readily while legs tend to sink. The importance of observing and analysing the density of the person undertaking hydrotherapy becomes apparent and should form part of the assessment of that person. Some disabilities, such as paraplegia or Guillain–Barré syndrome have marked alterations in density of body parts which have to be taken into account in treatment.

Metacentre

The metacentric principle is concerned with balance in water. A body immersed in water is subjected to two opposing forces – gravity and buoyancy. Gravity acts in a downwards direction, buoyancy in an upwards direction. If these two forces are equal and opposite to one another then the body is balanced and no movement takes place. However, if the forces of gravity and buoyancy are unequal and unaligned, then movement occurs and that movement is always one of rotation. The rotation continues until the two forces are once more in alignment.

When these forces are applied to the human body it can be seen that, when floating, the body is balanced and in equilibrium. However, if a part of the body is taken above the surface of the water the balance of the body is upset as the forces of gravity and buoyancy are no longer equal and directionally opposite. The body will rotate until the two forces are aligned once more.

Any movement of the limbs, trunk and head which alters the body shape, whether above or below the surface of the water, will produce rotational effects, as will any alteration in shape due to disability. Thus control of the rotations that occur is an important factor during activity in water. The physiotherapist needs to observe and analyse the shape of the person entering water for hydrotherapy and be able to instruct in regard to the appropriate actions to be taken to counteract the rotational effects. It must be understood that these can occur in the vertical as well as the horizontal positions.

Turbulence

Bernoulli's theorem is concerned with the relation between fluid pressure and fluid velocity along a streamline in the steady flow of a frictionless fluid which has a constant density. Part of the theorem is an expression of energy. The total energy of a particle of water of any moment is the sum of its energies, which are:

- pressure energy
- potential energy
- kinetic energy.

Turbulence is the term which denotes the eddies that follow in the wake of an object moving through a fluid. The degree of turbulence will depend on the speed of the movement. If the movement is slow then the flow of the particles is almost parallel to the object and proceeds in smooth continuous curves. Faster movements produce eddies and the energy in

these eddies is dissipated, reducing the pressure and increasing the drag on the body. The shape of the body greatly influences the production of turbulence.

Since any movement creates turbulence it may be used in hydrotherapy both to assist and resist movement. The physiotherapist needs to understand the effects of turbulence not only in relation to the patient, but also in relation to her movements around the person being treated in order not to cause a loss of balance. Coping with the effects of turbulence demands balance and coordination and this can be used to develop these skills as part of a treatment programme.

Reynolds' Theorem

Reynolds' work on flow indicates that there are two types of flow:

- laminar flow
- turbulent flow.

In the former the flow is of streamlines of molecules in even and regular patterns. In the latter case the movement of the molecules is rapid, random and not streamlined; this type of flow creates return movements and eddies. Activity in water can be made more difficult by changing from a streamlined movement to unstreamlined movement (Skinner and Thomson, 1983). For some disabled persons the inability to change the body shape may mean that work is taking place in the more difficult unstreamlined situation. The work of Reynolds helps with appreciating the theory of boundary layer which follows.

Prandtl's Theorem

When a fluid is flowing past a body or surface, a layer of fluid can be seen adjacent to the surface and the velocity of this fluid in relation to the surface is reduced so as to be nonexistent. This region is called boundary layer. Much of the theory of boundary layer is based on the work of Prandtl and others who undertook flow research in the earlier part of this century. The importance of this from the therapist's point of view is mainly that techniques for exit from a pool or river incorporating this theory can be taught, thus ensuring the person's complete safety. For instance, the fastest flow in a river will be at its centre. As the water gets close to the banks, the rate of flow is slowed until close to or against the bank there is an area of little or no flow. In exiting from the river, the person must learn to keep in this area and to lift the legs high and clear of the water as the forward movement over the side is carried out, otherwise they may find the body being dragged back into the water. To a lesser extent, the same situation arises in the pool. Turbulence created by the movement of the water equates with that of the river, and there is an area of little or no flow against the side of the pool. The technique of getting out of the water can be taught in the pool situation thus ensuring the safety of the swimmer.

Froude–Zahm's Experiments

The work of these two scientists was directed towards the measurement of skin friction of a body passed through water and through air. The results of their work showed that under similar conditions skin friction was proportional to the densities of the two fluids. Skin friction was found to be 790 times greater in water than in air. The amount of energy required to perform movement in water is in a ratio of 790:1. This impedance to movement in water has an important part to play. It provides a situation where more active exercise can be undertaken. Along with turbulent effect, it damps down involuntary movements and, if balance is lost, the falling movement is retarded and time allowed for the person to exert voluntary control to regain the original position.

Hydrostatic Pressure ✓

Pascal's law states that fluid pressure is exerted equally at any level in a horizontal direction, that is pressure is equal at a constant depth. An immersed body thus has fluid pressure exerted on all surfaces when at rest at a given depth.

However, pressure increases with depth and with the density of the fluid. Since the pressure is equal in all directions at a given depth it is felt evenly on all surfaces of the body. The increased pressure at greater depths may be used to reduce swelling more effectively if the part being treated is in as deep water as possible. This pressure also proves useful in smoothing out jerky movements and increasing coordination if activity is carried out well below the surface. A feeling of weightlessness is brought about through the lateral pressure that is applied combined with the effects of buoyancy.

INTRODUCING PEOPLE TO WATER

For all human beings – creatures of land — water is a strange element. Human development from an early apedal existence to bipedal locomotion takes place against gravity. On entering water for the first time the patterns of movement used on land are found to be of less use and the constant movement of the water, causing difficulties with stability, brings about gross postural confusion. Tension, anxiety and fear may also be present. The loss of datum points known on land and the seeming restriction of breathing only add to the anxiety. It follows therefore that time and effort should be spent on helping the person to adjust to the new environment and activities presented in such a manner that adjustment both mentally and physically can take place.

Adjustment to Water

Balance problems arise because the human body is not in perfect symmetry. For the able-bodied this asymmetry is small, and balance and stability are more readily acquired. But for the disabled asymmetry is much more severe, and balance becomes a serious problem. In addition to a natural anxiety and fear, the disabled will have a number of other problems with which to contend. Due to the disability, asymmetry in shape and/or density may be markedly altered. There may also be an acute fear of falling, difficulties with respiration, communication and comprehension, an inability to create movement as required, or an inability to control involuntary movement.

The asymmetry of the body shape and density needs to be observed and analysed. The importance of this should not be underestimated. It has a bearing on the mental adjustment of the person undertaking activity in water, on their security in the medium, on their willingness to cooperate with the physiotherapist in carrying out the activities and on the therapeutic and/or recreational programme itself.

Shape and Density

Normal

Water reacts to the shape and density of any object placed in it, and floats the object according to these factors. This also applies to the human being when in water, and the variations in shape and density of different parts of the body account for the many and varied balance positions.

All human beings are asymmetrical to a greater or lesser degree and will have a balance problem in water. The majority float since the sum of the relative densities of the bones, tissues, teeth, organs and so on usually add up to a density less than the weight of water. Since body changes occur throughout life, there are times when it is easier to float than others. Babies and young children and the middle and older age groups float easily, while teenagers and younger adults, especially the tall and lean, find it hard to float.

The person who has a disability will have varying degrees of alteration in shape and/or density. However slight this may appear to be it must be considered, as water is *so* critical of shape and density. The physiotherapist should observe the person's shape anteriorly, posteriorly, laterally on both sides and longitudinally. The latter is most easily performed with the person supported in supine lying in the water. From such observations and armed with knowledge of what happens to the various shapes and densities, programmes of activity can be developed to provide opportunities to achieve mental adjustment to water and to acquire the skills for balance restoration.

Provided the explanations of the effects of altered shape and density can be comprehended it is possible to commence mental adjustment prior to entering the water. Explaining what will occur to the shape as a result of buoyancy and metacentric action and detailing the actions needed to counteract the effects reassures the person and helps decrease anxiety.

Before discussing mental adjustment further it may be useful to study shapes – both geometric and human – in relation to stability in water.

Certain shapes are less stable than others in water (Table 3.2) and in practice it is found that the long thin shape is less stable, whereas a

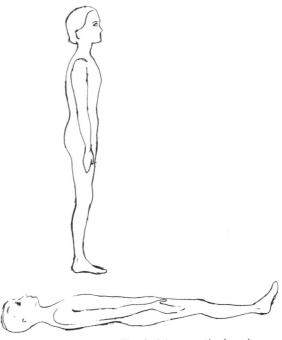

Figs 3.1a and 3.1b   *The 'stick' – vertical and horizontal*

curled-up shape is more stable. The long thin shape (or 'stick') is unstable both in the vertical and horizontal. In the former it can be disturbed easily in all directions, and in the latter readily rotated around the longitudinal axis (Figs 3.1a and b).

If the feet are placed wide apart sideways in the vertical position, some stability is provided laterally, but anteriorly and posteriorly the body is still easily displaced (Fig. 3.2).

If the body assumes a cube shape – a sitting posture with the legs apart and right-angles at hips, knees and ankles with the arms forwards – then increased stability is acquired and the head and arms can be used to assist the maintenance of this position against any disturbing influences. Thus the body has become more stable in balance (Fig. 3.3).

When the body is collapsed further into a 'ball' shape with the hips and knees flexed against it and the hands held around the knees, it is immediately adjusted by the water, and floats curled up over the centre of buoyancy (Fig. 3.4). This shape, though it may be easily disturbed, is the most stable in water, always returning to flotation over the centre of buoyancy with the thoracic spine showing above the

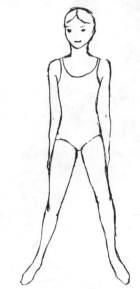

Fig. 3.2   *Triangular shape*

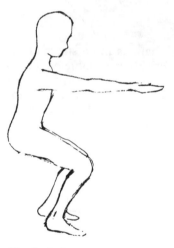

Fig. 3.3   *The 'cube'*

blind and the deaf will, in common with the able-bodied population, present minimal alterations in shape and/or density. Their disability will need particular attention for reasons related to their individual sense problems. The majority of other disabilities will have (to varying degrees) alterations in shape and density. The most common shapes seen are those listed in Table 3.3.

Complications following from these shapes include markedly altered density, such as is found in spina bifida, and further asymmetry of shape due to being affected more in one part or side of the body, as in spastic quadriplegia or hemiplegia. The person with congenital abnormalities or absence of limbs and the amputee will have alterations in both shape and density.

Since it is easier to bring about alterations in shape in water, and because it is important for the balance of the person, activities which will encourage a more equal shape or teach control of the altered shape and density should be introduced immediately. Thus it can be seen how necessary it is for the effects of shape and density to be understood.

Table 3.2   Stable and unstable shapes in water (adapted from unpublished lecture material, J. McMillan, 1975)

Stable shapes
Cube
'Ball'
Unstable shapes
'Stick'
   vertical
   horizontal
Triangle – antero-posteriorly, some stability laterally

surface. The precise floating position is always dependent on the individual's density, and some variations are seen in the size of the area of the back showing above the water.

Alterations in shape and density in the disabled (Table 3.3)

Those people whose disability does not affect their anatomical structure, for instance the

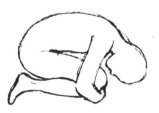

Fig. 3.4   *The 'ball' shape*

Table 3.3 Common alterations in body shape due to disability

1. Unequal quadrilateral
2. Triangular
3. 'Sitting' or wheelchair
4. Adducted or 'scissor'
5. Extended
6. Higher centres of buoyancy and gravity
7. Neutral equilibrium

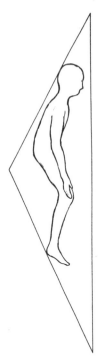

Fig. 3.6a   *Triangular shape*

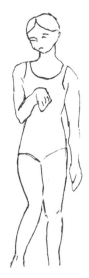

Fig. 3.5a   *An unequal quadrilateral*

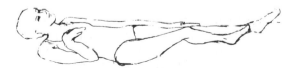

Fig. 3.5b   *An unequal quadrilateral in a horizontal position rolling to the altered side*

1. *The unequal quadrilateral* (Fig. 3.5a). This is most commonly seen in the hemiplegic and activities that will increase extension on the affected side and introduce symmetry should form part of the activity programme from the start. The hemiplegic will tend to be shorter on the affected side and, when placed in water, will rotate to that side due to the greater quality of upthrust beneath the unaffected side (Fig. 3.5b). The degree to which the body rolls is dependent on the degree of shortening on the affected side.

A similar rolling action may occur in quadriplegics where one side is considerably more affected than the other, or in those persons whose loss of density (particularly in the lower limbs) may be much more marked in one leg than the other.

2. *The triangular shape* (Fig. 3.6a). The triangular shape is frequently seen in children with spastic diplegia where there is flexion at hips and knees and plantar flexion at the ankle. Adults who have Parkinson's disease usually present a similar flexed posture, as do some people who have back pain or arthritic conditions especially of the hips.

Some spastic quadriplegics who have insufficient flexion and who half-lie on a chair acquiring a high dorsal kyphosis can also be considered triangular in shape (Fig. 3.6b). Other rarer conditions may bring about a marked increase in hip flexion resulting in a similar triangular shape.

In water a triangle will float with its point downwards, and so it can be seen

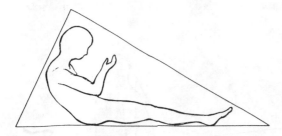

Fig. 3.6b   *Triangular shape*

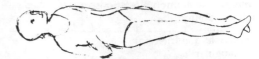

Fig. 3.8   *The adducted or 'scissor' shape*

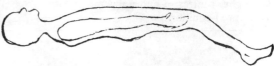

Fig. 3.9   *The extended shape*

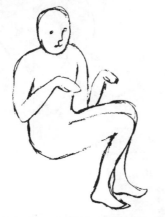

Fig. 3.7   *The wheelchair shape*

that these people should work in the vertical or supine lying position in the early stages of activity in water. To put the triangular-shaped person face downwards in water means that they not only have to cope with water which is trying to turn them over, but they may well have insufficient extension in the cervical and thoracic spine to get the face clear of the water. Rotational control is also important since such persons are likely to be more affected on one side than the other.

3. *The sitting or wheelchair shape* (Fig. 3.7). The disabled person who has had to spend a considerable amount of time in a wheelchair may have contractures of hips and knees. In cases where spasticity is part of the condition, there may also be flexion contractures of the upper limbs. By virtue of the flexion contractures of the lower limbs, there is a more stable posture for activity in water, but such activity will be limited. For the person's

own well-being and greater independence in water, active extension must be encouraged. Again, they will probably have an asymmetrical distribution of contractures and once again rotational effects will need attention, together with the teaching of control.

4. *The adducted or scissor shape* (Fig. 3.8). Where there is marked adduction or even 'scissored' legs, the rotation around the longitudinal axis is most obvious; therefore teaching control of lateral rotation should be commenced immediately, and activities which will alter shape through abduction of the legs need to be encouraged.

5. *The extended shape* (Fig. 3.9). Many disabled people present with a marked extensor pattern and can be described, when supine, as taking the shape of an inverted saucer. Such a shape, when supine in water, will be extended over the centre of buoyancy. Density may be different at one end of the body from the other, and the body will tend to sink at the heavier end. Again, if the distribution of the disabling condition is asymmetrical, rotation about the longitudinal axis will be present.

6. *Higher centres of buoyancy and gravity.* Certain disabling conditions mean that the person's centres of gravity and buoyancy are higher than is normal. Such people may be hydrocephalic or have a condition such as spina bifida or cerebral palsy where the upper trunk and arms are more developed than the lower trunk and legs. In these people it is important that control of vertical rotation is emphasized so that any movement of the head anteriorly

or posteriorly, however slight, is controlled, and no untoward loss of balance from the vertical occurs.

Neutral equilibrium

Some disabled people by virtue of their shape and density, may float in a state of neutral equilibrium. They float easily in both supine and prone, but the latter position may impede respiration. They may have rather large bodies with shorter arms and legs than normal, and lateral rotation around the longitudinal axis is difficult for them since the short levers give little assistance to rotation of the increased body size back to a safe breathing position. Density (as with shape) varies with each individual, but the person who is disabled is likely to have marked changes in this factor. Areas that are less dense will float more easily, whereas those that are more dense will have a tendency to sink.

Density equals weight divided by volume, and a significant reduction in weight rather than in volume has a greater effect on density.

Where limbs are atrophied due to disease, they are less dense and float easily. Those persons with spina bifida, paraplegia, anterior poliomyelitis, Guillain–Barré Landry syndrome and similar conditions will find that their limbs will rise to the surface. Since in most instances the lower limbs are more affected than the upper limbs, the upswing of these limbs can be disturbing, emphasizing the need for early control.

It has been shown that the head controls the feet and therefore teaching vertical rotational control is essential. Additionally, when supine in water, these people should extend the head in order to depress the lower limbs, thus the body is arched over its centre of buoyancy and can work more effectively.

Those who have congenital absence or deformities of limbs or who are amputees have both altered shape and density to a degree dependent on their disability, and control of the rotational effects must be effectively taught by use of the head and limbs.

The shape of the body can also be subjected to changes that are less obvious. Actions such as gripping, holding the breath and shutting the eyes tightly create tension which in turn alters the shape. These actions are frequently brought about by fear and anxiety, and the resulting tension is transferred to the body as a whole. In conditions such as athetosis, where control of involuntary movements is not possible, changes of shape occur frequently.

It should now be evident how critical shape and density are when taking the disabled into water. The physiotherapist must not only study the person's shape and density, but be able (through knowledge of the properties of water) to predict what will happen to that shape and therefore plan a suitable programme which will provide the most advantageous activities. These activities will be designed to teach control of rotational effects, and develop mental adjustment to water within a therapeutic and recreational programme.

Mental Adjustment

Having observed and analysed the person's shape and density and where possible commenced mental adjustment on the poolside, once in the water, and at an appropriate depth – the person's condition has a bearing on this – further mental adjustment can take place.

The ability to blow the water away from the mouth adds to security of mind. Facing each other the physiotherapist demonstrates the blowing action. With their hands on the physiotherapist's shoulders for support the person demonstrates a similar action repeating it several times until it has become a more automatic response.

An understanding that water has weight and can be leant on and used as a force against which work can take place helps in furthering mental adjustment. To develop this knowledge the physiotherapist adopts a similar position facing the person whose hands are on the physiotherapist's shoulders. The physiotherapist's hands are on either side of the person's waist with the fingers pointing away. The first action is to lean to one side with the shoulders and head and then to lean to the other side. The shoulders must be beneath the surface of the water. Once the feeling of being able to push against the water has been established it can be further stressed by taking several steps, if possible in a sitting position, first to one side and then the other, the head and shoulders leading the movement.

Balance Restoration

The ability to restore the body's balance should be developed around the two rotations that occur in water – vertical and lateral.

Vertical rotation. This occurs in a forward and backward direction around the body's centre of buoyancy and incorporates the ability to recover to the upright position from either supine or prone lying. It is a skill that is required for total independence in the water and demonstrates the ability to recover to a safe breathing position.

To achieve supine lying, the head is taken slowly backwards and the feet will slowly rise to the surface, the feet moving forward and upwards. Recovery from this position requires strong flexion of the cervical spine, trunk, hips and knees, with flexion of the shoulders in abduction followed by precise balance of the head over the body to maintain the upright position.

To achieve prone lying, the head is taken slowly forwards, while the legs move backward and upward to the surface. Recovery from this position to the upright may be achieved by laterally rotating onto the back and then effecting a forward recovery. Alternatively, the head may be strongly extended, the hips and knees flexed, and when the body is vertical the legs then extended and the body balanced precisely by the head in the upright position.

Apart from the feeling of security, the ability to perform vertical rotation proves useful when placing patients on a submerged plinth, or in flotation equipment. It also has implications for developing balance and coordination in a variety of conditions, such as the head injured and the paraplegic patient. Additionally, the ability to create vertical rotation can be used in a number of specific exercises.

Lateral rotation. This takes place in two planes. The rotational movement occurs around the longitudinal axis of the body. In the vertical position by using the head and arms the human being is able to create a lateral or turning movement in the upright position. When lying in the water the head, arms and legs, either singly or collectively, can be used to create a lateral or turning rotation around the longitudinal axis of the body.

Instruction in the techniques of creating or controlling lateral rotation in both positions aids the mental adjustment of the person, giving a sense of security and confidence. If such instruction follows on the acquisition of vertical rotation described above, lateral rotation and vertical may be combined so that the person can always return to a safe breathing position. Should the person fall forward in the water it is possible to rotate on to the back and then perform vertical rotation to achieve the upright position once more. When teaching the skill of lateral or turning movement it is essential that rolling is taught in both directions, that is to the right and left sides. It can also be developed in an extended as well as flexed pattern.

In extension the movements of the horizontal body are to turn the head to the side to which the roll is being directed while the arm and leg on the opposite side are brought across the body. If rotating in a flexed posture the head and arms repeat the action for the extended posture while both the legs may be flexed and rotated towards the side to which the head is turned. The amount of flexion in the legs can vary from leg to leg depending on the condition being treated. For example, while treating a patient with a low back pain problem recently it was found advantageous to teach rolling as this action presented considerable difficulty in bed. With considerable lack of mobility in the whole back and a marked tendency to hold the spine extended it was found that encouraging this rotation from one arm of the physiotherapist to the other arm (Reid Campion, 1991) in a flexed posture, broke the extended pattern demonstrated by the patient and developed some gentle rotation between the shoulder and pelvic girdles without any detrimental effects.

Extremes of Physical Dimension

The extremes of physical dimension are total flexion and total extension. The smallest shape – a 'ball' is when the body is curled up in full flexion – and the longest shape – a 'stick' represents full extension.

As a 'stick' the body if standing vertically is on a relatively small base and may be disturbed easily in any direction. If the 'stick' is lying in water it can again be easily disturbed and the movement which occurs is one of rotation around the longitudinal axis of the body. As a 'ball' the body balance is more stable and considerable effort is required to change the shape. Outside forces can disturb the shape, but simply cause it to rotate around its centre of buoyancy, and as these forces decrease or cease, the body returns to its floating position over the centre of buoyancy.

Thus it can be appreciated that the long thin shape of the 'stick' is the least stable, and the round shape of the 'ball' the most stable in water.

All early activities in water, therefore, should be carried out in shapes in which the body is more flexed and stable and as ability in water improves more extended postures which demand greater degrees of control may be employed.

Some activities are designated 'ball' or 'stick', others involve changes of shape from one extreme to the other.

With the acquisition of the skills of vertical and lateral rotation and awareness of the extremes of posture, the person is well adjusted to water and consequently exercises in a more effective manner. If possible a floating position should be developed. This can be achieved by altering the shape of the person through changing the positions of the legs and arms thus altering the centre of gravity and buoyancy. An extension of this would be to encourage independent bilateral movement through the water. A sculling action is recommended for the arms and a modified back stroke kick for the legs.

Armed with a knowledge and understanding of water and the actions to take if the body's balance is disturbed for any reason, the patient is reassured and has a greater pleasure in the use of water in the rehabilitation programme.

REFERENCES

MacDonald F. (1973). *Mechanics for Movement*, London: G. Bell and Sons.

Massey B.S. (1979). *Mechanics of Fluids*, 4th edn, New York: Van Nostrand Reinhold Company.

Reid Campion M. (1985). *Hydrotherapy in Paediatrics*, Oxford: Heinemann Medical Books.

Reid Campion M. (1991). *Hydrotherapy in Paediatrics*, 2nd edn, Oxford: Butterworth-Heinemann.

Skinner A.T. and Thomson A.M., eds (1983). *Duffield's Exercises in Water*, 3rd edn, London: Baillière Tindall.

Smith D.W. and Bierman E.L. (1973). *The Biological Ages of Man – From Conception Through to Old Age*, Philadelphia: W.B. Saunders.

4

Assessment and recording

Margaret Reid Campion

It is common practice to assess patients for physiotherapy treatment programmes on land and to record details of the treatment session in the patient's records. However, such practices are less regular when hydrotherapy treatments are undertaken. Frequently, the land assessment is considered adequate information on which to base the water programme (Harrison, 1980). In such instances no account is taken of the nature of the medium or of the special effects that result from the fact that on entering the water the body is acted upon by two forces simultaneously – namely, gravity or downthrust and buoyancy or upthrust.

As Davis and Harrison (1988) so rightly stress, translating dry land procedures to water denies the uniqueness of the medium and fails to capitalize on this factor for the benefit of the patient. An assessment carried out on land cannot take into account the effects of buoyancy on a movement. For instance, a patient with a problem involving the shoulder joint may only be able to abduct the arm from the side to 40° on land, but in the pool with buoyancy assisting the movement may obtain a greater range. This additional range may be achieved on land as an assisted active movement or with the limb in suspension, but is still not applicable as a baseline for the hydrotherapy programme.

All programmes, hydrotherapy programmes included, should have realistic aims, but such aims must be related to the medium in which activity is to take place.

A land assessment is essential and the details should be noted by the physiotherapist taking the patient for treatment in the water. An assessment based on the same format should be carried out for water, but a number of additional points with particular relevance to activity in water being taken into consideration.

ASSESSMENT

This assessment procedure follows the system in use at the School of Physiotherapy, Curtin University of Technology in Western Australia.

The format is based on the SOAP assessment (Weed, 1971), but has been expanded to SOAPIER (L. Hastings, 1983, personal communication). It is used for land and water assessments.

Method of Recording Physiotherapy Assessment and Treatment

The initials SOAPIER are derived from the following:

S: Subjective assessment – information given by the patients about themselves.
O: Objective assessment – examination of the patient.
A: Analysis of the above information – diagnosis and medical history and S and O to formulate a problem list.
P: Plan of action – for each of the problems.
I: Intervention – treatment of the patient.
E: Evaluation – evaluation of the intervention; what occurred as the result of treatment.
R: Review – the next treatment session and any proposed treatment changes.

These details are suitable for both land and water, but certain factors must be elicited that relate specifically to water.

S: Subjective assessment – must include the patient's attitude to water, information as to their perceived ability in water, and details of previous hydrotherapy or other water activity such as type, place, date and results.

O: Objective assessment – takes into account the shape and density of the patient as well as any contradictions to hydrotherapy.

A: Analysis – the analysis of shape and density is vital and forms part of the problem list.

I: Intervention – will also include the teaching of mental adjustment, balance restoration and rotational control.

For ongoing management the SOAPIER format is used as appropriate and is divided into two parts.

1. The acute/short-term patient.
2. The chronic/long-term patient.

For the acute/short-term patient a daily SOIER is conducted and a new A and P formulated as the S and O alter. For the chronic/long-term patient IER is carried out and a full SOAPIER takes place weekly.

Specific items that need to be used in assessment for water activity include the following:

- shape and density
- suitability for group activity
- goniometry
- Oxford Scale of Muscle Power modified for water
- percentage weight-bearing
- muscle tone
- breathing control.

Assessment of Shape and Density

The importance of shape and density and the effects on the person's balance in water and on their rehabilitation programme cannot be too strongly emphasized (p. 17).

When assessing shape, especially if the person is to be taught independent dynamic movement in water, the physiotherapist must note the person's ability to make a flat surface of the hands and feet. It is the large flat surfaces of the open hand, with adducted digits, and mobile

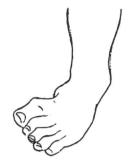

Fig. 4.1   *Equinus deformity of the foot*

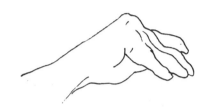

Fig. 4.2   *Flexion deformity of the hand*

feet that play an essential role in propelling the body through the water (Counsilman, 1968).

In some disabling conditions, the hands and feet are affected in such a way that is not possible for a flat surface to be created – for example, the equinus deformity of the foot in muscular dystrophy, the flexor synergy of the hand in cases of hemiplegia, and the flexion of the metacarpophalangeal joints and ulnar deviation of the hand in the person suffering from rheumatoid arthritis (Figs 4.1 and 4.2).

Analysis of the altered shape and density provides the physiotherapist with information as to the rotations and rotational control required which forms part of the water activity programme and acts as a guide to mental adjustment of the person (p. 21).

Hydrotherapy/Recreation Balance Analysis

All participants in activity in water must learn to create and control the patterns of rotation – vertical and lateral – as well as a combination of these two; combined rotation ensures the safety of the person.

Table 4.1   Hydrotherapy/recreation balance analysis

Vertical rotation	Lateral rotation	Combined rotation
Anxious/nervous (causing flexion or extension of the neck & trunk)	Orthopaedic conditions (of hips & shoulders causing adduction)	Orthopaedic conditions
Poor posture	Hemiplegia	Neurological conditions
Paraplegia	Scoliosis	Rheumatic conditions (congenital or acquired producing cross-lateral problems)
Spina bifida	Amputee – unilateral (or bilateral when marked discrepancies in leg lengths)	Athetosis
Diplegia		Mental retardation
Anterior poliomyelitis	Asymmetrical Diplegia	
Mental retardation	Quadriplegia	
Obesity	Other neurological conditions	
Hydrocephalus		
Parkinson's		
Head injury	Athetosis	
Myopathies	Head injury	
Bilateral amputee	Mental retardation	

Table 4.1 indicates the most likely rotation to occur in various conditions and therefore the rotation(s) to be taught first.

Suitability for Group Work

In assessing the individual for group work the physiotherapist considers the person's:

- condition
- age
- attitude
- mobility
- need for support or assistance in water.

The *medical condition* may or may not be suitable for group work, at least not initially, though in due course the person may be able to participate in a group with advantage. Those with injuries, spinal injuries and severe rheumatic conditions may best be treated individually at first, but inclusion in a group may well be advantageous at a later stage, not least for the psychological and motivational benefits.

The *age* of the person has to be taken into account. Very young children being introduced to water activity with their mother can form part of a group, the mother being the main participant. Children from approximately six months of age are much more aware of others and begin to be involved. The frail, older person can be part of a group but special considerations are necessary such as the need for one-to-one attention and gentle activity where the amount of turbulence is kept to a minimum so as not to disturb their balance unduly.

The *attitude* of the participant to group work has a bearing on whether or not they are assessed as suitable. It may well be that at the commencement the idea of group work is an anathema to them but this frame of mind can change so a flexible approach is advocated. The attitude to water itself and the person's ability to balance in water must be considered.

The amount of *support and assistance* required may determine whether or not it is advisable for the person to participate in a group. As progress in treatment takes place the need for help will diminish and the situation should be reviewed regularly.

Goniometry ✓

Goniometry is important especially when treating joint conditions. Frequently the use of the goniometer is overlooked because of the difficulty in reading under water. However, assessing joint range with a goniometer in water is possible with the plastic variety and with care being taken to hold the instrument firmly as it is lifted from the water to read the degrees of range having measured the joint.

Percentage Weight-Bearing

The research carried out by Harrison and Bulstrode (1987) on percentage weight-bearing at different levels related to anatomical landmarks on male and female subjects has proved valuable.

By referring to Table 4.2 and the person's weight the physiotherapist can gauge the

Table 4.2 Percentage weight-bearing when immersed in water

Level	Female	Male
C7	8%	8%
Xiphisternum	28%	35%
ASIS	47%	54%

amount of weight bearing at any depth and the correct level for each activity for the individual.

Oxford Scale for Muscle Power Modified for Water

This scale is provided for water but it is limited to the assessment of muscles which retain little power but good range of movement (Skinner and Thomson, 1983).

The scale of muscle power on land is graded from 0 to 5, with 0 equalling no contraction and 5 as normal. In water the scale commences at 1 and continues to 5 but it must be recognized that grade 5 in water is not normal as such function cannot be tested in there (Skinner and Thomson, 1983).

In addition to adding floats at grades 4 and 5 the lever arm can be lengthened.

Table 4.3 Scale of Muscle Power modified for water

1	= Contraction with buoyancy assisting
2	= Contraction with buoyancy counterbalanced
2+	= Contraction against buoyancy
3	= Contraction against buoyancy at speed
4	= Contraction against buoyancy and light float
5	= Contraction against buoyancy and heavy float

Muscle Tone

Measurement of muscle tone is a complex procedure and may take many forms ranging from simpler processes to complicated methods.

Carr, Shepherd and Ada (1995) stress the importance of retraining motor function in neurological conditions and advocate the use of motor assessment scales as well as other measures.

In water where warmth and support tend to alter the tonal state, such measurement becomes more difficult. The physiotherapist should assess tone on land by the method usually employed, whether this is by observation of movement or of the effects of tonic reflexes, by handling or by any other means.

Reassessment should take place in water allowing for the effects of temperature (p. 7), the supportive factor and the anxiety level of the person in regard to water activity. While each treatment session is in progress it is necessary for the physiotherapist to monitor tone constantly.

Breathing Control

Whether dealing with adults or children it is important to assess their breathing control (p. 38). On land the physiotherapist checks the ability to blow out and once in the water the level at which this can be achieved is assessed. Is the person able to blow regularly onto the water, into the water, beneath the surface or exhale through the nose under the water or hum? Humming is the acceptable alternative when exhalation through the nose is difficult.

Without adequate assessment hydrotherapy programmes tailored to the individual's needs are not possible. Continuous assessment ensures progression and improved and faster recovery of the condition.

The progression of exercise in water is markedly different from that on land and fine progressions of techniques are possible (Skinner and Thomson, 1983). This applies not only to buoyancy-assisted, buoyancy-neutral and buoyancy-resisted exercises, but to other procedures such as Bad Ragaz patterns, hold-relax, repeated contractions and exercises based on the combined effects of buoyancy, turbulence and metacentric principles, or each of these used separately.

RECORDING

Detailed recording of hydrotherapy treatments is as important as documentation of other treatments. The following items should be included:

- the length of the treatment
- the temperature of the water
- the depths used
- the exercises, patterns included in the programme
- any progressions of the exercises

- any improvements in the patient's condition and activity
- any untoward effects
- individual and/or group treatment.

Some hospital departments and centres may have other items they specifically need included in their records of treatment.

There is no doubt that only by accurate and comprehensive assessment and recording will it be possible to prove the effectiveness of hydrotherapy. Currently, there is a dearth of evaluative material, most of the comments about the value of hydrotherapy treatments are subjective. If careful and conscientious assessment and recording is carried out they will not only enhance the programmes themselves, but enable physiotherapists to promote hydrotherapy and ensure it takes its place in the overall rehabilitation of the many conditions treated in water.

A format for the assessment and recording of hydrotherapy treatment for children should reflect their age, the skills required and the therapeutic and recreational aspects.

The SOAPIER method of obtaining data can be used for essential information but the 'P'lan of action and 'R'eview would take into account the skills of entry, level of breathing control (p. 24), vertical balance and later vertical rotational control, lateral rotational control, combined rotational control, balance in all positions especially lying, the ability to float in supine and prone, advance skills such as somersaulting, stoking and exit. Progress through these skills could be recorded by the dates on which various levels are reached. These could be defined as 'engages and grips', 'engages without gripping', 'engages partially' and 'performs independently'. Entries and exits could be recorded as 'with support', 'with partial support' and 'unaided'.

The activities which develop the above-mentioned skills can be found in the paediatric section of this book and it is the responsibility of the physiotherapist to ensure that the therapeutic needs of the child are stressed within the recreational framework of the programme.

GROUP WORK

Working in groups has been shown to have considerable advantages and these apply to groups for adults and children. Many of the

benefits are similar for both ages but there are differences.

A group usually provides the child with a first community and socialization. It is probably more fully motivational to a child and provides greater opportunities to learn motor and behavioural skills.

Motivation, socialization and the ability to work longer with great concentration are among these advantages (Cotton and Kinsman, 1983) and these are brought about by classwork in the water just as in group work on land.

- the patient gains confidence from working with others
- a feeling of fellowship develops
- patients take some responsibility for their own treatment
- patients become more extrovert
- patients concentrate less on their own problems and tend to set standards for each other.

The suitability of a patient to participate in classwork should form part of the original assessment and later evaluation. Classwork may not be appropriate initially for some patients, but as they progress it may be possible for them to be included. Some of the techniques of exercise, for example the Bad Ragaz patterns, are not suitable for group work due to a lack of the one-to-one relationship required and to the space factor. Where staffing is a problem group work often means more patients can be treated by one or two physiotherapists.

There is a place for both individual and group treatment and many patients can benefit from both during each session of water activity. In the author's experience it is useful to gather the patients together as they enter the pool and conduct some general exercises all together at the beginning of the session. If these exercises are conducted to music the activity becomes more pleasurable. Individual treatment can be carried out following the early group work and gathering together again towards the end of the session as a 'wind down' is valuable. On the whole patients should be able to manage on their own in the water; this is important where there is only one physiotherapist to a group. However, judicious positioning of the more able patients in relation to those who are less able frequently eases the situation. The disadvantages of too large a group are familiar and regulating the number of participants in a group must be uppermost in the physiotherapist's mind. Too large a group can disadvantage all. Precise and accurate movement should not be sacrificed in classes; if there is a large number of participants it is difficult to monitor everybody's actions.

Group work is suitable for most conditions but probably more so for orthopaedic and rheumatic conditions, for antenatal and postnatal women and for general fitness. Patients with neurological problems can also enjoy participation in group work although the more severely disabled, such as the head-injured, require a one-to-one basis with a physiotherapist within the group situation. In the ensuing chapters group work for different conditions is discussed and the various criteria established for the particular conditions exercising in water.

With some ingenuity on the part of physiotherapists, classes can be conducted for a wide range of conditions exercising simultaneously. It is not necessary to have all participants suffering from a similar disorder. A wide range of techniques can be utilized and recreational activities introduced to increase the participation for the individual and their enjoyment.

THERAPY AND RECREATION

Water is fun! For the majority of people it holds a fascination; no age group being exempt.

In practice, when participating in hydrotherapy programmes there is an ever present recreational element. The ease of movement, the relief of body weight, the reduction of pain, the opportunities for relaxation contribute to the psychological benefits as well as the physical and bring about pleasure from the diversion for both adults and children.

Programmes that combine both therapeutic and recreational aspects are especially appropriate for children since hydrotherapy in the strict sense of remedial exercise may prove boring to them. It has been found that children, especially younger children, rarely respond directly to treatment techniques whether on land or in the water (Reynell and Martin, 1965). However, water is an element that children enjoy from a very early age and from which they gain a variety of learning experiences.

Water is a medium in which many disabled – adults and children – achieve total independence and can compete with their able-bodied counterparts on equal terms. For those who spend long periods in a wheelchair or can only walk with an aid, independent ambulation in water can become a reality, in addition to all the rolling and tumbling activities which must be of delight to the performer who is so confined on land.

To get out of one's wheelchair and to change one's wheelchair shape, to cast aside one's calipers and walking aids and find freedom of movement and independence brings about physical and psychological well-being which cannot be achieved to the same extent elsewhere or in any other activity.

If, then, both therapy and recreation in water are based on the same principles and method, they become complementary to each other and provide a broader framework for the overall rehabilitation of those undertaking water activity.

Traditionally, therapeutic techniques are used on a one-to-one basis and this is essential when Bad Ragaz patterns, spinal mobilizations, hydrodynamic exercises and other specialized techniques such as hold-relax, stabilizations and repeated contractions are employed.

As the reader peruses the later chapters it will become apparent that in the treatment of neurosurgical and neurological conditions there are patterns advocated that have been developed from the approach of the Halliwick Method – thus therapy and recreation are combined, and require a physiotherapist to work with a person individually; this can also take place within a group situation and the beneficial effects of group activity can provide the optimum situation for activity, motivation and progress. Furthermore swimming forms part of the rehabilitation programme for many conditions and the basis of the approach to stroking advocated by Halliwick is a sound one from which to include swimming in the treatment programme.

PROGRAMMES

Activity in water is usually undertaken for exercise and/or swimming. When planning programmes for either adults or children setting goals is vital and careful and detailed planning is required so that progress proceeds steadily for each individual. Ideally all skills should be acquired regularly and accurately so that ultimately each is performed automatically and safety is assured. Some severely disabled persons may not achieve the final goal of being mentally adjusted to water, physically balanced, safe under all conditions and totally independent in the medium. However, every effort should be made to ensure that the skills are developed in such a way that any weakness in ability is minimized.

The changes of shape and density of each person are variables to be considered when planning a programme of activity and defining the specific objectives of exercise in water. For instance, where an arthritic condition produces marked flexion of the hips resulting in a triangular shape, the initial stages of the programme would be conducted in the vertical and supine lying positions. The specific objectives of exercises in water would be the reduction of pain and muscle spasm, the maintenance and increase of the range of movement of the joints, the strengthening of weak muscles, improvement in posture, gait retraining and an increase in mental and physical adaptability.

The organization of the water activity programme should then include the objectives, an outline of work which is flexible and can be easily modified and adapted as necessary and a list of the required achievements. All this should be recorded (p. 27) and reviewed. Progress in precise objectives such as joint range and muscle power must be measured and recorded. Similarly, where a game is being played whether for its therapeutic or recreational value, improvement can be gauged by performing the activity at the advanced level or by choosing another game not previously used but which demands the same skill.

Feedback is important but must always be appropriate if the ultimate goal of total and safe independent activity in water is to be attained. The physiotherapist cannot be satisfied with less than accurate and automatic skills so that feedback when given praises correct actions and where actions are incorrect constructive comment and assistance are provided so that the patterns of action reflect the person's increasing competence.

Many of the activities provided in the paediatric section of this book are readily adapted for use with adults, who despite popular opinion thoroughly enjoy games and playing in water.

Most activities need no adaptation as far as the purpose and appreciation are concerned. The formation is varied in relation to individual or group work, holds remaining the same although support may not be needed to the same degree and disengagement proceeds more rapidly. Instructions are commonly changed particularly in relation to the songs and rhymes.

The use of adult songs changes the focus and makes the activity more acceptable. For instance, walking sideways in a circle to 'There was a crooked man' for children could be altered to 'Tea for two'. A 'Snake' usually played by the children singing 'Puffer train' or 'Hedi, hedi, ho' can be used by adults without a song or enacted as a 'conga'.

It is important to adhere to the principles of the activity and to maintain rhythm, so simply humming may be useful. In this author's experience most adults are happy to sing and usually know many of the older songs which have rhythms better suited to activity in water than modern 'pop' music.

REFERENCES

Carr J.H., Shepherd R.B. and Ada L. (1995). Spasticity: research findings and implications for intervention, *Physiotherapy*, **81(8)**: 421–429.

Cotton E. and Kinsman R. (1983). *Conductive Education for Adult Hemiplegia*, Edinburgh: Churchill Livingstone.

Counsilman J.E. (1968). *The Science of Swimming*, New Jersey: Prentice Hall.

Harrison R.A. (1980). Hydrotherapy in rheumatic conditions. In *Physiotherapy in Rheumatology* (S.A. Hyde, ed.), Oxford: Blackwell Scientific Publications.

Harrison R. and Bulstrode S. (1987). Percentage weight bearing during partial immersion in the hydrotherapy pool, *Physiotherapy Practice*, **3**: 60–63.

Skinner A.T. and Thomson A.M., eds (1983). *Duffield's Exercises in Water*, 3rd edn, London: Baillière Tindall.

Weed L.L. (1971). *Medical Records, Medical Education and Patient Care*, Chicago: Year Book Medical Publishers.

Section II
Practice of Paediatric Hydrotherapy

Margaret Reid Campion

INTRODUCTION

The unborn child exists in a liquid environment and after birth appears to have no fear of water. Babies find pleasure in the warmth of their bath and the feel of the water. Later, as the ability to move actively develops, kicking and splashing make bathing a happy part of the daily routine. Playing with toys while in water is also a source of pleasure, activity and learning in the child's life. Swimming, however, is a skill that has to be learnt.

The teaching of swimming is begun now at an early age for many reasons, not least as a protection against the risk of drowning. Other benefits gained are both psychological, physical, recreational and social.

If enjoyment of water and learning to swim are part of the able-bodied child's life so they should be part and parcel of the life of the disabled child. Water allows all of us to achieve marvellous feats of movement which can be performed on land only with difficulty, if at all. For the disabled child water may be the only environment in which total independence can be attained.

All children need to experience active movement if they are to develop. The lack of such movement for disabled children may well be an important factor in retarding their development. Water as a medium for activity is a most useful means of widening the experience of such children.

Hydrotherapy, in its strictly accepted sense of exercise in water, as being purely remedial may lose its value when taking children into water, because they could find the exercises as such boring. However, if the exercise can be hidden in an activity that is fun, the programme for the child becomes of interest and both the therapeutic and recreational aspects have been incorporated.

With this in mind the ensuing chapters have been written. It is hoped they will prove useful to physiotherapists and also to swimming teachers who work with disabled children, so that like their able-bodied peers, disabled children can not only cope with the risks attendant on being in water, but also benefit from its physiological, psychological, social and recreational aspects and can extend their horizons into many aquatic sports adapted for the disabled person who has acquired the skill of swimming safely under all conditions.

The chapters are based on the ideas and techniques of the Halliwick Method devised and developed by the late James McMillan. The functional value of the many activities and games is apparent, but the fun, laughter and pleasure should not be overlooked in the effort of providing function.

The promotion of functional activity is the essence of rehabilitation and an essential feature of Conductive Education. This global method devised and developed by Professor Petö in Hungary has similarities with the Halliwick Method. Both methods are used in the rehabilitation of children and adults with motor disorders and a chapter has been included in the text comparing and contrasting the two approaches, aiming to bridge the paediatric and adult sections of the book and to encourage physiotherapists to appreciate how the activities may be adapted for use by all age groups.

5

Activity in water – ways and means

Margaret Reid Campion

GENERAL PRINCIPLES

Activity in water is usually for two reasons: to exercise and/or to swim. As indicated earlier (p. 32) pure exercise may prove boring to children, less productive of effort and less effective for treatment outcomes.

Games and activities that are fun and interest the child are more likely to develop the skills required. The ingenuity and imagination of the physiotherapist will be taxed in devising programmes that meet the objectives of exercise in water as well as combining successfully both the therapeutic and recreational benefits.

CHILD–PHYSIOTHERAPIST RELATIONSHIP

A child's progress in activity in water is in some measure directly attributable to the child–physiotherapist relationship. It is important, therefore, that certain aspects of this are understood.

For many children, the initial introduction to water is a matter of anxiety. A physiotherapist who is unsure of the properties and characteristics of water, who lacks stability and balance and is reluctant to submerge is unlikely to be able to give reassurance. Poor handling and holds can also mar the experience for the child. Thus precise holds, careful handling and the ability of the physiotherapist to cope with their own body are of first concern in establishing a good water situation.

Inventiveness and creativity in developing games and activities, the use of rhythm, the voice and other factors described in the development of games (p. 52) assist in easing a tense situation.

It is possible for a child to become too dependent on one physiotherapist, and in most instances this should be avoided. A change of physiotherapist can be readily achieved in a group where the activities require the children to move from one physiotherapist to the next. In certain conditions, however, it can be advisable for the same physiotherapist to continue working with one child. For instance, where a problem of communication exists and the physiotherapist has established a rapport and an effective means of communicating with the child, the relationship should be maintained throughout treatments.

Achievement should always be acknowledged. The acquisition of a skill, whether blowing a bubble or retrieving a submerged object, needs to be recognized and praised if performed correctly. In this way a happy child–physiotherapist relationship is also developed.

INDIVIDUAL AND GROUP ACTIVITIES

Advantages

Where such a working situation as described above can take place within a group many benefits accrue. Group work has been discussed elsewhere (p. 28); however, there are some aspects particularly relevant to children in this setting.

The opportunity to work on a one-to-one basis with a physiotherapist within a group provides the optimal situation for children.

Many of the activities described in the text can be taught individually as well as in a group, and where a precise action requires particular attention and training, individual work may be used to advantage. However, in a one-to-one child–physiotherapist relationship within a group such training may also be achieved. At the same time the child benefits from the other advantages of working with others and is provided with the opportunity to acquire the required skills without undue attention being drawn to their absence.

While the advantages of group work – motivation, socialization, longer working spans and greater concentration remain the same for adults and children, the latter are affected by other factors.

For the children this may well be the first community they experience. Opportunities to develop initiative, to find security, to learn motor and behavioural skills and for increased repetition and reinforcement are essential.

Unlike the adult, children, certainly the younger ones, are not likely to take responsibility for their treatment and do not set standards for other group members.

A group is disadvantaged when all the children within it have the same disability. Progress is slowed, incentives are not developed and motivation is harder to establish. Socialization is diminished when the children are not given the opportunity of meeting others outside their usual environment.

Group Size

Too great a discrepancy in age between the children in the group tends to disadvantage the younger and smaller children, particularly during more energetic activities.

The number considered most suitable for a group is six or eight swimmers. But the size of the group will to some extent be determined by the size, depth and shape of the pool. It has to be remembered that six or eight children require the presence of six to eight physiotherapists and helpers, and the size and shape may not allow for 12 to 16 persons. It requires considerable ability to control a group of this size in activities, especially to raise the voice above the general noise level concomitant with such group activity and to maintain the group as a cohesive unit.

Group Function

Many disabled children have, of necessity, a considerable amount of attention and treatment and are set apart in some respects, isolated and insulated from experiences and activities able-bodied children develop naturally and take for granted. In a group this situation is altered. The disabled child is no longer special but part of a unit involved in activities with others.

In fact the group usually forms the first community the child experiences. It may not be possible for the child to participate fully in the group at first but the ability and appreciation of the other group members is stimulating, thus incentives are provided and increased participation follows. Opportunities to develop initiative, to find security, to learn motor and behavioural skills and for increased repetition and reinforcement are crucial. Motivation and socialization are valuable elements of groups, and the ability to concentrate and work for longer periods of time is enhanced by the group situation.

Groups provide a secure environment in which to perform activity and such security can be increased enormously by the ability and personality of the group leader and by advanced planning. A happy atmosphere is beneficial to all and promotes the appropriate conditions for achieving therapeutic and recreational aims.

The ability of the various children in the water should be fairly similar, but some disparity allows for the development of incentives and aids the swimmer's progression from dependence to independence in the water.

WATER ACTIVITY FOR THE YOUNG CHILD, 0–4 YEARS

As a means of stimulating development and widening movement experience, activity in water for the young child, whether able, at risk or disabled, is valuable. The ideas discussed concern the able-bodied; modifications for the disabled are given where appropriate.

Infants and young children will have experienced water in the bath, but the transition to a pool and a much larger expanse of water may, of course, give rise to anxiety.

The preterm infant and those who have a high risk for neurological impairment or developmental delay may have experienced hydrotherapy in an intensive care unit. A technique of waterbed flotation (Korner *et al.*, 1975) or immersion in warm baths may have been used; the latter being immersion only or immersion combined with hydrotherapy techniques (Sweeney, 1983).

Early intervention programmes for the preterm infant have been widely advocated and following an intervention programme of sensory motor facilities for very preterm, very low birth weight infants (Cole, 1988), children have participated in water activity groups for the developmentally delayed and those with frank disability. Infants as young as two to three months of age are involved with their mothers in the water programmes.

The teaching of swimming is considered by many authorities to be most appropriately begun when the child is about four years of age. At this time the ability to reason is developing (Gesell and Bates, 1974) and the child is becoming ready for school. However, this does not imply that children under four years of age should not be taken into water. Water-familiarization programmes have been developed by many people as a preparation for learning to swim (Elkington, 1978; Blanksby and Roberts, 1981; Bullock, 1982). Holt (1975, p. 13), discussing Piaget's contribution to child development, says that the child's 'sensori-motor stage has equipped him to explore further as he does in constant play'.

Play and games have a major role in a child's development (p. 52). From the early days of life the infant interacts with and relates to the parents or care-giver, observing and imitating behaviour and actions. Thus the provision of suitable opportunities and equipment is an essential part of the caring environment for young children whether able-bodied or disabled. In fact, group activity for this 0–4-year age group has been found valuable for both parent and child. But an essential ingredient when considering water activity for young children is security. Security is found in the parent's arms and in contact with the body. It is found in the sensation of the fluid environment, experienced prenatally, and now re-experienced in the warmth of the water. Security is

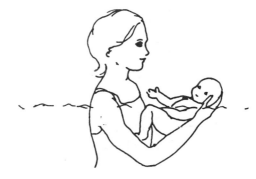

Fig. 5.1 *Supporting the head and body*

further enhanced if initially the child is kept mainly in the upright position. The hold should be at the child's waist level, and any movement of the head with a resultant swinging action of the feet can be controlled by the parent. A watchful parent can help the child appreciate the effect of movement of the head on the body by allowing the body and feet to swing in one direction or the other when the head is taken forwards or backwards, and facilitating return to the upright position. In this way the need for head control is instilled in the child from the very beginning.

With infants of two to three months, the parent holds the child in various ways to provide support for the head and body. When the child is facing the parent, the child's head is supported by one hand, and the arm and hand support the back and lower limbs (Fig. 5.1).

When a little more flotation is required, the infant's head may be cradled in the crook of the parent's elbow, and the forearm and hand of that arm can be used to provide further support if needed. In this position, the lower trunk and limbs will experience buoyancy and it allows for active movement of the lower limbs (Fig. 5.2).

Alternatively, the parent may have the child's head on the shoulder and support the body with the forearms, freeing the hands to facilitate leg movements (Figs 5.3 and 5.4).

With the baby curled up into a 'ball', a totally flexed position, the child may be rocked forwards, backwards and sideways to develop head control (Fig. 5.5).

The prone position may facilitate head and thereby trunk extension in the young child who has no difficulties, whereas for a child with a

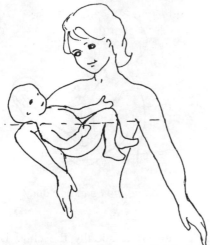

Fig. 5.2   *Cradling the head and allowing increased body flotation*

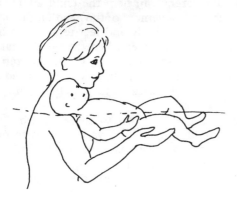

Fig. 5.3   *Facilitating leg movements – supine*

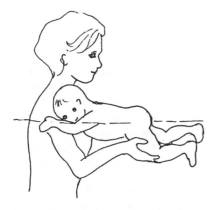

Fig. 5.4   *Facilitating leg movements – prone*

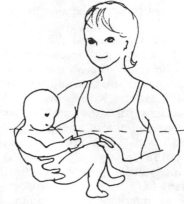

Fig. 5.5   *A 'ball'*

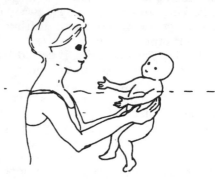

Fig. 5.6   *A waist hold when some head control is present*

disability, especially when a flexor synergy is present, being placed prone will not be advantageous as flexion is dominant in this posture and head and trunk extension are not facilitated.

Where the child's head control is beginning to be established, the child may be held at waist level and rocked in a similar manner (Fig. 5.6).

When introducing the very young child to water activity, the parent, holding in the ways described above, moves gently through the water in various directions to suitable music or rhythmical singing. As the child develops head control and arm and leg movements, the activities can be extended and progressed.

In addition to providing security within the parent's arms, colourful floating toys and objects which interest and attract the child should be used not only to break up the surface of the water and lessen the apparent vastness of the expanse, but as a means of introducing activity. Small ducks, fish, boats and quoits are usually of interest, even to quite young children, and they try to reach for them, thus bringing the hands to midline and encouraging reach and grasp.

Midline activity is vitally important and is a skill that may be affected in the preterm infant or in the developmentally delayed child. Holding a coloured quoit with two hands (it is possible to get various sizes) is one means of bringing the hands together and, since the child usually looks at the object and often mouths it, a forward movement of the head is obtained.

A ball floated on the water towards the child also develops head and arm control in midline reach, the opening of the hands and grasping. Learning to push the ball back to the therapist develops social behaviours as well as release.

By encouraging the child to leave the parent's hands and come to the physiotherapist, reaching is further promoted in addition to the prone position. The physiotherapist places the child in the upright position and, by asking 'Where is Mummy?', or by asking the parent to call out the child's name, ensures head turning which brings about body rotation. Placing the child prone again, the physiotherapist takes the child back to the parent, at the same time encouraging arm and leg movements. Once again behaviour is affected.

In games such as passing toys around the circle, reach, grasp and head control are increased and the child learns to part with the toys. Music and rhythm play an important role.

Although children under the age of 12 months are unlikely to be able to blow regularly into or onto the water, imitation of playful vocal sounds by adults occurs from approximately nine months of age. The parent should demonstrate blowing in a noisy fashion to attract the child's attention and encourage imitation. In this way emphasis is laid on the essential skill of breathing control. Toys that can be blown over the surface of the water prove helpful and, in bringing the head towards the object, head control is improved. Where a child has poor eye contact, focusing on the parent's vocal blowing sound helps gain better eye contact and head control.

Time spent in explaining to parents certain points about water activity is never wasted. If parents understand the reasons for particular holds and why certain actions are encouraged, the responses of the children will be enhanced.

Explanations need to cover the following points:

1. Why the body of a young child floats.
2. Why the child under five months of age 'swims'.
3. The importance of breathing control.
4. The importance of a forward head movement towards the water.
5. The importance of correct holding and gradual disengagement.
6. The need for control of the limbs.
7. The need for learning rotational skills.
8. The need for active movement.

This author believes it is of such importance that parents are made aware of the facts, that space is devoted here to the explanations. Armed with this knowledge parents become very effective handlers of their children and this has a bearing on the child's future water activity.

Why the Body of a Young Child Floats

The relative density of the body of the infant and young child is approximately 0.86 and therefore in the ratio of 0.86 of the child to the relative density of water which is 1, the child will float. Flotation may occur in both the face upwards or face downwards position, but the latter is totally unsafe. The child may in some instances instinctively rotate the body from the face-down position, but is unlikely to do this automatically until able to reason. Therefore the importance of total vigilance at all times when a child is near or in water becomes evident.

Why the Child Under Five Months of Age 'Swims'

Several authorities describe reflex swimming movements seen in children as young as 11 days old when held in or over water (Cratty, 1979). Since a child of this age has no head control, the head must be supported otherwise the face will submerge. The movements are more rhythmical than the crawling pattern which results from eliciting the crawling reflex. The reflex swimming movements have usually disappeared by five months of age.

Such reflex action should not be interpreted as proof that the child is swimming and, by implication, that the child is therefore able to swim enough to prevent drowning should a fall into water occur.

The Importance of Breathing Control

The importance of breathing control has been discussed earlier in the text but is reinforced by the manner in which blowing bubbles forms part of water-familiarization programmes (Elkington, 1978; Bullock, 1982). The ability to control respiration is vital when learning different swimming strokes (Counsilman, 1968; Elkington, 1978; Blanksby and Roberts, 1981). Blowing bubbles forces the water away from the nose and mouth and helps avoid taking water into the lungs or into the eustachian tubes and facial sinuses.

Many authors (for example Bullock, 1982) conclude that blowing bubbles is of first importance and can be regarded as an exercise leading to progressive submergence. The value of personal demonstration by the parent to the child is stressed and can be started at home in the bath. Appropriate toys such as fish, ducks, boats and balls that can be blown across the surface of the water may prove useful. Pouring water from teapots and jugs into other containers may be valuable in teaching manipulative skills on land. However, such items are not appropriate in a pool where a child might be encouraged to drink from them.

The Importance of a Forward Head Movement Towards the Water

Two points need to be understood in relation to forward head movement. First, if the head is extended when submerging, water may be forced up the nose if the child is not blowing. The infant and young child who has not established a regular blowing action is at great risk, especially if a fall into water occurs or the child is tossed into the air and allowed to submerge. A study of anatomy of the head and neck shows how the meninges of the brain dip down

through the cribriform plate at the base of the skull just above the upper part of the nose. Water forced up the nose may come into contact with the meninges – a possible site for infection (see Appendix). Water forced up the nose may also produce infections of the eustachian tubes and in the middle ear. In addition, in the neonate and infant the tympanic membrane is close to the surface, the growth of the external auditory meatus gradually affording protection as the child develops. This, however, is not complete until the fifth year of life (*Gray's Anatomy*, 1973). Since pressure on the ears is greater in water than in air, prolonged underwater activity should be avoided in the young child (see Appendix).

The second point relates to head posture and balance. If the head is brought forward, vertical balance can be maintained and such action is important for head control.

The Importance of Correct Holding and Gradual Disengagement

The manner in which this point can best be explained to parents is by using the parents as models. The parent is encouraged to lie back on the physiotherapist's hands using the backing hold described (p. 48). The parent is then instructed how to lie back and recover forward as for vertical rotation (p. 22). No physical assistance is given by the physiotherapist in the creation of the movement, and after several repetitions the physiotherapist transfers the supporting hands to the parent's scapulae. The lying back and recovering actions are repeated. In addition to the lesser degree of control with this hold, the altered position of the body in the supine lying position can be appreciated. When the hold is at the scapula level and the body is lying supine, there is a marked tendency for the feet to drop and the body to lie at an angle of 40°–45°. The parent then takes the physiotherapist's place and acts as the support for the physiotherapist in order that the parent realizes the difference between the two holds in the degree to which control of the supported body is achieved.

Disengagement has been discussed (p. 52), but it is important to ensure that the parents understand the need for gradual disengagement as the child acquires a skill.

The Need for Control of the Limbs

Control of the limbs is important in water not only for swimming with rhythmical movements of the arms and legs, but also in its relation to metacentric effects (p. 14). Parents come to a quicker understanding of this point if encouraged to experience the effects. This can be demonstrated by walking from shallow to deep water with hands clasped behind the back. When submerged in water up to the nostrils, the parents turn round and try to walk back to the shallow end of the pool. This is virtually impossible until the arms are raised above the head. Gravitational effects will to some extent then overcome buoyancy effects. The heels will drop to the floor of the pool and, with generation of a frictional force between the soles of the feet and the floor, it becomes possible to walk to shallow water. Alternatively, the parents can be asked to sit with the ankles, knees and hips at right-angles, the feet placed hip width apart and flat on the floor of the pool. The shoulders should be just below the surface of the water. One or both arms can be raised above the surface and held elevated while gravitational effects are appreciated. Another way in which metacentric effects can be experienced is by lying supine in the water in a 'stick' shape and raising one arm above the water towards the ceiling. The body will roll to the side on which the arm is lifted, rotating until it finds its point of balance face down in the water. If both arms are raised simultaneously, the body will sink first and then roll to whichever side is denser or shorter.

From these experiences, the need to keep as much of the body as possible in the water becomes evident, and so the need for control of the limbs is obvious.

The Need for Rotational Control

It will be recalled that two planes of rotation are possible in water. Most parents appreciate the necessity of being able to recover to a safe breathing position, but how to achieve this without the data points or points of resistance present on land needs to be explained and demonstrated. When taking young children into water, it is frequently found that rotation occurs as part of the normal pattern of development. The parent should be encouraged to allow both vertical and lateral rotation to occur, facilitated and/or controlled by them.

The Need for Active Movement

The reasons for active rather than passive movement are explained to the parents. A certain amount of passive movement may be necessary to show the child the action required, but it should cease immediately the child achieves the movement or attempts it.

A programme for the infant or young child includes activities such as blowing bubbles, trying to blow toys across the surface of the water, riding a bicycle, swinging as in the primary activity in 'Bells', splashing with fingers, hands, arms and legs, making waves and lifting the water through the fingers and also with a cupped hand.

Objects lighter than water can also be pushed under the surface and released so the child can watch them rise again. In this way the effect of buoyancy is introduced at an early stage and can be related to the effect on the human body later. With this age group and with those children whose head control and eye contact are poor, the parents are encouraged to dance to music in the water with the children held in the arms facing them and in contact with the body, thus providing security, tactile stimulation, body awareness and head control. In addition, the music provides a means of encouraging an appreciation of rhythm.

As the children progress, extension of the programme is made by using the activities and games for older children and progressing from the primary to the advanced aspect of each.

ACTIVITIES AND GAMES

Entry and Exit

There is a marked tendency among those working with disabled persons to use hoists, ramps and special wheeled chairs to get disabled swimmers into and out of the water. In the author's experience there is little need for this, as in most cases even the most severely disabled can be got into water over the side of the pool. All mechanical means of entry and exit place the disabled in an invidious position: already set apart by disability, a further handicap is placed upon them. Instead, the disabled should be enabled to participate in as normal a manner as possible so that integration, participation and socialization may become a reality. The earlier these aspects can be incorporated into water activity, the greater becomes the realization of these goals.

A method of entry and exit should be devised and developed so that in due course the disabled child enters and leaves the water independently. If the integration of disabled persons – whether children or adults – into normal life is desired, this is essential.

While appreciating that a few extremely disabled children may not achieve such independence, the author suggests that the following methods of entry and exit offer an appropriate means of help in the majority of instances. The most severely disabled may not progress beyond the first or second stages of entry and may never achieve exit over the side without assistance. But every effort should be made to try to obtain the greatest possible independence. These methods of entry and exit can be learned by anyone, and thus attendance at local swimming clubs and pools need not be a barrier. The able-bodied members can assist in entry and exit, be helped to understand the nature of the disability and how to overcome the problems relating to it. It is reiterated that it is unfortunate that the emphasis in the literature is on dependence on mechanical aids rather than on encouraging the use of the mobility and motivation of the disabled person.

Focal points

Certain other factors, in addition to those discussed in the 'Introduction', have to be taken into account when first introducing children to water.

Even a small expanse of water can seem vast and frightening to a child. To avoid distress, the physiotherapist should always be in the water

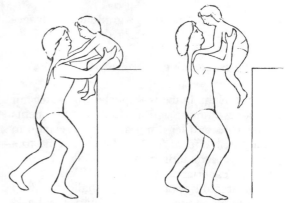

Fig. 5.7   *Sitting entry*

waiting at the side, at an appropriate depth, to receive the child. The physiotherapist then acts as a focal point when the child is placed in the sitting position on the poolside prior to entry. The physiotherapist and child can communicate easily, and encouragement and instructions can be given to the child, as well as physical support. If the distance from the poolside to water surface appears too great from the perspective of the child, the presence of the physiotherapist in the water can help to reduce this effect.

Entry

On entering the water the physiotherapist should move gently and avoid splashing. By ducking down, getting wet and blowing bubbles, it can be demonstrated to the child that water is a pleasant and enjoyable medium. Even if the water is cooler than desired or expected, the child must not become aware of this fact. Every child is probably anxious about entering water, so it is important that the physiotherapist shows no anxiety and that the water should not be cold (Reid, 1975).

The physiotherapist may work across a corner or use the shortest distance of the pool to provide a focal point, and the surface of the water will be broken up by a selection of interesting toys. In these ways, anxiety is lessened and active participation encouraged.

The sitting position has already been shown to be a stable one in water and thus a 'sitting' entry from the side ensures the child enters from a position of stability (Fig. 5.7).

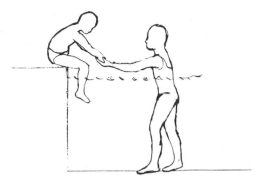

Fig. 5.8 *Entry – hands on hands*

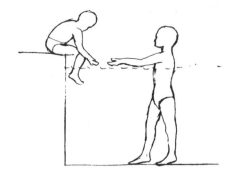

Fig. 5.9 *Sitting entry – a gap between the child's hand and those of the therapist*

The child is encouraged to reach forward and place the hands on the physiotherapist's shoulders. The physiotherapist's hands are placed on the child's back just below the lower border of the scapulae. The stance adopted by the physiotherapist is important. Step standing with the toes of the forward foot touching the wall ensures that a step backwards can be taken as the child enters the water. Talking to the child, encouraging a blowing action as the entry is made, reduces anxiety and assists in bringing the head forward towards the water. At no time should the child be allowed to place the feet against the wall or on a rail, nor extend the head and trunk as entry is made. To ensure that this does not occur, the physiotherapist can exert pressure through the hands, bringing the child into the pool with a forward action.

Once the child is in the water, it is advantageous to commence activity immediately, thus distracting the child's thoughts and avoiding anxiety about being in water, or about the water temperature. The best activities are those that keep the child in a stable 'ball' shape, such as 'Bicycles' or 'Bells' performed individually, or a jumping action which allows partial extension into a 'stick' shape. In all cases it is the 'blowing' that is important and this should be introduced rhythmically from the start.

As the child progresses and is more confident of entry, a 'hands on hands' hold is employed (Fig. 5.8). The physiotherapist's stance is similar to that for the previous hold, but the child now places the hands palm downwards on the upturned hands of the physiotherapist. Later a gap can be left between the child's hands and those of the physiotherapist. The latter picks up the child's hands as the water is entered (Fig. 5.9).

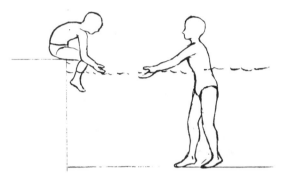

Fig. 5.10 *Independent entry – falling forward*

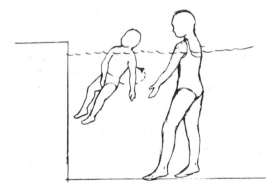

Fig. 5.11 *Independent entry – lateral rotation on to the back*

The final progression is independent entry, first using forward rotation (Fig. 5.10), and then lateral rotation to a supine lying position (Fig. 5.11) and either recovering forwards to the side of the pool or swimming away.

Forward and lateral rotational movements may be combined to produce another and more

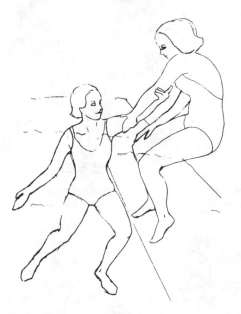

Fig. 5.12   *Entry – combined rotation*

advanced method of entry (Fig. 5.12). The child sits on the poolside and the physiotherapist takes up a stance in the lunge position diagonally to one side of the child. The child's arm on the side opposite to that on which the physiotherapist is standing is taken by the physiotherapist using the arm closest to the child. A hold is made by the physiotherapist's cupped hand placed under the upper arm of the child. The latter then places the hand on the physiotherapist's arm. Where necessary, support may be given to the child's legs by the physiotherapist's outer arm, or it may be held just below the surface of the water ready to provide support under the back as the child enters the water. The child's arm which is not being held must be placed on the lap. To obtain combined rotation it is essential that the child is instructed to look at the physiotherapist throughout the entry. As the child's body comes forward and rotates onto the back, the physiotherapist sweeps the child out into the water ensuring that the legs do not come into contact with the wall of the pool.

The important points to watch in all entries described are:

1. that the child comes forward towards the water and at no time extends the head and trunk.

2. that the child always blows as the forward movement towards the water occurs so that no water enters the mouth.

3. that the child's feet hang free of the bar and side of the pool.

It is useful for the child to be talking or singing a song or nursery rhyme when entering. Air is being expelled and water is less likely to enter the mouth. It is also a means of distracting the child, especially if it is a favourite song.

The above entries may have to be modified for some children, but it must be borne in mind that the aim is a method of entry and exit that the child can ultimately use independently.

Method of entry for the severely disabled

If the disabled child can sit, even though requiring support, the following method of entry may be used. The physiotherapist is in the water standing in a lunge position. The forward foot is close to the wall and bears the body weight. The child is brought towards the edge of the pool by a rocking movement in which the body weight is transferred from side to side. As the body weight is taken off one hip, so the physiotherapist facilitates a forward movement of that hip and leg. Once the child is close to the edge, the knees are placed high up on the therapist's shoulders on either side of the head. The child is instructed to place the hands over and behind the physiotherapist's shoulders so that they are over the latter's scapulae. The child is further instructed to lean the head to one side of the physiotherapist's head, but moving in the opposite direction (Fig. 5.13). To achieve entry the physiotherapist continues the gentle rocking movement until the child's hips are clear of the wall. Still supporting the child at the hips, the body is lifted and lowered into the water as the physiotherapist steps back, bending the knees to permit entry as soon as possible so that water takes most of the body weight. Only momentarily does the physiotherapist have the full weight of the child on the shoulders and, as this force is directly over the physiotherapist's centre of gravity, the weight is translated correctly through the body and entry achieved with a minimum of effort.

Exit

Many disabled children *can* exit from the water over the side, and this should be encouraged for reasons of independence. The basis of the exit described below is connected with the theory of boundary layer (Shapiro, 1961).

The child places, or is assisted to place, both hands on the wall (Fig. 5.14a). The physiotherapist holds the child on the lateral sides of the thighs just below the greater trochanter of the femur and helps the child to move onto the wall so that the body is lying on it. The hips remain flexed, thus keeping the legs close against the poolside (Fig. 5.14b). This is an important point for the child to appreciate, for if the hips and legs are extended and trailing in the water and if the water is flowing swiftly or is turbulent, the child could be dragged back into the pool.

The physiotherapist then assists the child to lift the legs quickly high and clear of the water as the child works forward pushing on the hands (Fig. 5.14c). Once the hips are over the pool edge, a rolling action is created by the child (Fig. 5.14d). This can be facilitated by the physiotherapist crossing the child's legs at the ankles and assisting sitting up through rotation by taking the child's arm across the body (Fig. 5.14e).

Any mobility the child has should be used

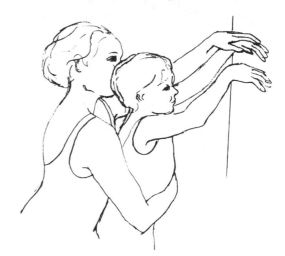

Fig. 5.14a *Exit over the side – hands on the poolside*

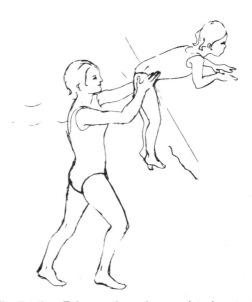

Fig. 5.14b *Exit over the side – assisted on to the poolside, the child's legs are kept close to the wall*

increasingly until the exit can be made independently.

Severely disabled children with poor head control and little use of their arms can use this form of exit. However, more assistance is needed, and another person on the bathside, if present, can control the head and arms. In the case of smaller children, the physiotherapist can manage to control and assist them alone.

The modification of this exit for the child with spina bifida is described on p. 142.

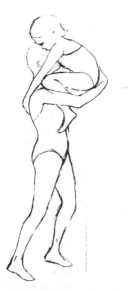

Fig. 5.13 *Entry for a severely disabled person*

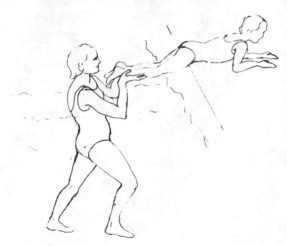

Fig. 5.14c *Exit over the side – the legs lifted together, high and clear of the water*

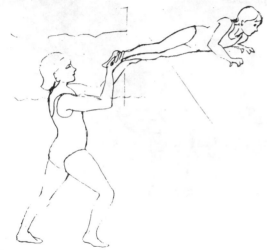

Fig. 5.14d *Exit over the side – the child is helped to wriggle forwards over the poolside and then to rotate*

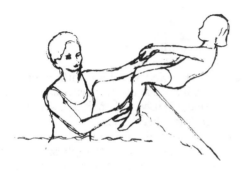

Fig. 5.14e *Exit over the side – assistance is given to sitting up with rotation*

Exit for the severely disabled child

A few severely disabled children may not be able to exit over the side of the pool in the manner described and require lifting from the water. Two or three people, depending on the size and weight of the child to be lifted, will be required in the water and one on the bathside. Small children may be lifted out by one person but it is still essential to have another person on the bathside.

The lifters stand in a line, shoulder to shoulder, facing the poolside and supporting the child on extended arms with the palms facing downwards. If three lifters are used, the person at the child's head and upper trunk places one arm under the neck, the other under the back at the lower angle of the scapulae. The lifter in the middle places one arm under the back against the first lifter's arm and the other under the child's thighs. The third lifter places one arm under the thighs against the previous lifter's arm and the other under the ankles.

It is important that the child remains still, with the hands crossed at the wrists and resting as low on the body as possible. Working in unison, standing in a lunge position, all with the same leg forward, the command 'up' is given and the child's weight is thus taken onto the extended arms of the lifters. The weight is taken off by the water as the lifters lower the arms on the 'down' command. This 'up–down' action is repeated three times, and on the fourth 'up' the lifters step forward placing the child on to the poolside, still on the arms. The lifter controlling the head and upper trunk starts to move the shoulders away and upwards from the poolside, the assistant on the poolside taking over to facilitate sitting up. The lifter controlling the pelvis rotates the hips towards the water, at the same time facilitating the sitting position. The legs and feet are moved towards the water by the third lifter, so that the final outcome is a supported sitting position for the child on the poolside with the feet in the water.

When using this lift the following points must be remembered:

1. The shape and density of the body to be lifted and the appropriate positioning of the lifters according to ability and strength to lift along the child's body. For example, where the hips and pelvis of the

child are the largest and densest part of the body, the strongest person should be the middle of the three lifters in the water.

2. All lifters should have a lunging stance with the same foot forward.
3. The arms supporting the child should be palms downwards and extended. Fingers should be extended, with the fingertips just touching the side of the pool. Fingers should not be holding the bar or any other projection.
4. Lifting should be done in unison, therefore one person should issue the commands.
5. The child being lifted should remain still and the arms kept on top on the body. Where the arms cannot be placed as suggested due to the disability, the assistant on the bathside must control the arm closest to the side of the pool and ensure that no friction occurs as the body is lifted on to the side.

Suggested songs and rhymes for entry

Many songs and rhymes are suitable for entry into the water. A few suggestions are given here.

'Jack and Jill'
'Humpty Dumpty'
'Green bottles'
Counting.

In a group which consists of boys and girls, 'Jack and Jill' provides a good rhyme for entering the water. At the words 'Jack fell down', the boys enter the water, and the girls follow at the words 'Jill came tumbling after'. The next two verses of this nursery rhyme can be utilized to practise jumping and blowing, and the group can move into the formation required for the next activity.

'Humpty Dumpty' can be used individually or in a group situation. It may be advantageous when first introducing a child to water to substitute the words 'blow' for 'fall'. The remaining lines of the rhyme may be used to practise jumping and blowing.

Using the song 'Green bottles', the number of bottles should match the number of children and all the bottles can 'fall' into the water together.

When using counting, each child is given a number and enters the water when the number is called. This is a useful method of entry in a group where some children are happier to enter the water than others.

Whatever rhyme or song is used, the purpose is to encourage a forward entry freely and confidently. The physiotherapist is concerned that a correct forward action and blowing are developed.

Some swimmers prefer to enter and exit from the water by the steps or ramp when these form part of the construction of the pool. This preference can be allowed, but the physiotherapist should bear in mind that the swimmer, at some point in the future, may participate in aquatic activities in a pool or other place where steps and ramps are not available. If entry is carried out in this manner, the physiotherapist should walk backwards in front of the swimmer and provide any appropriate assistance. When the exit is made by means of the steps or ramp, the physiotherapist should be behind the swimmer providing support if necessary, and should not leave the person until safely on the bathside.

Principles of holding

The manner in which the child is held contributes to confidence and to the degree of activity and progress that is achieved. It is essential that the holds are accurate, and constant observation is necessary in order that alterations and modifications of the holds are made commensurate with the child's progress in the skills being taught. Appropriate holds also provide the child with tactile stimulation and improved body awareness (Campbell, 1975). The points of resistance against which the human being works on land are removed in water. The new point of resistance – or datum point – is the centre of balance of the body. This is just below waist level and therefore holds should be made at or around this point. Effective control of the body is then obtained and a feeling of security imparted. Whatever position the physiotherapist takes up in relation to the child, this principle applies.

The amount of support given should be kept to a minimum so that maximum control of the body can be achieved. Holds should be relaxed and gripping avoided. Gripping may produce discomfort, increase tension and induce a

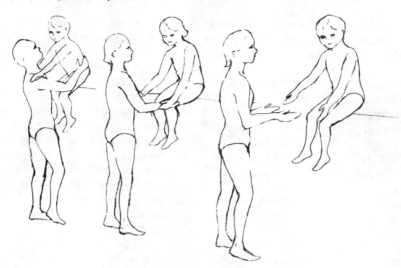

Fig. 5.15   *Group entry – showing the three progressions of 'sitting' entry holds*

change in shape with consequent alteration in balance, however small. The stability of the physiotherapist providing support to the child is vital. Whatever hold is used, the physiotherapist should have a wide stance, be well balanced and keep the shoulders at water level. The stability of this stance provides the necessary stable support for the child and also ensures that work takes place at the level of the child in the water. Thus the balance is not disturbed and communication can take place easily.

In cases of severe disabilities where marked alterations in shape and/or density are present, or where one side of the body is considerably more affected than the other, modifications of holds may need to be made. It should be borne in mind, however, that the ultimate aim is the independence of the child, and modifications that have been made should be reduced and ideal holds slowly introduced so that eventually the removal of all support becomes possible.

It is inadvisable to hold the child's head. Since the head controls the body and feet, holding of the head by another person removes the ability to produce that control independently. It has also been found to be alarming to children to be held by the head and towed through the water. This could well occur because the feeling of control over the body by movement of the head is lost. An exception to this is described under cerebral palsy.

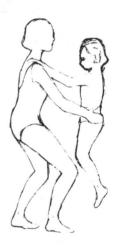

Fig. 5.16   *First facing hold*

Holds – facing

Since entry is made with child and physiotherapist facing each other, it is simple to commence activities in this position.

If entry is made with the child's hands on the physiotherapist's shoulders (Fig. 5.16), the first face-to-face engagement is achieved.

1. The child faces the physiotherapist, whose hands are placed on the child's waist, fingers pointing away. The child is then encouraged to extend the arms and place the hands on the physiotherapist's shoulders (Fig. 5.16).

   Modifications of this hold may be required when the child is unable to

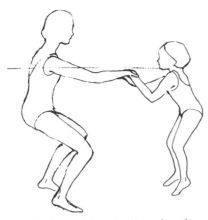

Fig. 5.17 *Facing hold – hands on hands*

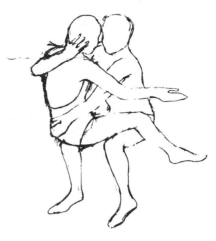

Fig. 5.18a *Holding a severely hypotonic child*

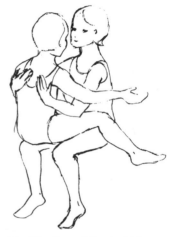

Fig. 5.18b *Modification of the hold for a hypotonic child*

extend the arms. Support is then given under the axilla, allowing the child's arms to rest on those of the physiotherapist.

2. 'Hands on hands' hold is achieved by the child placing the open hands palm down on the upturned palms of the physiotherapist (Fig. 5.17). The arms should be extended as much as possible. This hold may be progressed to a one-hand or fingertip hold.

   If work is taking place in a water depth where the child cannot touch the bottom of the pool, or if the child is small and a base is required, this can be provided by the thighs of the physiotherapist.

3. If a child has marked hypotonicity, the following hold, which gives adequate support and allows participation in many activities, can be used. The child's legs straddle those of the physiotherapist who is in the stable 'sitting' position. The physiotherapist's hands support the lumbar spine and the neck and lower part of the occiput of the child, the arms passing under the child's arms which can float free, be placed on the physiotherapist's shoulders or, when taking part in an activity in a circle, can be held by the persons on either side (Fig. 5.18a). When using this hold in a group activity, the physiotherapist will work with the back into the circle so that the child can observe the activity of the rest of the group and be part of it.

   When some degree of head control is present, this hold may be modified to support the child between the scapulae with one hand, or with both hands, one behind each scapula (Fig. 5.18b).

Holds – backing

The physiotherapist works from behind the child in the ensuing holds.

1. When the child has a severe disability the following hold may be employed. The child sits on the physiotherapist's thighs, with arms forward and supported on those of the physiotherapist. The child's elbows are outside the physiotherapist's and the hands are on top of the physiotherapist's hands (Fig. 5.19). The progression for this hold is the placing of the

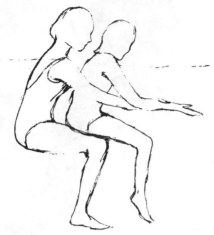

Fig. 5.19   *Hold for a severely disabled child*

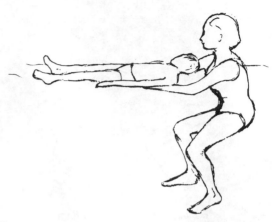

Fig. 5.21   *Backing hold – horizontal position*

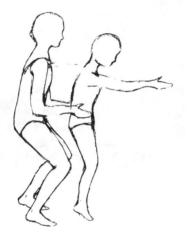

Fig. 5.20   *Backing hold – vertical position*

child's waist, the fingers pointing downwards over the child's buttocks. The child can then lie back on the flat hands of the physiotherapist (Fig. 5.21). To attain the vertical position the child creates a forward recovery and the supporting hands do not alter their position. Should the child overbalance forwards in trying to gain the upright position, the physiotherapist can readily move the fingers to a forward-pointing position and steady the child with the fingertips over the anterior superior iliac spines.

4. For activities where a line with alternate swimmer and physiotherapist (one behind the other) is required, support is given by the physiotherapist in one of two ways:

(a) Forward under the swimmer's arms around the waist of the physiotherapist in front. Where the swimmer has difficulty bringing the arms forward, the physiotherapist may hold the swimmer's arms and take them forward around the waist of the physiotherapist ahead.

(b) Around the waist of the swimmer, who holds around the waist of the physiotherapist in front.

In due course, as ability increases, the swimmer may be placed behind the physiotherapist. At all times safety of hold and the effects of turbulence must be understood and appreciated.

The **bicycle hold** has several progressions. With severely disabled children the backing

child's elbows inside the physiotherapist's arms. At times it is necessary for the physiotherapist to hold the child's forearms rather than hands to facilitate extension of the arms forward and maintain them close to the surface. Further progressions for the severely disabled child follow the lines of the backing holds for other children.

2. When requiring stabilization in the vertical position, the physiotherapist supports the child at the waist, fingers pointing forwards (Fig. 5.20).

3. When moving from the vertical position to horizontal supine lying, the physiotherapist supports the child in the upright position with the heel of the hands in the

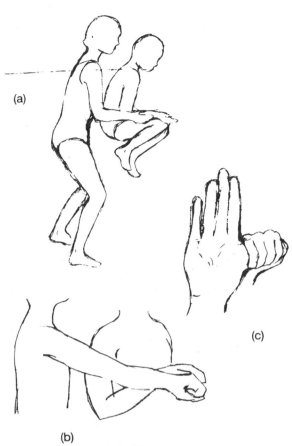

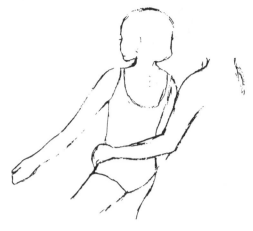

Fig. 5.23   *Across the back hold*

Fig. 5.22a   *Bicycle hold*
Fig. 5.22b   *Modification of bicycle hold –*
clenched fist
Fig. 5.22c   *Modification of bicycle hold – thumb*
hold

hold first described (Fig. 5.19) can be used. As progress is made the normal cycle holds are employed.

1. The child faces away from the physiotherapist, who supports the child's forearms with the arms held outside those of the child (Fig. 5.22a).
2. To decrease support, the child places the palms downwards on the physiotherapist's clenched fists, the elbows being inside the physiotherapist's arms (Fig. 5.22b).
3. The physiotherapist's extended thumbs give less support to the child who clasps them. Again, the child's elbows are inside the physiotherapist's arms (Fig. 5.22c).
4. During the development of lateral rotational control in the vertical position,

certain activities require a hold that provides a degree of independence but prevents the loss of balance. The physiotherapist's arms form a circle around the swimmer's body under the arms. This allows the swimmer freedom of movement within the encircling arms. Furthermore, the swimmer is able to use the physiotherapist's arms as a support and a means of facilitating lateral rotation.

Holds for line or circle activities

1. An across the back hold is formed by the physiotherapist placing the child to one side and taking the arm nearest to the child, across the child's back at waist level. The physiotherapist's hand is placed over the front of the pelvis just above the hip joint and the child held in contact with the physiotherapist's body (Fig. 5.23). This hold is used when the child's disability prevents the use of an arm for holding. When both arms are involved the physiotherapists on either side of the child embrace the child in the same manner. The forearms and elbows can be used to maintain the required position of the child's body in an activity and facilitate or control swinging actions.
2. A short arm hold is one in which the upper arm of the physiotherapist is placed under that of the child and the latter's

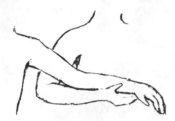

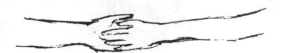

Fig. 5.24   *Short arm hold*

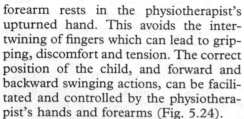

Fig. 5.25   *The position of the hands in a long arm hold*

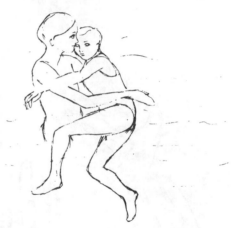

Fig. 5.26   *The hold for rolling from arm to arm*

forearm rests in the physiotherapist's upturned hand. This avoids the intertwining of fingers which can lead to gripping, discomfort and tension. The correct position of the child, and forward and backward swinging actions, can be facilitated and controlled by the physiotherapist's hands and forearms (Fig. 5.24).

3. The long arm hold provides a hand-on-hand situation. The arms of the child and those of the physiotherapist are extended sideways. To provide the child with a support that can be pushed against, the physiotherapist's open hands are sloping upwards and inwards while the child's hands are placed on them sloping downwards and outwards (Fig. 5.25). This hold is a progression on the short arm hold and is used when a greater degree of control is acquired by the child.

Holds for rolling in the horizontal

Rolling can be taught in several ways. When developing rolling on to the bar, the third hold described under 'Holds – backing' would be used (p. 47).

1. Rolling arm-to-arm hold. The child is placed in supine lying at a right-angle to one side of the physiotherapist, who supports the child at the level of the inferior angle of the scapulae with the arm on that side. To create a roll through 360° in front of the physiotherapist, the child turns the head towards the physiotherapist and brings the outer arm and leg across the body (Fig. 5.26). As the child's outer arm is brought across the body, the physiotherapist's free arm supports and guides it as it moves, without contacting the child's thorax. When the rolling action is complete the child will again be at a right-angle to the physiotherapist, supported as described above but on the side of the physiotherapist opposite to that on which the rolling movement commenced.

2. As a progression towards developing independent rolling, the following hold is used. The physiotherapist stands facing the child, the hands at the child's waist. A step is taken to one side and the child then lies back in a supine lying position. The physiotherapist places the leg nearest to the child directly below the centre of balance of the child's body and bends the knee, keeping the foot flat on the floor of the pool. The outer leg is abducted and extended (Fig. 5.27). The physiotherapist is now in a lunge position. The only further action the physiotherapist makes as the child rolls is to pat the child's body round, the hands remaining at waist level. For safety, the roll must take place toward the physiotherapist. In order to roll in the opposite direction, the physiotherapist moves around the child's head to the other side. During this manoeuvre the physiotherapist's hands maintain support at the centre of balance of the body.

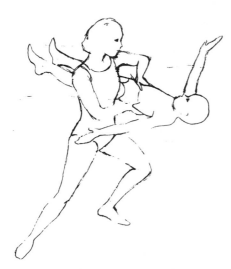

Fig. 5.27   *Rolling hold – starting and finishing position*

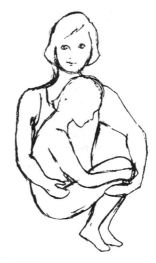

Fig. 5.29   *'Bells' hold*

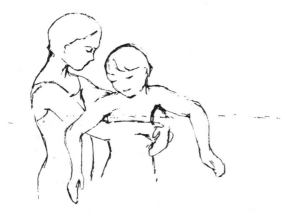

Fig. 5.28   *'Walking in space' hold*

The hold used for activities where the child requires some support but can turn round within the encircling arms is also used for those which develop lateral rotation in the vertical plane, such as 'Walking in space' (Fig. 5.28).

Modifications of holds

Modifications of holds are necessary with some children, and such modifications are acceptable, but the ideal holds described and the principles of holding, particularly of holding at or close to the centre of balance of the body, should be borne in mind at all times.

The following are some of the more useful modifications:

1. Holding at the elbows when working in a circle with a group. In this instance the child may not be ready to transfer from a short arm to a long arm hold.
2. If a child has poor head control and is working with a group in a line or circle, creating a swinging action of the body forward and backward around the centre of buoyancy, it may be necessary to adapt a short arm hold. In this case the physiotherapist's holding arm is externally rotated, bringing the child's arm into internal rotation, and the hand is held cupped ready to support the child's chin as the head comes forward. This can prevent sudden and frightening submersion of the face. If blowing is also not established as an automatic response, such action on the part of the physiotherapist avoids difficulties which may arise from inhaling water. As soon as the child shows a degree of head control in prone, this modification should be withdrawn.

Holds for individual activities

The hold used for the activity 'Bells' when working individually with the child is as follows. The child is held in front of the physiotherapist, supported around the waist with one arm, while the other hand is placed over the child's hands, which should be placed on the anterior aspect of the flexed legs just below the knees (Fig. 5.29).

It is essential that the child is held away from the physiotherapist's body, otherwise appreciation of the swinging action of the body is not experienced and the need to use the head to control or create the swing not learnt. Where the child has difficulty in bringing the arms forward and maintaining this position, the physiotherapist may need to assist the forward movement and hold the child's hands firmly on the knees. Alternatively, the physiotherapist may place the child's hands under the knees between the thighs and calves, and hold the child's legs firmly flexed, the hand being placed halfway between the knees and the ankles.

As the child gains control of vertical rotation, progression to a wider swing with extension of the body follows (as in the activity 'Rag dolls'), and a hold at the waist is used when working on an individual basis. The child is placed at the side of the physiotherapist, the arm nearest to the child being placed across the back at waist level. The other arm is across the front of the physiotherapist's body to the side of the child nearest to the physiotherapist, again at waist level. As the physiotherapist walks forwards, the child's body moves into the prone lying position. As the physiotherapist walks backwards, the child flexes the entire body, extends the head and as the body rotates backwards it is extended to the supine lying position. When the child experiences difficulty in creating the movement from prone to supine, the physiotherapist can facilitate the movement by using the forearms and elbow of the arm across the back in a downward and forward direction on the lumbar spine of the child.

Other holds for individual work with a child, some facing and backing, have already been described (pp. 46–7).

Disengagement

A major aim in water activity is total independence in the element if possible, and an important factor in the child's progress in learning the necessary skills is correct holding. However, if total independence is to be achieved, holds must be withdrawn gradually as the child becomes proficient in a skill and is able to perform it automatically and independently.

The art of knowing when and to what extent the hold can be withdrawn comes with experience. Constant observation and a feel for the child's ability within each activity act as a guide to disengagement. The most difficult point of disengagement is the final letting go. Frequently the child demands a hold, even if it is only by a fingertip. It appears to be a real hurdle to some children, despite mental adjustment and the ability to submerge at will.

Games

The significance and value of games and learning through play are well known and have been discussed by many authors (Freud, 1955; Erikson, 1963; Piaget, 1963). The word 'play' is applied to all the things children do for the joy of it, and it is suggested that for the child, play is a most important and serious activity (Stallibrass, 1977). A young child will begin to play spontaneously once the dependence on the early primitive reflexes disappears. The gradual integration of the child into the environment and the environment into the child is fostered by innate urges to develop relationships with other human beings and to acquire everyday skills through play (Sheridan, 1977). Sheridan also suggests that in play a child experiments with everything that is around, both people and things, and from this is able to develop concepts, language, intellect, emotional and social behaviours, and to control and adapt these to groups and society. Thus play provides a strong impetus towards growing up (Jolly, 1975) and is important to the optimal development of the child.

Disability frequently prevents the acquisition of skills because movement is impaired and development in some or all of its aspects is retarded, so the necessity for the provision of opportunities for play for disabled children needs to be recognized. Physiotherapists can use play in treatment to achieve desired responses and there are the additional advantages of avoiding lack of interest, boredom and antagonism towards treatment sessions (Reynell and Martin, 1965).

The author has found that in some instances the difference in a child's attitude to therapeutic activity on land and in water has been so marked that it has been advisable to cease physiotherapy on land temporarily and concentrate on activity in water. In this medium the children were happy, interested and responding. In due course it became possible to reintroduce land-based treatment sessions.

This approach applies to activity in water. Water tends to bring us all to the same level and provides an excellent means of widening the experience of the disabled child in many ways – physically, intellectually, socially and emotionally. Playing games helps to destroy the idea of 'treatment' and assists in the production of a greater response from the child. Where games are played in a group, the child is motivated by others in the group and provided with opportunities for socialization.

Games should incorporate both therapeutic and recreational aspects. Many of these are similar and thus easily combined in an activity. The emphasis may be placed in one direction or the other throughout an activity or programme or may alternate between the two. If, for therapeutic reasons, emphasis needs to be placed on a joint or joints to increase range of motion and strengthen the muscles around the joints being exercised, an activity which provides the required movements would be chosen or the physiotherapist would use ingenuity to develop such a game. Because each game has a particular aim or aims directed towards achieving recreational objectives and skills, games should never be selected randomly.

When developing games, the following points need to be considered:

(a) the objective or skill required,
(b) the appreciation by the child of the skill,
(c) position for the activity or transition from one position to another,
(d) the formation for a group and changes of formation,
(e) the movements involved,
(f) rotational control,
(g) control and/or movement of the limbs,
(h) head control,
(i) breathing control,
(j) the means of progression.

Development of the games should occur in such a manner that the skill being taught becomes gradually automatic and is performed correctly and independently. The method of development of games can be readily seen in the examples which follow in the text.

Other psychosocial factors requiring attention when constructing an activity are:

(a) degree of participation,
(b) the development of water confidence and mental adjustment,
(c) the provision of opportunities for the expression of personality and enjoyment,
(d) the use of songs, music and rhythm.

Explanations of the game should be short and explicit. Equipment may be used to encourage movement, to add to enjoyment, or to facilitate the acquisition of learning skills. When used it should be as simple as possible. The atmosphere and pace of an activity can be increased or decreased by the use of the physiotherapist's voice, tone and manner, and in the choice of song, music or rhythm. The child's interest and knowledge can be developed and extended by story telling, drama and the use of environmental factors. The development of breathing control, control of the head, trunk and limbs, and the creation of appropriate movement of these body parts not only assists in the recreational skill of swimming, but considerably enhances body image, spatial relationships and an awareness of the body as a whole unit.

In view of the similarity of both therapeutic and recreational goals, it is not intended that the description give more than a brief indication of the purpose of each activity. The physiotherapist will be aware that the encouragement of:

(a) relaxation,
(b) movement,
(c) head control,
(d) balance control,
(e) rotational control,
(f) the extremes of posture and increased range of movement,
(g) body image and spatial awareness,
(h) breathing control,

is present to a greater or lesser degree in each activity, and so can develop these in either a therapeutic or recreational direction as required.

Breathing control forms a basis for all activities and is as necessary for swimming as it is for helping respiratory control. The acquisition of lip closure, pursing the lips and blowing appears to improve the development of speech and feeding patterns.

Mental adjustment to the element of water involves aspects of perceptual and learning skills in addition to the acquisition of gross and fine motor skills.

The ability to restore the body's balance and maintain it against any disturbing forces has implications for head control, balance and coordination. In addition, rotational control assists the child therapeutically, as well as allowing for the achievement of swimming with all the implications that pertain to acquiring the art.

Many of the activities described in the following pages have been drawn from the Halliwick Method. Some of these activities have been included in books such as *Duffield's Exercise in Water* (Skinner and Thomson, 1983) and *Swimming for People with Disabilities* (Association of Swimming Therapy, 1992). All the games have been designed to teach the skills required of the swimmer and are closely interwoven with the ten-point programme of the method. Price (1980), discussing swimming for the physically handicapped child, cites the ten-point programme as developing the following:

1. Mental adjustment.
2. Disengagement.
3. Vertical rotation control.
4. Lateral rotation control.
5. Combined rotation.
6. Use of upthrust.
7. Balance in stillness.
8. Turbulent gliding.
9. A simple progression.
10. A basic movement.

The programme also describes the tasks involved in each stage. Since, in the Halliwick Method, each game has a teaching point related to the above stages, an orderly progression takes place from total dependence to the total independence of the person in the water.

For clarity, the games and activities in this text have been divided into sections related to their main purpose. In some instances more than one skill is required and such games will be listed under each heading.

The sections for activities are as follows:

1. Mental adjustment and disengagement.
2. Development of rotational control.
3. Development of balance and coordination.
4. Dynamic activity.

Although the activities have been categorized in this manner, it does not mean that the child must be able to carry out all the skills in one section before passing on to the next. For instance, mental adjustment and disengagement occur on a continuum throughout the activities though the need for mental adjustment lessens as skills are acquired. It may be necessary to support the child as each new skill is tackled, but disengagement is more rapidly achieved as the child progresses. Similarly, activities that develop rotational control will overlap with those for balance and coordination, and all lead into dynamic independent activity.

Activities for mental adjustment and disengagement

Activities under this heading provide the means by which the child can progress from the initial stages of dependence on the physiotherapist to becoming adjusted to the element of water and able to work either alone or with minimal support.

When a new skill is introduced it may be necessary for the physiotherapist to provide some support again. However, the length of time that this support will be required will be reduced and disengagement takes place more rapidly than hitherto.

It is important that an activity follows immediately upon entry. For instance having used 'Humpty Dumpty' as a means of entry, encouraging the child to come forward towards the water, entering on the physiotherapist's words 'had a great fall', the next two lines should proceed smoothly into jumping and blowing activities as the physiotherapist and child move away from the side of the pool. In this way the child's attention is distracted and any anxieties about being in water allayed.

Table 5.1 Activities for mental adjustment and disengagement

1. Jumping
2. Here we go round the mulberry bush
3. Stepping stones; Giant strides; Fairy strides
4. Clocks and watches
5. Ring a ring o' roses
6. There was a crooked man
7. How wide, how tall
8. Hickory, dickory dock
9. We reach up tall together
10. Come with me
11. Blowing objects along the surface of the water
12. I'm forever blowing bubbles
13. Walking around and across the circle
14. If you're happy and you know it
15. I hear thunder
16. Here's the sea
17. Puffer train (or Hedi, hedi, ho)

Jumping

A 'stick' and 'ball' activity suitable for a group and also the individual. Jumping in this form should be used immediately following entry.

Jumping as an activity leads towards independence in water and can be adapted and used in various activities as part of a pattern of movement. Whether jumping forwards or backwards, the head should be kept forward. In the early stages of water activity it is more appropriate for the swimmer to jump forwards and the supporting physiotherapist to move backwards. Later, jumping backwards and even sideways can be introduced to the swimmer. Many rhymes and songs about jumping are available for use in this activity and encourage rhythmic movement and breathing control.

Therapeutic aims

1. To develop head control in the anterior/posterior direction.
2. To encourage movement of the body, especially flexion and extension of the body as a whole.
3. To encourage control of the upper limbs.
4. To improve balance and coordination.
5. To improve respiration and breathing control.

	Primary activity	*Intermediate activity*	*Advanced activity*
Purpose	Mental adjustment and vertical rotational control	As primary	As primary
Appreciation	The need for forward action of the head to maintain vertical balance	As primary	As primary
Formation	The swimmer is facing the physiotherapist with hands on the physiotherapist's shoulders and supported at the waist	As primary, but a hands on hands hold is used (p. 47)	As primary, except that no support is given to the swimmer
Instruction	'Jump and blow'. The swimmer is encouraged to bend the knees up to the chest when jumping and to extend the legs for landing, but to keep the head forward and blow onto the surface of the water	'Jump and blow – blow into the water'. The swimmer uses the upturned hands of the physiotherapist as a base from which to work. The hands must remain below the surface, otherwise the swimmer's balance will be disturbed	'Jump and blow – keep your head and your hands forward'. The physiotherapist walks backwards in front of the swimmer who is reaching forward with the hands towards the physiotherapist. At first the swimmer may only blow onto the water, but at the intermediate level the swimmer must be able to blow into the water and at the advanced level should be able to submerge, blowing strongly, and maintain balance totally independently

'Here We Go Round the Mulberry Bush'

A 'stick' activity played in a circle and suitable for a group of young children.

Therapeutic aims

1. To develop head control in all directions.
2. To improve and maintain the range of movement in the cervical spine.
3. To improve balance and coordination.
4. To develop body image and awareness.
5. To improve respiration and breathing control.
6. To increase the range of movement in the hip joints and of trunk-side flexion.
7. To develop awareness of skills of daily living.

	Primary activity	*Intermediate activity*	*Advanced activity*
Purpose	Mental adjustment	As primary	As primary
Appreciation	The weight of water and how to enjoy water activity	As primary	As primary
Formation	A circle is formed of swimmers and physiotherapists placed alternately using a short arm hold	As primary, except a long arm hold is used	As intermediate, but less support is given, the speed of activity increased, and changes in direction of the circle may be introduced at any time
Instruction (same for all three activities)	'We are all going to walk sideways like a crab and lean our heads and shoulders in the same direction. Push with your head and shoulders.' While singing 'Here we go round the mulberry bush', the circle moves sideways leaning against the water. A progression at this stage may involve the swimmer blowing into the water each time the word 'bush' is sung. Other skills involving mental adjustment and head control may be introduced as follows:		

1. 'This is the way we blow bubbles' – the swimmer bringing the head forward and blowing.
2. 'This is the way we wash our ears' – the swimmer side flexes the head, first to one side and then the other, taking the ears close to the water.
3. 'This is the way we wash our hair' – the swimmer extends the head and cervical spine to place the occipital region in the water and turns the head from side to side.
4. 'This is the way we nod our heads' – the swimmer takes the head forwards and backwards slowly and rhythmically.

The physiotherapist can introduce any variations the imagination and ingenuity suggest.

Stepping Stones

A 'stick' activity.

Therapeutic aims

1. To develop rhythmical movement towards independence.
2. To encourage balance, coordination and postural reactions.
3. To increase and maintain range of movement.
4. To improve gait.
5. To increase mental adaptability.
6. To improve respiration and breathing control.

	Primary activity	*Intermediate activity*	*Advanced activity*
Purpose	Mental adjustment and disengagement	As primary	As primary
Appreciation	The effect of forward action of the head on vertical balance control	As primary	As primary
Formation	The swimmer faces the physiotherapist with the hands on the physiotherapist's shoulders. The physiotherapist supports the swimmer at the waist	A hands on hands hold is used	The physiotherapist is behind the swimmer supporting at the waist or not, depending on the swimmer's ability. Alternatively, the physiotherapist may remain in front, no support being provided
Instruction	'We are going to step from one stone to another across the pool.' The swimmer is encouraged to take larger and larger steps	As primary	The swimmer is encouraged to jump from one leg to the other

Giant Strides

A 'stick' activity suitable for individual work. A group of swimmers and physiotherapists working in pairs could use this activity.

Therapeutic aims

1. To improve mental adaptability.
2. To encourage independent movement.
3. To encourage balance and coordination.
4. To improve head control.

Fairy Strides

This activity is played in the same manner as 'Giant strides'. The purpose, appreciation and formulation are the same as in 'Giant strides', but the instruction to the swimmer is to take as small steps as possible.

A greater degree of balance control may be required when working on a small base.

	Primary activity	*Intermediate activity*	*Advanced activity*
Purpose	Mental adjustment and disengagement	As primary	As primary
Appreciation	The effect of movement through the water on the body	As primary	As primary
Formation	The swimmer faces the physiotherapist, who uses a facing waist hold. If the swimmer's ability permits, a hands on hands hold may be employed	The physiotherapist stands behind the swimmer using the backing waist hold	As intermediate, but no support is given to the swimmer
Instruction	'We are going to walk like giants, with big steps across the pool.' The physiotherapist walks backwards encouraging the swimmer to take as large a step as possible	As primary. The swimmer may need to be reminded to keep the hands forward just under the surface of the water	'Walk with giant strides across the pool'

Clocks and Watches, or 'The Grand-father's Clock'

A 'stick' activity for groups or individuals.

Therapeutic aims

1. To improve and maintain head control laterally.

2. To encourage and develop balance and coordination.
3. To develop spatial awareness.
4. To improve respiration and breathing control.
5. To increase mental adaptability.
6. To heighten awareness of the ability to lean against water and use it as a force with which to work.

	Primary activity	*Intermediate activity*	*Advanced activity*
Purpose	Head control in a lateral direction; appreciation of the weight out of water	As primary	As primary
Appreciation	Water has weight and can be leant against	As primary	As primary
Formation	The swimmer faces the physiotherapist placing the hands on the physiotherapist's shoulders, support being given to the swimmer at the waist	A hands on hands hold is used	The swimmer is not supported and in the case of a child using the physiotherapist's thighs as a base, a fingertip hold is given
Instruction	'Let's tick from side to side slowly like a grandfather clock.' The swimmer moves the head to one side to initiate the ticking action and then leans and steps to the opposite side. These actions are repeated with an increasing range of movements of the head and abduction of the legs. When the swimmer is too small to have the feet on the floor of the pool, the physiotherapist's thighs provide a base (p. 6)	As primary, and this can be varied to include ticking faster like a watch	As intermediate

'Ring a Ring o' Roses'

A 'stick' activity suitable for a group.

Therapeutic aims

1. To improve head control laterally.
2. To improve abduction/adduction of the hips (if the child is able to reach the floor of the pool with the feet), and trunk-side flexion.
3. To improve and maintain balance and coordination.
4. To improve respiration and breathing control.
5. To increase mental adaptability.

A number of verses to this nursery rhyme may be found in *This Little Puffin – Nursery Songs and Rhymes* (Matterson, 1969).

Many songs and nursery rhymes may be used in a similar manner to 'Ring a ring o' roses'. All are 'stick' activities and develop the same skills. Variation in direction can be introduced as suggested, and disengagement and lateral rotation in the vertical developed if the swimmers are asked to disengage and turn to face out of the circle and back again. They must observe the direction in which the circle is moving, leaning the head and shoulders correctly whether facing out of or into the circle.

Examples of songs and rhymes are:

'Dr Foster went to Gloucester'
'There was a crooked man'
'Here we go round the mulberry bush'
'Baa, baa, black sheep'
'Waltzing Matilda'

The creative physiotherapist will find it possible to introduce variation into the activities described – particularly for older children, teenagers or adults – by the choice of contemporary songs. Many variations can be introduced in these activities and a few of these are described in the following text.

	Primary activity	Intermediate activity	Advanced activity
Purpose	Head control; water has weight	As primary	As primary
Appreciation	The weight of water and the fact that it can be leaned against	As primary	As primary
Formation	A circle is formed with alternate swimmer and physiotherapist, using a short arm hold	As primary, but a long arm hold is used	As intermediate
Instruction	'We are going to walk sideways like a crab taking a step and bringing the feet together.' 'Ring a ring o' roses a pocket full of posies A-tishoo, A-tishoo We all go blow.' At this stage it is inadvisable to use the phrase 'We all fall down'. The circle moves round, leaning with the head and shoulders in the direction of movement. Blowing is encouraged on to the surface of the water	As primary. Changes of direction can be introduced. The swimmers must develop head control and lean in the new direction without losing the rhythm and must continue to blow into the water	As intermediate, and the swimmer is encouraged to submerge, blowing. At this stage the words 'We all fall down' may be introduced

'There was a Crooked Man'

A 'stick' activity suitable for a group.

Therapeutic aims

1. To improve head control.
2. To improve balance and coordination.
3. To increase range of abduction/adduction of the hips.
4. To increase mental adaptability.
5. To improve respiration and breathing control.

	Primary activity	*Intermediate activity*	*Advanced activity*
Purpose	Head control laterally	As primary	As primary
Appreciation	Water has weight	As primary	As primary
Formation	A circle is formed of alternate swimmer and physiotherapist using a long arm hold	As primary	As primary
Instruction	'Walk round sideways like a crab.' To the words of 'There was a crooked man', in a very definite rhythm, the circle moves in one direction	Walk round sideways 'like a crab' and when the group leader says 'change', the circle changes direction. Physiotherapists must ensure that when 'change' is called, the swimmers push their heads in the opposite direction *without* losing their rhythm and that 'blowing' is automatic	Walk round sideways 'like a crab' changing direction at the instruction 'change' and jumping into the centre when saying the last line – 'And they all lived together in a little wooden house'. By introducing changes of direction both sideways and forwards, the swimmer is given more to do and think about while at the same time maintaining the rhythm. The physiotherapist watches for automatic reactions of head control and 'blowing'

How Wide? How Tall?

A 'stick' activity suitable for group or individual work.

Therapeutic aims

1. To develop body image and spatial awareness.
2. To improve balance and coordination.
3. To increase mental adaptability.
4. To increase and maintain range of movement in the shoulder and hip joints.

	Primary activity	*Intermediate activity*	*Advanced activity*
Purpose	Body image; spatial awareness and disengagement	As primary	As primary
Appreciation	How large the body is	As primary	As primary
Formation	The child faces the physiotherapist who stabilizes the upright position of the child at waist level	As primary	As primary, but no stabilization is given
Instruction	'Spread your arms sideways and see how wide you are.' 'How tall are you?' 'Stretch your arms above your head.' 'Cuddle me.'	As primary, but the child is encouraged to spread the legs as well as the arms apart, and to stand on tiptoe when reaching up	As intermediate. The instruction 'Cuddle me' can be altered to 'Put your hands on my shoulders' if desirable for any reason – for example, a child demonstrating a distaste for such an action or in the case of the adult

'Hickory, Dickory, Dock'

A 'stick' activity suitable for group or individual
work for young children.

Therapeutic aims

1. To improve head control.
2. To encourage balance and coordination.
3. To develop independent movement.
4. To increase mental adaptability.
5. To increase range of movement in the
   upper limbs and abduction of the hips.
6. To improve respiration and breathing
   control.

	Primary activity	*Intermediate activity*	*Advanced activity*
Purpose	Encourage disengagement, balance and head control	As primary	As primary
Appreciation	The need for head-forward position to maintain balance	As primary	As primary
Formation (same for all three activities)	The swimmer stands facing the physiotherapist. In the case of small children out of their depth, they may stand on the physiotherapist's bent knees. The physiotherapist holds the swimmer at the centre of buoyancy, i.e. about waist level, hands on hips		
Instruction	'We sing "Hickory, dickory, dock", ticking like a clock from side to side. Climb the clock by climbing up your physiotherapist as "The mouse runs up the clock"; clap hands over your head when "The clock strikes"; run down your physiotherapist and blow as "The mouse runs down"; repeating the ticking.' In the primary activity the physiotherapist will be giving maximum assistance	As primary. Now the swimmer must climb up and down with less assistance. When 'ticking', stabilization at waist level only should be required. There is a danger of falling forwards or backwards when in a triangular shape, which gives some lateral stability but none anteroposteriorly	As primary. To ensure lateral stability, the physiotherapist can push the swimmer gently, but firmly, from side to side in the 'ticking' and see if the swimmer restores to the triangular position and is controlling body forwards and backwards. All climbing should be done independently and, when standing on the physiotherapist's knees high out of the water, the swimmer should control the body's balance without assistance if possible. If not, minimum help is given by the physiotherapist. Blowing must be automatic when 'The mouse runs down'

We Reach Up Tall Together

A 'ball' and 'stick' activity.

Therapeutic aims

1. To encourage and maintain movement of the head, trunk and all four limbs.
2. To improve body image and spatial awareness.
3. To improve balance and coordination.
4. To improve respiration and breathing control.
5. To improve mental adaptability.

	Primary activity	Intermediate activity	Advanced activity
Purpose	Extremes of posture; disengagement; vertical rotation; head control; control of movement; balance and upthrust	As primary	As primary
Appreciation	The use of the head to control the body; body image	As primary	As primary
Formation	The physiotherapist supports the swimmer at the waist from behind	The swimmer is given less support throughout and in the second verse faces the physiotherapist using a hands on hands hold	The swimmer is given the minimum of assistance or no assistance
Instruction (same for all three activities)	*'Reach up tall'. The swimmer stretches the arms above the head while singing or saying:* 'We reach up tall together We reach up tall together We reach up tall together Like giraffes at the zoo.' *'Curl up small'. The swimmer curls the body up as small as possible while singing or saying:* 'We curl up small together We curl up small together We curl up small together Like pussy likes to do.' *'Lie still in the water'. The swimmer 'sits', extends the head and allows the body to float in the supine lying position, supported at the waist by the physiotherapist and with the head on the physiotherapist's shoulder, and sings or says:* 'We lie still in the water We lie still in the water We lie still in the water Like all good children do.'	*'Kick your legs'. The swimmer proceeds to kick the legs alternately in the supine lying position, singing or saying:* 'We kick our legs together We make it rainy weather We kick our legs together Until the skies turn blue.' *'Stand up'. The swimmer regains the upright position by flexing the knees to the chest, brings the head and arms forward until the body is rotated to the vertical and then remains standing, balanced, while singing or saying:* 'We stand up in the sunshine We stand up in the sunshine We stand up in the sunshine And blow our bubbles too.' *On the last line the swimmer demonstrates blowing*	

Come with Me

A 'stick' activity suitable for group and individual work. 'Swimming', 'paddling', 'floating', 'kicking' and 'rolling' are other actions that could be employed as the swimmer becomes more competent.

In the primary activity the swimmer would be supported in the supine lying position. In the intermediate activity, less support would be given. At the advanced level, the swimmer would be able to move independently through the water. Attaining the supine lying position and recovering introduce the extremes of posture and vertical rotational control.

Therapeutic aims

1. To encourage and develop movement and the control of movement.
2. To improve balance and coordination.
3. To develop body and spatial awareness and other perceptual skills.
4. To improve respiration and breathing control.
5. To increase mental adaptability.

	Primary activity	*Intermediate activity*	*Advanced activity*
Purpose	Mental adjustment, movement and control of movement, balance and rotational control	As primary	As primary
Appreciation	The head controls the feet; awareness of movement through water effects	As primary	As primary
Formation	The swimmer faces the physiotherapist with hands on the physiotherapist's shoulders. Support is given at the swimmer's waist. A line formation or free order is used	The swimmer and physiotherapist are facing using a hands on hands hold	The swimmer works independently. The physiotherapist is nearby, at first in front and later behind the swimmer. Finally the swimmer is able to achieve the actions alone
Instruction	'Come walking with me, Come walking with me, Over the highway and down to the sea, come walking with me.' Variations such as jumping, hopping, tiptoe and dancing may be used	As primary. A further progression may be introduced in which the physiotherapist supports the swimmer at the waist from behind	As intermediate, with minimal or no support

Blowing Objects Along the Surface of the Water

A 'stick' activity suitable for group and individual work.

Whether facing or backing holds are used, the child should be kept in front of the physiotherapist as vertical rotational control is also developed in this activity.

Therapeutic aims

1. To develop head control.
2. To develop and maintain breathing control.
3. To increase balance and coordination.
4. To improve mental adaptability.

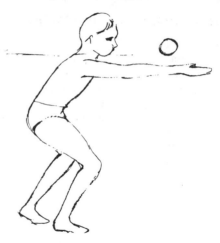

Fig. 5.30 *Blowing an object across the water*

	Primary activity	*Intermediate activity*	*Advanced activity*
Purpose	Head and breathing control	As primary	As primary
Appreciation	The effect of blowing on the head and body	As primary	As primary
Formation	The swimmer faces the physiotherapist and places the hands on the physiotherapist's shoulders. The physiotherapist supports the child at the waist. A bath toy is placed between the faces on the surface of the water	The swimmer faces away from the physiotherapist, who supports the child at the waist	As intermediate
Instruction	'Blow the duck (fish, table tennis ball, "poached egg", etc.) to me and I will blow it back to you.' The physiotherapist should remain stationary at first as any movement backwards will cause the object to move away from the child's face due to turbulent effect. However, as a progression, such action can take place and the author has found that towing the object away in this manner may focus the child's attention, and bring the head, eyes and often the hands (if they are not on the physiotherapist's shoulders) to midline	'Put the duck on the water in front of you; keep your arms forward and blow the duck across the pool.'	As intermediate. An incentive, such as a race, will increase the speed and depth of the blowing action. The aim is to encourage the blowing to proceed from blowing regularly on to the surface to blowing regularly into the water

'I'm Forever Blowing Bubbles'

A 'stick' activity suitable for a group. As an individual activity, walking sideways across the pool may be used.

It is possible to alter the words to make the activity more appropriate for water – for example, exchange the word 'sea' for 'air'. Other lines can be made to rhyme by the use of words such as 'whirl' and 'swirl'.

Therapeutic aims

1. To encourage and maintain head control in the vertical.
2. To improve balance and coordination.
3. To encourage the movements required in walking sideways and forwards.
4. To improve and maintain respiration and breathing control.

	Primary activity	*Intermediate activity*	*Advanced activity*
Purpose	Head control	As primary	As primary
Appreciation	Effect of head movement on body; water has weight	As primary	As primary
Formation	A circle with alternate swimmer and physiotherapist using a short arm hold	As primary, but a long arm hold is used	As intermediate with swimmers inside the circle
Instruction	'Walk sideways and whenever the word "blowing" is said, blow into the water.'	As primary	'Walk anywhere in the circle or across it singing and blowing.'

Walking Around and Across the Circle

A 'stick' activity suitable for a group.

Therapeutic aims

1. To improve head control.
2. To encourage active movement and increase the range of movement.
3. To improve mental adaptability.
4. To increase respiration and breathing control.
5. To improve balance and coordination and spatial awareness.

	Primary activity	Intermediate activity	Advanced activity
Purpose	Mental adjustment and disengagement	As primary	As primary
Appreciation	Increasing ability to move in water independently	As primary	As primary
Formation	The swimmer faces the physiotherapist and places the hands on the physiotherapist's shoulders. A circle is formed by all the physiotherapists joining hands	As primary	As primary
Instruction	'While we stand still, walk your hands along our arms all the way round the circle to the right (or left).' The swimmers must all go in the same direction, and are verbally encouraged to move round the circle passing each physiotherapist in turn. If a swimmer's feet do not touch the floor of the pool, dependence on the arms and hands is greater and head control to maintain the vertical position must be well developed. Crossing the hands and arms while moving around the circle is inadvisable, especially when the child's condition produces strong flexion, adduction and medial rotation of the shoulders with extension at the elbows. However, in circumstances where crossing the body's midline is to be encouraged, such an action can prove helpful	'Walk round the circle close to us but do not hold on.' Alternatively, the swimmers could hold the physiotherapists' arms and move around the circle while the circle itself moves in one direction and then another. This would require greater control from the swimmers, especially against the turbulence created by the physiotherapists' movements	'Walk around and across the circle without holding on.' Some swimmers may choose to jump across, others will attempt to swim. For the child who cannot touch the bottom of the pool, swimming across is encouraged. In this case a physiotherapist may choose to come into the centre of the circle to assist any swimmers who may be uncertain of their ability. A further progression could be made by having the swimmers walk round the outside of the circle

'If You're Happy and You Know it'

A combined 'ball' and 'stick' activity suitable for individual and group work. Any therapeutic activity can be introduced into the words of the song.

Therapeutic aims

1. To encourage head control.
2. To improve balance and coordination.
3. To improve and maintain respiration and breathing control.
4. To improve body image and spatial awareness.
5. To develop control of the limbs and encourage awareness of the head for control.
6. To encourage active movement of the trunk and limbs.
7. To improve mental adaptability.

	Primary activity	*Intermediate activity*	*Advanced activity*
Purpose	Head control; disengagement; control of the limbs and balance	As primary	As primary
Appreciation	The effect of movement of the head, arms and legs on the balance of the body	As primary	As primary
Formation	This may vary from a circle with alternate swimmer and physiotherapist to the swimmer either facing the physiotherapist or facing away	This may be altered to encourage disengagement. A circle may change to the swimmer facing the physiotherapist	The swimmer works independently, little or no support being provided
Instruction	To perform the action required by following the physiotherapist's instructions. For example, 'If you're happy and you know it, bend your knees' or 'blow some bubbles' or 'make some waves'. The physiotherapist will give the appropriate support to allow the swimmer to achieve the required action	As primary	As primary. More advanced skills, such as submerging when blowing bubbles or mushroom floats (p. 112) or rolling, can be introduced

'I Hear Thunder'

A 'stick' game suitable for group and individual activity.

Therapeutic aims

1. To develop movement of the upper and lower limbs.
2. To develop control of the upper and lower limbs.
3. To develop balance and coordination.
4. To increase and maintain head control.
5. To improve respiration and breathing control.

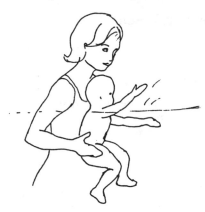

Fig. 5.31 *'I hear thunder'*

	Primary activity	Intermediate activity	Advanced activity
Purpose	Vertical rotation control and limb control and movement	As primary	As primary
Appreciation	The need for control of the limbs and balance control	As primary	As primary
Formation	The swimmers stand in front of the physiotherapist facing into the circle, supported by the backing hold – vertical position (Fig. 5.20, p. 48). The arms are stretched forwards	As primary but less support is given	As intermediate, except that less support is given and more energetic movement is encouraged for the thunder and even smaller ones for the raindrops, so that the swimmer appreciates the contrast and acquires control of the limbs
Instruction	'I hear thunder, I hear thunder. Oh don't you, Oh don't you.' The swimmers make large splashing movements with each arm alternately up and down in front of them. 'Pitter patter raindrops, pitter patter raindrops, I'm wet through, so are you.' The swimmers make small movements with their fingers to create raindrops	Larger arm movements are encouraged for the thunder, developing increased splashing and the need to cope with the effects of these actions and not take the head back and away from the splashing. The swimmers then lay back on the physiotherapist's hands and repeat the actions with their legs. Large splashes for the thunder and small kicks for the raindrops	As primary with additional words to encourage the larger movements and control the finer ones

'Here's the Sea'

A 'stick' activity suitable for a group.

Therapeutic aims

1. To develop head control and encourage active movement.
2. To improve and maintain balance and coordination.
3. To encourage flexion and extension of the whole body.
4. To increase mental adaptability.
5. To improve respiration and breathing control.

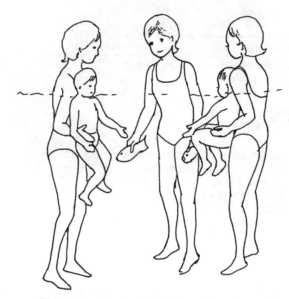

Fig. 5.32   *'Look at the fishes down below'*

	Primary activity	*Intermediate activity*	*Advanced activity*
Purpose	Vertical rotation and lateral rotation in the horizontal	As primary	As primary
Appreciation	The effect of head movement on the body	As primary	As primary
Formation	The swimmer stands in front of the physiotherapist facing into the circle. The physiotherapist uses the backing hold for the horizontal position (Fig. 5.21, p. 48)	As primary but less assistance is provided	As primary, assistance only being given to the swimmer to attain the lying position and also to help balance in the vertical if necessary
Instruction	'Sit in your chair, arms forward, let your head go back until you are lying in bed'. The physiotherapist sways the swimmer from side to side with the words 'Here's the sea, the wavy sea.' The physiotherapist rotates the swimmer tilting the body from side to side during the second line 'And this is a boat'. At the words 'And this is me', the swimmer recovers forwards to the upright. 'Look at the fishes down below' – the swimmers bring their heads forward to look at toy fish held below the surface. When the words 'Wiggle their tails' are said, the swimmers kick their legs and on the words 'Away they go', the physiotherapist rolls the child into the prone position and encourages the swimmer to 'swim away'	As primary	As primary

'Puffer Train' or 'Hedi, Hedi, Ho'

A 'stick' activity suitable for group work.

This activity should be taken slowly and gently at first, especially with young children, with whom it is a great favourite. As an alternative to the train, 'Hedi, hedi, ho' can be sung and the elephant's trunk tries to catch the tail.

Therapeutic aims

1. To improve mental adaptability.
2. To increase head control.
3. To encourage balance and coordination.
4. To improve and maintain respiration and breathing control.

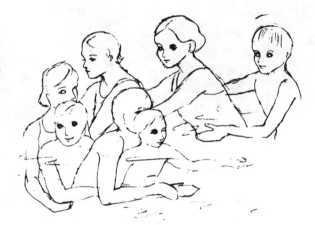

Fig. 5.33   *Line formation for 'Puffer train'*

	Primary activity	*Intermediate activity*	*Advanced activity*
Purpose	Mental adjustment; head control and balance	As primary	As primary
Appreciation	Water has weight and can be leaned against; turbulent effect	As primary	As primary
Formation	Alternate swimmer and physiotherapist in a line behind each other. The first physiotherapist in the line may circle the swimmer with the arms or use a forearm bicycle hold. The next and all other physiotherapists take the arms forward *under* the swimmer's arms and grasp the physiotherapist in front *around* the waist. The line is closely linked in this way and each child is secure and feels safe. Where a swimmer has strongly extended arms or marked lack of control of these limbs, the physiotherapist may hold the wrists and take the swimmer's arms forward and around the waist of the physiotherapist in front, maintaining them in this position	As primary, except that the hold is changed to each swimmer holding around the waist of the physiotherapist in front and each physiotherapist holds around the swimmer's waist	As primary, but the swimmer is placed behind the physiotherapist
Instruction	As we sing 'Puffer train', the line will move around the pool in any direction the leader chooses. At the end of the verse the 'driver of the train' tries to catch the 'guard' at the end. The physiotherapists at the end of the line must encourage the swimmers to lean away from the direction in which the 'driver' is approaching. Once the 'guard' has been caught, a new swimmer takes the lead and the activity is repeated. Each swimmer is the responsibility of a physiotherapist and it is essential that the swimmer is observed to ensure that breathing control is encouraged and that the swimmer does lean from side to side appropriately	As primary. It is important that the physiotherapist watches the swimmer's hold and encourages the appropriate actions at all times	As primary. The turbulence in this activity is considerable and the swimmer may be dragged off by it. The physiotherapist must be aware of this possibility and watch carefully to cope with this contingency should it arise. Initially the swimmer's hands may be held by one of the physiotherapist's, therefore the other arm and hand of the physiotherapist connect with the swimmer in front

Activities for the development of rotational control

Activities for the development of rotational control can be divided into the following:

1. Vertical rotational control.
2. Lateral rotational control in the vertical and horizontal planes.
3. Combined rotational control.
4. Control of buoyancy or upthrust effects.

Notes related to each of these divisions precede the descriptions of the activities (see also Table 5.2).

VERTICAL ROTATION

The activities contained in this section are designed to help the child create and control all movements around the centre of buoyancy of the body in a forward and backward direction. The child is able to maintain the upright position and move from it either to supine lying or prone lying and recover to the vertical or upright posture.

Table 5.2 Activities for the development of rotational control

Vertical rotation
1. Bells
2. Little boy blue
3. Catch an object (ducks, fish in the pond, catching toes, reach for the bar, eggs for breakfast)
4. Rag dolls or swinging backwards and forwards
5. Wind, sun and rain
6. Bicycles
7. Charlie is over the water
8. The Grand Old Duke of York
9. Here we go Looby Loo
10. The wheels of the bus
11. Red red robin
12. Over the arches; Under the arches
13. Walking in space (see also Lateral rotation – vertical plane, p. 94)
14. Little boats are on the sea
15. Pop goes the weasel

Bells

A 'ball' activity suitable for group and individual work.

At this level of activity a further progression could be that of encouraging the swimmer to extend the body in the supine and prone lying position, curling up to create the swing from one position to the other. Good head control is required at this stage to ensure that no sudden upswing of the legs occurs.

When using this activity on an individual basis, the physiotherapist uses the hold described on p. 51. As the swimmer progresses to the advanced level the physiotherapist can support at the waist. This support can be removed gradually until the swimmer is performing the activity independently.

Therapeutic aims

1. To develop head control.
2. To encourage active flexion and extension of the whole body.
3. To develop awareness of the extremes of posture and body image.
4. To improve coordination.
5. To increase mental adaptability.
6. To improve respiration and breathing control.

	Primary activity	*Intermediate activity*	*Advanced activity*
Purpose	Vertical rotational control	As primary	As primary
Appreciation	The effect of the movement of the head on the body position in the water	As primary	As primary
Formation	A circle is formed of alternate swimmers and physiotherapists using a short arm hold	As primary	As primary except that a long arm hold is used
Instruction	'Swimmers, bend your knees to your chests, heads back slowly, heads forward and blow.' When necessary, facilitation and/ or control of the body swing can be provided by the physiotherapist through the supporting arms	'Let's sing "Ding dong bell" as we swing forwards and backwards.' A slow rhythm is important and the physiotherapist watches for head control and breathing control while giving less assistance to the body swing	As intermediate

'Little Boy Blue'

A 'ball' and 'stick' activity suitable for group or individual work.

Therapeutic aims

1. To improve head control.
2. To improve and maintain balance and coordination.
3. To encourage body and spatial awareness.
4. To increase mental adaptability.
5. To improve respiration.
6. To encourage flexion/extension patterns of the whole body.
7. To increase the range of abduction/adduction in the hip joints.

Catch an Object

Included under this title are activities such as 'Eggs for breakfast', 'Reach for the bar' and 'Catching toes'.

Therapeutic aims

1. To develop flexion/extension patterns of the whole body.
2. To encourage and maintain balance and coordination.
3. To improve rotational control in the anterior/posterior direction.
4. To improve control of the arms, reach and grasp symmetrically and asymmetrically if required.
5. To develop body image, spatial awareness and laterality.
6. To improve respiration and breathing control.

	Primary activity	*Intermediate activity*	*Advanced activity*
Purpose	Vertical rotation, head control	As primary	As primary
Appreciation	Effect of head movement on the body	As primary	As primary
Formation	A circle is formed of alternate swimmer and physiotherapist using a short arm hold	As primary	As primary but using a long arm hold
Instruction	'Blow when the word "blow" is sung. Put the ear to the water to "hear the horn". Keep still when singing "fast asleep".'	As primary except lie back, remain still and go 'fast asleep'	As intermediate but the circle moves round, first in one direction and then the other, progressing further by frequent change of direction

	Primary activity	*Intermediate activity*	*Advanced activity*
Purpose	Vertical rotational control	As primary	As primary
Appreciation	The effect of head movement on the body	As primary	As primary
Formation	The swimmer in front of and facing away from the physiotherapist. The backing hold (Fig. 5.20, p. 48) is used	As primary but less support and assistance are given	As intermediate but support is only given to the floating position. The circle may be widened further and a competitive note introduced if one object is removed each time the activity is played
Instruction	' "Sit" in your chair, hands forward, head back slowly until you are lying in bed, your head on my shoulder and go to sleep. When the bell sounds, you bend your knees up to your chest, bring your head and hands forwards, blow and get a "fish".' Ducks, eggs, rings, the bar or other swimmers' toes may be used as the objects to catch. If reaching for the bar, the swimmer and physiotherapist should be facing the side of the pool and when the swimmer lies back, the toes should rest just touching the wall. At no time should a swimmer be permitted to catch the toes behind the bar as this may prove dangerous as the recovery action is made. The bell rings and the swimmers create a forward recovery and take an object. This activity is known as 'Eggs for breakfast' in the Halliwick Method but can also be developed as 'Ducks for dinner', 'Fish for lunch', 'Reach for the bar', 'Catching toes' and so on	As primary. The circle can be widened so that the swimmer has to reach forward a greater distance on recovering	The physiotherapist must ensure that the swimmer controls the movement from the vertical to lying position with the head. This action should occur slowly as flotation is required. The correct starting position with the arms forward can be developed if the swimmer places the object in the centre of the circle and holds the object there until ready to lie back. When recovering forward, the swimmer will only be interested in reaching for an object whereas the physiotherapist's concern is with ensuring the correct movement pattern is created together with breathing control

Rag Dolls or Swinging Forwards and Backwards

A group or individual activity involving the 'ball' and 'stick' pattern of movement.

Therapeutic aims

1. To encourage and maintain head control in the anterior/posterior direction.

2. To improve the flexion and extension pattern of the whole body between the two extremes of posture.

3. To improve respiration and breathing control.

	Primary activity	Intermediate activity	Advanced activity
Purpose	Head control in a forwards and backwards direction; the extremes of posture	As primary	As primary
Appreciation	The effect of head movement on the body; body image	As primary	As primary
Formation	**Group activity:** a line of alternate swimmers and physiotherapists is formed, all facing the same way, using a short arm hold. An extra physiotherapist, if available, should work at the end of the line where a swimmer would be unsupported on one side. If an extra physiotherapist is unavailable, the physiotherapist supporting the child at the end of the line places an arm across the back at the waist as described on p. 49 **Individual activity:** the physiotherapist places the swimmer to one side using the across the back hold (p. 49) with the other hand at the waist on the nearest side and facilitates the swinging action by walking forwards and backwards and by applying pressure on the lumbar spine using the arm which is in contact with the swimmer's back	As primary except that a long arm hold is used	As intermediate with a minimum of support or fingertip hold and no facilitation is provided
Instruction (same for all three activities)	'As we walk forwards, let's all blow. Let your legs go up behind you. When we walk backwards, bend your knees up to your chests, put your heads back and lie out long.' The instructions are repeated as the line moves forwards and backwards. Where necessary, the swinging movement of the swimmers can be facilitated by the arms of the physiotherapists		

The Wind, Sun and Rain

A group activity using the 'ball' and 'stick' extremes of posture.

Therapeutic aims

1. To improve head control.
2. To increase body image and awareness.
3. To improve mental adaptability.
4. To improve respiration and breathing control.
5. To encourage active movement.

	Primary activity	*Intermediate activity*	*Advanced activity*
Purpose	Vertical rotational control	As primary	As primary
Appreciation	Effect of the movement of the head on the body and awareness of the extremes of posture	As primary	As primary
Formation	A circle with alternate swimmer and physiotherapist using a short arm hold	As primary except the hold is changed to a long arm hold	As intermediate
Instruction	'All blow like the wind towards the middle of the circle.' The circle moves inwards and as the sun comes out, the swimmers are instructed 'Put your heads back slowly, let your legs float up and lie out in the sun.' The physiotherapists move backwards and widen the circle, still retaining the short arm hold. The blowing and floating is repeated several times as the circle moves in and out. Finally, the swimmers, while lying supine, are encouraged to 'make some rain' by kicking their legs. When it 'rains' the swimmers should blow away the splashes, at the same time keeping the eyes open. The physiotherapist should set an example	As primary. The swimmer has to control the body swing to a greater extent and the physiotherapist should ensure that the head is controlling this, that the correct vertical rotation action is used and that blowing with the eyes open occurs	As intermediate, but less facilitation is given to the swinging action if the physiotherapists remain stationary. The activity and forward and backward movements of the circle could also be speeded up, thus demanding control against increased turbulence. The swimmer's reactions should be completely automatic at this stage

Bicycles

A 'ball' activity that can be used individually or in a group.

Variations of this activity can be introduced and a range of songs used. Bicycling is enjoyed by the children and may form part of an activity as, for example, in 'Here we go Looby Loo' or 'The wheels of the bus'. Alternatively, it may be used as an activity on its own and progressed to a competitive level.

The physiotherapist must ensure that the child is not lifted out of the water and that head control and breathing control are developed. Therapeutically, strong flexion of the body is achieved in addition to head control, balance and flexion/extension movements of the lower limbs.

Therapeutic aims

1. To improve and maintain head control in anterior/posterior direction.
2. To encourage active movements of flexion/extension in the lower limbs.
3. To encourage control of the upper limbs symmetrically.
4. To improve respiration and breathing control.
5. To develop and maintain balance and coordination.
6. To develop flexion of the body as a whole.
7. To improve mental adaptability.

	Primary activity	Intermediate activity	Advanced activity
Purpose	Vertical rotational control	As primary	As primary
Appreciation	The head controls the feet	As primary	As primary
Formation	The swimmer in front of the physiotherapist, facing away. A bicycle forearm hold is used (p. 49)	As primary but the bicycle fist hold is used (p. 49)	As primary but a bicycle thumb hold is used (p. 49)
Instruction	'Bend your knees up to your chest and make your legs go round and round like riding a bicycle.' The swimmer uses the head to maintain the curled-up body in the vertical position while alternately flexing and extending the legs as if riding a bicycle. Verbal facilitation in regard to head control may be given. If the swimmer's legs come up towards the surface in front, then the instruction is directed towards a forward head movement. Should the swimmer's body go too far forwards, the instruction is to extend the head until the body is vertical again. Manual facilitation may be given by the physiotherapist to the swimmer's forearm. The hold is not altered or lost	As primary but the activity is played more energetically	As primary but it is played extremely energetically and may take the form of a race across the pool

'Charlie is Over the Water'

A 'ball' activity suitable for a group. This is a variation on 'Bicycles' and is played to the rhyme:

'Charlie is over the water
Charlie is over the sea
Charlie caught a blackbird
But he can't catch me.'

Therapeutic aims

1. To improve and maintain head control in an anterior/posterior direction.
2. To encourage control of the upper limbs.
3. To develop active flexion and extension of the lower limbs.
4. To improve respiration and breathing control.
5. To encourage flexion of the body as a whole.
6. To increase mental adaptability.

	Primary activity	Intermediate activity	Advanced activity
Purpose	Vertical rotational control	As primary	As primary
Appreciation	The effect of the head movement on the body	As primary	As primary
Formation	One physiotherapist and swimmer act as 'Charlie', using a bicycle forearm hold. The remaining physiotherapists and swimmers, using the same hold, form a circle around 'Charlie'	As primary, but the hold is changed to the second bicycle hold (Fig. 5.22b, p. 49)	As primary, except the bicycle hold using the thumbs is used (Fig. 5.22c, p. 49)
Instruction	As the group repeats the rhyme, the circle bicycles around in one direction, and on the last line 'Charlie' bicycles after the other swimmers, endeavouring to catch someone. The swimmer who is caught then becomes 'Charlie', and the activity is repeated	As primary, but the game is played more vigorously	As primary. The speed of the game is increased further

'The Grand Old Duke of York'

A 'ball' activity suitable for group or individual work.

Therapeutic aims

1. To improve and maintain head control in an anterior/posterior direction.
2. To encourage control of the upper limbs.
3. To develop active flexion/extension of the lower limbs, and flexion of the body as a whole.
4. To improve respiration and breathing control.
5. To improve spatial awareness.
6. To encourage mental adaptability.

	Primary activity	*Intermediate activity*	*Advanced activity*
Purpose	Vertical rotational control	As primary	As primary
Appreciation	The effect of the head in controlling the body position	As primary	As primary
Formation	The swimmer is in front of the physiotherapist, facing away and supported by a bicycle forearm hold (p. 49)	As primary, but the hold is changed to a bicycle fist hold (p. 49)	As primary, but the hold is changed to a bicycle thumb hold (p. 49)
Instruction	'Bend your knees up to your chest and make your legs go round and round like riding a bicycle.' As the swimmer moves the legs the physiotherapist walks around. Both swimmer and physiotherapist sing the nursery rhyme. 'The Grand Old Duke of York'. At this stage of the activity it is inadvisable to lift the swimmer out of the water when singing 'he marched them up to the top of the hill' as strong control of the head and body is required	As primary. If the swimmer is to be lifted out of the water at the appropriate words, a further instruction to 'keep the head forward' must be given	As primary and intermediate. Lifts above the surface of the water can be made higher, thereby demanding greater head and body control to keep the body vertical in a 'ball' in both the buoyancy- and gravity-dominated situations

'Here We Go Looby Loo' or 'The Hokey Cokey'

A 'ball' and 'stick' activity.

The chorus and first verse used for this activity are as follows:

Chorus:
Here we go Looby Loo
Here we go Looby Li
Here we go Looby Loo
All on a Saturday night.

1st verse:
I put my right arm in
I put my right arm out
I shake it a little, a little
And turn myself about.

Therapeutic aims

1. To encourage and improve balance and coordination.
2. To improve body image, spatial awareness and laterality.
3. To develop head and trunk rotation.
4. To improve respiration and breathing control.
5. To increase mental adaptability.

	Primary activity	Intermediate activity	Advanced activity
Purpose	Vertical rotation, lateral rotation in the vertical plane; laterality; turbulent effect	As primary	As primary
Appreciation	The effect of head movement on the body; body image; right and left	As primary	As primary
Formation	The swimmer is in front of the physiotherapist, facing away. The holds vary throughout the activity (see bicycle hold, p. 49)	As primary, but the hold is changed to a bicycle fist hold (p. 49) and less support is given when performing the actions of the arms and turning	As primary, but the hold is changed to a bicycle thumb hold and no support is given when performing the arm and leg actions and turning
Instruction (same for all three activities)	Varies from verse to verse. *Chorus* (p. 49): using a forearm bicycle hold, the circle of swimmers and physiotherapists moves round in one direction, the swimmers flexing and extending the legs as if riding a bicycle, and using the head to maintain the vertical position. *1st verse* (p. 48): the swimmers and physiotherapists face into the circle and the hold is changed to the waist. The swimmers follow the action in the verse, but if unable to turn themselves about, the physiotherapist either 'turns about' with them or facilitates the turn. The chorus is repeated in between every other verse. The actions follow according to the verse that is being used, i.e. *2nd verse*: 'I put my left arm in', *3rd verse*: 'I put my right foot in', *4th verse*: 'I put my left foot in', *5th verse*: 'I put my whole self in'		

'The Wheels of the Bus'

A 'ball' and 'stick' activity mainly suitable for a group.

1st verse:
The wheels of the bus go round and round,
round and round, round and round.
The wheels of the bus go round and round
Down the busy street.

2nd verse:
The people on the bus go up and down,
up and down, up and down.
The people on the bus go up and down
Down the busy street.

3rd verse:
The driver on the bus goes toot toot toot,
toot toot toot, toot toot toot.
The driver on the bus goes toot toot toot
Down the busy street

4th verse:
The windscreen wipers go swish swish swish,
swish swish swish, swish swish swish.
The windscreen wipers go swish swish swish
Down the busy street

As an alternative and to introduce further appreciation of vertical and lateral rotation, lateral sway and drag effect, the following form may be used.

A circle is formed by alternate swimmer and physiotherapist using a short arm hold. The swimmers are instructed to sit in their chairs and put their heads back slowly until lying out long. The circle of physiotherapists then moves round in waterwheel fashion. As the verse finishes, the swimmers are instructed to 'recover forwards', that is, to bend the knees up to the chest, heads forward, blow and stand up.

Therapeutic aims

1. To improve head control antero-poster-iorly.
2. To encourage active movement of the limbs, and flexion of the body as a whole.
3. To develop head and trunk rotation.
4. To increase balance and coordination.
5. To develop control of upper limbs.
6. To improve respiration and breathing control.
7. To increase mental adaptability.
8. To improve body image and spatial awareness.

	Primary activity	Intermediate activity	Advanced activity
Purpose	Vertical rotation; body image; spatial relationships; lateral rotation in the vertical plane	As primary	As primary
Appreciation	The effect of head movement on the body; awareness of body parts and the body in space	As primary	As primary
Formation	Varies from verse to verse	As primary, but a bicycle fist hold is used and less support and assistance given to any of the actions. If the waterwheel formation is used, the hold would change to a long arm hold	As primary, but the bicycle thumb hold is used and little or no support is given in the other formations. In the final verse, if a waterwheel formation is used, the wheel could change directions and a kicking action of the legs be introduced
Instruction (same for all three activities)			

1st verse (p. 49): the swimmer is in front and facing away from the physiotherapist, who is using a bicycle forearm hold. A circle of swimmers and therapists moves around 'bicycling' and singing.

2nd verse (p. 48): the swimmers and physiotherapists turn to face the middle of the circle. The physiotherapist supports the swimmer at the waist, while the swimmers jump up and down rhythmically, blowing as they come down towards the water.

3rd verse (p. 49): the swimmers and physiotherapists turn to face in one direction, using the bicycle forearm hold. As the words 'toot toot toot' are sung and the swimmer brings the head forward and blows into the water, the circle moves round.

4th verse (p. 48): the swimmers and physiotherapists face into the middle of the circle. The swimmer is instructed to clasp the outstretched hands together while the physiotherapist supports at the waist. The swimmer then moves the arms through the water from side to side.

5th verse: This is a repeat of the 1st verse, and the actions can be the same.

'The Red Red Robin'

A 'ball' and 'stick' activity suitable for a group.

Therapeutic aims

1. To develop rotational control in an anterior/posterior direction, including head control.
2. To improve body image and spatial awareness.
3. To develop balance and coordination.
4. To improve respiration and breathing control.
5. To increase mental adaptability.
6. To increase range of movement, especially abduction/adduction.
7. To increase active flexion/extension of the body as a whole.

	Primary activity	*Intermediate activity*	*Advanced activity*
Purpose	Vertical rotational control	As primary	As primary
Appreciation	The effect of head movement on the body	As primary	As primary
Formation	A circle is formed with alternate swimmer and physiotherapist using a short arm hold	As primary, but a long arm hold is used	As intermediate
Instruction	'Bend your knees, put your head back and let your legs come up and lie out long. We will all sing "The red red robin" and when we say "get up, get out of bed", bend your knees up to your chest, bring your head forward, blow and stand up.'	As primary	As primary but 'Now we are going to walk sideways, slowly lie back and stand up as before, then continue walking.' The circle moves round and the swimmers have to control vertical rotation on the move. Some lateral rotational control in the horizontal is introduced when the swimmers are lying supine and being moved round in the circle by the physiotherapists

Over the Arches

A 'ball' and 'stick' activity suitable for a group. It may be used in conjunction with 'Under the arches'.

Therapeutic aims

1. To encourage movement, balance and coordination.
2. To develop body image and spatial awareness.
3. To develop and maintain head control.
4. To improve respiration and breathing control.
5. To increase the range of flexion/extension in the body as a whole.
6. To increase mental adaptability.
7. To improve gait.

	Primary activity	*Intermediate activity*	*Advanced activity*
Purpose	Vertical rotation, head control and extremes of posture	As primary	As primary
Appreciation	The effect of head movement on the body	As primary	As primary
Formation	A circle of alternate swimmer and physiotherapist using a long arm hold which **must** be maintained throughout the activity	As primary	As primary
Instruction	A swimmer with physiotherapists on either side walks forward across the circle towards an 'arch' formed just below the surface by two of the group. The swimmer who is instructed to 'sit, put your head back slowly, and lie out long', is pushed over the arch, and told to, curl into a ball and stand up'. The 'ball' and 'stick' actions are repeated as the swimmer is drawn backwards by the physiotherapists, all walking back to the original position. NB. The correct actions for vertical rotation must be encouraged throughout the activity. When walking backwards in water the swimmer is instructed to 'keep your head forward and stick your bottom out' – thus the upright position is maintained	As primary. To increase the difficulty, this activity can be done more rapidly and with less assistance for the swimmer	As intermediate

Under the Arches

A 'ball' and 'stick' activity suitable for a group. It can be used in conjunction with 'Over the arches'.

Therapeutic aims

1. To encourage movement, balance and coordination.
2. To develop body image and spatial awareness.
3. To improve and maintain head control.
4. To improve respiration and breathing control.
5. To increase active flexion/extension in the body as a whole.
6. To increase mental adaptability.
7. To improve gait.

	Primary activity	*Intermediate activity*	*Advanced activity*
Purpose	Upthrust, rotational control, mental adaptability	As primary	As primary
Appreciation	Buoyancy of the water	As primary	As primary
Formation	A circle of swimmers and physiotherapists is placed alternately using a long arm hold	As primary	As primary
Instruction	Without a break in the circle, a swimmer walks across the circle to 'duck' under the arch made by a swimmer and physiotherapist's arms just below the surface. The swimmer is instructed to 'bend the knees', go under the arch blowing and stand up on the other side. The physiotherapists continue to hold the swimmers' hands throughout the action. To return into the circle, the swimmer bends the knees and comes backwards under the arch blowing, standing up prior to walking backwards to the original position	As primary. The progressions are made by lowering the level of the arch and finally allowing the swimmer to perform the activity independently	As intermediate

Walking in Space

A 'stick' activity suitable for a group or an individual.

This activity can be progressed even further by increasing the rocking action, the speed and thereby the turbulent effects. This demands greater head control, increased ability to hold the physiotherapist and/or move around the physiotherapist without holding. In the latter instance the swimmer is paddling independently.

Therapeutic aims

1. To encourage and maintain head control.
2. To encourage movement of head, trunk, upper and lower limbs.
3. To encourage balance and coordination.
4. To improve respiration and breathing control.
5. To increase mental adaptability.
6. To improve spatial awareness.

	Primary activity	*Intermediate activity*	*Advanced activity*
Purpose	Vertical and lateral control in the vertical	As primary	As primary
Appreciation	The effect of head movement on the body	As primary	As primary
Formation	The swimmer in front of the physiotherapist, facing away. A hold for lateral rotation in the vertical plane is used (backing holds p. 47 – No. 2 p. 48)	*Phase 1*: As primary but the physiotherapist now rocks from side to side *Phase 2*: As primary and phase 1, but the physiotherapist also moves sideways *Phase 3*: As primary and phases 1 and 2. If the child circles the physiotherapist in a clockwise direction, the physiotherapist then pivots counterclockwise on the longitudinal body axis	As primary and intermediate phases 1, 2 and 3, but the physiotherapist now turns in the same direction as that taken by the swimmer when proceeding out of the arms and around the physiotherapist
Instruction	'Turn round and face me. Touch the side of my head with one arm to open the doors. Turn round and face out of the doors. "Walk" down my arms and out and around my back. Walk up my arms and close the doors by touching the other side of my head. Turn around and face away from me.'	As primary	As primary

'Little Boats are on the Sea'

A combined 'ball' and 'stick' activity suitable for a group, but which can be adapted for individual work. The song is taken from *This Little Puffin – Nursery Songs and Rhymes* (Matterson, 1969).

Therapeutic aims

1. To improve head control.
2. To encourage flexion and extension of the body as a whole.
3. To improve and maintain respiration and breathing control.
4. To develop awareness of body image, the extremes of posture and the body in space.
5. To improve mental adaptability.

	Primary activity	*Intermediate activity*	*Advanced activity*
Purpose	Vertical rotational control	As primary	As primary
Appreciation	The effect of movement of the head on the body	As primary	As primary
Formation	The swimmer is in front of the physiotherapist, supported as in the back lying hold (p. 48)	A circle is formed with alternate swimmer and physiotherapist using a short arm hold (p. 50)	As intermediate, except that the hold is changed to a long arm hold (p. 50)
Instruction	'Lie still and relax until we sing "loudly the wind begins to shout", then bend your knees to your chest, head and hands forwards, blow and stand up. As the wind dies away, lie back again.'	'Swimmers, bend your knees, head back slowly and lie out long.' The physiotherapists move the circle two or three steps in one direction and then in the other until the words 'loudly the wind', when the swimmers recover to the vertical and blow, lying back again as the wind dies and the circle continues moving	As intermediate. As the swimmer progresses, the speed and tossing movements can be increased. At all times the physiotherapist must observe the swimmer's recovery action for the correct components of movement

'Pop Goes the Weasel'

A 'ball' and 'stick' group activity.

Therapeutic aims

1. To develop head control in the upright position.
2. To maintain and improve breathing control.
3. To increase balance and coordination.
4. To appreciate the extremes of posture.
5. To increase mental adaptability.

	Primary activity	*Intermediate activity*	*Advanced activity*
Purpose	Vertical rotational control	As primary	As primary
Appreciation	The effect of head movement on the body and turbulent effects	As primary	As primary
Formation	The swimmers and physiotherapists form a circle, the swimmer in front and facing away; forearm bicycle hold	As primary, but one swimmer with a physiotherapist acts as the weasel and another pair act as the monkey. Use the bicycle fist hold	As intermediate, using a bicycle thumb hold
Instruction	'Bicycle your legs and when we sing "Pop goes the weasel" jump up and down and blow.'	'All swimmers bicycle your legs while the monkey chases the weasel in and out of the circle, and jump up and down and blow.' (Let each swimmer take a turn at being either the monkey or the weasel.)	'All swimmers bicycle your legs, move in any direction around the pool, jump up and down and blow on the last time "pop goes the weasel".'

Lateral rotation – vertical plane

The following activities are primarily concerned with lateral rotation in the vertical plane and follow sequentially. Partial lateral rotation in the vertical may already have been introduced in activities such as 'The wheels of the bus' during the windscreen wiper section, and in 'Here we go Looby Loo', for example, a complete turn has taken place. This turning action in the upright can be further developed in the ensuing activities (Table 5.3).

Table 5.3 Activities for the development of lateral rotational control in the vertical plane

Lateral rotation – vertical plane
1. Passing the ring
2. Walking in space (see Vertical rotation, p. 91)
3. Rotating around the circle in the vertical
4. This is the way we roll around
5. Turning in the circle
6. Jumping on the spot

Passing the Ring

A 'stick' activity suitable for a group and which must be played in both clockwise and counter-clockwise directions.

Objects such as balls, fish or ducks may be used instead of the ring. Where manipulation is difficult or impossible, the object can be made to move on to the next swimmer by turbulence. In this case the swimmer rotates the body towards the next swimmer, and the object which has been floating on the opposite side will be drawn across by the turbulent effect.

As the swimmer's control of lateral rotation improves, this activity can also be played in the supine lying position, when it is advanced in the same manner as described earlier. The critical element is the ability of the swimmer to roll the body in both directions using the head and limbs. Finally, the swimmer will be able to perform a complete 360° roll independently, and for this the following activity may be used.

Therapeutic aims

1. To improve and maintain head and trunk rotation.
2. To improve laterality, body image and spatial awareness.
3. To improve balance and coordination.
4. To improve control of the limbs.
5. To improve respiration and breathing control.

	Primary activity	*Intermediate activity*	*Advanced activity*
Purpose	Lateral rotational control in the vertical plane	As primary	As primary
Appreciation	The effect of turning the head and taking the arm across the body on the body position	As primary	As primary
Formation	The swimmer stands in front of the physiotherapist, supported at the waist, facing into the circle	As primary, but the circle is widened a little	As intermediate, but the circle is widened further
Instruction	'Pass the ring which is in your right hand across the body to the swimmer on your left and look at them. Once the ring has been taken from your hand, turn your head back in the opposite direction until your body is in a flat position.'	As primary	As primary. At no time must the swimmer change the ring from one hand to the other in front of the body. Such action defeats the purpose of the activity

Rotating Around the Circle in the Vertical

A 'ball' game suitable for a group.

Therapeutic aims

1. To develop head control especially rotation.
2. To encourage arm and trunk movement.
3. To develop balance and coordination.
4. To maintain breathing control.
5. To increase mental adaptability.

	Primary activity	*Intermediate activity*	*Advanced activity*
Purpose	Lateral rotation in the vertical	As primary	As primary
Appreciation	The effect of head movement on the body	As primary	As primary
Formation	A circle with the swimmers, sitting on the physiotherapists' laps, facing into the circle	As primary but the circle is widened to increase the rotation	As primary but no assistance is given to the swimmer
Instruction	'Take your right arm across your body and reach for the right arm of the physiotherapist on your left, and turning your head rotate your body to sit on the next physiotherapist's lap.' The swimmers continue to rotate around the circle when instructed to avoid any collisions and allowing them to settle between rotations. Singing an appropriate song to maintain a rhythmic and smooth rotary movement is important	As primary	As primary

It is essential the swimmer learns to rotate in both directions
When a hoop is used, or in the Advanced activity, a physiotherapist may be on the far side of the hoop (or arch) to ensure the swimmers rotate safely
This activity is undertaken largely under water

'This is the Way we Roll Around'

A 'stick' activity suitable for a group.

Therapeutic aims

1. To encourage head control.
2. To improve balance and coordination.
3. To develop rotation around the longitudinal axis of the body.
4. To improve body image and spatial awareness.
5. To increase mental adaptability.
6. To improve respiration and breathing control.

	Primary activity	*Intermediate activity*	*Advanced activity*
Purpose	Lateral rotation in the vertical and horizontal positions	As primary	As primary
Appreciation	Effect of turning the head on the body	As primary	As primary
Formation	The child stands in front of the physiotherapist facing into the middle of the circle	As primary	The child lies supine on the physiotherapist's hands, feet into the middle of the circle
Instruction	'Turn around and face your physiotherapist. Now turn and face into the circle again, singing "This is the way we turn around, turn around, turn around. This is the way we turn around, when in the pool we play".' This can be progressed to a complete turn in front of the physiotherapist	'Jump right round in front of your physiotherapist, turning your head and taking an arm across your body.' In jumping and turning to the right, the left arm is taken across the body. The jump can be started in half turns and progressed to the full turn. Watch that the swimmer blows, singing as above	'Half roll to the right and back flat.' Repeat to the left, singing as in primary. This is progressed to a complete roll in front of the physiotherapist or can be used to roll around the circle from physiotherapist to physiotherapist as in 'Rolling around the circle'

Turning in the Circle

A 'stick' game suitable for a group.

Therapeutic aims

1. To develop rotation of the head and trunk.
2. To improve control of the limbs.
3. To encourage movement, balance and coordination.
4. To increase mental adaptability.
5. To improve respiration and breathing control.

	Primary activity	Intermediate activity	Advanced activity
Purpose	Lateral rotational control in the vertical plane	As primary	As primary
Appreciation	The effect of turning the head on the body with upper limb involvement	As primary	As primary
Formation	The swimmers stand with their hands on the physiotherapists' shoulders in a face-to-face position. The physiotherapists complete the circle formation by using a long arm hold with each other	As primary	As primary
Instruction	'You are all going to walk and turn all round the circle. Take your right hand off the shoulder and in to the middle of the circle and continue to take it back and out towards the next physiotherapist's left shoulder. Let go with your left hand and bring it round to the physiotherapist's right shoulder so that you are facing a new physiotherapist.' This rotatory action is repeated right round the circle and performed in the opposite direction	As primary but 'Now you must only use your fingertips to touch the shoulders.'	'This time take your feet off the bottom as you rotate round the circle and hold as lightly as you can.' At this level the swimmers are rotating at an angle of 45°

Jumping on the Spot

A 'stick' activity suitable for individual or group work.

Therapeutic aims

1. To develop rotation of head and trunk and encourage active movement.
2. To improve and maintain balance and coordination.
3. To improve respiration and breathing control.
4. To encourage control of the upper and lower limbs.
5. To increase mental adaptability.

	Primary activity	*Intermediate activity*	*Advanced activity*
Purpose	Lateral rotation in the vertical plane	As primary	As primary
Appreciation	The effect on the body of turning the head	As primary	As primary
Formation	The swimmer stands back to front of the physiotherapist and encircled around the chest by the physiotherapist's arms. There is no contact other than that of the swimmer's arms on top of those of the physiotherapist (p. 51)	As primary, but the swimmer is only supported at the waist	As primary, but no support is given to the swimmer
Instruction	'Turn round and say "Hallo" to me; you can use my arms to help you round.' Once the swimmer is facing the physiotherapist, the instruction is to turn and face away again. Turning in both directions must be developed as it is an essential skill for safety	'Jump round and face me', then 'Jump round and face away.' The swimmer must turn the head in the direction of the movement and may also take the arm on the opposite side of the body across the chest to facilitate the jump	'Jump all the way round and face away from me again.' The same action of the head and arm is required and the swimmer must regain a stable position on landing

Lateral rotation – horizontal plane

The following activities take the child from turning in the vertical plane to rotating in the horizontal. A halfway stage is possible if required, and is achieved by the child rotating around the circle of physiotherapist's arms with the feet off the bottom, as in the activity 'Rolling round the circle'.

It should be remembered that the ability to create or control a roll around the longitudinal axis of the body is dependent upon the use of the head and limbs. The activities described below encourage the use of these body parts. In developing the rolling action, the physiotherapist must ensure that the child is able to rotate in both directions, that is, to the right and to the left.

Table 5.4 Activities for the development of lateral rotational control in the horizontal plane

---

Lateral rotation – horizontal plane
 1. Seaweed
 2. Hallo
 3. Rolling on to the bar
 4. Resisted rolling
 5. The wheel
 6. Passing the ring
    (see Vertical plane, p. 9)
 7. Rolling arm to arm
 8. Rolling through 360°
 9. Rolling around the circle
10. Rolling down the river

Seaweed

A 'stick' activity suitable for an individual and a group.

Therapeutic aims

1. To encourage relaxation.
2. To improve balance and coordination in the horizontal.
3. To encourage control of upper and lower limbs.

	Primary activity	*Intermediate activity*	*Advanced activity*
Purpose	Lateral rotational control in the horizontal position	As primary	As primary
Appreciation	The effect of lateral sway and drag on the body	As primary	As primary
Formation	The swimmer is supported by the physiotherapist in supine lying, held under the waist	As primary, but less support is given and, provided no adverse response occurs, a widening of the swaying action	As intermediate, but less support is given and the relaxed body of the swimmer is drawn backwards by the turbulence created by the movement of the physiotherapist
Instruction	'Lie still and relax; be like a piece of seaweed floating in the water.' The physiotherapist walks backwards swaying the swimmer from side to side so that the legs and lower trunk relax	As primary	As primary

'Hallo'

A 'stick' activity suitable for a group or an individual. It is similar to 'Seaweed'; the differences relate to the swing of the floating body and the turn of the swimmer's head.

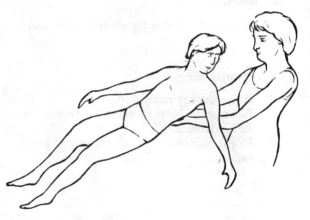

Fig. 5.34   *'Hallo'*

Therapeutic aims

1. To improve and maintain head control and rotation of the cervical spine.
2. To improve and maintain balance and coordination.
3. To improve respiration and breathing control.
4. To increase body awareness, especially of the lower limbs.

	Primary activity	*Intermediate activity*	*Advanced activity*
Purpose	Lateral rotational control in the horizontal plane	As primary	As primary
Appreciation	The effect of lateral sway and the drag of the body; the effect of head turning on the body	As primary	As primary
Formation	The swimmer is supported by the physiotherapist in supine lying, held at the waist	As primary, but the speed of the swing from side to side is increased	As primary and intermediate, with increasing speed and swing
Instruction	'When you are swayed out to the side, turn your head and say "Hallo" to me.' The physiotherapist walks backwards, swaying the swimmer from side to side so that the arms are extended and the swimmer's body is at arm's length from the physiotherapist	As primary	As primary. The physiotherapist requires the development of head turning independently of the rest of the body as a means of creating and controlling lateral rotation

Rolling onto the Bar

A 'stick' activity suitable for a group or individual. It is a progression from the 'Seaweed' and 'Hallo' activities and can be incorporated in them and others which involve the supine lying position and movement through the water, such as 'Speedboats'.

Therapeutic aims

1. To encourage movement in rotational pattern for head, trunk and limbs, and control of the head and limbs.
2. To reduce truncal spasticity.
3. To improve respiration and breathing control.
4. To improve balance and coordination.
5. To increase mental adaptability.
6. To increase body image and spatial awareness.

	Primary activity	*Intermediate activity*	*Advanced activity*
Purpose	Lateral rotational control in the horizontal plane	As primary	As primary
Appreciation	The effect of turning the head on the body	As primary	As primary
Formation	The swimmer is supported by the physiotherapist in supine lying, held under the waist	As primary, but less assistance is given in creating the roll on to the bar and greater speed encouraged	As intermediate, but no assistance is given to creating the roll on to the bar
Instruction	'Relax and let me sway you through the water. When we reach the other side of the pool, turn your head to the left, reach for the bar with your right hand, then your left hand, bring your legs up underneath you and stand up.' If the swimmer rolls to the right, the head is turned in that direction and the left hand reaches for the bar first	As primary	As primary

Resisted Rolling

A 'stick' activity suitable for group or individual.

Therapeutic aims

1. To develop, maintain and improve cervical rotation.
2. To create a change in shape, especially when extension is required on one side of the body.
3. To improve coordination.
4. To encourage mental adaptability.

	Primary activity	Intermediate activity	Advanced activity
Purpose	Lateral rotational control in the supine lying position	As primary	As primary
Appreciation	The effect of the movement of the head on the body	As primary	As primary
Formation	The swimmer stands in front of the physiotherapist, facing away. The backing hold for the vertical position is used by the physiotherapist (p. 48)	As primary	As primary
Instruction	'Sit in the chair, hands forwards, put your head back on my shoulder and let your legs go out long.' 'When you are rolled to the left, turn your head to the right and feel how your body comes flat again.' 'If you are rolled to the right, turn your head to the left to bring the body flat.' The physiotherapist rolls the swimmer manually, first to one side and then to the other, and allows the body of the swimmer to return to the supine lying position when the swimmer turns the head away from the roll	As primary. The physiotherapist gives resistance to the uppermost side of the swimmer's body and prevents, to some degree, a return to the flat position. The swimmer has to work harder in turning the head and extends and abducts along the side of the body to which the head is now turned	As intermediate. Progression is brought about by increasing the amount of resistance given to the counter-rotational action

The Wheel

A 'stick' activity suitable for a group.

Therapeutic aims

1. To improve balance and coordination.
2. To increase and maintain mental adaptability.

	Primary activity	*Intermediate activity*	*Advanced activity*
Purpose	Lateral rotational control in the horizontal	As primary	As primary
Appreciation	The effect of movement of the head on the position of the body	As primary	As primary
Formation	A circle is formed with the swimmers and physiotherapists placed alternately, using a short arm hold (p. 50)	As primary, except that the short arm hold is changed to a long arm hold (p. 50)	As intermediate
Instruction	'Swimmers, bend your knees and hips and sit; put your heads back slowly and lie out full length.' The physiotherapists then walk sideways in one direction and the swimmers relax and allow their bodies to be moved through the water. When the physiotherapists change direction of the circle, the legs of the swimmers will tend to swing away from the centre of the 'wheel'. The swimmer is then instructed to turn the head to prevent this lateral movement of the legs and feet	As primary. The progression is achieved by the change of hold and more frequent alterations in direction of the circle	As intermediate, with further progression achieved by increasing the speed and frequency of the changes in direction

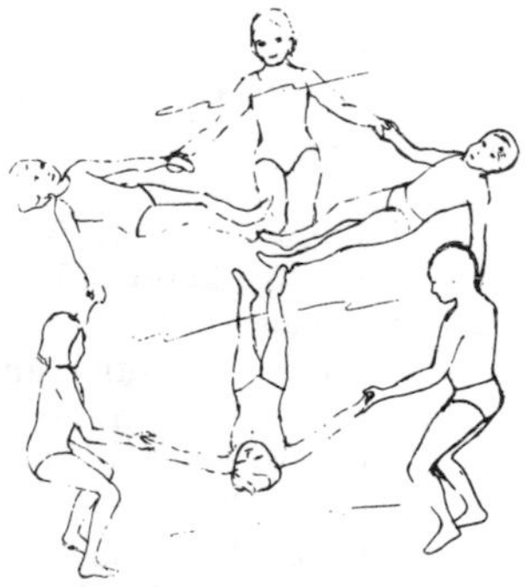

Fig 5.35 *'Water wheel' formation using a long arm hold. A short arm hold may also be employed*

Rolling Arm to Arm

A 'stick' activity suitable for groups and individuals.

Therapeutic aims

1. To develop rotation of head and trunk.
2. To develop control of the limbs.
3. To improve balance and coordination.
4. To improve respiratory and breathing control.
5. To increase body image and spatial awareness.

	Primary activity	Intermediate activity	Advanced activity
Purpose	Lateral rotation in the horizontal	As primary	As primary
Appreciation	The effect of rotation of the head on the body	As primary	As primary
Formation	The hold is described on p. 50	As primary	As primary
Instruction	'Turn your head towards me; bring your outer arm over my arm and the outer leg across the other; blow as you roll.' The position of the swimmer above the surface of the water as the roll occurs can be controlled by the physiotherapist. At first the head and shoulders are above the surface. The finishing position after each roll is on the opposite arm of the physiotherapist to that from which the roll was commenced. After each roll, the swimmer's leading arm will be behind the physiotherapist's shoulders	As primary. Progression is achieved by providing less assistance and allowing the roll to occur lower in the water	As primary. Progression is achieved by allowing the roll to occur virtually unaided at the surface. Any suitable rhythmical music may be used to develop the rolling action

Rolling through 360°

A 'stick' activity suitable for individual work, but a group could be formed with each physiotherapist working with a swimmer. The movement can be taught with an extension or flexion pattern according to the condition of the swimmer.

Therapeutic aims

1. To improve head control.
2. To encourage active movement.
3. To increase mental adaptability.
4. To reduce muscle spasm in the trunk through the rhythmical rotatory action.
5. To improve respiration and breathing control.
6. To improve balance and coordination.

	Primary activity	*Intermediate activity*	*Advanced activity*
Purpose	Lateral rotation in the horizontal	As primary	As primary
Appreciation	The effect of head, arm and leg movement on the body	As primary	As primary
Formation	Swimmer lying horizontal beside the physiotherapist who uses the second rolling hold (p. 51)	As primary	As primary
Instruction	'Bring your outer arm and leg across your body; turn your head towards me; blow as you roll and lift on the elbow of the other arm as you come round.' The physiotherapist pats the waist of the swimmer to facilitate the action	As primary. The progression is obtained by the physiotherapist giving less assistance	As primary. Little or no support is provided by the physiotherapist. Independent rolling through 360° in both directions should be possible at this stage. It is important that all rolling should be carried out rhythmically

Rolling round the Circle

A 'stick' activity suitable for a group.

The rolling action must be developed to both the right and left. Most swimmers have a preferred direction but, in the interests of safety, must learn to create and control lateral rotation in both directions.

Therapeutic aims

1. To develop rotational patterns of head, trunk and limbs, encouraging creation and control of rotation.
2. To reduce truncal spasticity.
3. To encourage active movement.
4. To improve and maintain respiration and breathing control.
5. To increase body image and spatial awareness.

	Primary activity	*Intermediate activity*	*Advanced activity*
Purpose	Lateral rotational control in the horizontal plane	As primary	As primary
Appreciation	The effect of creating a roll and controlling the body	As primary	As primary
Formation	The swimmer stands in front of the physiotherapist, facing into the circle	As primary, except that the circle is widened a little	As intermediate, with further widening of the circle
Instruction	'Bend your knees, hands forward, head back slowly until you are floating.' The physiotherapist gives support at the waist to stabilize the swimmer's floating position. 'You are rolling to the left. When the instruction "roll" is given, turn your head to the left and bring your right arm and leg across your body, blow, and roll on to the next physiotherapist.' As the swimmer leaves the physiotherapist's hands, the physiotherapist prepares to receive the next swimmer. It is advisable to wait at this point until all swimmers have completed the roll and are lying in the supine position on the hands of the next physiotherapist	As primary. A suitable song may be introduced to develop a more rhythmical pattern of rolling as well as to control the timing of each roll. The physiotherapists give less and less support to the swimmers	As primary and intermediate. Assistance is only given when required

Rolling down the River

A 'ball' and 'stick' group activity.

Therapeutic aims

1. To develop head control.
2. To acquire rotational control – vertical and lateral.
3. To experience the extremes of posture.
4. To develop coordination and balance.
5. To maintain breathing control.
6. To improve mental adaptability.

	Primary activity	*Intermediate activity*	*Advanced activity*
Purpose	Vertical, lateral rotation control, extremes of posture	As primary	As primary
Appreciation	The effect of head movement on the body	As primary	As primary
Formation	A circle; swimmer and physiotherapist face to face using the 'floppy hold' (p. 47, Fig. 5.18b). One extra physiotherapist without a swimmer is required in the circle	As primary	As primary
Instruction	All physiotherapists turn to the left and face out of the circle, swimmers lie back and are assisted to float on to the next physiotherapist who supports at the centre of balance and the physiotherapists continue to turn to allow the swimmers to recover forward to a 'floppy' hold with the next physiotherapist. The process of the instructor turning and swimmer recovering and lying out continues round the circle	As primary; add singing – 'Rolling down the river'	As the swimmer lies back they roll on to the next physiotherapist

Combined rotation

Combined rotation is concerned with linking vertical and lateral rotation to ensure the swimmer's safety. The combination of the two rotational movements permits a swimmer to fall forwards, turn on to the back and recover forward again to the upright position if desired (Table 5.5).

Table 5.5 Activities for the development of rotational control

---

Combined rotation

1. In and out the windows
2. Mushroom float
3. Beyond the vertical
4. Fishes in the net
5. Rolling under an arch or through a hoop

In and Out the Windows

A 'ball' and 'stick' activity suitable for a group.

Therapeutic aims

1. To increase mental adaptability.
2. To improve respiration and breathing control.
3. To improve balance and coordination.
4. To encourage active and independent movement.
5. To increase spatial awareness and directionality.

	Primary activity	*Intermediate activity*	*Advanced activity*
Purpose	Lateral rotation and upthrust	As primary	As primary
Appreciation	The effect of head movement on the body to produce rotation and upthrust effects	As primary	As primary
Formation	Swimmers holding hands in a line inside the circle formed by the physiotherapists who hold each other's hands to form arches at the surface of the water	As primary	The swimmers do not hold hands
Instruction	'Follow the leader under the arch; come up outside the circle and move on to another arch. Go under the arch coming inside the circle. Move all the way round the circle and don't forget to follow.'	As primary, but 'The circle is going to move round slowly so watch for the arches.'	As primary, but 'Do not hold hands this time.'

Mushroom Float

A 'ball' activity suitable for individual activity, but a group of swimmers and physiotherapists may be formed. It is a prerequisite for combined rotation and the appreciation of upthrust.

Therapeutic aims

1. To improve flexion and extension of the body as a whole.
2. To increase respiration and breathing control.
3. To improve mental adaptability.
4. To improve balance and coordination.

	Primary activity	*Intermediate activity*	*Advanced activity*
Purpose	Combined rotation and upthrust	As primary	As primary
Appreciation	The effects of upthrust and the value of rotational control	As primary	As primary
Formation	The swimmer stands in front of the physiotherapist, facing away. Support is given at the swimmer's waist by the physiotherapist	As primary	As primary
Instruction	'Bend your knees up to your chest; hold your knees with your hands, head forward and blow.' The physiotherapist controls the forward action of the body that will occur as the 'ball' shape is achieved, so that the swimmer's body does not rotate forwards too rapidly	As primary. Progression is achieved by the lessening of the support and control provided by the physiotherapist	As primary, but stress that the flexion of hips and knees should be performed slowly to aid flotation. No assistance is given to the swimmer by the physiotherapist

Beyond the Vertical

A 'stick' and 'ball' activity suitable for individual work which can be performed in a group.

Therapeutic aims

1. To improve flexion, extension and rotation of the body as a whole.
2. To improve head control.
3. To increase respiration and breathing control.
4. To improve mental adaptability.
5. To increase balance and coordination.

	Primary activity	*Intermediate activity*	*Advanced activity*
Purpose	Combined rotational control	As primary	As primary
Appreciation	The importance of rotational control for recovering to a safe breathing position and restoring balance	As primary	As primary
Formation	Swimmer stands in front of the physiotherapist, facing away. Support is given at the swimmer's waist	As primary	As primary
Instruction	'Sit in your chair with your hands forward; put your head back slowly and lie out long. Bend your knees up to your chest, head and hands forward; blow, and go forward beyond the upright position. Then turn on to your back and recover forwards to me.'	As primary. Less facilitation and support is given. The physiotherapist should be the focal point to which the swimmer recovers after rotating in the horizontal	As primary. Objects floating on the water or under the water can be retrieved by the swimmer and presented to the physiotherapist. This will encourage greater movement and provides interest in the activity

Fishes in the Net

A 'ball' and 'stick' activity for a group.

Therapeutic aims

1. To maintain rotational control, balance and coordination.
2. To improve respiration and breathing control.
3. To encourage active movement through-out the body in all directions.
4. To increase body image and spatial awareness.
5. To improve mental adaptability.

	Primary activity	*Intermediate activity*	*Advanced activity*
Purpose	Combined rotation	As primary	As primary
Appreciation	The effects of buoyancy; rotational control and the combination of vertical and lateral rotation required to gain a safe breathing position	As primary	As primary
Formation	A circle is formed by the physiotherapists using a long arm hold (p. 50) around the swimmers who stand independently in the middle of the circle	As primary	As primary
Instruction	'Swimmers, you are fishes in the net and you can get out of the net by going under the arms, and come back in over them. You can hold the arms to assist you if you wish.' The swimmers proceed out of the circle under the arms and, once clear, rotate onto the back and recover to the upright position. This pattern is repeated as the swimmers return into the circle	As primary, but the swimmers must not use the physiotherapist' arms to assist exit and entry of the circle	As primary, but the circle is going to move round in one direction or the other and may change from time to time. The skill of keeping the eyes open under water is also encouraged since the swimmers must watch for the spaces to exit and enter the circle

Rolling under an Arch or through a Hoop

A 'stick' game suitable for group and individual activity. It is essential the swimmer learns to rotate in both directions. When a hoop is used, or in the Advanced activity, a physiotherapist may be on the far side of the hoop (or arch) to ensure the swimmers rotate safely. This activity is undertaken largely under water.

Therapeutic aims

1. To develop rotational movements of the head, trunk and limbs.
2. To develop respiration and breathing control.
3. To develop balance and coordination.
4. To provide vestibular stimulation.

	Primary activity	*Intermediate activity*	*Advanced activity*
Purpose	Combined rotation	As primary	As primary
Appreciation	The effects of head, arm and leg movement on the body; recovery to a safe breathing position	As primary	As primary
Formation	Two physiotherapists form an arch with their arms low over the surafce of the water. The swimmers are supported by their physiotherapists in the vertical position on one side of the arch. A weighted hoop may be used instead of the arch	As primary but less assistance is given	As primary but no assistance is given to the swimmer
Instruction	The swimmer lies in the prone position held at the waist by the physiotherapist. Together they proceed under the arch, the swimmer being rotated onto their back as they reach the far side of the arch and the swimmer recovers forwards to the upright position once through the arch	As primary	As primary

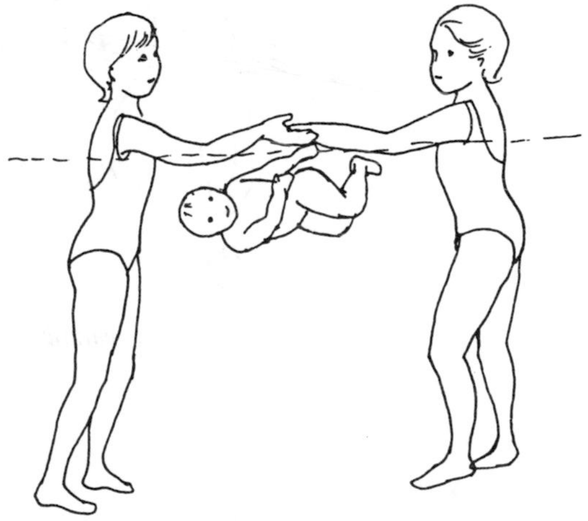

Fig. 5.36 *Rolling under the arch*

Upthrust

Activities in this section are designed to help the swimmer appreciate the effects of buoyancy or upthrust. The swimmer is encouraged to go to the bottom of the pool, which is difficult due to upthrust effects. True appreciation of these effects reassures the swimmer, and a change of attitude develops when it is clearly understood that water acts as an upward force rather than a downward one (Table 5.6).

Table 5.6 Activities for the development of rotational control

Upthrust

1. The big ship sails through the Alley Alley O
2. Oranges and lemons
3. Pieces of eight
4. Sitting on the bottom

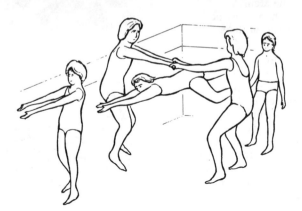

Fig. 5.37 *Swimming through underarms*

'The Big Ship Sails through the Alley Alley O'

A 'stick' and 'ball' activity suitable for group work.

'The big ship sails through the Alley Alley O,
Alley Alley O, Alley Alley O;
The big ship sails through the Alley Alley O,
On the last day of September.

The captain said "It will never, never do,
Never, never do, never, never do,"
The captain said "It will never, never do,"
On the last day of September.

The big ship sank to the bottom of the sea,
The bottom of the sea, the bottom of the sea,
The big ship sank to the bottom of the sea,
On the last day of September.

We all dip our heads in the deep blue sea,
The deep blue sea, the deep blue sea,
We all dip our heads in the deep blue sea,
On the last day of September.'

Therapeutic aims

1. To improve respiration and breathing control.
2. To increase mental adaptability.
3. To improve head control in the anterior/posterior direction.
4. To encourage flexion and extension of the body as a whole.
5. To encourage independent walking.
6. To increase balance and coordination.

This activity can also be used to facilitate 'blowing' and breathing control early on as another game under those for mental adjustment and disengagement in programmes for the young child.

An arch may be formed by the physiotherapist's arm held touching the wall high above the surface of the water or by holding an object against the wall to increase the width of the arch, the height of the arch is lowered as the children's skills progress.

The parents or those working with the children, using an upright facing hold, walk backwards ducking down and demonstrating 'blowing' as they pass under the arch. As a progression the children are held facing away from their carer. Gradually the children are encouraged to go deeper in the water as their 'blowing' becomes more regular and automatic.

	Primary activity	Intermediate activity	Advanced activity
Purpose	Upthrust control and vertical rotation	As primary	As primary
Appreciation	The effects of head movement on the body and the effects of upthrust	As primary	As primary
Formation	The swimmer in front of the physiotherapist, facing away. A backing waist hold (or, in severely disabled cases, sitting in the physiotherapist's lap (Fig. 5.19, p. 48)) is used	The swimmer faces the physiotherapist using a hands on hands hold, the physiotherapist walks backwards	The swimmer now proceeds independently. The physiotherapist is close by if help is required
Instruction	The pairs follow the leader through the Alley O (i.e. a physiotherapist making an arch with the arms towards the side of the pool, or two people hold hands facing each other). The swimmer blows going under an arch. Repeat instruction for second verse	As 'The big ship sank to the bottom of the sea', swimmer and physiotherapist submerge to the bottom, moving under the arch. Also during the fourth verse	The swimmer passes under the arch independently. The physiotherapist can at first be on the other side of the arch to receive the swimmer

'Oranges and Lemons'

A 'stick' and 'ball' activity suitable for a group.

Therapeutic aims

1. To improve respiration and breathing control.
2. To encourage general relaxation.
3. To encourage movement, especially total flexion and extension.
4. To improve and maintain balance and coordination.
5. To improve head control, especially in the anterior/posterior direction.

A modified form of this activity, similar to 'The big ship sails through the Alley Alley O', may also be used in early programmes.

	Primary activity	*Intermediate activity*	*Advanced activity*
Purpose	Breathing control and upthrust	As primary	As primary
Appreciation	The need for breathing out when submerging; buoyancy effects	As primary	As primary
Formation	One swimmer and physiotherapist make an arch with both arms just below the surface. Other swimmers are supported at the waist, facing away from their physiotherapist, and follow each other under the arch	As primary	As primary
Instruction	'We're going to sing "Oranges and lemons" as you go under the arch below.' The game of 'Oranges and lemons' can be played as on land or simply modified by going under the arch. The important points are breathing control and the willingness on the part of the child to submerge with the head forward rather than extended. Swimmers and physiotherapists submerge under the arch, surfacing on the other side, and follow the leader to repeat the process	As primary. Less assistance is given at the waist, thus allowing greater appreciation of the upthrust effect; alternatively, the swimmer can be placed behind the physiotherapist	No assistance is given, the child submerging and proceeding under the arms independently. The physiotherapist may move round to the other side of the arch to receive the swimmer

Pieces of Eight

A 'stick' activity more suitable for a group but which may be played between two people.

Therapeutic aims

1. To improve respiration and breathing control.
2. To encourage and maintain balance restoration and rotational control.
3. To encourage movement at the surface and below the water.
4. To develop eye–hand coordination.
5. To provide perceptual stimulation aurally.

	Primary activity	*Intermediate activity*	*Advanced activity*
Purpose	Buoyancy effects and breathing control	As primary	As primary
Appreciation	The effects of buoyancy	As primary	As primary
Formation	A circle is formed with the swimmer in front of the physiotherapist, who supports the swimmer at the waist	As primary, but less assistance is given to the swimmer	As primary, except the swimmer works independently
Instruction	'When I say "go", you all go under the water for these objects. Don't forget to blow.' The physiotherapist may assist submersion if necessary and aids control of buoyancy and rotational effects	'Wait 'till I say "go".' The objects are pushed further under before the order 'go' is given. If the objects are of different colours, each colour can be given a number and the swimmers encouraged to go for the objects with the higher points. The physiotherapists keep the score for individual swimmers. However, the important factors are that the swimmer is blowing out under water and keeping the eyes open. A variety of objects, some which sink more slowly than others, should be used	As primary and intermediate, but now the objects are allowed to sink close to or right to the bottom of the pool. This activity can be carried out in other formations or on an individual basis, although in the latter situation, competition cannot be introduced

Sitting on the Bottom

A 'ball' and 'stick' activity.

Therapeutic aims

1. To encourage extremes of posture, body image and spatial awareness.
2. To improve balance and coordination.
3. To improve respiratory control.
4. To increase mental adaptability.

	Primary activity	*Intermediate activity*	*Advanced activity*
Purpose	Upthrust and rotational control	As primary	As primary
Appreciation	The effects of upthrust	As primary	As primary
Formation	Swimmer and physiotherapist facing each other, the swimmer's hands on the physiotherapist's shoulders. The physiotherapist holds the swimmer's waist	A hands on hands hold is used	A circle of alternate swimmers in physiotherapist' long arm hold can be used as a further progression
Instruction	'We will jump up and down three times and then go under the water blowing. See if I am blowing bubbles.'	As primary	The swimmer submerges independently as in the primary activity

Activities for balance and coordination

The development of balance control and coordination has already commenced in the activities described in the previous sections. However, the activities in this section (Table 5.7) may be used specifically to increase balance control and stability against the movement of the water, that of the swimmer, and that of other persons in the water.

In these activities the swimmer can obtain a fine degree of balance control against any disturbing factors and should do so in the standing, sitting, kneeling and lying positions.

Turbulence – a strongly disturbing force – may be used deliberately by the physiotherapist around the swimmer to teach such balance control combined with coordination.

Table 5.7 Activities for balance and coordination

1. Twinkle, twinkle little star
2. Making waves
3. Stars and stripes
4. Speedboats
5. Roundabouts
6. Turbulence deliberately placed around the swimmer

Activites 1–5 are undertaken in the form of a game. Activity 6 is in the form of a technique that aids the development of balance control.

'Twinkle, Twinkle, Little Star'

A 'stick' activity for younger children in a group or individually.

Therapeutic aims

1. To encourage active movement, especially abduction, adduction of the legs and arms, and elevation of the arms.
2. To develop flexion and extension of the body as a whole.
3. To improve control.
4. To develop body awareness.
5. To develop balance and coordination.
6. To improve respiration and breathing control.

	Primary activity	*Intermediate activity*	*Advanced activity*
Purpose	Balance control in the vertical and supine lying positions	As primary	As primary
Appreciation	The effect of the use of the head to control the body position	As primary	As primary
Formation	A circle is formed, all facing inwards, the swimmers in front of the physiotherapists, supported at the waist in the vertical	As primary	As primary
Instruction	'As we sing "Twinkle, twinkle, little star, how I wonder what you are", slowly raise your arms out of the water and over your heads.' 'As we sing "Up above the world so high, like a diamond in the sky", make your arms reach as high and as wide as you can.' 'Wave your hand and wiggle your fingers when we sing "Twinkle, twinkle, little star", and bring your arms down into the water when singing "how I wonder what you are".'	'Lift your arms out of the water as we sing "Twinkle, twinkle, little star". Curl up into a ball and lie back slowly and put your legs out long as we sing "how I wonder what you are, up above the world so high ". Spread your arms and legs as wide as you can while singing "like a diamond in the sky". Bring your arms and legs together, curl up and stand erect while singing "Twinkle, twinkle, little star, how I wonder what you are".'	As intermediate. The progression is made by increasing the speed of the activity and by the physiotherapist gradually disengaging the hands

Making Waves

A 'stick' activity suitable for group and individual work. It can be used as an activity on its own or as a component of other games such as 'If you're happy and you know it' or 'Simon says'.

Therapeutic aims

1. To increase the range of movement and muscle strength in the arms and legs.
2. To improve balance and coordination.
3. To increase awareness of body image and spatial relationships.

	Primary activity	*Intermediate activity*	*Advanced activity*
Purpose	Balance control in the vertical and horizontal positions	As primary	As primary
Appreciation	The effect of the head movement on the body and turbulent or drag effect on moving limbs	As primary	As primary
Formation	The swimmer stands in front of, and facing away from, the physiotherapist who provides support at the waist. The swimmer's shoulders should be in the water	As primary	As primary
Instruction	'Stretch your arms forward, hands flat, and swing your arms out sideways, then bring them together again.'	'Stretch your arms forwards, the palms of your hands facing each other; swing your arms out sideways and then bring them together again.'	'Stretch your hands forwards, head back on the shoulder and lie out long. Let's make waves with arms and legs going in and out.' Progressions are made by decreasing the support given and by increasing the speed of the activity

Stars and Stripes

A 'stick' activity.

Therapeutic aims

1. To improve and maintain the range of abduction/adduction in the hip and shoulder joints.
2. To encourage control of the limbs.
3. To develop rotational control, balance and coordination.
4. To develop body image and spatial awareness.

	Primary activity	*Intermediate activity*	*Advanced activity*
Purpose	Balance control in supine lying; lateral rotational control	As primary	As primary
Appreciation	The effect of head control on rotation; buoyancy effects	As primary	As primary
Formation	The swimmer stands in front of the physiotherapist, facing away. The physiotherapist places the hands in readiness to support the swimmer in the supine lying position (p. 48)	As primary, less support and assistance being given to the lying position and to recovery. Increasing the speed of the movement increases the degree of control required	The swimmer is not supported, lying back, floating and recovering independently
Instruction (same for all three activities)	'Sit in your chair with your arms forwards; put your head back slowly until you are lying in bed. Part your arms and legs and make a star. Close your arms and legs and make a stripe'		

Speedboats

A 'stick' activity.

A greater degree of rotational control may be introduced by encouraging the swimmer to roll on to the bar (p. 103) as the side of the pool is reached.

Therapeutic aims

1. To encourage movement and control of the limbs.
2. To encourage head and rotational control.
3. To improve balance and coordination.

	Primary activity	*Intermediate activity*	*Advanced activity*
Purpose	Movement and control of the legs leading to independent movement in the supine lying position, involving rotational control	As primary	As primary
Appreciation	Ability to control rotation during movement through the water	As primary	As primary
Formation	The swimmer stands in front of the physiotherapist, facing away. The swimmer proceeds to lie back on the physiotherapist's hands	As primary, but providing less support	As primary. The physiotherapist only supports if necessary to get flotation in the supine lying position, the swimmer then proceeds independently
Instruction (same for all three activities)	'Kick your legs.' The physiotherapist walks backwards supporting the swimmer during the kicking action. If this activity is played in a group, a line of swimmers facing a wall can be formed and in addition to 'Kick your legs', encouragement to move actively can be given by adding a competitive note: 'Who is the fastest speedboat?'		

Roundabouts

A 'stick' activity suitable for a group which could be modified for working with an individual.

Therapeutic aims

1. To develop and maintain balance control and coordination.
2. To improve and maintain postural reactions.
3. To develop control of the limbs, especially that of the arms.
4. To encourage the development of body and spatial awareness.

	Primary activity	*Intermediate activity*	*Advanced activity*
Purpose	The development of balance and coordination; postural reactions and an increase in mental adaptability	As primary	As primary
Appreciation	Turbulent effects with the consequent loss of balance and the need for head control	As primary	As primary
Formation	The swimmers stand back to back in the middle of the circle formed by the physiotherapist. A hands on hands hold is used for each swimmer	As primary	The physiotherapists form a circle around the swimmers using a long arm hold
Instruction	The swimmers remain standing as the physiotherapists walk sideways round the circle, removing the hands from the first swimmer and picking up the hands of the next swimmer. A beat or number is used in order that all physiotherapists move from one swimmer to the next at the same time and the swimmers are only without support momentarily	As primary, but the moving circle may change direction when instructed and the swimmers are given less support	The circle of physiotherapists walks sideways in one direction and then the other with increasing speed. Each swimmer must stabilize the body against the turbulence and remain balanced, 'sitting' with the head and hands forward, the legs hip-width apart, the hips, knees and ankles flexed, the feet on the floor of the pool

Turbulence Deliberately Placed Around the Swimmer

An activity suitable for individual work; the factors are the same for all levels of this activity.

The progression is made by increasing the amount of turbulence placed around the swimmer. Turbulence may be created in the manner described in the instruction below or may be increased by the movement of the physiotherapist around the swimmer. This movement may be slow and gentle at first but may be gradually increased in speed and thus cause greater turbulent effects. Further progressions are achieved by creating turbulence around the swimmer in sitting, kneeling and supine lying.

Therapeutic aims

1. To improve balance and coordination, particularly fine balance.
2. To increase mental adaptability.

Purpose	Balance control and coordination
Appreciation	The effects of turbulence on the body and the manner in which control can be acquired
Formation	Swimmer standing facing the physiotherapist
Instruction	'Try to stop me making you fall.' The physiotherapist, using the extended arms, creates gentle turbulence in front of the swimmer. This is done by holding one arm above the other in order that the hands may pass over each other. The hands should be shoulder-width apart and pass laterally to the same distance, crossing in midline and back again. If the action is repeated a number of times, turbulence will build up in front of the swimmer. If the turbulence is created low on the swimmer's body, the resulting loss of balance will occur more rapidly. The physiotherapist may need to instruct the swimmer as to how to control the body balance. When the body is falling forwards, the swimmer should lift the arms forward to shoulder level, keep the head forward and at the same time adopt a sitting posture by flexing the hips and knees. Additional stability is obtained if the legs are abducted to just beyond the width of the hips.
	Turbulence may also be created in the same manner behind the swimmer. In this case the tendency would be for the swimmer's body to fall backwards. In order to counteract this falling action and to stabilize the body, the swimmer should flex the hips and knees slightly, bringing the head and arms forward.
	If turbulence is placed behind the swimmer and to one side, the swimmer's body will tend to fall backwards and to rotate to the side on which the turbulence has been placed. To avoid a loss of balance and to maintain a position of stability, the swimmer adopts a sitting position, at the same time taking the head and arms forward and away from the direction in which the body would fall and rotate

Dynamic activities

The activities included in this section (Table 5.8) lead directly on to swimming, and many of them may be found in books and manuals concerned with the teaching of swimming. However, it must be appreciated that such activities have been devised for the able-bodied swimmer and may need modification for the disabled.

The advanced levels of activity in many of the preceding pages are appropriate dynamic activities, and it is not proposed to set out in such detail those activities listed here. Once the swimmer has reached the level of ability to cope with dynamic activity, progression through a series of stages, such as has been developed in the games so far, is not necessary.

Swimming strokes frequently need to be modified for each disabled swimmer, and such modifications are dependent almost entirely on the mobility of the swimmer.

An unorthodox approach to stroke techniques is provided.

Table 5.8 Dynamic activities

Gliding on turbulence

Pushing off and gliding

Mushroom float

Prone float

Log roll

Corkscrew

Washtub

Somersault forward

Somersault backward

Diving for objects

Rowing boats

Swimming through legs

Swimming

Gliding on Turbulence

The swimmer floats supine and is moved through the water on turbulence created by the physiotherapist. In shallow water the turbulence may be created by the arms. In deeper water this may be done by the physiotherapist's legs as the supine position is adopted. At all times the turbulence should be placed under the swimmer's trunk at the lower border of the scapulae. The swimmer should control with the head any rolling action of the body that may occur.

Pushing Off and Gliding

The swimmer pushes off from the side of the pool in either supine or prone, and glides as far as possible without moving the limbs. The hands may be kept at the sides of the body or extended forwards with the thumbs entwined. The legs should be adducted and extended. At the end of the glide the swimmer adopts the erect position.

Mushroom Float

This float is also called the jellyfish float. The swimmer bends the knees to the chest and places the hands on the knees. The body rotates forwards and the swimmer floats with the thoracic spine visible above the surface of the water. The face is immersed and the swimmer should slowly be blowing air out of the mouth. This is a useful skill to acquire as it is a prerequisite for somersaulting and is a simple way in which to progress to prone floating.

Prone Float

A prone float requires the swimmer to be face down in the water, the arms and legs extended and abducted, thus making a star shape. This position can be altered in several ways and is helpful in teaching the breast stroke action (p. 132).

Log Roll

The body is fully extended, the arms stretched above the head. The body is rotated on the surface of the water without the use of the limbs.

Corkscrew

The corkscrew action is similar to the log roll, but the arm position is altered, one arm remaining extended above the head, the other held at the side.

Washtub

The body is extended in supine lying on the surface with the arms at the side of it. The knees are drawn up to the chest, the thighs being held vertical and the lower leg parallel to the surface of the water. A flat sculling of the hands at the sides rotates the body through 360°. The head remains steady and the eyes looking upwards throughout the activity.

Somersaults – Forward and Backward

The ability to somersault is of importance to any swimmer, especially when swimming in the sea. Many disabled people can attain this skill, though in some instances somersaulting in either direction may be physically impossible. In such cases it is important for the person's safety that any modified somersault is built on the necessary basic skills performed automatically, and at an advanced level.

The prerequisites for somersaulting are:

(a) the ability to keep the eyes open under water,
(b) the ability to exhale strongly through the nose,
(c) the ability to perform a mushroom float.

Somersaults may be taught in several ways. The simplest method is for two physiotherapists to assist the swimmer: they stand on either side and provide support with their hands.

Forward somersault

The physiotherapist on the swimmer's right places the right clenched hand for support of the swimmer's right hand, and the left hand is placed palm up under the swimmer's thigh. This is reversed for the physiotherapist on the swimmer's left.

Backward somersault

The physiotherapist on the swimmer's right now places the right hand under the swimmer's shin, while the clenched left hand offers support for the swimmer's hand. Again the position is reversed for the physiotherapist on the swimmer's left.

Alternatively, when two physiotherapists are working with a swimmer, they can link hands; the swimmer holds the arms and creates a somersault around them.

When working on an individual basis with a swimmer, the forward somersault can be facilitated by a hand placed on the back as the swimmer curls up into a ball shape. The other hand is placed under the thighs. A backward somersault may be facilitated by support provided by two clenched hands beneath the centre of balance of the body. As the swimmer's body is curled up and the head extended, the physiotherapist moves the hands upwards and laterally to assist the swimmer's action.

When a swimmer has the ability to prone float with the arms extended beyond the head and can push off and glide, somersaulting independently can be achieved. The swimmer adopts the prone position described, pushes off from the side of the pool and at the end of the glide moves the arms to the abducted position, takes the head downwards at the same time flexing the hips and adopting the tuck position. The body rotates around the shoulder joints, having converted linear velocity into angular velocity. If a swimmer is unable to push off from the side of the pool due to a lack of power in the lower limbs, the physiotherapist holds the legs extended, one hand under the thighs, the other on the soles of the feet, and pushes the swimmer through the water, thus providing the motive power for the glide. The swimmer uses the arm and body actions already described to achieve the somersault.

Diving for Objects

This activity is an extension of the game 'Pieces of eight' (p. 119). Any object that sinks may be recovered, and these can range from items such as bricks, dive rings, discs and sticks, to coins. This action ensures that the eyes remain open under water, and the swimmer should exhale slowly throughout the time the body is submerged.

Rowing Boats

Rowing boats is a team activity and one in which a competitive spirit can be engendered. Two or three swimmers stand behind each other, facing the side of the pool. The person nearest the wall remains standing while the second and third lie back in the water and place their legs around the waist of the person in front. All the swimmers use a bilateral arm back stroke, taking the timing from the first person who has now adopted the supine lying position and kicks with the legs also. The boat tries to reach the other side or end of the pool without sinking.

Swimming through Legs (Fig. 5.38)

This activity can be carried out in both a group and individual situation. When working with a group, either a line or a circle formation may be used. If a circle is formed, the physiotherapists hold hands and stand with their legs wide apart sideways. The swimmer goes under one 'arch' and may pull and push against the physiotherapist's leg to move through and round to the next 'arch'. By keeping the body close to the legs, curling around them, the swimmer may be able to increase the number of 'arches' traversed.

If a line formation is used, the physiotherapists stand with a wide stance at arm's length,

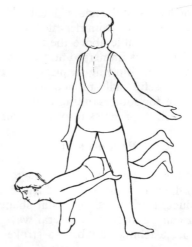

Fig. 5.38   *Swimming through legs*

one behind the other, all facing in the same direction. The gaps provided allow a swimmer to emerge in between the physiotherapists should the necessity arise.

SWIMMING

Activity in water is considered to be the finest form of exercise for all. For the disabled, water offers an excellent medium for therapeutic exercise and recreation for a wide range of disabilities and for people in any age group. Swimming is a skill that has to be learnt and is the natural progression from water-familiarization programmes.

Hydrotherapy is the concern of the physiotherapist with a specialized knowledge of disease and disability, of movement and of rehabilitative techniques. However, the teaching of swimming skills has also become part of the physiotherapist's work due to the desirability of the disabled maintaining fitness through recreational activity in water. General teaching techniques and details of specific strokes can be found in books on this subject such as *Swimming: A Handbook for Teachers* by Helen Elkington (1978).

It must be clearly understood that the application of these methods of teaching swimming strokes is not always successful because allowances for the disability are not made or the handicap understood. Adaptations and modifications are needed and, due to lack of mobility, the strokes produced by a disabled person may not resemble the classic strokes produced by the able-bodied. It seems logical, therefore, to look to a different and less orthodox approach for teaching swimming strokes to the disabled.

The necessity for the acquisition of breathing control has been stressed throughout the text, as well as the important effects it has on relaxation and balance, and the swimmer's breathing ability should be of first concern. This is closely linked with the ability to achieve and maintain safe breathing positions in the water. It is around these points that the swimmer's strokes can be developed. This approach is in contrast to the orthodox method in which the swimmer is taught the technique of the strokes while holding the breath. When the arm and leg actions have been learnt, attempts are made to fit the breathing into the strokes.

There will be certain prerequisites for the various strokes, and these will include the following abilities.

1. To submerge and control exhalation.
2. To keep the eyes open in the interests of safety and in order to swim in a straight direction.
3. To float in both the supine and prone positions.
4. To push off and glide in both the supine and prone positions.
5. To regain and maintain a vertical position from both prone and supine positions.
6. To rotate the body from the supine lying position to prone lying and back to supine again.

Specific strokes will then require the practice of specific actions. These actions vary from stroke to stroke, and the manner in which the progressions may be made is given for back crawl, front crawl and breast stroke. It is advisable to commence with back crawl swimming, for the majority of disabled persons, affected more often and more severely in the lower limbs, can use the upper limbs to maximum advantage to propel the body through the water in the supine position. The face is also clear of the water and any anxiety about breathing is largely removed. This point is reinforced by Elkington (1978), who states that most beginners manage better in the supine position. However, the semi-sitting position, described by her for use initially with disabled persons who have high-floating legs due to loss of density in those limbs, would interfere with the suggestions made below. The high flotation of the lower limbs in cases of spina bifida and paraplegia and the manner in which this may be controlled have already been discussed (p. 17).

Back Crawl Stroke

Prerequisites: the ability to back glide, the body extended with toes pointed and the arms by the side.

Training begins with the addition of the leg action, and this is practised to a high level of competence before the arm action is added. During practice with the legs, the arms may be placed in any one of a number of different positions. For example, they can be placed on the abdomen, behind the head with the elbows depressed, held extended above the head with thumbs locked, or folded across the chest.

The leg action also needs to be practised, not only in supine but also in prone and side lying with the arms extended and close to the body. This adds variety and prepares the swimmer for other strokes. When the swimmer is proficient with the leg action, arm movements can be introduced, at first bilaterally simultaneously and then alternating.

In achieving a bilateral movement the swimmer is directed to push backwards, at the same time reaching back 'over the water' with both arms, bringing the hands into the water and pulling strongly under the water back to the side of the body. When reaching back, the arms should be kept low above the surface. When introducing an alternative arm action, the non-reaching arm is inhibited by having the swimmer hold it close to the body. As the swimmer progresses through the water using the leg and *one* arm, the head controls the rolling action of the body. This sequence is repeated with the opposite arm.

When the alternate action of *both* arms is begun, each arm cycles continuously, moving 'over the water' from the thigh, into the water, and back to the thigh again. The full back crawl (as with all strokes) should initially be practised at a slow pace to reduce errors and conserve energy.

Front Crawl Stroke

Prerequisites: as for back crawl but with the addition of competence in performing the back crawl stroke.

Gliding in the prone position with the body, arms and legs extended and as flat as possible in the water, is the first action to be practised. This should be repeated frequently at all stages of acquiring the front crawl stroke. The same sequence used in practising the leg action is followed.

It is necessary to introduce breathing control, and initially the swimmer is taught to stop swimming and stand up prior to running out of breath. Later the swimmer is instructed to roll on to the back prior to requiring another breath and to proceed swimming using the back crawl stroke leg action. In the next progression the swimmer lies on the side, with the head turned towards the surface so that the nose and mouth are just clear of the water. The crawl leg action is used to propel the body in this position. It is advisable to commence this lying first on one side and then the other. Once this has been achieved, the swimmer is instructed to lie on one side and extend the arm on that side forward. The other arm is kept close to the body. This is repeated on the other side. The leg action will help to control the balance, but the position of the head is critical. The weight of the head must be taken by the water. Should the swimmer lift the head, the body position is altered to such an extent that all efforts to remain afloat will be sabotaged.

The arm action is introduced as the body moves in the prone glide following the commencement of the leg action. The swimmer moves as far as possible before breathing control is lost and should then stop swimming and stand up. The same sequence used in practising the leg action is followed – that is, the swimmer learns to roll from prone to supine, to breathe, and continues across the width of the pool in this position.

To develop the arm stroke further, the swimmer is instructed to arrest the progression of one arm in full forward extension while the other arm remains at the side. Thus further propulsion is achieved solely by leg action. The arresting procedure alternates between arms and is followed by a slow lazy roll to the side to breathe. The swimmer is told to stay on the side for as long as desired before completing the front crawl stroke with the face in the water. It is now essential that the swimmer learns to keep the arms moving, but turning the head to the left when the left arm is pulling through the water and has reached a point where the hand is immediately below the left shoulder. The face should turn into the water before the hand in its over-water recovery action reaches a line with the shoulder. This is practised in the same manner to the right. It may prove valuable to perform front crawl with continuous leg action, but with only the right arm propelling while the left arm is extended forward and kept still – breathing taking place to the right. This should be practised to the opposite side. Another helpful variation is to swim a mixture of front and back crawl, rolling on every third arm pull. The swimmer should be encouraged to swim widths or lengths at both slow and fast speeds.

Breast Stroke

The prerequisites for this stroke are as follows.

1. The ability to float prone for at least 6 seconds in the following positions:

   (a) prone float with the arms extended, the hands touching with the palms facing downwards; the head should be in the water between the arms; the knees are bent so that the heels are close to the hips and the feet everted;

   (b) prone float as above but the legs are extended and abducted with the feet everted;

   (c) prone float as above but the legs are extended and adducted and the feet are pointed backwards.

   The body must remain flat and any rolling action caused by body asymmetry corrected if possible.

   The swimmer progresses the prone float by slowly changing the body shape, moving through the three stages (a), (b) and (c) above. This results in a symmetrical leg action for breast stroke. This should be practised until the movements are habitual, and the arm actions are not introduced until this is attained.

2. The swimmer should be able to jump forwards unaided.

3. The swimmer should be able to dive through an arch provided by two physiotherapists or through the physiotherapist's legs. This latter skill simulates the arm action of breast stroke as the swimmer passes through the arch of the physiotherapist's legs. Once submerged, the hands are parted to hold the physiotherapist's on either side or, in the case of going through the legs, the calves of the physiotherapist, against which the swimmer now pulls and then pushes to pass through the arch. The breast stroke leg action is not employed when passing under the arch because it may result in someone being kicked. If a leg action is required, that of the front crawl stroke may be used.

The coordination of the arm and leg actions is most quickly achieved with the swimmer submerged. A long arm pull with the hands finishing at the thighs is encouraged. When performing breast stroke at the surface, the chin should be kept at the surface and the arm pull should become smaller, the hands never passing beyond the shoulder, and the action of the limbs should be within the body line. The pattern of movement for a continuous stroke is 'pull, kick', 'pull, kick' but for a more leisurely stroke the pattern of movement is 'pull, kick, glide'. Where coordination is not maintained, an examination of the action of the limbs is necessary. The fault usually lies with an imbalance in the reciprocal action of arms and legs, one pair of limbs having a larger action than the other. Accordingly, modification of either the kicking or pulling action is needed.

The coordination of breathing can be performed in two ways. The first is carried out in shallow water, the swimmer adopting a prone float with the head raised to allow the arms to be extended forwards parallel with the surface of the water. The head is raised enough to allow the feet to sink. The face remains submerged at eyebrow level and the feet drag on the floor of the pool. While floating in this position, the arms are pressed backwards and slightly downwards on the water. Such action will cause the face to clear the surface of the water automatically. The swimmer is instructed to exhale while the face is submerged, inhalation occurring as a reflex action as the face clears the surface. Breast stroke swimming can take place with the face immersed, the eyes looking forwards and the breathing coordinated with the arm action as indicated.

The second approach to breathing coordination is through a combination of head-up breast stroke and also swimming submerged. One complete stroke with the face immersed is followed by one with the head up. This results in breast stroke with alternative breathing – that is, breathing on every other stroke. From this the swimmer should proceed to breathing on every stroke.

Techniques and Modifications of Strokes

Techniques and modifications of strokes for specific conditions have been dealt with in the section concerned with disability. However, many of the progressions already cited lend themselves well to the teaching of strokes in particular disabilities. For instance, when instructing a swimmer who is only able to use one arm, the progression for front crawl stroke – where side floating, breathing and one arm action are involved – would prove effective. Adaptations of strokes have been advocated by other authors (Elkington, 1978; Price, 1980) along with the use of flotation equipment. This author discourages the use of such equipment, however, for a number of reasons.

First, marked alterations in shape and density make it extremely difficult for the physiotherapist to know precisely where the flotation equipment should be placed on the body or limbs. The swimmer will undoubtedly alter the body shape while working in the water, and this tends to nullify the value of the flotation apparatus and causes the swimmer to become unbalanced.

Second, swimmers who become dependent on flotation equipment may resist its removal. Therefore, they are distinguished always from their able-bodied or less dependent peers by the flotation equipment, which must always be securely attached to them. They thus fail to achieve the aim of independence in water.

Third, with the exception of some makes of life-saving jackets, no flotation equipment offers complete safety in all circumstances. The vigilance of the care-giver is still required constantly, and if this is so, the swimmer would be better served by learning to cope with the balance and rotational problems of the body without the false sense of security engendered by aids.

Finally, the disabled are living in a world made special by virtue of the disability and its needs. Many of these needs involve the use of aids and appliances to assist movement. In water, movement becomes easier and is more readily obtained, and total independence can be achieved. The disabled person discards the aids and appliances used on land and is able to enjoy the freedom of movement water provides. Why then are aids and appliances advocated for water? Surely this is denying the joys and delight of such freedom of movement and independence.

Many of the ideas provided in the section on dynamic activities form part of the build-up to swimming and independent movement and furnish the swimmer with activities that supplement those of strokes. They all demand propulsion, and thereby competence in that area is attained. Additionally, changes of shape, speed and direction are required and this provides extra awareness of body image and of the body in space.

The swimming programme should be made as varied and interesting as possible and the potential of any swimmer developed to the level the swimmer desires. This may include swimming for recreation, fitness, competition, synchronized swimming, or may provide for participation in other aquatic sports.

The aim for all disabled must be that they swim in safety. However, for some disabled persons this will not be achieved, and activity in water for them must always be supervised.

REFERENCES

Association of Swimming Therapy (1992). *Swimming for People with Disabilities*, 2nd edn, London: A. & C. Black.

Blanksby B.A. and Roberts D.M. (1981). *Guide for Teachers of Swimming*, Perth: University of Western Australia Press.

Boyle A.M. (1981). The Bad Ragaz ring method. *Physiotherapy*, **67(9)**: 265–268.

Bullock K. (1982). *Waterproofing Your Child*. Australia: Rigby.

Campbell W.R. (1975). *Aqua Percept*, Pointe Claire: Wendy R. Campbell.

Cole J.H. (1988). *The Evaluation of An Intervention Programme of Sensory Motor Facilitation for Very Preterm, Very Low Birth Weight Infants*. Doctoral Thesis submitted to the Department of Physiotherapy, University of Queensland.

Counsilman J.E. (1968). *The Science of Swimming*, New Jersey: Prentice Hall.

Cratty B.J. (1979). *Perceptual and Motor Development in Infants and Children*, 2nd edn, New Jersey: Prentice Hall.

Elkington H. (1978). *Swimming – A Handbook for Teachers*, Cambridge: Cambridge University Press.

Erikson E.H. (1963). *Childhood and Society*, 2nd edn, New York: W.W. Norton.

Freud S. (1955). *Beyond the Pleasure Principle*, standard edn, Vol. 18, London: Hogarth.

Gessell A., Ilg F.G. and Ames L. Bates (1974). *Infant and Child in the Culture Today* (revised edn), London: Hamish Hamilton.

Gray's Anatomy (1973). Hartwick R. and Williams P.L. (eds), London: Longman.

Holt K.S. (1975). How and why children move. In *Movement and Child Development*, London: Heinemann Medical/Spastic International Medical Publications.

Jolly H. (1975). *Book of Child Care*, London: George Allen & Unwin.

Korner A.F., Kraemer H.C., Haffner M.E. and Cooper L.M. (1975). Effects of waterbed flotation on premature infants: a pilot study. *Pediatrics*, **56(3)**.

Matterson E. (1969). *This Little Puffin – Nursery Songs and Rhymes*, Harmondsworth: Puffin.

Piaget J. (1963). *Play, Dreams and Imitation in Childhood*, New York: Norton.

Price R.J. (1980). *Physical Education and the Physically Handicapped Child*, London: Lepus Books.

Reid M.J. (1975). *Handling the Disabled Child in Water – an Introduction*, Association of Paediatric Chartered Physiotherapists.

Reynell J.K. and Martin M.C. (1965). The response of children to physiotherapy. *Physiotherapy*, **51(6)**: 186–189.

Shapiro A.H. (1961). *Shape and Flow, the Fluid Dynamics of Drag*, London: Heinemann Educational.

Sheridan M.D. (1977). *Spontaneous Play in Early Childhood from Birth to Six Years*, Slough: NFER.

Skinner A.T. and Thomson A.M. (eds) (1983). *Duffield's Exercise in Water*, 3rd edn, London: Baillière Tindall.

Stallibrass A. (1977). *The Self-respecting Child – A Study of Children's Play and Development*, Ringwood: Penguin (Australia).

Sweeney J.K. (1983). Neonatal hydrotherapy: an adjunct to developmental intervention in an intensive care nursery setting. In *Aquatics: A Revised Approach to Pediatric Management* (F.M. Dulcy, guest ed.) *Phys. Occ. Ther. Pediatr.*, **3(1)**.

6

Specific paediatric disabilities and their handling

Margaret Reid Campion

The disabilities discussed in this section are specific disorders seen in childhood and have been grouped into five sections:

1. Disorders of bones, joints and muscle.
2. Neurological and developmental disorders.
3. Sensory disorders.
4. Mental retardation and behavioural disorders.
5. Respiratory disorders.

DISORDERS OF BONES, JOINTS AND MUSCLE

Juvenile chronic arthritis
Muscular dystrophy
Congenital abnormalities
Spina bifida
Osteogenesis imperfecta
Burns

Juvenile Chronic Arthritis

This is the name by which juvenile rheumatoid arthritis is more commonly known today. There are inflammatory changes involving soft tissues in and around the joints and bones and articular cartilages. The joints most usually affected are those of the knees, hips, ankles, wrists, metacarpophalangeal and cervical spine. The condition may affect a single joint or many joints.

The onset of the condition usually occurs at an early age and thus most patients will undergo treatment for a prolonged period of time. These are the formative years when normal physical, intellectual, social and emotional development will be disrupted. For these reasons it is important that the child leads as normal a life as possible and that treatment is made a pleasurable time.

Joint range and function must be maintained, and programmes of active daily exercises are provided. Not only affected joints must be exercised, so activities should be used which offer the opportunity to achieve as full a range of movement as possible in all joints and allow the child to gain socially and emotionally as well.

Hydrotherapy provides these ideal conditions, particularly when therapeutic exercises can be hidden in a programme of games and activities that are fun and which lead on to swimming – a sport which the child will be able to use throughout life and which provides social contacts.

The warmth of the water provides relief of pain and muscle spasm, and buoyancy relieves the strain on joints, particularly the weight-bearing joints.

The aims of hydrotherapy are to:

- relieve pain
- aid relaxation
- increase range of movement and muscle strength
- decrease deformity
- improve functional ability.

The children may be referred for hydrotherapy while still on bed rest as they are able to exercise in a non-weight-bearing situation and stand and walk partially weight-bearing. In the chronic stage, hydrotherapy is an excellent medium for rehabilitation.

The physiotherapist must observe the child's shape and density. Alterations in the former will come about due to the pain, muscle spasm and joint changes. Density may be altered due to the loss of muscle bulk which can result from the decrease in use caused by pain. In practice, it is advisable to introduce the child to the water gently and quietly at first, observing all the points of handling and entry mentioned earlier in Chapter 5.

The young child in pain will be anxious about going into water and may exhibit fear. A one-to-one relationship within a group situation is desirable, but at first care should be taken to avoid joining a group that contains other extremely active children.

Games which attract the child's attention and divert the thoughts from the anxieties and pain should be introduced immediately following entry, and the physiotherapist should be using activities in both a therapeutic and recreational manner. An awareness of which joints are most affected is important, and activities directed towards exercising them and strengthening the muscles surrounding them must be used. As with all children and all water activity, it is advantageous to encourage blowing on to and into the water from the earliest time. In addition to the effects on respiration, such action induces the forward movement of the head and encourages flexion of neck and trunk. The range of abduction and adduction of the hip joints may need to be increased and muscle power strengthened. If the child is non-weight-bearing due to pain in the hip joints, these can be exercised in supine lying supported by the physiotherapist at the centre of balance of the body, with the head resting on the physiotherapist's shoulder, when 'Twinkle, twinkle little star' could be used for the younger child and 'Stars and stripes' for the older age group. However, if partial weight-bearing is possible, and as a progression, walking sideways as in any of the circle games could be used. It is important that the child does not cross the legs, that a step is taken to the side and the other leg brought to it, otherwise the effect of overcoming turbulence and leaning against the water, together with the necessity of increasing the size of the steps, is lost. Circle games also have the advantage of making the child aware of the weight of water and that it can be leant against. Lateral head control is required, which means that some cervical side flexion and,

incidentally, trunk side flexion occurs, particularly when the circle direction is changed and turbulence has to be overcome. Cervical flexion and extension and side flexion can be encouraged if the playing of 'Here we go round the mulberry bush' is extended to include verses such as 'This is the way we blow bubbles' (flexion), 'This is the way we nod our heads' (flexion and extension), 'This is the way we wash our ears' (side flexion), and 'This is the way we wash our hair' (extension with some rotation). Rotation is encouraged in all activities that include lateral rotation, either in the vertical or horizontal plane, for example 'Space ships', 'Looby Loo', 'The hokey cokey' or 'Passing the ring'.

Fingers, wrists, ankles, knees and hips can be exercised in the game 'If you're happy and you know it'. The child can make rain with the fingers and hands and good 'splashes' with the legs when lying supine, the emphasis being laid upon whichever joints require most attention. Saying 'hallo' and 'goodbye' to the toes and feet exercises the metatarso-phalangeal and ankle joints; taking the heels down and toes up to catch a fish and bring it to the surface encourages knee flexion and hip extension. Passing a light plastic beach ball held between the feet around a circle in the supine lying position increases muscle work and range of movement in all joints of the lower limbs. Ball games played with the upper limbs in the upright position do the same for these. Making waves with the arms unilaterally or bilaterally increases shoulder movement and muscle strength in addition to trunk rotation. The child should at first stretch the arms out in front and clasp the hands. Later, as a progression and to increase the muscle work, the child should hold the hands and arms shoulder width apart. For total flexion and extension of the body with shoulder movements involved, the teaching of vertical rotation in such activities as 'Catch an object' or 'Reaching for the bar' is excellent. Vertical rotation requires precise balance in the vertical position against turbulence, which improves balance and coordination. 'Bells', where the child uses flexion and extension of the cervical spine to swing the body in a 'ball' shape, can be extended to total flexion and extension in 'Rag dolls' and 'The wind, sun and rain'.

Bicycle riding is advocated as an interesting activity on land to maintain movements in the ankles and knees to encourage knee extension especially, and to improve and maintain muscle strength. 'Bicycles' in the water is great fun also; it is incorporated in many of the activities and can be used to teach vertical rotational control. A modified bicycle forearm hold is valuable where there are any changes in the shoulder and cervical joints causing pain. The child is supported by the physiotherapist using the bicycle forearm hold, the modification being that the child is held close to the physiotherapist, who uses a stable sitting position with legs widely spaced. Undue pressure on the shoulder, acromio-clavicular and cervical spine joints is avoided in this modification of the hold. The child is held so that the feet are clear of the bottom of the pool, but must not be lifted too high out of the water as this will increase the downward effects of gravity on the child and prove tiring for the physiotherapist. To increase range of movement in the hip joints, the child is asked to abduct the legs 'to let the boats go through' and adduct them 'to close the lock gates', keeping the knees extended. Combined hip and knee flexion, either alternately or together, can be likened to a 'lift going up and down'. If the scissor action of flexion and extension of the hips with straight knees is required, the child should be held to one side of the physiotherapist, close to the body with the same arm hold.

An imaginative physiotherapist can devise many ways in which to divert the child and provide a pleasurable means of exercise, at the same time familiarizing the child with the element of water and leading the activities towards swimming.

For the child with juvenile chronic arthritis who may have involvement of the thoracic spine, breathing control is as essential as for any other child. The physiotherapist should ensure not only that the skill of blowing on to, into and out under water becomes an automatic one, but that activities specifically designed for teaching breathing control are included in the programme.

Although specific swimming strokes are advocated by some writers, the children's degree of mobility should be the guiding factor in their selection. In the author's experience, the children frequently 'paddle' off in activities such as 'The big ship sails down the Alley, Alley O' using what mobility they have. They should be encouraged to improve stroking in the classic styles of crawl, back stroke and breast stroke, the last of which may be restricted by limited abduction of the legs. Side stroke can be used to advantage with some children.

Muscular Dystrophy

There are a number of clinical descriptions of muscular dystrophy, a disease characterized by progressive degenerative processes in the skeletal muscles. That most commonly seen is the Duchenne-type muscular dystrophy. The activity in water described in this section is applicable not only to this type, but also to other diseases demonstrating muscle weakness, such as spinal muscular atrophy.

Duchenne-type muscular dystrophy is an inherited disorder usually seen in males. It is sex linked and transmitted by an unaffected female.

In the first four years of life the early signs become apparent. The child finds increasing difficulty in walking, enlargement of muscles occurs, together with muscle weakness which begins proximally in the pelvic and shoulder girdles and progresses until the child is unable to walk. Despite weakness in the shoulders and arms, some hand function is retained until a later stage.

The increasing muscle weakness in the flexors and extensors of the hip and the extensors of the knee, combined with that of the trunk and pelvic girdle, creates difficulties in maintaining the erect posture against gravity, with resultant hip and knee flexion, scoliotic and lordotic deformities.

Respiratory function is affected by the disease, more markedly if there is spinal deformity.

Due to the progressive muscle weakness, resultant deformity and changes in muscle tissue, shape and density will be considerably altered in these children. The alteration will be increasingly marked as the disease progresses, and the physiotherapist will need to be alert to the changes when taking the child into the water.

The advantages of activity in water for these children are:

(a) water mobility is encouraged and can be maintained long after activity on land has become extremely difficult,

(b) stamina and endurance can be encouraged,

(c) respiratory function is enhanced,

(d) a social and recreational activity is established that can be enjoyed with others, enabling a happier and more interesting active life to be maintained.

The aim of activity in water should be to teach the child to swim. For this, mental adjustment, breathing and balance control must be developed. In the early stages of the disease while the child is still ambulant, these skills should be acquired as quickly as possible so that there is a long period of time in which the child can enjoy swimming and take part in other aquatic activities if desired.

By the choice of appropriate games, specific activities to maintain range of movement, the erect posture and walking can be incorporated in the child's programme. As the disease progresses these will have to be modified. Emphasis is placed by the physiotherapist on the component of movement required at any point in the activity.

Effective stretchings are not easily carried out in water as it is difficult to acquire sufficient stability of either the child or the physiotherapist. Modified movements of the Bad Ragaz Ring method (Davis, 1967; Boyle, 1981) can be introduced for early stretching of some joints, but in time the increasing muscle weakness renders the use of these techniques impractical. Where a scoliosis is presenting, it is possible to get some active contraction on the side of the convexity and stretching of the concave side by the use of the technique described on p. 147 under the heading of Hemiplegia.

Certain general points need to be considered:

1. The increasing muscle weakness.
2. The increasing deformities.
3. The involvement of the respiratory muscles and the risk of respiratory infections.
4. The child's personal attitude to the disease and the anxiety that develops with the progressive weakness.

Increasing muscle weakness

The child is less and less able to create movement in the water, particularly those movements of vertical and lateral rotation. Consequently the child is at greater risk and care must be taken to ensure safety. Facilitation of rolling and forward recovery eventually becomes necessary.

As muscle changes take place, so the density of the child alters and there will be a tendency for those parts which have become less dense to float higher. Floating is usually easy for the child but, for comfort, happiness and safety, floating should be in the supine position. In the later stages of the disease the child may have little strength to maintain the head at water level in the supine position, the nose and mouth being all of the face that is above water. If the child is anxious about this situation, some means of flotation for the head may be of value. Since flotation collars are often restrictive, a large swimming cap, inside and at the back of which a plastic bag filled with the required number of polystyrene balls can be appropriately placed may be useful.

Increasing deformities

The increasing deformities will alter the shape of the child, and adjustments to body position, balance and rotational control will need to be made. The alterations in shape will occur slowly and the physiotherapist should be constantly alert for them. While specific work to maintain a reasonable range of movement and prevent deformity may be possible in the early stages, as the disease progresses it is unrealistic to continue stretchings or other specific exercises. Walking in water can be continued after it has ceased to be possible on land, even if it is achieved only by rotation of the shoulders in the vertical. Support will gradually be required and should be given by the therapist from in front as in the facing hold (see Fig. 5.16), especially as the ability to control the head decreases and the child's fear of losing balance in the vertical grows.

Involvement of respiratory function

The involvement of the muscles of respiration makes inspiration and expiration increasingly ineffective. In the early stages, 'blowing' and encouraging the good breathing control required for swimming will aid respiratory function. It will be necessary to ensure, at all times, that the child is not exposed to extra risk of infection through activity in water. Changing areas should be free from draughts and appropriately heated, and adequate drying of the body and hair is essential. The child should not participate if feeling unwell, since this suggests an infection could be present.

The child's attitude to the disease

The child with muscular dystrophy needs constant encouragement. The condition will place a growing number of restrictions on the ability to achieve, however hard the child tries. The continual failure causes depression, and negative attitudes develop. Water is one environment in which movement and enjoyment can be maintained for longer. However, the child does become aware of the ability to move less and less well in the water. With the loss of control due to muscle weakness, there is the fear of losing balance and of being unable to recover to a safe breathing position. This affects the attitude to water activity. The physiotherapist will need to encourage the child but must avoid activities which are too difficult. More and more manual support has to be given and should be at the centre of balance of the body whatever the hold. The exception is for the vertical position in the later stages when the 'floppy hold' (see Fig. 5.18a and b) may be used. At all times, the emphasis should be on independence, but the child must not be faced with frequent failure.

Congenital Abnormalities

When the child with a congenital abnormality is introduced to activity in water, the altered shape and density of the child's body must be studied. These factors will be different in each child and so an individual programme must be devised to assist the child in coping with the particular problem.

All activities are appropriate as a means of teaching the child the skills required for swimming. However, the alterations in shape and density will almost certainly produce problems with rotational control laterally and vertically. Therefore early acquisition of this control is essential to the child's progress in water and should be emphasized at all times.

In particular, where a child has been born lacking full development of all four limbs, it is of paramount importance that rotational control is learned early and rapidly. The child will be dependent on head control both to create a forward and backward movement around the centre of buoyancy and to control very precisely the swing of the body, which will be a rapid one. This is so because in normal development the weight of the lower limbs has a braking effect. Without strong and accurate head control, the phocometic child may well be disturbed by this rapid movement.

In the same way, the child may fall forward in the water and need to rotate onto the back before creating a forward recovery to the upright position. The head must create the roll over the body by initiating strong lateral rotation. The act of rolling will also be prolonged in relation to the normal, so mental adjustments must be made and good breathing control established.

Once these children have mastered the necessary skills, they are able to move through water with a dolphin-like action and take considerable pleasure in the activity.

Rotational skills are equally important with either partial absence or deformity of a limb or limbs. But in these cases control of lateral and vertical rotation can be taught simultaneously. The ability to achieve the upright position may at times depend on a combination of gravitational and rotational effects, much as in the spina bifida child.

Children who have absence of limbs can become excellent swimmers and may participate in many advanced aquatic skills.

Spina Bifida

Spina bifida refers to a congenital abnormality in which there is a failure of closure in the midline of neural, bony or soft tissue (Carmel, 1974). It is among the commonest major congenital abnormalities and is often associated with others such as hydrocephalus, congenitally dislocated hips, and talipes equino varus.

Spina bifida is usually classified as being of two main types:

(a) spina bifida occulta,
(b) spina bifida cystica,

and under the last heading meningocele and myelomeningocele are described.

It is the child with myelomeningocele who most concerns the physiotherapist (Shepherd, 1995). Such cases would be the ones more frequently treated in water, since the milder forms of spina bifida rarely present problems, and activity in water for this group would almost certainly follow that for the able-bodied.

The child with a myelomeningocele will have marked alterations in both shape and density, and this will be a major consideration when undertaking activity in water. Other considerations relate to hydrocephalus, if present, incontinence, lack of sensation, social and psychological factors.

The need to study the shape and density of the spina bifida child in relation to activity in water cannot be too strongly emphasized. As a background to this, the hydrodynamic principles, characteristics and properties of water and all aspects of rotation must be fully understood.

Alterations in shape and density in spina bifida

These vary considerably with each individual child, but the common and frequent complications are:

(a) the loss of density in the lower limbs leading to high floating of these limbs,
(b) the ease with which vertical balance can be disturbed or lost,
(c) the rotational problems occurring due to asymmetric distribution of muscle power and deformity.

The child affected by spina bifida must learn the effect of head movement on the body, particularly anteriorly and posteriorly, and thereby appreciate how the head controls the body position and the feet. Any action that takes the head back and away, or forward and away, from the vertical will cause a quick upswing of the legs and trunk with rotation. This loss of balance is a disturbing experience and usually causes the child to cling to the physiotherapist, the bar or the side of the pool in an effort to maintain the vertical position.

In the early stages, control of vertical rotation must therefore be strongly emphasized until it becomes an automatic response. Instruction should begin in the 'ball' shape and at first only small rocking movements should be permitted.

These movements can be widened as control is gained. 'Bells' provides an excellent means of teaching such control and should be done on a one-to-one basis, progressing to less support with a short arm hold between two therapists and eventually to a 'Rag dolls' swinging action.

The 'bicycling' action and hold employed in a number of activities, such as 'Bicycles', 'Looby Loo' and 'The wheels of the bus', encourage a fine degree of vertical rotation control, and when this has been gained progress can be pursued through activities which involve the extremes of posture from 'ball' to 'stick', such as in 'Eggs for breakfast'.

Vertical or forward recovery requires a quick movement, since a 'sinking' action is required if the legs are to go down and the upright position be obtained. To create forward recovery, the knees must be flexed towards the chin as much as possible, the head and arms stretched forward to rotate the body from supine lying to the vertical. To facilitate the forward head movement and to encourage breathing control, the swimmer should blow out as the head is brought forward. Where high-floating legs make the 'sinking' action difficult, the arms may be carried up above the water, thus increasing the gravitational effect and, therefore, the 'sinking' action. Since the paralysis may not be equally distributed in both legs, there will be a tendency for one leg to float higher than the other. In this instance the arms need to be taken above the water surface and carried to the side on which the higher floating leg is. This causes rotation over that side and enables the swimmer to regain the vertical position. Balance is then maintained by appropriate head control and the forward position of the arms.

'Rag dolls' and other activities designed to encourage the swimmer to move from the supine to the prone position in the water are a natural progression as the degree of head control is developed and lessens anxiety. Such progression has to be steadily but surely developed as the child will have considerable anxiety about the changes of body position anteriorly and posteriorly.

Encouragement of the supine lying position from the vertical is the first progression, and when such control has been achieved, moving to prone from the vertical is next, then progressing to swinging actions between supine and prone.

When vertical rotational control is achieved, the child will be more mentally adjusted to water and physical balance will be better controlled. However, problems of lateral rotation may have to be considered and this control should be taught along with vertical rotational control. The need for consideration of lateral rotational control will have been evident when observing the asymmetry of the child's body along the longitudinal axis in supine. All rotational alterations, however small, will be seen and the importance of teaching lateral rotational control obvious. Such control is taught in the vertical, half lying, and finally in the horizontal positions. The child learns to control any longitudinal rotational effects by turning the head away from the side rolling under the water. Activities which teach lateral rotation firstly in the vertical plane and through to the horizontal plane should be developed. Examples of such activities in the vertical are 'turning' and 'Jumping on the spot' and they also form part of activities such as 'Looby Loo' or 'The hokey cokey', 'Space ships' and 'Passing an object around the circle'. Games such as 'Seaweed', 'Hallo' and 'Rolling on to the bar' assist in the progression towards horizontal lateral rotation. Complete rolling through 360° follows with the physiotherapist 'patting' the body around to facilitate the roll until the swimmer is able to produce the roll to either side independently, blowing as the face goes towards and is submerged in the water.

When vertical and lateral rotation have been achieved and the swimmer can roll horizontally in both directions and recover forward from lying to a safe breathing position, it is necessary to combine both rotations for final control prior to underwater activity and 'paddling off'.

The author is convinced that it is the disturbing effect of loss of balance that causes much anxiety in the spina bifida child. This is most evident in the prone position which produces marked degrees of trunk and cervical extension. This troubles the child excessively and it appears that activities carried out in the vertical and supine positions are best adhered to at first until a considerable degree of vertical rotation control has been acquired. Lateral rotation should be introduced and then a combination of both rotations until the child progressively develops skills which lead to complete mental adaptability and balance control.

Due to the frequency of losing balance in the backward or, more frequently, forward direction, the child is often forced into the prone position. To counteract this the head is usually extended strongly, and encouraging the child to get the head forward and blow into the water is difficult.

If the size of the child's head is increased, it will mean that the centre of buoyancy will be higher in the body than in children not suffering from this problem. This will compound the difficulty of vertical rotational control, as even the slightest movement of the head forwards or backwards will increase to a marked degree the loss of balance and quick upswing of the legs in either direction.

These two points emphasize the importance of teaching vertical rotational control.

Children who have hydrocephalus associated with spina bifida will almost invariably have had surgery with the insertion of a shunt or valve to control the condition. Care must be taken not to press on the valve, which will be *in situ* behind the ear. Heads should not be held, but in these children there is the added problem of the shunt. The abnormal head size, even in those children whose hydrocephalus has been arrested, makes the development of head control an onerous task. Balance is slow to develop and will need attention, but all activities in water have, inherently, a balance component.

Due to difficulties in maintaining the vertical position, the spina bifida child has a great need to cling either to the physiotherapist or the bar, and disengagement is another step in progress that needs strong emphasis. Activities that encourage such disengagement are 'How wide? How tall?', 'Hickory, dickory, dock', 'Looby Loo', 'Space ships', 'walking' round the circle and all those other activities which have the child facing away from the physiotherapist, such as 'Eggs for breakfast', 'Bicycles' and 'Space ships'.

Swimming becomes a reality for the child only when it has acquired all rotational control, is able to disengage and appreciates upthrust.

Therapeutically the child will have acquired much activity for head, trunk, legs and arms, and through independent mobility will have

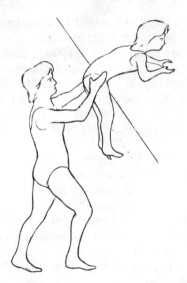

Fig. 6.1a   'Normal' exit over the side

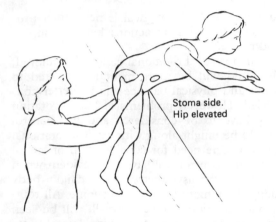

Stoma side.
Hip elevated

Fig. 6.1b   Modification of exit over the side for spina bifida child with stoma and bag

worked those muscles which have some power.

Entry and exit

The child with spina bifida and/or hydrocephalus can enter over the side. The problem in entry is the fear of loss of balance and lack of trunk control as the hands are placed on the physiotherapist's shoulders. This may be overcome by secure handling, verbal reassurance, frequent repetition of the mode of entry, and, for entry to the water, the choice of a rhyme or song that appeals to the child.

The form of exit from the pool can be over the side, but if the child has had a urinary diversion which involves the wearing of a bag attached to a stoma, the hip on the side of the stoma must be lifted well clear of the side of the pool as progress from the water and 'wriggling' along the poolside take place. Thus the bag is not disturbed (Fig. 6.1a and b).

Incontinence

Children with myelomeningocele will have bowel and bladder incontinence. The former is usually managed by appropriate diet and training and, if managed well, is not a problem during activity in water, though it should be ascertained that the bowels have been evacuated that day (Trussell, 1971; Skinner and Thomson, 1983). Bladder incontinence presents a different problem, but does not act as a total contraindication provided suitable precautions are taken.

If the spina bifida child is being trained by expression of urine, this must be attended to prior to entering the water. If a bag of any type is worn, it should be emptied before the child enters the water and the tap secured in a closed position.

The wearing of plastic pants under the swimwear, especially those fastening at the side with press studs, is an added precaution. Plastic pants with elasticated openings may prove tight and uncomfortable and cause pressure on skin that has no sensation and poor nutrition, and should only be used provided such problems do not arise.

If at any particular time the spina bifida child appears to be, or is confirmed to be, 'off colour', water activity should be avoided until the child is well again as an infection may be developing.

Social and psychological factors

Social and psychological factors may be associated with the problems of incontinence. This presents a difficulty only where such children swim in public facilities. Appropriate and tactful handling can minimize these factors.

For the spina bifida child, learning to swim – which many ultimately do extremely well –

offers the same beneficial social and psychological effects as in any other condition.

Osteogenesis Imperfecta

Although osteogenesis imperfecta is a rare disease, it is one that can ideally receive physical treatment in water.

In the severe congenital form, frequent fractures are caused by minor trauma and the prognosis is poor. In the milder form the future is less bleak. For all the children, movement in water is easier than on land and there is less danger of fractures. Following surgery, especially of the long bones to correct deformity, weight-bearing in water in the upright position can be gradually introduced, provided the child is handled appropriately.

Great care must be taken when introducing the children to water, and it is preferable that severe cases are treated individually. The child with a milder form may benefit from group activity, but the physiotherapist must guard against the child coming into sharp contact with other persons in the group or with the sides of the pool. It is advisable that the child does not jump into the water, nor land heavily on the feet, and diving is best avoided – although the author has worked with two children who had a very mild form of osteogenesis imperfecta and who eventually engaged in all such activities.

Growth is retarded and all the children will be small in stature, but not all are confined to wheelchairs, though this may be so in adult life.

Osteogenesis Imperfecta Congenita

This severe form may be seen in children's hospitals, and physical treatment may be requested both preoperatively and postoperatively.

Entry into the water can be effected in several ways but is best achieved with the child lying supine on a stretcher. In the case of the very young, small child, a tray made of suitable splinting material with sides and canvas handles may prove invaluable (Fig. 6.2). The child can remain on this throughout the treatment. The physiotherapist supports the tray and can angle it so that the buoyancy of the water floats the limbs to be exercised off the tray, thus allowing free movement.

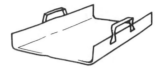

Fig. 6.2 *Tray used for treatment of child with osteogenesis imperfecta congenita*

The child is invariably terrified at entering water, and it takes a long time, many pool sessions and much patience, to overcome the very real fears. The same situation will recur following surgical treatment, even though the child is aware that the warmth of the water is comforting and movement easier.

Shape and density are important, particularly where deformities are marked, but until the child is actively exercising off the tray they are of lesser concern to the physiotherapist.

Post-surgical treatment usually involves obtaining the upright position with the gradual introduction of weight-bearing in standing and walking. In addition, general mobilizing and strengthening exercises for the limbs are introduced. Water depth is critical. The child should be taken to a sufficient depth so that in the vertical position the feet are initially clear of the floor of the pool. As weight-bearing is gradually permitted, the child is taken into less deep water. To ensure that the progression into shallower water is carefully graded, it is essential to record the exact depth at each treatment. Close cooperation with the surgeon in charge of the case in relation to the progression of weight-bearing is important.

The child will need to be made aware of how important head control is in maintaining the upright position. If the head is kept forward, the feet will remain down. The physiotherapist should sit in a stable position supporting the child at the waist from in front. The child's arms should be forward and just under the surface, or resting on the physiotherapist's arms (Fig. 6.3).

Cervical flexion and extension begun in a very small range are then encouraged. The movement in each direction should be slow so that the child can appreciate the swing of the body and counteract the movement with the head.

Gentle, active movement of the legs is encouraged in this position – flexion/extension, abduction/adduction of the hips with the knees

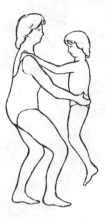

Fig. 6.3   *First facing hold*

straight, and hip and knee flexion. These movements can also be performed in supine lying when the child is supported by the physiotherapist's hands lightly held under the waist, with the child's head resting gently on the physiotherapist's shoulders. The physiotherapist must be in a stable sitting position with the shoulders under the water. In both positions active arm movements can be encouraged. From supine lying, forward recovery will not only encourage flexion and extension but also stress head control.

As further weight-bearing is allowed, activity is carried out in progressively shallower water. Weight transference should be encouraged from side to side – 'tick, tock' as the pendulum of a clock. This activity may be introduced before weight-bearing is permitted, and will develop lateral flexion of head and trunk. As with all activities, it is commenced in a small range at first. Step-standing weight transference is introduced next and then walking small steps, gradually extending the length of the stride. The walking pattern can be varied, walking with hip and knee flexion or with the knees extended. The physiotherapist will support the child at the waist from in front at the commencement of all progressions – that is, in each new depth – and will gradually disengage by removing the waist support and allowing the child to hold on to the physiotherapist's outstretched arms, working towards a hand hold, fingertip hold and total independence.

While working in front of the child, the physiotherapist has good eye contact and communication is easy. For progression and further disengagement, the physiotherapist walks behind the child with arms stretched forward so that the child's hands or arms can rest on them.

All movements should be slow and rhythmical. Any sudden movement may cause trauma and must be avoided. These children therefore require a one-to-one basis for hydrotherapy. If other help is available, it can be very useful. However, it depends on the nature of the child – parent relationship and attitude as to whether parents are used in this assistant role. In the author's experience, the parents' help should be at the bathside, in dressing and undressing, lifting and handling into and out of the pool – daily activities they are used to performing.

Milder forms of osteogenesis imperfecta can be treated on similar lines to those of other orthopaedic conditions. However, the treatment sessions should be handled cautiously and progressions made more gradually. The child progresses well towards swimming, and provided awareness of the precautions to be taken are instilled, this should present no difficulties. It is essential that rolling is taught, especially rolling on to the bar, so that when swimming back stroke and nearing the end of the pool, no sudden hard contact occurs with the walls of the pool. The ability to keep the eyes open when taking part in water activity is essential.

Burns

Hydrotherapy, in the strictest sense of the word, has a part to play in the treatment of burns. Behrend (1963) points out the value of the Hubbard tank with water in motion for debridement, and an appropriate temperature of about 38°C (100.4°F). Shepherd (1995) indicates that debridement may be carried out non-traumatically in the bath, the whirlpool effects and active movements helping the process, facilitating the removal of dressings and reducing infections. Capillary ingrowth is also improved. The temperature suggested by Shepherd (1980) is three degrees lower than that advocated by Behrend (1963). Shepherd (1995) gives useful advice on general procedures for the burnt child and her book should be consulted if it is planned to use hydrotherapy in these cases. It should be noted that the effects of burns on a child's emotional well-being are enormous, and the child may be in a highly anxious state at the prospect of hydro-therapy. Bernstein (1976) cautions as to the possible effects on the child and others of the burned parts of the body and the sight of charred flesh becoming detached in the water.

If at all possible, the child should not only be gently informed as to all the procedures undertaken and their purpose, but diversions such as toys and music should be available to relieve anxiety. At all events, the child must be treated with consideration and allowances made for extreme swings in behaviour and attitude during the bath sessions.

Later, when newly grafted sites have healed, gentle active movements in water may be permitted. Very much later, when healing has taken place and the child is returned to living as normal a life as possible, swimming may form part of the activities the child engages in and which help not only to maintain function generally, but also to institute obvious social and psychological recovery.

NEUROLOGICAL AND DEVELOPMENTAL DISORDERS

Cerebral palsy
Head injury
Epilepsy
Infections of the central nervous system

Cerebral Palsy

Cerebral palsy is one of the more common handicapping conditions, varying a great deal in degree of severity, distribution and in its effect on intellectual ability.

'The cerebral defect commonly results in disorders of movement and tone referred to as spasticity, rigidity, flaccidity, athetosis and ataxia' (Shepherd, 1995), and these are frequently accompanied by associated disorders of vision and hearing, intellectual retardation and perceptual problems. All these will have a bearing on the child's activity in water and must be taken into account when working in the water with such a child.

It is beyond the scope of this book to discuss in detail the aetiology and characteristics of types of cerebral palsy, but categorizing the children according to the distribution of the motor involvement is helpful when considering taking them into water. The distributions most commonly met with are hemiplegia, diplegia and quadriplegia. The alterations in body shape and density that occur as a result of the motor involvement need to be studied carefully and the programme for each child developed accordingly.

The major concerns confronting the physiotherapist when taking cerebral palsied children into water are:

(a) altered shape and density,
(b) an inability to create voluntary movement readily due to spasticity,
(c) an inability to control the involuntary movement of athetosis and ataxia,
(d) poor respiration,
(e) difficulties with comprehension and communication.

The problem can be further compounded by perceptual disorders, difficulties with head control, poor postural tone and lack of rotation within the body axis.

The problems will be discussed under the major categories of distribution.

The hemiplegic child

The hemiplegic child will have altered shape and possibly altered density, though the latter may only be slight or more evident in older children. Asymmetry of posture is noticeable in both the young child and older child, and a pattern that involves flexion and abduction of the leg is found, while the arm tends to be retracted, flexed and abducted. Alternatively, the arm may show signs of extension when the head is turned towards the affected side due to the influence of the asymmetrical tonic neck reflex. Most hemiplegic children dislike the prone position because the affected arm remains flexed and is often caught under the child's chest. This can also occur if the child is placed prone in the water. It is then impossible to bring the arm forward and reach out. There may be difficulty in extending the head to keep the face clear of the water, and to achieve this the child may turn the head to one side. If the influence of the asymmetrical tonic neck reflex is strong, arm movements may be further inhibited. Add to this an overall anxiety about being in water and it will readily be seen that these children should be kept in the vertical position for their early activities, progressing later to supine lying.

The alteration in shape with 'shortening' of the affected side can be described as having the form of an unequal quadrilateral. The child will then tend to roll to the affected side (see Fig. 3.5b).

Correction of this rotation can be obtained by encouraging the child to rotate the head away from the affected side, whether in the vertical or horizontal supine position. The movement of the head will help to bring the body flat, thus developing a balanced position. The rotation of the head should be limited to that required to bring the body to a flat position. The head should not be allowed to turn so far as to affect the limbs if the asymmetrical tonic neck reflex is present.

In trying to equalize the unequal quadrilateral shape of the child, activities that involve swaying, 'Seaweed' which reduces tone, and those that involve lateral rotation in the vertical and horizontal planes are valuable. These activities include 'Lobby Loo' and 'Space ships' where lateral rotation in the upright position is one pattern of movement in the total activity. Games such as 'Seaweed', 'Resisted rolling' and 'Rolling onto the bar' encourage lateral rotation in the horizontal plane.

A useful activity to increase symmetry is manual rolling to the affected side. The physiotherapist supports the child, who is in supine, by placing the upturned hands just below the child's waist. The child is requested to turn the face to the side opposite to which the body is being rolled. The physiotherapist then resists this induced counter-rotation so the child must work harder to restore the flat position, and extension occurs on the affected side.

Once improved symmetry is obtained, other skills will be acquired more easily. If the child is markedly 'shorter' on the affected side and the roll cannot be corrected solely by a turn of the head in the supine position, then the affected leg may be crossed over the unaffected leg, either at the ankle or knee, depending on the amount of roll that requires correcting. The nearer to the centre of balance of the body the limbs are crossed, the greater the effect. If turning the head and crossing the legs are not sufficient to counter the roll to the affected side, the affected arm can be taken across the body when the additional weight will assist in controlling the higher-floating unaffected side.

Once the body has found a balanced position, activities that will encourage a more equal shape should be emphasized.

The hemiplegic child may tend to swim in circles at first. This is largely due to an inability to equalize arm movements but may also be the result of an asymmetry of shape.

When acquiring swimming strokes, therefore, the hemiplegic must learn to move the limbs in as equal a range as possible, gradually extending the range. If the child starts swimming on the back, arm movements should be equal and bilateral and the arms should initially be kept in the water. The back crawl leg action should be modified so that each leg acts equally. There is a tendency for a total flexion pattern of the affected leg to occur, the knee coming too far out of the water, and metacentric effects result, with rotation of the body to the affected side with each kick.

Another way in which a flat position for swimming may be achieved in supine is by the child using the unaffected arm in an extended position underneath that side. By creating turbulence beneath the unaffected and potentially higher-floating side, the child can independently roll the body flat. The affected arm is used in a paddling action at the side of the swimmer.

If the child swims in the prone position, 'dog paddle' is probably the easiest stroke to commence with. This can be gradually progressed to breast stroke, again ensuring limb movements of the affected and unaffected sides are kept equal in range.

Side stroke is frequently useful. However, it is essential that the child has the affected side lowest in the water and that both arms and both legs are involved in the action. All too frequently one sees the hemiplegic swimming side stroke with the affected side uppermost, the limbs of that side moving into abnormal patterns as the unaffected side makes increasing efforts to propel the child through the water.

Although time and patience are required, it is not only desirable but possible to achieve swimming in a straight line. As the strokes used become more proficient, competitive swimming can be undertaken should the child so wish.

The affected arm and hand require particular attention if these outcomes are to be achieved. Additionally, it is essential that the upper limb – more likely to be neglected by the child – should be stimulated.

Already it has been appreciated that vertical balance in water requires that the head and arms should be kept forward. This must constantly be encouraged in the hemiplegic in walking, jumping and hopping. Activities which have as their teaching point vertical rotation not only develop patterns of total flexion and extension and precise balance, but can encourage bilateral arm action if a bar is reached for, toes caught, larger objects retrieved or, in 'Eggs for breakfast', the child has an 'egg' for each hand.

In any activity which requires a bicycle hold, symmetry and awareness of the affected arm can be enhanced by the use of a 'handle bar' or 'steering wheel'. A 1-foot long (30 cm), 1-inch diameter (2.5 cm) stick, either wood or electric wiring conduit, makes a useful handle bar and a quoit, 9–12 inches (23–30 cm) in diameter, a good steering wheel. The 'stick' provides a pronated grasp and the hoop a grasp in mid position between supination and pronation.

This equipment can also be used in activities such as 'Seaweed', 'Hallo' and 'Speedboats', when the child should be encouraged to aid symmetry by holding it as low on the body as possible with both hands while being swayed through the water, or towed while kicking the legs.

Awareness of the affected limbs, especially the arm, can be obtained in activities that require large movements. Making waves, splashing with the hands and kicking require balance control whether performed in the vertical or horizontal position. At first the physiotherapist will need to assist with balance control, holding at the child's waist from behind, gradually reducing the amount of support as the child gains such control.

Since the hemiplegic child has a tendency to contract the trunk on the affected side, trunk and postural work are important. Resisted rolling (p. 104) is valuable to produce contraction of the trunk extensors and side flexors of the unaffected side.

The physiotherapist can also hold the child in supine lying by standing with the child's legs abducted either side of her waist, supporting along the lateral border of the thighs and pelvis with the forearms and hands. Swaying the child gently from side to side gradually induces relaxation. The speed of the swaying has to be adjusted to each individual's needs. Too fast a swing may produce an inappropriate response. Water going onto the face may also cause such a response. In this position both trunk flexion and limb flexion with rotation can be employed. The child is asked to sit up towards the physiotherapist, the arms reaching towards the physiotherapist's shoulders. To introduce rotation the child brings the body and arms forward towards the opposite shoulder of the physiotherapist. In lying back the child must control the head and body action. It is important that the physiotherapist bends her knees and 'goes down' as the child comes forward, rising again as the child lies back.

In order to work the trunk side flexors on the unaffected side, the child is held in the same position, but the body is swayed to the unaffected side and the child instructed to bend to that side when sufficient turbulent or drag effect has been created. To return to the starting position, a gentle passive swing without side flexion is used.

The diplegic child

The child who has spastic diplegia has altered shape: this will be triangular due mainly to the pattern of flexion at hip and knees. Since water floats triangular shapes point downwards, these children should begin water activity in the vertical and supine positions and not be placed prone at first, as in the prone position they will have to contend with this effect of the water. Additionally, the child may not have sufficient cervical and trunk extension to lift the face clear of the water to breathe, thus causing anxiety, tension and a further alteration in shape.

The diplegic child finds it difficult or impossible to balance in the upright position due to a narrow standing or walking base. In water, where stability and balance are at first less easily obtained, and the establishment of a wide base for stability is important, the diplegic child faces considerable problems. Abduction is difficult and it is therefore not possible to walk sideways. So activities which will gradually enable the child to change the shape, control balance and stabilize the body position must be part of the programme.

The distribution of the diplegic's spasticity is rarely symmetrical, so the additional problem of rotation to the more affected side is present.

As with the hemiplegic child, rotation of the head away from the side rolling under the water will counter this effect.

To alter shape in the diplegic child, extension of the lower limbs should be encouraged along with abduction. Activities in the vertical position which are helpful are the circle games in which not only is the child made aware that water has weight, but, in walking sideways 'like a crab', abduction is increased. 'Hickory, dickory, dock', 'Clocks and watches' (or 'The grandfather's clock') or walking sideways with the physiotherapist across the pool and back, the head and arms forward, have the same effect.

In supine lying, swaying the child from side to side with some rotation so that drag effect breaks the flexion pattern may prove helpful in creating more extension. The speed at which the child should be swayed can only be ascertained by working with each individual. A reversion to the flexion pattern on the part of the child means that one has swayed too fast and too hard.

Rotation in supine lying, as suggested for the hemiplegic, encourages extension and a more suitable shape for activity in water for the diplegic, but rolling to both sides must be employed. Where there is a marked asymmetry of the distribution of spasticity, more emphasis would be placed by the physiotherapist on rotation away from that side, and resistance, when introduced, would be greater in order to bring about more extension in that side of the body.

The diplegic can be introduced by degrees to the prone position as favourable alterations in shape occur, and breathing control and the ability to submerge improve.

Among the therapeutic efforts of activity in water are the relief of muscle spasm, development of relaxation and an increase in the range of joint movement. If activity takes place in a buoyancy-dominated situation where the effects of gravity are diminished, an increase in the creation of voluntary movement can be achieved. Therefore, all activities described under Ways and means (p. 33) are of value, and changes of pace, of atmosphere and of mood are as important to the diplegic as to the child with any other condition.

Poor respiration and difficulties with communication are less likely to present problems in the diplegic child, but comprehension varies and perceptual problems may be present. However, the teaching of breathing control will improve respiration and mouth closure. Repetition of activities may be necessary where comprehension is poor. If the perceptual problems are those of poor body image and spatial awareness, these can be improved by those activities which involve extremes of posture and large movements of limbs. For example, 'Eggs for breakfast', 'Rag dolls' and other games where vertical rotation is the teaching point should be used, and for larger movements of the limbs 'Stars and stripes', 'Speedboats' and 'Making waves' are valuable.

All activities that have lateral rotation either in the vertical or horizontal plane as their teaching point will assist rotation around the longitudinal axis.

Individual work as well as group activities can be used with the diplegic child. Specific work on adductor spasticity and rotation can be introduced by the physiotherapist standing between the child's legs as described for the hemiplegic child. 'Stepping stones' and 'Giant strides' will assist with improving gait. The use of turbulence to encourage stability against this disturbing force aids the diplegic with balance and counter-rotational control, but (as in other conditions) turbulence can be used to aid mobility.

The quadriplegic child

In children suffering from quadriplegic cerebral palsy, it is necessary to differentiate between those with spasticity and those with athetosis. While both will have alteration in shape, it will tend to be more fixed in the spastic and to fluctuate in the athetoid. The spastic quadriplegic child will therefore require activities which will assist in equalizing dimensions of shape as much as possible. Strong adductor spasticity resulting in crossing of the legs will cause marked problems of lateral rotation and rolling around the longitudinal body axis. To control this rotation, the head, arms and legs can be used in activities directed at control in the vertical and horizontal planes. Examples of these activities are 'Passing the ring' (in the upright position and lying), 'Seaweed', 'Hallo', 'Rotating around the circle' (vertically, half lying and horizontally), 'Rolling onto the bar', 'Rolling from arm to arm', 'Resisted rolling' and 'The wheel'.

The athetoid whose posture, and therefore shape, is constantly fluctuating, needs to learn good blowing reactions and control of the head, arms and legs as soon as possible, thus giving the child a degree of control over the rotational movements that occur.

Respiration is usually explosive and poorly controlled in these children, and when head control is also poor, good blowing reactions will take a long time to acquire. Blowing should be in the background of all activities for all children, at all times, but acquires additional urgency with these children. Blowing is a means of bringing the head forward and therefore is an essential precursor to head control. For this action, games such as 'Bicycles', 'Bells', 'Eggs for breakfast', 'Charlie is over the water', 'Jumping', 'Rag dolls' and 'The wheels of the bus' are a few examples. Some of these activities bring in head control in the more stable 'ball' shape, others use the extremes of posture from 'ball' to 'stick', and all bring the head forward towards the water at some point in the activity when blowing can be encouraged.

Control of the arms and legs is needed, as, should any of the limbs come out of the water unexpectedly, the water will immediately try to balance the child's body according to the new shape. Thus though good head control is essential, if the arms and legs can be controlled, rotational problems are less likely to occur.

Awareness of and the need for control of the limbs can be achieved through activities such as 'lifting' water with hands and kicking it with the feet. Learning to splash with hands and feet or to make waves, stopping on command and staying still, is excellent for teaching this control. 'How wide? How tall?', patting the water in time to a song and jumping, walking sideways in a circle, 'Stepping stones', 'Giant strides' and 'Fairy strides' are further examples.

Spasticity and movement creation

In water, particularly in a buoyancy-dominated situation, or when the feet are not in contact with the bottom of the pool, the effect of gravity is diminished and therefore so is its effect on the postural mechanism. As a result, spasticity presents less of a problem.

The support of water helps relieve muscle spasm and gives freedom of movement not possible on land. However, responses to the demand to create a movement are slow and it is important that the child is given time to respond, whether this is to a blowing action or to the movement of limbs or trunk. Activities should, to a reasonable extent, be performed at the speed at which the children *can* respond. Changes of speed, atmosphere and pace are important in the programme, but time must be given for action on the part of the child.

Awareness of affected limbs can be assisted through turbulent or drag effect. This effect is appreciated most at the distal end of the limbs, and consequently large movements which create greater turbulence are useful.

Since it is important that the child appreciates the necessity of keeping as much of the body in the water as possible, encouraging the child to 'lift' water in the cupped hand upwards through the water and feel the difference between below the surface and above is a useful means of introducing this concept.

Reduction of spasticity

Apart from the advantages of working in a buoyancy-dominated situation, rhythmic swinging, swaying and rolling actions reduce spasticity. Examples of activities that incorporate rhythmic swinging and swaying are 'Bells', 'Rag dolls', 'Seaweed', 'Hallo' and 'The grandfather's clock'. Those that incorporate rolling are 'Rolling from arm to arm', 'Rolling onto the bar' and simple gentle manual rolling facilitated by the physiotherapist as in 'Little boats are on the sea'.

Reflex-inhibiting patterns assist in the reduction of spasticity and are easily incorporated into many activities. For instance, the child who has a predominantly extensor pattern of spasticity can be flexed into a 'ball' shape and held by the physiotherapist. The child is held away from the phsyiotherapist's body and gently rocked forwards and backwards. As with all activities, the child must be encouraged to blow as the face goes towards the water. Head control can also be acquired or improved in this exercise.

Where adductor spasm is a problem, the physiotherapist can part the child's legs and stand between them as close to the knee level as possible. Support is given on the lateral side of the child's thighs and hips by the forearm and hands of the physiotherapist. The child can

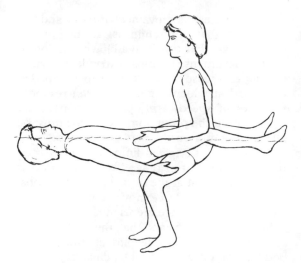

Fig. 6.4 *Hold for a child with adductor spasm*

then be swayed from side to side and also gently rotated (Fig. 6.4).

Adduction can be overcome by 'pendulum rocking'. The child is in the vertical position, facing the physiotherapist, with outstretched hand on the physiotherapist's shoulders. The physiotherapist stabilizes the child at the waist. The child is encouraged to part the legs sideways as far as possible and weight is transferred to one leg by a movement of the head and trunk to one side and then to the other in a rhythmic manner. Increasing abduction occurs as the child and physiotherapist lean from side to side overcoming turbulent effect and leaning against the water. Where a child is unable to touch the bottom of the pool, the physiotherapist's thighs provide a platform in the stable 'sitting' position and working at the same level as the child.

Where flexion is the predominant pattern of spasticity, every effort should be directed towards increasing extension through activities such as 'Rag dolls' and 'The wind, sun and rain' – in fact any which involve the extremes of posture moving from a long unstable 'stick' position to a stable 'ball' shape and then to a 'stick' again in supine lying. This pattern rhythmically repeated is valuable. The prone floating position, which might seem of use, presents formidable problems. It has been seen already that when the body is flexed, the tendency is for water to rotate that shape forwards and float it face down. Thus the flexed child in prone is

likely to be rotated forward, and since extension of the head and spine will be limited, it is difficult for the child to achieve extension.

Athetosis, ataxia and control of movement

Water has a damping-down effect on movement, and for children with athetosis and ataxia this can be helpful. Keeping as much of the body in the water as possible is even more essential for these children, and teaching awareness and control of the limbs is extremely important.

Stability in water – always difficult to achieve – presents a special problem to the athetoid and ataxic. Involuntary movements further compound the difficulties, so the use of activities that begin in the more stable 'ball' shape and control the limbs are recommended, for example 'Bells' and 'Bicycles' performed on a one-to-one basis. As control develops, unrolling of the body can be employed, as in 'Rag dolls' and 'The wind, sun and rain'.

Frequently when taking the athetoid into water, head control and arm control are poor, especially in lying supine. The tendency is for the arms to be abducted asymmetrically and one arm or both to be above the surface of the water. Symmetry and control of the arms by the side of the body are desirable and are not achieved by the child without considerable difficulty.

It may be necessary to hold the head of the athetoid for brief periods to allow the child to get the arms to the side. As this movement is experienced it becomes easier to achieve and gradually the need to hold the head decreases. Once the arms are down, the child can be encouraged to hold a 12-inch (30 cm) wooden stick with both hands, keeping this as low on the body as possible. If the child has difficulty in maintaining the grasp on this stick, the physiotherapist can assist with the hands. Once more, if the hold is close to the centre of balance of the swimmer's body, symmetry can be maintained. The child's head rests on the physiotherapist's shoulder and, should it have a tendency to turn to a particular side, the shoulder of choice will be the one on which the physiotherapist's own head can control the tendency to turn.

When symmetry and control of the arms have been achieved in this manner, movements of the legs can be encouraged in rhythmical patterns. Demands to stop and lie still help gain control of the lower limbs. Impaired or absent head control requires constant attention and can be slowly and steadily improved in activities that encourage side-to-side, forward and backward and rotational head movements. Moving sideways in 'circle' games and appreciating that water has weight and can be leant against encourage side-to-side head movements. 'Bells', Bicycles', 'Eggs for breakfast', 'Reach for the bar' or 'Catching toes' will assist forward head control and control of the upper limbs. Turning or lateral rotational activities in the vertical and horizontal planes, such as 'Space ships', 'Turning in the arms', 'Passing a ring or ball' around the circle, 'Rolling from arm to arm' and, finally, moving around the circle independently will all demand head control, and so the child obtains the necessary skill in controlling the body.

Respiration and communication

It must be stated again that 'blowing' needs to be in the background of all activities and, with constant emphasis, the child may gain degrees of control.

Where the child has a poor cough reflex with a mouth constantly 'gagged open' and limited head control, the vertical position facing the physiotherapist and supported by her below the axillae is the one of choice. To increase the child's control, the arms should be stretched forwards and the hands placed on the physiotherapist's shoulders. This is often difficult for the child to achieve, but by modifying the hold the physiotherapist can facilitate the position of the arms. Gentle assisted active kangaroo jumps with the commands 'jump' and 'blow' can introduce rhythm and control.

As mouth closure and head control improve, the child can be held vertically facing away from the physiotherapist. It is important that the child stretches the arms forwards. Attainment of the supine lying position is gradually introduced, followed by recovery forwards to the vertical position.

Mario, an athetoid with marked fluctuations of tone but predominantly extensor in pattern, had poor head control and respiration, a mouth that gagged open and a depressed cough reflex. He was treated as suggested, and within six months it was possible, holding him in the vertical, to proceed through 30 feet (9 metres) of water with it lapping his mouth without his lips opening or his mouth filling with water. The speech therapist remarked on the ease with which he was now closing his mouth for speech and in feeding, and noted that his head was more controlled. It was almost two years before his breathing was such that taking him underwater was suggested. Mario was delighted. He was instructed to take a breath as he 'jumped' upwards and to 'blow' out as he submerged. These actions were achieved successfully several times without any coughing or problems with his respiration. A major milestone had been achieved and, since nothing succeeds like success, Mario was spurred to greater effort and the physiotherapists were encouraged to develop his skills.

Postural tone

Poor or absent postural tone may be improved through activity in water. Water is a supportive medium and in the appropriate buoyancy-dominated situation – that is, a water depth over two-thirds a person's height – it is possible to encourage a more upright posture. Since shape can also be more readily altered in water and with less adverse stimulation of the antigravity muscles, improved posture can be obtained.

If turbulence is then introduced, the resultant actions taken by the swimmer to maintain stability become apparent in tone and posture. If the swimmer is required to move, a pause between each part of the pattern of movement demands greater postural control, balance and stability, and coordination can be developed.

Rotation

Many people with neurological problems lack rotation, particularly of the trunk, and this is a common problem in cerebral palsy. Lateral rotation around the longitudinal axis is easy to create in water and if it is facilitated, lateral rolling and rotation may be improved. Performed rhythmically both in the vertical and horizontal planes, rolling is a valuable adjunct to both therapeutic aims and the recreational aspects of water activity.

Head Injury

The number of people sustaining head injuries has increased steadily in recent years. These injuries can arise from accidents on the road, during participation in sport, in the home and in industry (Jennett and Teasdale, 1981). Whatever the cause or type of head injury, people who survive the accident are frequently left with a number of problems that affect function and require prolonged treatment.

Head injury in both adults and children presents similar problems and the resulting difficulties are numerous, complex and tend to change in nature over time. They can be physical, emotional, intellectual and behavioural and may include changes in personality, difficulty in controlling emotion and varying degrees of intellectual impairment. In particular, physiotherapists and others taking head-injured adults and children into water need to be aware of the sudden and sometimes violent fluctuations in emotion which can occur. In spite of this hydrotherapy has a part to play in the treatment of the head-injured.

Hydrotherapy for the head-injured adult has been discussed elsewhere in this book (p. 189). While the indications, contraindications and untoward effects are the same, some aspects of treatment for children differ from those for the adult and are presented below.

The approach to hydrotherapy for the head-injured child should in the author's opinion combine both therapeutic and recreational aspects. When planning such a programme the physiotherapist will have taken into account the child's altered shape and density, will be aware of the importance of the basic skills of breathing control, head control and rotational control and must ensure a fine balance between relaxation and movement.

The method of entry to the water may differ for the child from that of the adult or teenager. Whereas the latter will utilize a hoist, smaller children may be carried into the water or enter over the bathside being passed from one physiotherapist to another already in the pool.

When head control is poor the physiotherapist may feel it necessary to place a horse-shoe shaped flotation collar around the neck prior to entry. Due to the smaller size of younger children an experienced physiotherapist may find it possible to dispense with this; it is somewhat restrictive and can hamper teaching head control. However, when other flotation equipment is needed the head being supported allows the physiotherapist to attach other floats more readily.

Children, especially if the work is to take place within a group, prefer to conform; wearing flotation equipment may single them out and mar their response to the programme of activity.

At all times, even to the youngest, explanation of and the reasons for each activity should be provided. This will encourage participation. Acknowledgement of achievement, however small, must always be made.

The goals of hydrotherapy for the head-injured child and adult are similar and can be listed as:

- to reduce tone and promote relaxation,
- to encourage movement and increase the range of weak movement,
- to improve head control, breathing control and voice production,
- to retrain and stimulate righting reactions,
- to retrain rotational patterns of movement,
- to retrain reciprocal patterns of movement,
- to re-educate functional movements patterns,
- to treat orthopaedic complications,
- to provide opportunities for recreation, socialization and their psychological effects.

Following assessment, especially of the child's altered shape and density due to the asymmetrical distribution of increased tone and the decision as to which rotational pattern needs particular emphasis, the early stages of the programme would be to reduce tone and induce relaxation. This may be achieved by swaying the body laterally. The hold will be the backing hold but may require the physiotherapist's hands to be placed beyond the waist towards the hips and for them to be placed on the sides of the body. This gives the physiotherapist better control and leverage as the body is swayed from side to side through the water. The swaying movement is a lateral one, but at times a rotational component may be added towards the end of each swaying action. There are no firm guidelines for the speed, direction and manner of this swaying action. The physiotherapist must work this out on the basis of individual responses, which will be specific to the person on any particular day. Thus, it requires constant observation and evaluation of the effects of the swaying action. Any adverse responses which occur, such as an increase in spasticity, indicate that the swaying action needs to be modified or temporarily withdrawn; they may also result from poor handling on the part of the physiotherapist.

The upper trunk may be swayed from side to side and rotated to reduce spasticity. The physiotherapist stands between the child's legs. The elbows are placed on the outer side of the child's knees, the forearms along the lateral borders of the thighs and the hands over the hips. The head is supported by the inflated collar. Once again the range of sway, the speed and the particular direction are adjusted to the individual being treated. Small automatic postural effects can be induced by the judicious and appropriate use of this swaying action. This swaying technique is an adaptation of 'Seaweed' and later, combined with the activity 'Hallo', can improve head control. As always, 'blowing' whenever the face goes near water or the water near the face must be developed. The word 'blow' should be the one most frequently heard in the pool. 'Blowing' is in the background of every activity in water but in the case of the head-injured needs constant repetition and reinforcement.

A large proportion of head-injured children demonstrate problems of extension; others may have a pattern of flexion. Although it might seem unwise to place the child in supine lying, the position in which increased extensor tone is present (Brodal, 1981; Heiniger and Randolph, 1981), the buoyancy of the water and reduced effects of gravity make this position less inappropriate. Where flexion is the problem, extension can be developed in the supine lying position using the modified backing hold and swaying the body laterally with rotation so that the legs cannot be maintained in such marked flexion against the weight of water and the drag effect of turbulence.

Following induction of some degree of relaxation, it is then necessary to develop breathing control. This is not an easy task and requires time and patience from the physiotherapist and the head-injured child. Instruction should begin with the first session and be practised throughout all future sessions. The physiotherapist must communicate to the child the role that breathing control has in achieving and maintaining balance, relaxation and safety, as well as in respiratory function, oro-facial function and speech. The first sounds may result from the attempts to blow, closure of the mouth against the water may become habitual and improved respiratory function may result when the movements of the chest are alternately facilitated and resisted by the pressure of the water around the chest. The speech therapist plays a large part in the rehabilitation of the head-injured and, in the author's experience, it has proved invaluable to consult with the speech therapist and, when possible, attendance at the pool sessions, especially in the early stages of rehabilitation, on the part of the speech therapist enhances this aspect of treatment.

Breathing control is important when lying supine in the water but it is extremely difficult to teach when the child is in this position. A sitting position is required initially and this may be achieved from the supine lying position in two ways. If the child already has some ability to sit on land, the physiotherapist may remain behind the swimmer, supporting at the waist, and instruct the child to bring the head and arms forward at the same time as flexing the hips and knees. If the physiotherapist's body has been stabilized against the wall of the pool and a stable sitting position has been adopted, the child can sit on the physiotherapist's thighs. In the second method the physiotherapist should move to the side of the child and support under the trunk just below the lower border of the scapulae with one arm and under the thighs with the other. The child is given the same instruction as previously, but in this position the physiotherapist is able to facilitate the action. If a second physiotherapist is available, it is possible for one to work from behind or at the side and the other to be a focal point for the child to work towards. A rail at the side of the pool can also be useful when working alone. A small floating object that can be blown across the surface helps the child to focus in midline and encourages the blowing action. As some control is gained, attempts may be made to blow into the water. Children will be happy to blow objects such as plastic ducks, fish or 'eggs' across the surface of the water and as expiration improves may find it fun to blow items such as trumpets or suitable whistles into the water.

Gross patterns of flexion and extension of the whole body are gained in teaching the child to come to the sitting position and lie back again. The emphasis should be on the control of the head, both in coming erect and lying back. With a child demonstrating marked extension, the pattern of flexion and the sitting position would be accentuated – the reverse where flexion was predominant.

Head control, as already seen, can be introduced while reducing tone but can also be developed when stimulating movement. This can be done with the child in supine lying but using objects of interest and attractive to the child to encourage more effective movement. With the child curled into a 'ball' and supported by the physiotherapist (Fig. 5.5) not only may extensor tone be decreased but head and breathing control developed. The extent to which the child is rocked forwards and backwards is controlled by the physiotherapist and these movements may range from minute to larger ones depending on the level of the child's head control and whether it is necessary to provoke a reaction. By turning the child to face away from the physiotherapist and rocking the body from side to side lateral flexion of the head can be promoted as well as breathing control.

Retraining rotational patterns of movement commences in the earlier techniques used to decrease tone but is extended as the emphasis on teaching lateral rotation is developed. Head control is an important component of these activities. While rolling through 360° is not usually possible in the early stages head control can be encouraged in the manner described in 'Resisted rolling' (p. 104). 'Rolling onto the bar' (p. 103) and 'Rolling arm to arm' (p. 106) are the best activities to employ when commencing teaching rolling through 360°.

To retrain reciprocal patterns of movement any residual movements of the limbs should be encouraged. Minimal changes in tone can affect reciprocal movements. If the child is well supported by flotation equipment and permitted to move freely concentration on coordinating the movement rather than on moving is possible. Where one arm or leg moves more easily than the other, the child will tend to progress in circles. Therefore the action of the better limbs should be modified, and passive, then assisted active, movements applied in the appropriate range to the more affected limbs, especially the arm, by the physiotherapist.

Activity in the vertical should be developed. However, it is essential to introduce the upright position carefully, particularly in those children who are generally recumbent or semi-recumbent. Standing either supported by the physiotherapist from in front or behind, or holding on to the rail, should be undertaken in deeper water. Transference of weight sideways and later walking sideways should be commenced first. Later, step-standing, transference of weight forwards and backwards and walking forwards are introduced.

If increased spasticity should occur during any activity while treatment is taking place, it is advisable to return to the supine lying position and begin lateral swaying to regain relaxation. This may be required several times in any one pool session.

As the person progresses, an increasing number of activities are introduced, especially those described under the sections for rotational control and balance and coordination.

In the later rehabilitative stages the goals of treatment remain the same but are extended. Previously the work may have taken place on a one-to-one basis between child and physiotherapist and not within a group because of the severity of the condition and the need for the child's attention to be focused on the activities.

Children adapt much more readily to group work – adults usually fighting shy of the situation, especially those in their teens and early twenties – but the author has seen interesting and dramatic advances in the acquisition of skills for adults when persuaded to join in group activities.

The group provides greater motivation and stimulation, but it also encourages socialization. All of the activities described in the text are of value at this stage, and every effort should be made to ensure that the head-injured person's activities are directed towards independent functioning in the water: this includes safety in swimming, on the poolside and in the changing areas.

For those head-injured whose consciousness has returned but who remain severely affected – chairbound in either sitting or half-lying – activities should be carried out in groups. The person may have been discharged home or into care, and water activity in the hydrotherapy pool may no longer be possible on a regular basis. The swimming club that caters for the disabled can offer a suitable alternative, especially the club that numbers a physiotherapist among its members. The physiotherapist can act as an adviser to those who would work in the water with the person to the advantage of both swimmer and club helpers.

The author has seen marked changes in attitude and effort on the part of the head-injured when enabled to work in a group and club situation. Whenever possible, independent floating and swimming with whatever mobility the person possesses should be developed. The joy and freedom of independent movement that can be achieved in water when such movement is difficult or impossible on land should not be denied those who remain severely disabled.

Epilepsy

Epilepsy is described as a disturbance of cerebral function produced by recurrent abnormal discharges of neurons. It takes a number of different forms, and is frequently accompanied by loss of consciousness (Lance and McLeod, 1975). The clinical effects depend on and are determined by the location and duration of the discharge.

Farmer (1975) indicates that the most frequently seen seizure in children is that of a febrile convulsion which occurs in association with fevers and acute systemic infections. Epileptic attacks, however, can occur in people of any age, any background and any level of intellect. Epilepsy is frequently found in conjunction with other conditions such as cerebral palsy – approximately half of the children having this condition, particularly those who are hemiplegic or quadriplegic, also suffer from epilepsy. Differing views are held as to whether activity in water is suitable for those with epilepsy. Burden and Schurr (1976) indicate that epileptics can be allowed to swim as long as appropriate supervision is provided. In the case of children, the agreement of the parents and the child's doctor should be sought prior to commencing swimming. The adult swimmer should also have medical permission. The author does not wish to argue for or against the inclusion of the epileptic in water activity programmes, but does suggest that if approached to take a known epileptic into the pool, certain factors must be ascertained and precautions taken.

For the person who is an epileptic and has no other complicating factors, swimming can be taught by any method. However, the instructor must have obtained the following information.

1. Are there any warning signs when a seizure is about to occur?
2. Is the swimmer on any medication for the seizures?
3. Are the seizures well controlled by this medication?
4. How frequently does the swimmer take the medication and what are the times of administration?
5. The state of health of the swimmer at each attendance.

The warning signs or aura should be known to all concerned. If the swimmer is on medication, the instructor should check when the last dose was administered and ascertain the state of health at each attendance. Should the swimmer have failed to take the prescribed drugs or indicate in any way that the general state of health is lower than is usually the case, then activity in water should be postponed on that day.

It is interesting to note that epileptic seizures are uncommon in water. The author, in discussion with specialists in the treatment of epilepsy, has been informed that provided undue excitement and tension are avoided, and any factors such as flickering lights and reflections on the water are eliminated, a fit is unlikely to occur.

It is also important that facilities are available for coping with an attack and that experienced personnel are on hand to assist in the event of a fit occurring. It is essential that all personnel should be aware of the measures to be undertaken. Although appropriate measures have been laid down by a number of statutory bodies, these do tend to vary throughout the world.

At all times the swimmer suffering from epilepsy should be carefully watched. The author believes this can be carried out diligently but unobtrusively. It would appear more advantageous to allow the epileptic to swim under controlled conditions with efficient and knowledgeable personnel on hand than to refuse to allow such a person to swim. In the author's experience, such a refusal has led to a situation where the person has chosen not to divulge the presence of the condition in order to be permitted to join in a swimming class. This is potentially dangerous for the sufferer and could lead to serious or even fatal consequences.

The epileptic who, between convulsions, is usually fit and normal, will not present marked alterations in shape and density. The problem of balance in water will be slight, just as it is in the able-bodied population. However, when epilepsy is associated with cerebral palsy, the altered shape and density due to the primary condition must be taken into consideration.

When working on a one-to-one basis and with the knowledge not only that the swimmer suffers from epilepsy, but also the nature of the warning and of the aura, the situation can be managed well. Although the epileptic may be able to swim, the condition warrants a continued one-to-one ratio.

It is in the interests of safety for everyone that if the epileptic cannot swim the skill should be learned, since individuals, particularly children, already incur many restrictions in their lives. Much, however, depends on the type of fit and the frequency of the attacks. The social and psychological benefits of swimming have already been stated and are equally applicable to the epileptic. Risks are part of activity in water for all persons; for the epileptic it is the sudden and unpredictable nature of the attacks that adds to the risks (National Co-ordinating Committee on Swimming for the Disabled, 1975). If the precautions stated in the text are taken, the risks can be minimized and the epileptic gains in many ways from learning to swim.

Infections of the Central Nervous System

Infections of the brain, spinal cord and peripheral nerves may result from a variety of causes, and while many children do recover from the effects of the inflammation of these structures, some are left with permanent neurological damage. It is these latter children that the physiotherapist may be called upon to treat in the water. Examples of conditions in which hydrotherapy has a part to play in the stage of recovery include anterior poliomyelitis and Guillain–Barré-Landry syndrome.

Anterior poliomyelitis

This is an acute infection caused by a virus which destroys the motor cells of the anterior horn of the spinal cord and brainstem. The initial influenza stage of the illness is followed by paralysis of the muscles of a flaccid motor neuron type. The paralysis is usually widespread to begin with, but as considerable recovery takes place, the person is left with some residual asymmetrical paralysis of certain muscle groups.

The aims of treatment are to:

(a) prevent contractures,
(b) maintain the circulation,
(c) strengthen the affected muscles.

Activity in water will assist with all these aims. However, since pain is a symptom of the condition and the muscles have been tender to the touch, the child may be extremely anxious about movement when allowed out of bed. If the child can understand, it may be explained that the warmth and buoyancy of the water will make it easier to move. For the younger child, such explanations are not feasible and overcoming fear will require time and patience. In both instances the pool sessions should be conducted gently and made as enjoyable as possible.

There will in these children be marked alterations in shape and density due to the effects of the disease, the asymmetrical nature of the flaccid paralysis and the loss of density, all of which will produce rotational effects and body parts that will float easily. Careful observation of these effects must be made, and the treatment programme chosen will reassure the child and teach control of these effects.

Passive movements may be given to prevent contractures, and the warmth of the water will allow these procedures to be carried out more easily than on land, but great care must be exercised. Active movements should be encouraged and the fullest range of movement obtained. Buoyancy will both assist and resist movement and the exercise programme should be planned accordingly and the progressions carefully graded. As with all activity in water for children, the exercises are best carried out in the form of games.

Re-education of walking may be commenced in the water. The appropriate depth is important: the water should cover the child's shoulders in the vertical position as this assists the maintenance of an upright posture, the water providing support around the whole body. To encourage balance and stability, turbulence may be placed around the body (p. 127). Initially, however, the physiotherapist will need to use the facing hold. The procedures for re-educating gait have been described (p. 189), and may be followed for children with anterior poliomyelitis commencing with transference of weight sideways. An alternative method of teaching weight transference and walking sideways is that of working in a group in a circle formation. The preferred hold would then be across the back (p. 49), at least in the early stages of the activity.

Other activities such as jumping, hopping, skipping and dancing can be undertaken in deeper water, encouraging increased movement. The buoyancy of the water allows this without undue weight-bearing. In addition, these actions provide interest and psychological benefits for the child. As improvement occurs, the child should work in shallower water with increasing gravity effects. Balance and coordination can be increased if, instead of walking and jumping continuously, a pause is introduced between each phase of walking and between each jump. The turbulence created by the forward movement will disturb the body's balance. The child should pause for as long as is required to stabilize the body before moving again. The ways in which a stabilized position may be obtained are given in the description of the re-education of walking (p. 185).

The Bad Ragaz techniques may be of interest to the older child who can understand what is required and become intrigued by the patterns of movement. For the younger child, these techniques are of little value and the physiotherapist's ingenuity will be taxed to encourage similar movements in another form. As respiratory function may have been affected by the disease, the importance of breathing control and the need to improve respiration are evident.

As with all children in connection with activity in water, the physiotherapist must watch for signs of fatigue or the effects of cold. A warm pool is essential, but it should be neither too warm nor too cool. The former will be enervating and the latter will inhibit muscular activity. The temperatures already advocated are suitable for the treatment in water of the child suffering from anterior poliomyelitis.

Guillain–Barré–Landry syndrome and peripheral nerve lesions

This syndrome is a form of peripheral neuropathy, the cause of which is unknown although it may follow a viral infection of the gastrointestinal or upper respiratory tract. The disorder affects both motor nerves and those of sensation and the person may have difficulty in moving, breathing, swallowing, talking and smiling, as well as some numbness, paraesthesia and loss of sense of position. Pain is a feature of the condition and varying degrees of weakness and paralysis commence in the lower limbs and spread to the upper limbs. The person is hospitalized and management is symptomatic. Physical treatment is similar to that for poliomyelitis and would, in both the intermediate and ongoing stages of rehabilitation, include pool therapy.

The condition gradually resolves itself, the strength of muscles returning in an ascending order. Assessment of muscle power is carried out on land and the Modified Oxford Scale for Water can be employed for hydrotherapy evaluation. Pool programmes would follow that outlined for anterior poliomyelitis, but, owing to the symmetrical distribution, there is less likelihood of alterations in shape. Density will be affected but this will alter as recovery takes place.

The aims of hydrotherapy are to:

(a) increase muscle power,
(b) improve respiratory function,
(c) increase the range of movement,
(d) improve the circulation.

Passive movements may be given to all joints to prevent stiffness of contractures, though in the case of children such movements may be inappropriate. The anxiety engendered by the pain experienced in the early stages of the disease and the understandable fear of being handled make it more suitable to employ assisted active or active movements. Games that will encourage activity in as full a range of movement as possible should be used. The games provide a means of distraction for the child, who usually produces greater movement as a result, and this in turn may be of more value than Bad Ragaz or other very specific techniques. As recovery takes place, careful grading of the progression of exercise is essential.

The points made regarding fatigue and cold are as valid for this condition as for other peripheral nerve lesions. For all conditions where circulation may be affected – for example a peripheral nerve lesion, spina bifida and cerebral palsy – care should be taken that the feet are not damaged by dragging on the pool floor. The wearing of socks will help to prevent abrasions and injuries of this kind.

In dealing with peripheral nerve lesions, it should be remembered that the treatment programme and the progressions will vary with the extent of nerve involvement. Therapeutic exercise and recreational activity have considerable value in both the stages of recovery and final rehabilitation of these disorders.

SENSORY DISORDERS

The sensory disorders discussed below are those of blindness and deafness. Aquatic activities are not only possible for both conditions but are eminently suitable for both, particularly the blind and those who are partially sighted (Cordellos, 1976).

The Blind Child

One of the most serious handicaps of childhood is that of defective vision, especially when it is severe. On its own it leads to deprivation for the affected child bringing isolation from the environment, from everyday life, and from communication with everyone with whom the child has contact (Harcourt, 1977).

Visual defects may be found in neurological disorders, for example in cerebral palsy, and children who suffer from other physical and mental disorders.

While blindness itself, especially when severe, has a devastating effect upon the child's development, where deafness and blindness are associated then enormous difficulties in communication are presented.

The blind child will have delays in motor, language, cognitive, social, emotional and self-

care development (Olson, 1987). These factors will have a bearing on activity in water.

Studies have shown lags in motor and locomotion development. Olson (1987) cites a study by Fraiberg (1977) where, with assistance, that is with the hands held, most visually impaired children could perform the motor patterns of sitting, rolling, standing and stepping at about the same time as sighted children. The difficulties arose when the child had to move independently into space, and in moving between motor patterns and in dynamic activities, such as running and jumping.

Body image is frequently disturbed, and it is often difficult to promote. Having not seen their hands, feet or the body, it is unlikely the child can estimate the size, reach and span of the body parts or the body as a whole.

Posture is often affected due to the factors mentioned above, as well as the child holding the head and possibly the trunk in such a position to allow perception of the environment. This is especially the case in the partially sighted child. Certainly movement is more robot-like and does not flow, and there is a hesitancy in the gait.

Language, cognitive, social, emotional and self-care delay will have some bearing on movement in water but can be enhanced by activity in the medium.

Care must be taken with the analysis of shape and density. Although alterations in posture may not be great, it is essential that they are precisely assessed so that the correct strategies to control any rotational effects can be taught throughout each game and programme.

Prior to taking the visually handicapped person into the water, familiarization of the pool area is important. A route from the main entry to the pool complex to the changing rooms, and so to the immediate pool surroundings, should be devised and followed on every occasion. Tactile and auditory cues are used to orientate the swimmer, especially to the shallow and deep ends of the pool.

Importantly, the swimmers should have intact sensation so that, at all times, the child is able to indicate at what level the water is on the body in the upright position. The swimmer should also be made aware that two-thirds their height, that is xiphisternum level, is the point at which vertical balance becomes critical.

There is no doubt that a visually impaired person can enjoy activity in water as much as a sighted person, and movement can take place freely and adapted equipment is rarely required (Adams *et al.*, 1982). Personal experience has shown that the simple items used in the games shown in the preceding pages are all that are needed. By using descriptive language about the items of equipment, encouraging the child to touch the toy and explore it, tactile and other sensory inputs are developed. For example, when using the 'eggs' and blowing them across the surface of the water, the visually impaired swimmer is given the 'egg' to hold while it is described, then the physiotherapist blows onto the child's hand and then asks the child to blow on to the physiotherapist's hand. This is followed by the physiotherapist blowing partly into the water so that the child feels the bubbles; this should also be very vocal. The child repeats the action and this is followed by the 'egg' being placed on the water close to the swimmer's lips and blowing is encouraged.

The blind become familiar with water through the games and activities advocated in this book. In the process of learning to swim, the acquisition of the necessary basic skills remains the same for the blind child as for any other person. If a visual handicap is combined with a neurological condition, then the factors and approach to activity in water and finally swimming follow similar lines to those discussed under the heading of Cerebral palsy, (p. 145) with additional allowance being made for the limited vision.

Walking and jumping in all directions can be developed in water which supports the body and slows falling considerably. Body image, reach span and movement of the body as a whole are readily developed in the medium. Turbulence is created by every movement in water and it is at the distal portion of the limbs that it is most noticeable. This helps the blind swimmer to appreciate the length of the limbs and further enhances body awareness.

Through acquiring the skills of creating the rotations, the blind swimmer finds it easier to launch into space and improve dynamic balance.

Cognitive, language, social and emotional and self-care activities can be elicited and improved through water activity. The games develop cognition; singing the songs or saying the rhymes will assist the development of language, while emotions must be controlled within the group situation and within the medium of water where risk has to be respected and contained. Self-care activity can be trained in the changing room and on the bathside.

A frequent difficulty for the visually impaired swimmer is that of swimming in a straight line. Swimming alongside the pool wall, allowing the fingertips to touch the wall on each stroke, may solve the difficulty. Sounds – the beat of a drum or the ringing of a bell – may guide the swimmer's direction. Careful modifications of the swimming strokes may also assist the swimmer to move from one end of the pool to the other in a straight line.

The acquisition of swimming skills means that the visually impaired person can participate in other aquatic activities for recreation in safety.

The Deaf Child

The child with a hearing loss suffers from many deprivations. The inability to hear means that verbal thought and communication are denied the child as well as sharing with parents, other family members and all other humans the experiences of life which are 'mediated by spoken language' (Martin, 1977, p. 432).

Hearing loss ranges from the less severe but common condition arising within the middle ear to the rarer but profound deafness due to damage to the neural pathways. Where deafness is the sole handicap the child's shape may not be any more asymmetrical than would occur in normal circumstances. If the hearing loss is not total, then the child may well hold the head in such a position that allows the hearing of sounds. This position may become habitual and alterations in the posture of the trunk may result. Water will take these changes into account and, therefore, shape must be analysed in as much detail as for any other disability.

The water programme follows that for other disabilities. However, demonstration is important, especially for the profoundly deaf child. The advantage of working in a group is obvious as the child can see others participating and follow the actions. The physiotherapist would watch and correct any wrong or inappropriate action.

Importantly, any physiotherapist working with a hearing impaired child should be aware of the method of communication being employed for the child and every effort made to learn and follow the preferred technique. Where a physiotherapist has established a good rapport and an efficient means of communicating with a child, it is best to remain working with that child continuously. Changing the carer too frequently can prove very confusing for the child.

At no time should the swimmer need to turn or extend the head in order the see the physiotherapist's lips, thus disturbing the body's balance. The physiotherapist, therefore, has a responsibility to be properly placed at all times when working with a child with a hearing loss. Speaking clearly, naturally and in sentences which provide a context is better than single words and it is most important to remember that many children are excellent at lip-reading and will understand all that is said.

Activity in water and learning to swim should not prove difficult where hearing loss is the only handicap. However, the hearing impairment may be associated with other disorders.

Children suffering from cerebral palsy or mental handicap may have hearing impairment. In these instances, the teaching of the necessary skills is complicated by the hearing loss but the major disability, either cerebral palsy or mental disorder, will impact on the child's shape and thus becomes the first consideration. Ways of dealing with these are provided elsewhere in the text. The hearing loss complicates the learning process but should not impede it to any major extent if the above ideas are put into practice.

The Deaf Blind Child

In defining the deaf blind child, Griffiths (1977) quotes Davis (1961) who wrote that the condition is one 'whose combination of auditory and visual handicap is such that he cannot be educated adequately in a normal programme for deaf or blind children'.

The condition is rare but does present a formidable problem in relation to activity in water. However, such children should not be denied the experience of going into water. It is

an alternative to air and, with its unique properties, provides a learning experience for the child.

The deaf blind syndrome may be genetic in origin but may be acquired prior to, during or after birth. The sensory deficits may be associated with a more global handicapping condition. A rubella affected child may be deaf, blind, and suffer from motor and learning difficulties. Again, such children should not be denied experience of water. In addition to the benefits mentioned earlier, the child may well find movement easier and the warmth of the water will bring about relaxation.

For the deaf blind child with or without other disorders, it is necessary to facilitate the movement and activity required in the games described. The physiotherapist will need to implant the skills by moving the child through the patterns required. For instance, to develop vertical rotation the legs, trunk and head will need to be flexed, the arms brought forward till the upright position is obtained and then the legs extended and the body balanced.

Some may question the value of taking such severely affected children into water but, in the author's personal experience, it has been found valuable for the reasons described above, as well as in decreasing irritability of a cerebral nature. In one case, the child made a high pitched cry constantly. Only in the pool did this cease. During this time, the mother as the principal care-giver enjoyed some respite and an hour's peace which lessened her burden and allowed her to shop or have a rest.

Meningitis and encephalitis are infections that may bring about a deaf blind syndrome with accompanying physical problems. Again, water activity can help and movements commence. One such child showed their first pleasure when placed in the pool and developed active movement more readily in water.

The sensory disordered child can and does benefit from activity in water, and once the skills related to swimming and the art of swimming are learnt, the child is able to participate in a wide variety of aquatic activities.

Facilitation and demonstration are the two most important means of instructing these children. Communication with the blind child must be descriptive, and with the deaf child, by the method the child is using. For obvious reasons, hearing aids cannot be worn in the pool, and if the child who would one is not learning any of the methods, then the physio-therapist must create a simple method for communication related to water.

LEARNING DIFFICULTIES AND BEHAVIOUR DISORDERS

Severe learning difficulties
Mild learning difficulties and borderline normal
Autistic children
The hyperkinetic syndrome
Perceptual disabilities
The clumsy child

Children who have learning difficulties or have disorders of behaviour derive great benefit from activity in water and can learn many skills that carry over into their daily lives.

In the following pages, children with frank learning difficulties are separated from those who have combined mental and physical handicaps. Children with specific behaviour disorders are dealt with under individual headings.

The child with learning difficulties has suffered an arrest in development so that intelligence is impaired and there is difficulty in learning and in adapting to society. In addition, due to particular perceptual disabilities, the child may well have difficulties in processing incoming information. In various ways these problems may be improved by activity in water.

In general, the deficit has been present from birth and the children are usually classified as having profound learning difficulties, severe learning difficulties, moderate learning difficulties or mild learning difficulties, bordering on normal.

When taken into water, children with frank learning difficulties do not present with the marked problems of altered shape and density we have seen in other disabilities. Their shape and density may be altered through fear, anxiety, tension, hyperactivity or complete disregard or lack of awareness of water and its characteristics, but this alteration in shape will not be seen in such an obvious manner as in the physically disabled.

The real problem facing the physiotherapist is the level of comprehension of the swimmer. The individual's response to and translation of instructions will be directly related to enjoyment, effective use of water, and progress and safety.

The ultimate aim of water activity for these children must be, as in all disabilities, that the swimmer will be physically balanced, mentally adjusted and a safe participant in the medium. The best means of achieving this aim is through continuous repetition and reinforcement. The physiotherapist will need considerable patience in maintaining the child's contact and interest and in developing the concentration span. Often this is achieved more effectively by working in groups with a one-to-one basis of swimmer and physiotherapist or instructor.

Every skill must be learnt to a level at which it is performed completely automatically. This means that there must be a variety of activities used, all with the same teaching point, so that a splinter skill is not learnt. It is necessary that each skill is taught first in its primary form, then as a follow-up activity, and finally obliquely so that it is tested for the correct response. It must be demonstrated that the whole skill has been acquired and not just part of it.

Reactions to stressful conditions must be carefully observed. If the swimmer reacts appropriately, then the skill has been acquired. If an appropriate reaction is demonstrated, the teaching of the skill must continue until such time as the correct response is shown.

All the games and activities that have been set out previously are applicable to the child with learning difficulties. Similarly, groups can be utilized for working with these children. The following points, however, are particularly applicable.

The group

The group can be formed of those with mixed handicaps and not necessarily only of children with learning difficulties. Where it is not possible to combine physically handicapped children and children with learning difficulties, the group should be made up of children with differing levels of ability. Group members should stimulate one another and therefore the grouping of all children with severe learning difficulties together should be avoided, since interaction in such a group will tend to be poor and little progress can be expected.

Since some exceptions to grouping occur, these are discussed under the individual conditions.

Intellectual ability

The range of intellectual ability of the children who can benefit from and enjoy the water is enormously varied. The ability of the individual swimmer to translate instruction into action has to be understood, and the greatest care exercised by the physiotherapist in ensuring that the action is correctly performed.

Some of these children are over-eager to participate and may be considered irresponsible, with no awareness of their actions and the possible consequences, while others show a lack of willingness to become involved either in the group or in responding to instructions.

Relaxation

Relaxation has an important role to play when taking the intellectually impaired into the water. Any fear or anxiety about the medium and activity in it may create tension. An approach that lessens fear and anxiety includes mental adjustment and balance restoration (p. 21) can be enhanced by swaying – 'Seaweed' and 'Hallo' – swinging – 'Bells' and 'Rag dolls' – rolling – 'Rolling onto the bar' and 'Rolling arm to arm'. All three actions *must* be performed rhythmically, smoothly, calmly and slowly. To maintain these components the physiotherapist may find it helpful to hum or sing quietly.

Severe Learning Difficulties

Under this heading the ways in which children with profound, severe and moderate learning difficulties can be introduced to and taught basic skills in water are discussed.

The child who is profoundly affected will have gross retardation with delays in all areas of development. As the child matures, basic skills may develop and, with skilful training, the child may learn to use the limbs, walk, gain primitive speech and benefit from regular physical activity.

The child with severe learning difficulties will demonstrate obvious delays in motor development and communication but gradually develops motor skills, some understanding of speech

and some response. The child's needs will include continuing direction and supervision, but such children usually conform to repetitive activities and routine which, in water, can be developed in the group and by using a large variety of games which have the same teaching point.

Motor development and speech are noticeably affected in the child with moderate learning difficulties, but simple communication, manual skills and safety habits can be taught on land and in water and many achieve the ability to swim, although they may always require a degree of supervision.

All of these children invariably show extremes of reaction to the water. There may be fear or no fear at all. The latter is more dangerous, and the children have to learn to respect water and acquire survival skills in addition to all the other aspects of swimming. It is necessary to help them achieve an understanding of varying water depths, recovery to a safe breathing position at all times and under all circumstances, and to ensure that they appreciate other risks such as those incurred by running around the bathside, which is usually wet. Under controlled conditions with experienced instructors, respect for the medium can be taught, but it is a slow process and every care must be taken to ensure that nothing untoward occurs that may set the learner back.

Others, less happy and extrovert, may have a fear of water and will need a period of time spent watching other children at play in the water. Gradually these children move closer to watch and are finally ready to join in. Introduction to the water must be allowed to happen in this way and should not be rushed. Occasionally it becomes necessary to bring the child in from a sitting position on the edge of the pool. Almost certainly a fuss will be made in this instance, but rapid involvement in an activity which is performed to a song that the child knows usually attracts the child's attention and further protestation is avoided, at least for a while.

While these children benefit from group work, there is also a place for individual handling, particularly when acquiring balance in all positions – walking, jumping, submerging and swimming. This individual emphasis can be stressed even within the group by the physiotherapist who understands each child and any particular problems, so that the correct performance is ensured.

Mild Learning Difficulties and Borderline Normal

Children with mild learning difficulties are usually slower than their normal peers to walk, feed themselves and talk, but can achieve practical skills and useful levels of academic and social skills while gaining a level of adequate self-maintenance.

Borderline normal children are near average in the acquisition of physical and self-help skills and gain academic, social and vocational skills that allow them to undertake semi-skilled, skilled or service occupations.

These children benefit greatly from activity in water and can become good swimmers. However, it is again of the utmost importance to ensure that the skills learned become completely automatic under all conditions and in all circumstances. The physiotherapist must realize that there is a variation in understanding parts of the instruction, one part of a skill being readily absorbed, another part not understood. For example, in combined rotation the child may fall forward into the water and roll onto the back but fail to recover forward to a safe breathing position. It is then necessary to assist the child through the skill manually until certain that it has been acquired.

In the above example the physiotherapist would manually 'fold' the body into a ball and then 'assist' extension to the upright standing position. Repetition of combined rotation with this manual assistance would be necessary with less assistance in creating the movements and holding the child for longer periods in each position until the child made active attempts to do the action independently.

There is frequently good physical ability and the children are usually happy extroverts. A noticeable feature is their persistence in repeating an action or skill they have acquired or found easy to perform, while evading the learning of new skills or those activities they find less appealing.

An example of this persistence can be cited in the case of an 8-year-old boy with Down's syndrome who could swim, albeit underwater. He would jump in at the shallow end, swim three strokes when he then needed to stand up and breathe. This sequence was repeated across the pool until he reached the other side. He then climbed out and jumped back in again to repeat the whole process. To break this habit and to ensure progress, an experienced instructor jumped into deep water with the child. Only when he could not find the bottom of the pool when needing to breathe did this child begin to understand about varying depths of water. Six jumps later he was swimming on the surface and went on quickly to swimming lengths of the pool.

Such persistence of part of an acquired skill should not be allowed to continue indefinitely. Progress and development should be ensured, and under controlled conditions with experienced personnel who understand the child's problems as well as the requirements of water activity, this can be achieved.

These children enjoy close personal contact and love to cling. They will take every opportunity to clasp the physiotherapist closely, which impedes progress towards independence. Therefore entry and holds should be used at arm's length and clinging avoided.

Many of the children also avoid touching the bottom of the pool with their feet and, when participating in activities, will keep hips and knees flexed and hang on by the hands, thus being carried through an activity. By quickly dropping the hands, instructors can frequently bring about an effective reaction in the children, who lower their feet to find a point of contact with a surface and thus gain security. Without such attention to these details the children will not learn to disengage or control their bodies when acted upon by buoyancy and rotational forces, nor, indeed, will they learn to swim.

The responses of the Down's syndrome children need to be channelled appropriately and concentration maintained, and this is more readily achieved in a group situation. However, these children can quite unexpectedly disrupt the group and should be quietly withdrawn by their instructor to a part of the pool where the inappropriate behaviour can be channelled into activities such as vigorous 'kangaroo jumps' or kicking and splashing then stopping and lying still on command, repeated several times. This can bring the situation under control, thus allowing the swimmer and the instructor to rejoin the group.

Autistic Children

Autism is an uncommon developmental disorder of childhood. Stone (1976, p. 66) cites Leo Kanner in 1943 as first drawing attention to the disorder, which he termed early infantile autism. Kanner delineated three presenting clinical features:

1. A lack of awareness of people, an avoidance of ordinary contact with others, an 'alone-ness' which is what autism really means.
2. Abnormalities in the development of speech varying from unusual forms of syntax to the extremes of complete mutism.
3. An 'obsessional desire for sameness' – that is, a tendency to become acutely distressed when an accustomed arrangement is disturbed.

The label 'autistic' has been applied rather loosely to a variety of developmental disorders. Stone (1976) suggests that autism should be restricted to cases presenting the syndrome as described by Kanner, recognizing that this is not a common condition and that more frequently a variety of clinical states showing autistic features is encountered.

The 'alone-ness' is an aspect of these children that can be avoided by contact with the physiotherapist and by working in a group situation, though these ideals are not always easy to achieve.

The situation where the autistic child is left alone in water and ignored must be rigorously avoided. The author has seen such children left in this way with their hands close to their faces, rocking forwards and backwards, circling continuously and making their way into deeper and deeper water, 'alone' in their world and totally unaware of the danger.

They generally love the feel of water and have a good response to rhythm, thus the use of games and activities to music and, above all, singing which frequently brings about their first verbal responses, is an excellent way in which to work with them.

Like the Down's syndrome children, the autistic child can suddenly go wild and disrupt the group. This should be dealt with as it arises in the same was as for the Down's syndrome child.

The Hyperkinetic Syndrome

Graham (1977) suggests overactivity in children arises for a variety of reasons, and that the level of activity is partly determined as a temperamental characteristic. However, he states that severe overactivity may occur as part of a poorly differentiated cluster of symptoms in which, in the absence of severe social stress (and in addition to overactivity), there may be impersistence, lack of concentration, short attention span, distractibility, impulsiveness and lack of social inhibition.

Not all these problems are present all the time, and vary from situation to situation. Hyperkinetic behaviour can be improved through activity in water. Drag effect, the weight of water and the extra energy required to move in water have a dampening effect on movement for these children which can be used to advantage in teaching more acceptable behaviour.

Graham (1977) suggests that they are very responsive to environmental situations. People taking them into water should note the activities which suit the children best. These activities may need to change from individual to group work depending on the child's reaction at any time. Thus, the programme needs to be flexible.

The overall mastery of the act of swimming with controlled rhythmic movement appears to have a beneficial effect upon hyperkinetic children.

Perceptual Disabilities

The perceptual disabilities discussed here are spatial awareness, body image, difficulty in estimating size, distance, time and depth, perseveration and concentration.

Spatial awareness

Examples of activities that improve a child's ability to locate the position of objects in space and enable accurate movement are 'How wide? How tall?', 'Eggs for breakfast', 'Ring a ring o' roses', and similar circle activities, 'Kangaroo jumps' and 'Stepping stones'.

When working in a circle, it is not necessary to move continually sideways. The circle can be made smaller by walking or jumping towards the centre, and larger by moving backwards.

Comments on the size of the circle help reinforce spatial awareness, and emphasis on the position of the head when walking forwards or backwards is important. In order for the feet to remain down in the vertical plane, the head should be kept forward, whether walking forwards or backwards. The children, with the assistance of a physiotherapist, can at first make their way around the bar. Care must be taken that they become aware of the point at which their vertical balance becomes critical – at a water level of two-thirds their height. Thus they learn about gravity-dominated shallower water and buoyancy-dominated deeper water.

Body image

Children who have poor body image can be made increasingly aware of themselves through activities which involve the extremes of posture, which require control of their arms and legs, in which greater turbulence is created.

Activities which involve the extremes of posture are all the 'ball' and 'stick' games, that is those used for vertical rotation and consisting of total patterns of flexion and extension (Reid, 1976). 'Eggs for breakfast', 'Reach for an object', 'Rag dolls', 'The wind, sun and rain' are a few examples.

To encourage control of the limbs, 'How wide? How tall?', lifting up the water with the hands or kicking it with the feet, will help give an awareness of the weight of water. Splashing with hands or feet and stopping on command, making waves with the arms and legs in games such as 'Stars and stripes', in both standing and in lying, encourage control and awareness of the limbs. Turbulent or drag effect is most noticeable at the distal part, and the child can be made aware of the length of the limbs and the dimension of the body reach and span. 'Simon says' and games that involve hiding feet and hands in different ways are also useful. As the child acquires this control, the arm and leg actions for appropriate strokes may be introduced along with good breathing control – both requisites for swimming.

Size, distance, time and depth

Activities which will help reduce the difficulties in estimating size and distance are those that encourage the children to curl up in a 'ball' and extend to a 'stick', changing the circle size from small to large and changing from a short arm hold to a long arm hold as they move in and out. Games involving equipment, such as 'Pieces of eight' in which various sized objects are used, are valuable. Jumping from one object to another, 'Fairy strides' and 'Giant strides' are other useful activities.

Time estimation can be encouraged through rhythm and the use of songs and music and spoken rhyme where the beat is strongly emphasized.

Estimation of depth is involved in entry and exit, whether this is down the steps or ramps or over the side. It is reinforced also by working from shallow to deeper water and in submerging and trying to touch the bottom.

Perseveration

Children who have difficulty in changing from one task to another can be helped by appropriately planned programmes of activity in water. The programme should have changes of pace from slow to fast, changes of atmosphere from quiet to noisy, changes of mood from seriousness to laughter, and changes of shape, not only from 'ball' and 'stick' and their own body shapes, but in the formation in which the activities are performed and linked together in the programme.

Concentration

It may seem that children who are easily distracted, especially by sound or movement in their surroundings, are not suited to programmes of activity in water.

Pools tend to be noisy areas where shouting, laughter and splashing, combined with active movement on the part of the swimmers and the constant movement of the water, can have a distracting and disturbing effect. However, working in groups has been found to assist concentration over longer time spans. As the child's attention is focused on the group and the other children and their achievements, increased awareness and motive follow. This can be encouraged further by the introduction of more competition in the games.

The Clumsy Child

Clumsy children demonstrate problems in motor skills that are out of keeping with their general abilities. The majority also have learning difficulties, and the combination leads to the children failing in many areas. As a result, behavioural and emotional factors arise.

Programmes for the acquisition of motor skills have been used to help the clumsy child but these have been almost entirely land based.

Arnhem and Sinclair (1979) suggested that water activity introduced the clumsy child to a new dimension, and stated that if water was used appropriately, it could enhance the physical and perceptual training of such children. Campbell (1978) described a combined programme of land-based and water-based activities. The philosophy is based on the link between the prenatal fluid environment of the fetus and the similar fluid environment of the pool (especially where the water is warm) and all the other advantages of the medium such as buoyancy and ease of movement.

The games and activities which have already been described have proved valuable in the treatment of clumsy children and may be adapted to augment the programmes propounded by Arnhem and Sinclair (1979) and Campbell (1975). Such items as:

(a) breathing control,
(b) body image and spatial awareness,
(c) balance and coordination,
(d) sequencing,
(e) laterality and directionality,
(f) endurance and strength,
(g) swimming ability,
(h) social skills,
(i) speech and language,

should be included in the programme.

Activities can be developed by the use of equipment – balls, hoops, ropes, dive rings, discs, sticks and bricks, play tubes and other inflatable toys. Awareness of body image can be increased by adapting the activity 'If you're happy and you know it', by the use of 'Simon says' and similar games. Laterality may be taught in games such as 'Looby Loo' or the 'Hokey cokey', and directionality when moving around or to one side of objects. Ropes and other items are valuable when developing spatial awareness. The children can go over and under in many different ways. Obstacle courses, sequences for memorizing the retrieval of dive rings, the use of coloured hoops and other toys are just some of the ways in which

sequencing and memory skills may be trained.

Breathing control and swimming ability should be checked at the commencement of the programme and recorded. During the sessions these skills can be progressed by timing the children swimming either widths or lengths or interesting them in improving their own times. Endurance and strength will also benefit.

A programme of activity in water appeals to these children, and those who at first appear timid and lacking in confidence do develop skills in the water quite rapidly, with a resulting alteration in attitude. For many, an aquatic programme in itself is a morale booster. Water is a great leveller and thus they are able to participate with less awareness of their failings.

The manner in which land-based motor skill training programmes are conducted applies to the water activity sessions. The parents should be informed about all aspects of the activities and the author has found it invaluable to have mothers or fathers recording swimming times and other achievements on the bathside, as the presence of the physiotherapist is necessary in the water throughout the pool sessions.

The progress of the children can only be measured if accurate recording is undertaken on each occasion and the results transferred to appropriate charts which should be kept for each child.

The proper orientation of the children to the pool and pool area is important, and all safety rules should be both explained and enforced at all times.

Water has much to offer the clumsy child, just as for the vast majority of normal people. The appropriate and specific use of water can aid the development of a child who is falling behind his peers, and thereby confidence, self-respect and emotional behaviours improve in addition to gross and fine motor skills.

RESPIRATORY DISORDERS

Asthma

When swimming programmes for asthmatics were introduced some 20 years ago, it was known that exercise induced asthma in most sufferers. At that time there was no scientific evidence to prove that swimming was more or less likely to provoke an attack (Lindsay, 1979). Since then, research has been undertaken and has provided evidence both supporting swimming as an excellent activity for the asthmatic (Fitch and Morton, 1971; Fitch, 1978; Oseid *et al.*, 1978), and indicating that a re-examination of the results of swimming for asthmatics might suggest a need for the development of other types of exercise programmes (Phelan, 1980). However, the important psychological advantages accruing from swimming programmes have been noted by critics and advocates alike.

Oseid *et al.* (1978) suggest that the physical treatment of asthmatic children is directed towards controlling attacks through relaxation, breathing exercises, postural drainage and specific efforts to correct chest deformities. Oseid and his colleagues (1978) are not alone in indicating that appropriately planned programmes are beneficial and that improved exercise tolerance and breathing control can result (Fitch, 1978; Shepherd, 1995). Fitch (1978) maintains that swimming is an excellent exercise to restore and maintain fitness in many conditions, including asthma, and sees it as valuable not only for rehabilitation but also for recreation and sport. For the asthmatic child who requires treatment over a prolonged period of time, an activity that is of interest and stimulating, yet at the same time improves the physical condition, should prove valuable in several ways. Swimming programmes can include underwater activity, improve breathing control and physical development. The development of secondary chest deformities can also be prevented by performance of correct stroking techniques. Perhaps of equal significance though are the social and psychological benefits which undoubtedly improve the quality of life enjoyed by the asthmatic.

Physiotherapists who are deeply involved in the treatment of asthmatic children may well be faced with the task of taking such children into water. Familiarization with the element can be carried out in the manner already described. The emphasis on breathing control in all the activities is of major importance. The asthmatic child may learn to swim quickly, particularly as no marked changes in shape will be evident. However, small alterations may be present and these should be observed and evaluated and a balanced position developed. Correct positioning for stroking is critical, not only because the child may wish to participate in competitive swimming programmes, but also as a means of improving physical development and preventing deformities of the thoracic region.

REFERENCES

Adams R.C., Daniel A.N., McCubbin J.A. and Pullman L. (1982) *Games, Sports and Exercises for the Physically Handicapped*, 3rd edn, Philadelphia: Lea and Febiger.

Arnhem D. and Sinclair W. (1979). *The Clumsy Child – a Program of Motor Therapy*, 2nd edn, St Louis, Miss.: C.V. Mosby.

Behrend H.J. (1963). Hydrotherapy. In *Medical Hydrology* (S. Licht, ed.), New Haven: Elizabeth Licht, pp. 239–253.

Bernstein N.R. (1976). *Emotional Care of the Facially Burned and Disfigured*, Boston: Little, Brown.

Brodal A. (1981). *Neurological Anatomy in Relation to Clinical Medicine*, 3rd edn, Oxford: Oxford University Press.

Burden C. and Schurr P.H. (1976). *Understanding Epilepsy*, London: Crosby Lockwood Staples.

Campbell W.R. (1975). *Aqua Percept*, Pointe Claire: Wendy R. Campbell.

Carmel P.W. (1974). Spina bifida. In *Spina Bifida in the Child with Disabling Illness* (J. Downey and N. Low, eds), London: W.B. Saunders, pp. 131–154.

Cordellos H.C. (1976). *Aquatic Recreation for the Blind*. Washington DC: Physical Education and Recreation for the Handicapped. Information and Research Utilization Center.

Davis B. (1967). A technique of re-education in the treatment pool. *Physiotherapy*, **63**(2): 57–59.

Davis C.J. (1961). The deaf–blind child: diagnosis and evaluation. Proceedings of the Convention of American Instructors of the Deaf, pp. 40–69.

Farmer T.W. (1975). *Paediatric Neurology*, 2nd edn, London: Harper & Row.

Fitch K.D. (1978). Swimming, medicine and asthma. In *Swimming Medicine*, Vol. IV (B. Eriksson and B. Furburg, eds), Baltimore: University Park Press, pp. 16–31.

Fitch K.D. and Morton A.R. (1971). Specificity of exercise-induced asthma. *British Medical Journal*, **4**: 577.

Fraiberg S. (1977). *Insights from the Blind*, New York: Basic Books.

Graham P.J. (1977). A child psychiatric approach. Behaviour disorders. In *Neurodevelopmental Problems in Early Childhood* (C.M. Drillien and M.B. Drummond, eds), Oxford: Blackwell Scientific.

Griffiths M.I. (1977). The deaf–blind child. In *Neurodevelopmental Problems in Early Childhood: Assessment and Management* (C.M. Drillien and M.B. Drummond, eds), Oxford: Blackwell Scientific Publications.

Harcourt B. (1977). Visual disability and visual handicap. In *Neurodevelopmental Problems in Early Childhood: Assessment and Management* (C.M. Drillien and M.B. Drummond, eds), Oxford: Blackwell Scientific Publications.

Heiniger M.C. and Randolph S.L. (1981). *Neurophysiological Concepts in Human Behaviour*, St Louis, Miss.: C.V. Mosby.

Jennett W.B. and Teasdale G. (1981). *Management of Head Injuries*, Philadelphia: F.A. Davis.

Lance J.W. and McLeod J.G. (1975). *A Physiological Approach to Clinical Neurology*, 2nd edn, Sydney: Butterworths.

Lindsay D. (1979). *The Importance of Swimming to Asthmatics*. Paper presented to Water Safety Symposium. Sydney: Department of Sport and Recreation.

Martin J.A.M. (1977). Hearing loss. In *Neurodevelopmental Problems in Early Childhood: Assessment and Management* (C.M. Drillien and M.B. Drummond, eds), Oxford: Blackwell Scientific Publications.

National Co-ordinating Committee on Swimming for the Disabled (1975). *Swimming and Epilepsy*, London: The Sports Council.

Olson S. (1987). Early intervention for children with visual impairments. In *The Effectiveness of Early Intervention for At-Risk and Handicapped Children* (M.J. Guralnick and F.C. Bennett, eds), Orlando: Academic Press.

Oseid S., Kendall M., Larsen R.B. and Selbeck R. (1978). Physical activitiy programs for children with exercise-induced asthma. In *Swimming Medicine*, Vol. IV (B. Eriksson and B. Furburg, eds), Baltimore: University Park Press, pp. 42–51.

Phelan P. (1980). Asthma in children. *Medicine Australia*, Series 1, **23**: 1639–1647.

Reid M.J. (1975). *Handling the Disabled Child in Water – an Introduction*, London: Association of Paediatric Chartered Physiotherapists, p. 186.

Shepherd R. (1980). *Physiotherapy in Paediatrics*, 2nd edn, London: Heinemann Medical.

Shepherd R.B. (1995). *Physiotherapy in Paediatrics*, 3rd edn, Oxford: Butterworth-Heinemann.

Skinner A.T. and Thomson A.M. (eds) (1983). *Duffield's Exercise in Water*, 3rd edn, London: Baillière Tindall.

Stone F.H. (1976). *Psychiatry and the Paediatrician*, London: Butterworths.

Trussel E.C. (1971). *Guidelines for Teaching the Disabled to Swim*. Dudley: Netherton Printers for Swimming Teacher's Association.

7

The Halliwick Method and Conductive Education

Margaret Reid Campion

The Halliwick Method and Conductive Education have factors in common which make them complementary to one another; the former provides a valuable adjunct to the latter as a combined therapeutic and recreational activity for both children and adults with motor disorders.

The value of experiencing another medium than air is considerable and the opportunities afforded by water for enhancing movement should be exploited to the full especially where compatibility between land and water techniques exists.

To appreciate the two approaches and their integration it is necessary to explore their similarities and differences.

THE HALLIWICK METHOD

This method is a means by which anyone can be taught to swim but is particularly suitable for the disabled. Devised by the late James McMillan MBE in 1949 in London, it takes its name from the school for disabled girls where the work began. Based on scientific principles of hydrodynamics and body mechanics it has proved safe for people of all ages, with any disability and of any severity.

It differs from other methods of teaching swimming in that it appreciates the critical nature of water and applies that to the altered shape and density of the disabled person. Swimmers become mentally adjusted to the element of water, acquire the skills of balance restoration, head and breathing control – all requisites for independence in the water and swimming.

While the method's aim is a mentally adjusted, physically balanced safe swimmer the many physical and psychological aspects ensure that the confidence and self-esteem acquired in the pool carry over into life on land.

CONDUCTIVE EDUCATION

Conductive Education is based on a unified approach to the management of the motor disordered. Professor Andras Petö, who devised the method, recognized the confusion experienced by all affected by a motor disorder and developed a system that integrates therapy with education and deals with the person globally.

The neuropsychological basis of the method allows for the acquisition of skills in a manner which is different from the traditional neurophysiological approaches, such as the neurodevelopmental method used by the Bobaths and the conditioned reflex therapy of Vojta.

Conductive Education is concerned with the person as a whole, the psychological aspect being as important as any other. Both children and adults with motor impairment may participate in programmes using Conductive Education principles to their advantage and work towards their maximum functional potential.

THE ESSENTIAL COMPONENTS OF THE HALLIWICK METHOD AND CONDUCTIVE EDUCATION

There are several essential components of each method that have much in common.

Table 7.1 Essential components of the two methods

Halliwick method	Conductive education
The Group Leader	The Conductor
The group	The group
Vocalization/movement	Rhythmical intention
The work	The work

The Group Leader/Conductor

The Group Leader has an important role in planning programmes and conducting the group activities. Training for the role is to an advanced level and covers all aspects of the method, resuscitation and safety. A knowledge of the disabilities involved does not necessarily mean an in-depth understanding of the medical conditions. It does, however, demand that the essential points about the effects of a swimmer's disability and the necessary precautions are known. It is the leader's responsibility to pass on such information to the instructors working with individuals in the group. Work must take place at appropriate depths and be effectively and efficiently carried out in a suitable atmosphere – all of which is the group leader's responsibility.

The Conductor is vital to Conductive Education and to the conductive principle (Russell & Cotton, 1994). The role is a demanding one and the training, covering four years, is rigorous and comprehensive. The Conductor regulates the activities of the group, is responsible for the task series; is aware of each individual's needs and guides the group members throughout the day integrating each part of the day's programme so that a whole pattern of learning is created (Kinsman *et al.*, 1988).

The Group

Groups are an integral part of both methods. Homogeneous groups provide socialization, motivation, the development of initiative and concentration, security, the learning of motor and behavioural skills, repetition and reinforcement. Groups permit people to work for longer periods of time with greater attention and concentration spans. This is especially so if the work is conducted in a rhythmical manner (Russell & Cotton, 1994).

As far as possible groups should comprise people with similar disabilities and levels of ability. In Conductive Education selection for a group is largely undertaken by the conductor and is achieved by observation of the motor disordered person performing appropriate tasks as well as by a full assessment. The selection of swimmers for groups in the Halliwick Method is based on the ability of the swimmer in the water. An assessment using an Initial Ability Test involving skills such as breathing and rotational control is applied. The ability of the various swimmers should be fairly similar, but some disparity allows for development of incentives within the group.

The size of groups tends to vary between the two methods. At the Institute for the Motor Disabled in Budapest groups are quite large in number. The size of groups in other countries where programmes based on Conductive Education principles exist varies enormously. The selection processes of swimmers for water activity groups, the criteria and other factors have been discussed previously (p. 26) and are mentioned again here to stress the similarity between the two approaches.

The Halliwick Method advocates that groups be conducted at a speed to which the participants can respond. Changes of speed, atmosphere, mood and pace are important in the programme. This echoes Conductive Education, for the conductor must know the tempo for the group and for each individual. In response to the question 'How do you distinguish between spastics and athetoids in your work?' Professor Petö replied, 'It's a question of tempo – it is like andante and allegro' (Campion, 1979).

Rhythmical Intention/Vocalization and Movement

Rhythm may be considered as constant changes of strength, pace and duration and as affecting not only movement but also the sense of hearing, vision, touch and kinaesthesia (Holle, 1976). Patterns of movement that are synchronized produce efficient movement and when coordinated movement is required an exact sense of space, time and force is essential (Arnhem and Sinclair, 1979).

When a person performs a motor task alternate contraction and relaxation of muscles occurs. This action may be strong or weak, quick or slow, sudden or hesitant and of varying lengths of time. For the motor disordered there is frequently difficulty in synchronizing these factors; the use of different rhythms often assists motor control. Emotional and social aspects for the child and adult are aided by rhythm.

Rhythmical intention is the foremost facilitation in Conductive Education. Through it the person expresses the intention while moving actively towards the goal. Precise wording is important and movement takes place to slow and rhythmic counting or dynamic speech. In this way time, rhythm and an understanding of movement, body image and spatial awareness is acquired and memory aided. Conductive Education also emphasizes the use of rhythm in the performance of a pattern of movement in many different situations so that by repetition and reinforcement the rhythm of the day is established and re-established (Reid Campion, 1986).

Swimming – the propulsion of the body through water by the use of the limbs – requires rhythmical breathing and movement patterns. The Halliwick Method stresses the importance of rhythm and develops its use of songs, music and rhythmic verse or instruction. Thus speech is encouraged and breathing control developed. The importance of 'blowing' is constantly emphasized and in activities such as 'Kangaroo jumps' rhythmic breathing control is developed along with movement in and out of the extremes of posture combined with head control. The songs, rhymes or instructions – the intention – require action, thus movement takes place and body image and spatial awareness are acquired.

The Work

In Conductive Education the work is embodied in the task series, each task having an intention and a goal. Active movements related to function are required and the person learns that between the intention or idea and the goal is the means by which the goal is achieved (Russell, 1994). It is through active movement that learning takes place.

The work in the Halliwick Method is developed in games and activities that are enjoyable

Table 7.2 Facilitations

Conductive Education	Halliwick Method
Rhythmical intention	Manual facilitation
Motivation	Motivation
Continuity	Continuity
Self-facilitation	Vocalization
Manual facilitation	Self-facilitation

Source: Cotton and Kinsman, 1981.

and subtly teach the skills necessary for mental adjustment, balance restoration and swimming. The idea that pool activity is treatment is removed by the element of fun and enjoyment that is consistent with the method. While the 'fun' aspect may be more obvious in the Halliwick Method, there is no doubt that there is a fun element in Conductive Education. Programmes designed for function include pleasurable themes and the joy that accrues when a task or a skill is successfully completed acts as a great stimulus and motivational force.

In both methods the work should be interesting and allow time for trial, experimentation and success (Cotton and Kinsman, 1981).

FACILITATIONS

While Conductive Education employs a number of facilitations designed to assist the motor disordered achieve function facilitations have not been identified as such in the Halliwick Method. Nevertheless, the author believes they exist and can be pinpointed.

Manual facilitation must head the list of facilitations for the Halliwick Method. The necessity of supporting the swimmer in the water is of paramount importance initially, and whenever a new and more advanced skill is being learnt. As described earlier the support or manual facilitation given should always be the minimum amount to allow the swimmer maximum control of the body. The manner in which this support is given and its gradual withdrawal as skills are obtained contributes to the confidence of the swimmer and to the degree of activity and progress; thus appropriate holds are proportionate with the improvement in the skills being acquired. Suitable holds also provide tactile stimulation and improve body awareness.

Holds in the Halliwick Method take into account the new datum point – the centre of balance – the swimmer uses in the water when all the points of resistance available on land are removed. Holding the swimmer at this point provides security, allows facilitation of the body from one position to another, which with the gradual disengagement leads to independence in the water.

In Conductive Education manual facilitation is the last facilitation to be used as active movement by the child or adult is essential. When other facilitations have failed a *minimum* of manual facilitation is given to the person to help in the acquisition of a desired movement.

Rhythmical intention has been discussed as part of the essential ingredients of the methods and needs no further elaboration here (p. 170).

Independence on land and in the water is the ultimate aim of both approaches.

Motivation

This facilitation applies to both Conductive Education and to the Halliwick Method and is fostered to a large extent by working in groups. All the benefits of group activity (p. 33) accrue particularly if the work is conducted in a rhythmical manner. Rhythm is a vital component of the two methods.

Vocalization

The vocalization encouraged in the Halliwick Method has some similarity to rhythmical intention used in Conductive Education. They act as a stimulus to speech and are directed towards active movement. However, in Conductive Education rhythmical intention is more intensive and directive, while the Halliwick Method uses songs, rhymes and spoken rhythmic verse to lead towards active movement and speech as the swimmers respond to the words and instructions of the group leader, their individual instructor and their vocalization.

Continuity

Continuity is in the hands of the conductor and the group leader. The work in both approaches should be full of interest and allow time for trial, experimentation and success (Cotton and Kinsman, 1981). Continuity is more concentrated in Conductive Education due to the intense daily work whereas water activity sessions will be more episodic. Both methods plan their programmes carefully in order that the participants progress steadily through the work to independence.

Self-facilitation

Self-facilitation in Conductive Education is used once a task is understood and a movement attempted. Vision, pressure, gravity, correct starting positions, clasping of the hands and language may be incorporated.

The term self-facilitation is not one that has been used previously in the Halliwick Method but the author believes that it is related to rotational control which involves head and limb movement and control. Head control is vital for controlling the body position in water and counterbalancing the rotational effects brought about by altered shape and meta-centric effects (p. 14).

ADDITIONAL COMMON FACTORS OF CONDUCTIVE EDUCATION AND THE HALLIWICK METHOD

Both methods have therapeutic and recreational components. Conductive Education by comparison lays more emphasis on the therapeutic aspect while the Halliwick Method stresses the recreational approach in which therapy is subtly hidden.

Symmetry, Stability and Fixation

These three factors are among the most important similarities between the two methods. Symmetry is of great importance to both methods. Movement out of abnormal asymmetric postures is encouraged and is vital for function and control of the body in the water.

For instance, whether in lying on land or in water the value of having the head in midline, the arms by the sides and the legs straight will produce symmetry. In water this means a more balanced body and the 'cigar shape' is the most effective for swimming as it causes fewer wakes and eddies as the body moves through the water (Blanksby and Roberts, 1981).

Any means may be employed to develop a symmetrical shape; the facilitations – furniture and equipment used in Conductive Education – encourage this and equipment such as sticks, small hoops and rings and floating toys can be used in many activities to develop symmetry in water. An activity in supine lying such as 'Seaweed' may be cited to develop symmetry when the swimmer holds a stick or a ring with both hands as low as possible on the body. In 'Catching an object' or in 'Eggs for breakfast' the forward movement of the arms to grasp the object as the body recovers to the upright should be symmetrical to induce the even form.

Stability is more difficult to obtain in water due to the effects of buoyancy, turbulence and the metacentric principle. It can be achieved through the use of head and trunk to control rotation through activities that produce symmetry of the limbs and body and the shapes that give stability and balance, for example the 'sitting' position. The instructor's holds provide stability in the early stages.

Fixation is developed in Conductive Education through grasping initially. In supine lying on a slatted plinth grasping the slats at the sides of the body with the hands converts asymmetrical arm patterns to symmetrical ones. When sitting, grasping the rungs of a ladderback chair with both hands and straight arms facilitates balance and allows the person to achieve a more normal sitting position and in standing grasping either a ladder or leaning forwards to hold a slatted plinth provides stability as well as symmetry.

A wide range of disabilities participate in water activity. All locomotor disorders may take advantage of the medium, unless there are any co-existing contraindications. Most commonly the disabilities are:

- cerebral palsy
- neurological conditions, e.g. Parkinson's, CVA, multiple sclerosis
- orthopaedic conditions
- spina bifida
- paraplegics

- muscular dystrophy
- arthritic and rheumatic conditions
- amputees
- congenital abnormalities
- intellectual disorders
- spinal injuries
- head injuries.

Conductive Education provides programmes for the disorders of:

- cerebral palsy
- spina bifida
- muscular dystrophy
- CVA
- Parkinson's disease
- multiple sclerosis
- head injuries.

As many of these conditions have been presented in detail elsewhere in this book there is only need here to emphasize a few points that are specific to the methods discussed in this chapter. In other parts of this book the treatments suggested are therapeutic rather than recreational, however, physiotherapists are increasingly aware of the value of the specific skills and precise handling taught by the Halliwick Method. All the authors are influenced by these factors.

For all neurological conditions the importance of rotation is well reported (Sullivan *et al.*, 1982). Rotation and control of it is vital to Halliwick and is stressed when teaching vertical rotation, lateral rotation and combined rotation. Rotation appears to play a less dominant role in Conductive Education but is utilized in activities such as rolling from side to side and from supine to prone and back on the plinth.

Symmetry is a required component for both methods and in water may need increased emphasis as there are fewer opportunities to provide facilitation through the use of equipment so the ingenuity of the physiotherapist in choosing appropriate activities is most important, as is ensuring that each carer working with a swimmer constantly encourages symmetry.

Balance reactions can be developed in standing, 'sitting' and lying in the water in a manner not possible on land where overbalancing causes a rapid fall. Water, due to the impedance to movement by drag and the denser nature of the liquid, allows the person to react and restore their balance.

For the head-injured adult and child, activity in water offers a reduction in tone, stimulation of movement and the development of rotational and reciprocal patterns of movement. Functional movements are accessed, and breath control and voice production harnessed. Additionally there are the psychological effects and opportunities for recreation and socialization. The Halliwick Method, with its emphasis on the rotations, speech, singing, rhythm, symmetry, recreation and socialization has a considerable role. Young adults, the most affected age group, may resent working in a group; however, it does have value if they can be encouraged to participate. A 20-year old head-injured male, who was recovering motor skills well, was mouthing words but not producing sound. He was persuaded to join a group and, when walking sideways in a circle, singing sound began to materialize especially when the song chosen was from his native land. From that point on sound was used in speaking.

The value of the Halliwick Method in spinal injuries relates to the later phases of rehabilitation for recreation, socialization and the modification of swimming strokes, especially when the swimmer returns to the community and all the psychological effects that accrue.

CONCLUSION

The value of the two approaches for rehabilitation of disabled adults and children has been explored. The Halliwick Method and Conductive Education have similarities and serve as valuable adjuncts to each other.

Both the disabilities and the nature and effects of water on the immersed body need to be understood. Symmetry, rhythm, speech, active movement, balance, coordination, stability and function are important factors in both methods, and programmes should reflect and include these aspects if the maximum potential of each participant is to be achieved.

Physical and psychological benefits result from working in the water and with Conductive Education. In many ways the skills even the most disabled learn in the pool are carried over into their whole life; many who perhaps have malfunctioning limbs and a tendency to disregard them discover the body as a whole unit.

Conductive Education is concerned with the whole person and works globally for the rehabilitation of the motor disordered. Dysfunction becomes orthofunction, that is the best possible function with the minimum of aids, and is an aim specific to Conductive Education (Russell and Cotton, 1994). The Halliwick Method develops function in water without aids and works with the person as a whole.

REFERENCES

Arnhem D. and Sinclair W. (1979). *The Clumsy Child – A Program of Motor Therapy*, 2nd edn, St Louis, Miss.: C.V. Mosby.

Blanksby B.A. and Roberts D.M. (1981). *Guide for Teachers of Swimming*, Perth: University of Western Australia Press.

Campion M. (1979). Conductive education – The Peto method. *Australian Journal of Physiotherapy*, Paed. Mono., December: 47–50.

Cotton E. (1975). *Conductive Education and Cerebral Palsy*, London: The Spastics Society.

Cotton E. and Kinsman R. (1981). *Conductive Education for Adult Hemiplegia*, Edinburgh: Churchill Livingstone.

Holle B. (1976). *Motor Development in Children – Normal and Retarded*, Oxford: Blackwell Scientific Publications.

Kinsman R., Verity R. and Waller I. (1988). A conductive education approach for adults with neurological dysfunction. *Physiotherapy*, **74**(5): 227–230.

Reid Campion M. (1986). Conductive education and the Halliwick method. In *Hong Kong Physiotherapy Journal*, **8**: Special Issue – Conductive Education.

Russell A. (1994). *C.P. Entities: Research and Neurodevelopmental Overview: Philosophy, Principles and Practice*, London: Acorn Foundation Publications. (Available from Acorn Foundation Publications, 10 and 12, 88 Portland Place, London W1N 3HB.)

Russell A. and Cotton E. (1994). *The Peto System and its Evolution in Britain*, London: Acorn Foundation Publications. (Available from Acorn Foundation Publications, 10 and 12, 88 Portland Place, London W1N 3HB.)

Sullivan P.E., Markos P.D. and Minor M.A.D. (1982). *An Integrated Approach to Therapeutic Exercise: Theory and Clinical Application*, Reston, Va: Reston Pub. Co.

Section III

Practice of Adult Hydrotherapy

Margaret Reid Campion

INTRODUCTION

These chapters cover treatment techniques and a wide range of conditions which have been subdivided into:

- neurological and neurosurgical
- spinal mobilizations and spinal cord injuries
- rheumatic, orthopaedic conditions and sports injuries. Each chapter stands in its own right. Each subdivision has its own introductory notes.

A study of the historical background to hydrotherapy shows that even in ancient times and down through the ages the value of water in the treatment of all the above-mentioned conditions was recognized.

Hippocrates (c. 460–375 BC) not only advocated the use of water for the treatment of a wide variety of diseases, but taught that it could be employed as a tonic and a sedative. Homer suggested that warm baths were efficacious in overcoming fatigue. More recently it has been said that water enhances the ability to feel (Bennett, 1951) and physiotherapists will readily see the advantage this has when treating patients suffering from neurological conditions. In the fifth century BC the Greeks recognized the essential nature of a pool as an adjunct to their sporting activities and the Romans followed in the footsteps of the Greeks. In that same century a Roman residing in northern Africa used some modern concepts of physical treatment when he prescribed the use of natural waters, especially warm springs, for paralysed patients as a means of restoration. He advocated swimming in the sea or warm springs 'initially with an inflated bladder attached to the paralysed part to reduce the effort required in swimming'.

The tide ebbed and flowed in ensuing centuries but by the fifteenth, sixteenth and seventeenth centuries the use of water as a therapeutic measure was increasingly recognized. Sir John Floyer (1697) and John Wesley (1747) wrote about the value of water in the treatment of many diseases. The scientific background to hydrotherapy was promoted in the latter part of the nineteenth century and the early decades of the twentieth century. Hydrotherapy as we know it today really began in the 1920s and major developments with specific techniques are of much more recent times.

The influence of the Halliwick Method on water activity is marked. It has brought about refinements in hydrotherapy techniques, developed new means of exercise and shown that combined therapeutic and recreational programmes provide continual rehabilitation for all disabilities in both paediatric and adult fields allowing the maximum potential to be reached and the physical, psychological and social benefits to accrue.

8

Techniques of exercise in water and therapeutic swimming

Margaret Reid Campion

Hydrogymnastics as a systematic form of exercise in water began in the early part of the twentieth century (Kamenetz, 1963). The first Hubbard tank, made in 1928, was designed primarily for underwater exercise. Some years earlier, in 1911, Lowman was using such exercise for patients with spasticity, while others suffering from anterior poliomyelitis, including Franklin D. Roosevelt, were finding hydrogymnastics in warm water beneficial.

Harris (1963) stresses that hydrotherapy in water should only be conducted by physiotherapists who have been given practical instruction in the techniques of exercise in water. Bennett (1951, p. 513) proposes that 'unless exercise in water is carried out by trained personnel the advantages – motivation, pleasure, novelty and enhancement of movement – may become disadvantages and lead to poor patterns of movement and fatigue'.

It is vital that the physiotherapist appreciates the difference between exercises carried out on land and in water. It is totally inappropriate to use land-based exercise in water since the unique properties offered by the medium are neglected and water not used as a modality for rehabilitation in its own right. Exercises in water differ from similar exercises carried out on land. The difference lies in the dissimilarity of the physical properties of the two environments.

The uniqueness of water lies mainly in the presence of buoyancy. Buoyancy supports the body and diminishes the effects of gravity. An advantage accruing from this is that it induces relaxation and relieves pain, thus the movements a person can perform on land only with difficulty and considerable pain may be used in the hydrotherapy programme where pain is eased and where the weightlessness allows a greater freedom of movement. Other factors are cohesion, viscosity, turbulence and friction. Describing cohesion and viscosity Harris and McInnes (1963) state that these factors provide resistance to all movements in the water. Other authors use the term resistance (Bolton and Goodwin, 1974; Skinner and Thomson, 1983), while Davis and Harrison (1988) write of resistance but also refer to the bow wave effect impeding movement. For some years this author has advocated the use of the word impedance as more suitable than resistance.

Resistance implies the solidity of an object such as the resistances against which the human being works on land. For example, for a person to achieve the standing position from sitting the floor is used against which to thrust. Such resistance is not present in water, especially when in deeper water or in the horizontal position where there is no 'resistance' to thrust against, but movement is impeded by cohesion, viscosity, turbulence and frictional forces. The degree to which movement through water is impeded also depends on the speed of the action and the shape of the object.

In the author's opinion the physiotherapist should be in the water when treating patients (p. 6). For a number of reasons it is undesirable to expect patients to go into the water while the physiotherapist remains on land. Most techniques require that the physiotherapist is in the water with the patient; the exercises that can be taught from the bathside are usually carried out less effectively if the physiotherapist instructs from dry land. Risk factors are compounded when the physiotherapist is not in the pool. The advantages of the physiotherapist's presence in the water far outweigh the disadvantages.

THERAPEUTIC EFFECTS OF EXERCISE IN WATER

The therapeutic effects of exercise in water have been well documented (Skinner and Thomson, 1983; Davis and Harrison, 1988). It is recognized that an increase in muscle power and endurance, the mobilizing of joints, the reduction of spasticity, relaxation, improvements in balance and coordination, functional activity and recreation are among the most important of these effects.

Techniques of Exercise in Water

There are a number of techniques of exercise in water available to the physiotherapist. These include:

- buoyancy assisted, supported, resisted, exercise
- Bad Ragaz patterns
- hold–relax techniques
- stabilizations
- repeated contractions
- breathing exercises
- spinal mobilizations
- hydrodynamic exercises.

Buoyancy assisted, supported, resisted exercise

These are the most commonly used exercises carried out in the hydrotherapy pool. They are usually accomplished with the patient lying supported on a submerged plinth or in flotation equipment or in the sitting and standing position, when the patient may hold the rail for support and stability.

The starting position for each exercise is important as on this will depend whether the movement has buoyancy either assisting, supporting, or resisting it. In these exercises the physiotherapist endeavours to isolate the movement and this may be achieved by providing suitable floats above the joint being exercised or by the physiotherapist giving manual assistance. With the hands involved in this way the physiotherapist cannot give manual assistance

or resistance to the patient's movement which is frequently required.

The four main starting positions of standing, sitting, kneeling and lying can be varied enormously (Bolton and Goodwin, 1974; Skinner and Thomson, 1983). There is little advantage to be gained from reiterating the variations here, but it is important to stress that depending on the effects of buoyancy required these must be understood if this type of exercise is to be effectively executed and the progression of exercise obtained. Apart from the starting position the commands to the patient are important so that the correct movement takes place. It is all too easy to involve other body parts due to the difficulty of acquiring stability in water so attention to detail is essential. Progression in this type of exercise can be further obtained by altering the lever arm, adding floats, the speed and range of movement as well as the number of repetitions.

Bad Ragaz patterns

Bad Ragaz patterns were originally developed in Germany, but have been adapted and developed at Bad Ragaz in Switzerland. This technique utilizes the properties of water, for instance buoyancy is needed for flotation only, whilst the bow wave and drag effects provide the impedance to movement. The patterns themselves allow normal anatomical and physiological movements involving the joints and muscles concerned in the movements.

The bow wave effect demonstrates an increase in pressure ahead of the direction of movement while the drag effect occurs behind the direction of movement. By varying both the bow wave and drag effect, impedance to movement can be varied.

Bad Ragaz patterns can only be carried out if the physiotherapist is in the water handling and instructing the patient. There are three ways in which the physiotherapist acts in relation to the patient. They are:

- the physiotherapist provides fixation while the patient moves through the water – either towards, away from or around the physiotherapist
- the physiotherapist acts as the stabilizing factor but this moves and the patient is pushed in the direction of movement

which leads to an increase in impedance to the movement

- the patient holds a fixed position while being pushed through the water by the physiotherapist.

These points highlight the need for the stability and flexibility of the physiotherapist. To ensure these factors are developed the physiotherapist should not work in a depth greater than that of the level of the eighth thoracic vertebra.

Holds should be precise and capable of guiding the patient to work the required muscle groups of the mass pattern of a limb or trunk. Holds can also provide resistance to movement so that stronger components can be developed – irradiation or overflow carried over to the weaker muscle groups. It is possible to vary the hold from proximal to distal positions on the limbs. Proximal holds give the physiotherapist greater control and there is increased security for the patient, and such a hold would be employed when the pattern involves movement of a possible painful joint. Distal holds allow greater ranges of movement and encourage increased muscle work.

The starting positions for Bad Ragaz patterns are supine lying, side lying or prone lying. Patterns provide both isotonic and isometric muscle work and have been devised for the upper and lower limbs and trunk. The Bad Ragaz patterns allow the physiotherapist and patient to work together in enjoyable cooperation and the strength of the movement can be carefully monitored and graded.

As the individual patterns have been well documented (Skinner and Thomson, 1983; Davis and Harrison, 1988) it is not proposed to detail them here. More recently some of the patterns have been modified and appear to demand more specific movement and an increased workload for the patient. Additional patterns have been devised in which precise holds are used to bring about exact movements (Egger and Zinn, 1990). The patterns can be adapted and modified as the physiotherapist becomes skilled in their use and finds it possible to devise and develop individual variations.

Hold–relax techniques

Hold–relax techniques in water are similar to those carried out on land except that the patient must be positioned so that buoyancy assists movement into the required range.

Stabilizations

The freedom of movement which is possible in water is the only difference between this technique on land and in water. It is used to produce co-contraction of a joint which has implications for balance and coordination in addition to increasing muscle strength and improving the circulation to painful joints.

Repeated contractions

This technique involves isometric and isotonic work and when used in water movement and the 'holding' component can be developed against turbulent effect or a combination of turbulence and buoyancy. The activity which is repeated permits the weaker components of movement patterns to develop thus increasing the development of strength and stamina.

Breathing exercises

The freedom of movement available in water is used in this technique to develop lateral and posterior costal expansion. The technique involves careful monitoring of the patient's breathing and judiciously applied light stretch. Like all the other specialized techniques listed breathing exercises have been described in detail and the reader is referred to those authors (Skinner and Thomson, 1983; Davis and Harrison, 1988).

Spinal mobilizations

The development of specific spinal mobilizations in water is of a comparatively recent nature. They are used where there are difficulties with spinal mobility and utilize passive manual mobilization and passive mobilization using turbulent drag (Chapter 11). These techniques may be combined with other techniques such as Bad Ragaz patterns, hydrodynamic exercise, stretching and relaxation.

Hydrodynamic exercises

These techniques are based on the hydrodynamical principles of buoyancy, turbulence and balance in water. The techniques may use any or all three of the principles at any one time. They can only take place in water where the forces of gravity and buoyancy are present and act simultaneously on the body. In any situation balance, coordination, movement, movement control, body image, spatial awareness and reaction to positions, shape, buoyancy and turbulence may be involved.

As already seen water reacts to the shape and density of any object placed in it and floats the object accordingly (Reid Campion, 1985). The variations in the shape and density of human beings account for the myriad of balance positions.

General Principles

The general principles involved in these patterns are that from a position of stability a movement is made, then balance occurs against the turbulent effects created by the movement and further adjustments are made to balance the body in the new posture. Where movements are small and little or no turbulence is created buoyancy and balance are the two principles involved. Where the body is supported by the physiotherapist buoyancy plays a part. Involved as it is with the balance of the body in water as opposed to gravity, the alteration in shape, particularly if a part of the body is taken above the surface of the water produces a quick and massive rotational response. Controlling this response produces strong muscle work even when the alteration of the shape is small.

Turbulence is felt as a force along the surface of a limb behind the direction of movement, but mainly distally. Small slow movements will create little turbulence, but larger and more rapid movements will create greater turbulence with increased appreciation of the drag effect which impedes movement. This enhances awareness of body image and, with the necessity of controlling the body against the disturbing factor of turbulence, develops balance and coordination.

Marked alterations in shape and density which occur in disease and disability demand more control to counteract the rotational movement. Such control may be developed in the rehabilitation programme, but should be taught from the beginning. The importance of analysing shape and density has already been discussed. Reference to it has been made at this point to expand on its use as a means of teaching balance and coordination, as well as developing exercises and patterns of movement and control which require precise muscle work. The patterns can be conducted in the four main starting points – standing, sitting, kneeling and lying. The depth at which they are conducted in the first three of the above starting positions must be appropriate for the patient's condition, ensuring that the water level is not below the xiphisternum where approximately 30% of weight bearing occurs and preferably with the body positioned so that the shoulders are covered by the water so that approximately only 10% of the body weight is borne.

The following examples will serve to illustrate ways in which these techniques may be developed.

Changing body shapes

Changing body shapes mean that water will balance the body in a new position. For instance if the body is collapsed into its smallest shape, that of being curled up like a 'ball' (Reid Campion, 1985), water will rotate this shape forward and balance the body over its centre of buoyancy with the thoracic spine visible above the surface of the water.

If the physiotherapist holds the person's curled-up body by placing one arm behind and around the waist and placing the other hand over the person's hands which are clasped around the knees it is possible to control the forward movement created by the water (Reid Campion, 1985). The person's curled-up body should be held as low as possible in the water so that the shoulders are covered and where the neck is to be treated this should be immersed as deep as is practical. Gentle rocking of the body by the physiotherapist will promote flexion and extension of the cervical spine. It is essential that the water is blown away from the mouth as the head goes forward; this tends to increase the movement of flexion. Such breathing control has been described under mental adjustment and balance restoration.

Tilting the body

By tilting the curled body sideways, side flexion of the neck can be obtained.

In neurological conditions where extensor tone is increased in the lower limb(s) and flexor tone increased in the upper limb(s) the curled-up or 'ball' position (Reid Campion, 1985) will have the effect of reducing the extensor spasticity in the leg(s) and encourage protraction of the shoulder, extension of the elbow, the mid-position of the forearm and some extension of the wrist and fingers. If the physiotherapist, holding the curled-up body as described above, then rocks the person forwards and backwards slowly and rhythmically reduction of increased muscle tone is aided. When the person is required to come out of the curled-up posture this should be performed slowly and with the physiotherapist's support. If the erect position is required then the procedure of uncurling should take place in deep water so that as the person attains the erect position the minimum amount of gravity is placed on the patient. Should spasticity return or be a problem it is advisable to let the uncurling take place slowly into supine lying still supported by the physiotherapist.

Rotating the body

Rotation of the cervical spine, can be developed if the body is extended into its longest shape, that is lying with the hands by the sides of the body and supported by the physiotherapist using the horizontal backing hold (Reid Campion, 1985). The body is rolled first in one direction and then the other and the person instructed to bring the body to a flat position again by rotating the head to the opposite side to which the body is being rolled.

Use of turbulence

When retraining gait greater balance and coordination can be developed over and above that achieved with turbulence judiciously placed behind the patient to increase the difficulty of forward movement. This can be accomplished by instructing the person to pause and stabilize the body, not letting it be disturbed by turbulent effect created by the movement. If walking is performed in this way, the starting position is standing on one leg with the arms stretched forwards just below the surface of the water, with one leg raised in flexion at the hip, the knee extended and the foot dorsiflexed. The supporting knee should be extended. A step is

taken onto the forward leg and the original supporting limb is allowed to extend at the hip, the pelvis facing forwards, so that rotation of the pelvis and trunk does not take place. The steps taken may be small at first, but can be gradually increased. If maintaining balance is difficult in the pauses between each movement, the arms may be moved slowly sideways in abduction from the forward position, thus bringing the centre of gravity back within the body. Once a stable position is achieved, the arms are moved forward in a controlled manner and the next part of the pattern commenced. The extended leg is brought forward with a straight knee and is raised forwards as high as possible. Buoyancy assists the flexion at the hip. the body is stabilized again before the next step is taken.

This 'goose-step' demands considerable control throughout the body, particularly as the size of the stride increases, producing great turbulence. These movements can be extended till eventually the person may jump onto one leg, pause to stabilize the body, before continuing the pattern.

This method of gait retraining has, in the author's experience, proved valuable in many conditions, notably in the orthopaedic and neurological ones. The pattern is not easily learned, and careful instruction is necessary, but the majority of persons treated enjoy both the mental and physical exercise required in the acquisition of the skill. In one instance this gait retraining combined with other techniques developed on similar lines were of particular value in the rehabilitation of a ballet dancer who had suffered severe damage to one knee requiring surgery and prolonged rehabilitation. Progress was excellent and she finally returned to dancing on points with the ballet company.

The 'goose-step' can be varied to stepping and turning so that all the movements of the hips are involved in the pattern combined with trunk, shoulder girdle and head rotation.

Static muscle work

Static muscle work is developed in techniques that utilize a fixed position followed by changes of shape using the lower or upper limbs or both. It is usual to convert one shape to another by repositioning one lower limb and using the arms in varying patterns pausing after each movement to allow the body to be balanced.

Controlling the body shape after each movement produces muscle work that is fine yet strong.

To develop muscle work for the dorsiflexors and plantarflexors of the foot the person may be in the 'sitting' or 'cube' position (Reid Campion, 1985) with the arms forward and the feet about hip width apart, a right angle at the hip, knee and ankle joints. Stretching the fingers forwards will cause the body to rotate forwards and the heels will rise. When sufficient elevation of the heels has occurred extension of the head will bring the body back to the original starting position. To produce dorsiflexion the hips should be allowed to drop towards the heels; this action brings about rotation of the body in a backwards direction. Once sufficient dorsiflexion has been created a forward action of the head will bring the body to the upright 'sitting' position again. Slow rocking forwards and backwards in this position using the actions described, or the extended wrists and hands, just above the surface in a pulling or pushing type action will produce strong muscle work for the dorsiflexors and plantarflexors of the ankle. If only one muscle group is to be exercised then the action which produces the movement is done repeatedly, the person coming back to the original starting position between each movement.

Where knee extension with dorsiflexion requires re-education and training and as a strengthening activity for the quadriceps muscle the 'sitting' position may be utilized again. Extending first one knee and then the other towards the surface, but outside the forward held arms, at the same time dorsiflexing the foot and creating a 'bubble' on the surface. The foot should never break through the surface of the water. The body weight has to be transferred to the supporting side just prior to the kicking action. The person remains in the 'sitting' position with the arms forward all the time. The movements once learnt can be gradually speeded up so that the shifting of the body weight and the kicking action proceed continuously. As a useful lead into the back-stroke kick the kicking action may be brought closer to the arms and so into midline, the person gradually lying back as they do so.

The combined use of buoyancy, turbulence and balance in water adds a new dimension to activity in water. These patterns are unique to hydrotherapy as only in water is the body acted upon by two forces simultaneously – the forces of gravity or downthrust and buoyancy or upthrust. A wide range of patterns can be developed. They require that the patient and physiotherapist work closely together particularly where pain is present. In some instances the patient has to be supported by the physiotherapist. In others the physiotherapist must correct the patient's posture and this requires minute attention to the muscle work which changes with each alteration of shape. Reactions, balance, coordination and the enhancement of movement are developed strongly in these patterns.

It can be seen then that the physiotherapist being in the water with the person will produce the best results. Bad Ragaz patterns, successive induction, slow reversals and stabilizations, together with hydrodynamic exercise where the physiotherapist must observe the muscle action and correct any untoward alterations in shape, demand the presence of the physiotherapist in the water. This is also true where turbulent assisted and resisted activity is taking place. The physiotherapist is required to create turbulence in appropriate areas in relation to the person's body. Much is made of the time factor but in the author's experience the advantages of effective treatment far outweigh any disadvantages. A session for a number of persons being treated at the same time can be appropriately timetabled to include both group and individual work. It is sad to reflect that in some instances people are given a few instructions about exercise in water for their condition and are then left to carry them out with little or no supervision nor any attempt to evaluate and progress the programme.

THERAPEUTIC SWIMMING

In some countries hydrotherapy is considered to be a hydrotherapy treatment carried out in water by physiotherapists. When it comes to swimming there are those physiotherapists who see such activity as recreational and not their concern. This author believes that swimming is an integral part of hydrotherapy programmes and forms part of the patient's overall rehabilitation. As such it can be considered as therapeutic swimming and is best undertaken by the physiotherapist who has extensive training in movement and knows the pathology of disease. For physiotherapists who have also undertaken training in hydrotherapy techniques and in the recreational aspects of water activity, therapeutic swimming should certainly be their province.

Slade and Simmons-Grab (1987) suggest that therapeutic water programmes supervised by trained physiotherapists may be designed to cover exercise in water, instruction in appropriately amended swimming strokes and therapeutic recreational swimming. Involvement of personnel from other disciplines, such as swimming teachers who have trained in adapted aquatics through courses provided by tertiary institutions, is desirable.

There is little doubt that today water activity and swimming are favoured by the medical profession in treating a wide variety of conditions both medical and surgical. This is supported by the upsurge in the numbers of referrals for hydrotherapy, the suggestions made by doctors to their patients to swim to keep fit and the installation of an increasing number of pools. Swimming is a most useful activity (Kraus, 1973) because it can be so readily adapted to suit each individual's needs and capabilities – above bodied and disabled alike. This aspect of recreational water activity is an important part of the Halliwick Method of swimming for the disabled (Reid Campion, 1985). The method is suitable for all but especially for the disabled of any age with any disability and any degree of that disability. In fact, the more severely disabled benefit considerably (Reid, 1975).

The buoyancy of the water diminishes the effects of gravity and thus reduces the stress on the joints. It also allows easier movement and where muscles are weak this is a distinct advantage. In water it is possible to perform movements, patterns of movement and feats which may be difficult or impossible on land (Grove, 1970; Campion, 1983). At the same time the impedance to movement due to the density of the liquid, the turbulent effects and the need to expend more energy to move in water facilitates the strengthening of muscles and increases the range of motion and flexibility.

An important advantage, especially when considering functional training, is that the execution of exercises in water can be carried out in the erect position without strain due to the loss of weight in water. However, it is possible to exercise and swim in the horizontal position without the need to gain the upright posture. Upthrust or buoyancy, and the support of water make movement easier and provide motivation to move more. This is important for enjoyment, happiness and morale.

Slade and Simmons-Grab (1987) suggest rehabilitation for many patients is a long-term process and the reality is that much of this can take place in therapeutic swimming programmes within the community. A considerable advantage for many swimmers, however disabled, is that they are able to find total independence in water. On land many disabled persons have to use some form of aid. In the medium of water the swimmer discards the wheelchair or other aids and can learn to control his own body in the water without resorting to flotation equipment or other devices. In most instances once such independence is gained it is possible for the disabled person to join with able-bodied peers in a social activity and it may also offer the opportunity to compete with their normal counterparts (Campion, 1983).

Experience has shown that the teaching of vertical and lateral rotational control, breathing and head control as advocated by the Halliwick Method is valuable for everyone. When dealing with the head and spinal cord injured as well as with rheumatic, orthopaedic and other neurological conditions these skills are an essential part of the programme, whether this is a hydrotherapeutic exercise programme or for therapeutic swimming. In this way the goals of general health and fitness as well as mobility and flexibility are achieved and when the patient is discharged from hospital may be maintained by participation in community programmes based on treatment schemes.

The selection of swimming stokes is vitally important. This means that not only must the physiotherapist understand the patient's condition and mobility in detail, but must also have knowledge of the muscle groups involved throughout the body for each individual. A strong stable trunk is essential from which the upper and lower limbs must work as they propel the body through the water. This suggests that throughout the rehabilitation programme the whole person should be treated and not just the affected part, so that ultimately the patient can use therapeutic swimming as a means of remaining fit.

As Slade and Simmons-Grab (1987) indicate such therapeutic water activity has considerable potential for rehabilitation for many differing disabilities, many severe. Such programmes give considerable help both physically and psychologically to the patients and to their families and friends, and permit integration into the more normal aspects of living. The physiotherapist's role in this type of activity is an essential one because of their training and knowledge of disabilities and mobility. They can give the appropriate exercise and swimming activity and thus avoid some of the potentially dangerous movements. If swimming is to be adapted to the needs of the individual and based on that person's mobility then this should be considered as therapeutic swimming. As in all training programmes suitable exercises are used to improve movement, strength and stamina and so these should be included in any therapeutic swimming programme.

Orientation in the water plays an important part in group therapeutic exercise programmes advocated by Slade and Simmons-Grab (1987). They suggest walking in various directions be used as a means of orientation and extend this to prone kicking for cardiovascular exercise. In many centres in Western Australia walking forwards, backwards and sideways would be used as a warm-up and in some situations swimming laps might be used for the same purpose.

The teaching of mental, adjustment and balance restoration, which in Western Australia is considered part of the orientation process, has been found essential to the orientation of patients whether entering the water for hydrotherapy or therapeutic swimming programmes. It ensures that the person's anxiety is lessened and that activity in water is undertaken with a greater degree of confidence and cooperation. The two factors, mental adjustment and balance restoration, are thus essential preliminaries to any programme (p. 21).

Mental adjustment means that the swimmer appreciates the effects of buoyancy, turbulence, and the weight of water and has acquired a degree of breathing and head control. *Balance restoration* involves teaching the swimmer both vertical and lateral rotational control and a combination of these rotations. A combination of these two rotations ensures that the swimmer is always able to recover to a safe breathing position.

A balanced floating position that can be controlled against all disturbing forces and the ability to regain the upright position ensures the swimmer will be safe in water. Once mentally adjusted and physically balanced the person is able to work effectively in the water, cooperate with the physiotherapist and cope with the demands of the programme. Learning swimming strokes requires balance, buoyancy, flotation and relaxation. The external and internal forces acting on a human body and the effects produced by these forces are studied when the biomechanics of stroking is undertaken. The greatest barrier to good stroking is tension, an internal resistance. If the swimmer has been taught the basic skills relating to breathing, head control and rotational control and is thus mentally adjusted to and physically balanced in water, swimming will come easily.

In all this, the swimmer will gain an understanding of body function, body awareness, spatial awareness particularly through the 'feel' of water and turbulence of which one is most aware at the distal parts of the limbs (Reid Campion, 1985). Harmonious movement is developed as it is easier to shift between contraction or relaxation of muscles (Myrenburg and Myrenburg, 1982).

Whatever the patient's condition there will be physical and psychological advantages accruing from a therapeutic water activity programme. These effects cover a wide range from kinaesthetic stimulation, cognitive sensorimotor patterns, improved circulation, the reduction of pain and muscle spasm, improved metabolism, re-education of muscle groups and improved range of motion. Morale and confidence are boosted by recreational activity; functional abilities are improved along with balance and coordination.

When therapeutic swimming takes place in the community benefits common to group activities occur. These include motivation and socialization. Since some therapeutic swimming would take place as a home programme or within the community, a means whereby the patient can move into the community again is provided; thus the patient can experience all the benefits brought about by such an action.

Breathing control is vital for good swimming and it has important effects on relaxation and thus aids balance (Reid Campion 1985). Relaxation can be achieved by mental adjustment to the element of water; by the ability to regain and maintain a safe breathing position. With the other basic skills suggested previously the patient can participate in an activity which is a good method of keeping fit, improves endurance and stamina, produces a feeling of general well-being and provides social and psychological benefits that can be pursued throughout life.

RE-EDUCATION OF WALKING

The re-education of functional activities, especially walking, is a considerable part of activity in water. The reader will see that there are differing views as to the value of gait retraining in some chapters. The doubts usually arise because of distorted underwater vision and altered perception. However it is generally advocated by most authorities (Bolton and Goodwin, 1974; Skinner and Thomson, 1983; Davis and Harrison, 1988) for most conditions.

The attainment and maintenance of the upright position and the balance and coordination required have been described. Activities for the acquisition of vertical rotation are numerous, and the judicious placing of turbulence helps the person stabilize the body. A forward head and arm action ensures the feet remain on the floor of the pool, and this position should be adopted when commencing retraining the gait. If support from the physiotherapist is necessary then this should be provided from in front, using the facing hold (p. 46). Later, support is given from behind and gradually total disengagement is achieved.

The correct depth of water should be used – that is the water should just cover the shoulders and should not be lower than the axillae. This provides a buoyancy-dominated situation and support to the whole body. As walking skills improve, the person may gradually be taken into shallower water, walking forwards, backwards and sideways from a buoyancy-dominated to a gravity-dominated environment.

Transference of weight sideways should commence the re-education of walking. The feet are placed apart sideways as widely as necessary and the body weight moved over first one leg and then the other. Walking sideways can be carried out on a one-to-one basis, the person and physiotherapist working together, or in a group using a circle formation.

Weight transference is progressed in the step standing position and support may be provided in the same sequence, moving from a buoyancy- to a gravity-dominated situation. Walking forwards is developed from the forwards and backwards 'rocking' action. It· should be remembered that different muscle work is involved in walking in the water from that of walking on land (Skinner and Thomson, 1983) as buoyancy assists and resists the movements of the lower limbs. For example, buoyancy assists hip and knee flexion but resists the lowering of the leg. Throughout gait retraining, the person will need to lean forward against the build-up of pressure in front of the body. However, when walking backwards the head and arms should still be kept forwards, for if the head is taken back, a loss of balance in the upright position will occur.

Balance and coordination can be further improved during gait retraining by instructing the person to pause and stabilize the body, not letting it be disturbed by turbulent effect created by the movement (p. 15).

REFERENCES

Bennett R.P. (1951). Water as a medium for therapeutic exercise. *N.Y. St. J. Med.*, 51: 513.

Bolton E. and Goodwin D. (1979). *An Introduction to Pool Exercises*, Edinburgh: Churchill Livingstone.

Campion M. (1983). Water activity based on the Halliwick method. In *Duffield's Exercise in Water*, 3rd edn (A. Skinner, A. Thomson eds), London: Baillière Tindall.

Davis B.C. and Harrison R.A. (1988). *Hydrotherapy in Practice*, Edinburgh: Churchill Livingstone.

Egger B. and Zinn N.M. (1990) *Aktive Physiotherapie im Wasser, Neue Ragazer Methode mit Ringen*, Stuttgart: Gustav Fischer Verlag.

Grove F. (1970). Aquatic therapy: a first real step to rehabilitation. *Journal of Health, Physical Education and Recreation*, October, 65.

Harris R. (1963). Therapeutic pools. In *Medical Hydrology* (S. Licht, ed.), New Haven: Elizabeth Licht.

Harris R. and McInnes M. (1963). Exercises in water. In *Medical Hydrology* (S. Licht, ed.), New Haven: Elizabeth Licht; pp. 207–217.

Kamenetz H.L. (1963). History of American spas and hydrotherapy. In *Medical Hydrology*, (S. Licht, ed.), New Haven: Elizabeth Licht.

Kraus R. (1973). *Therapeutic Recreation Service, Principles and Practice*, Philadelphia: W.B. Saunders Company.

Lowman C.L. and Roen S.G. (1952). *Therapeutic Uses of Pools and Tanks*, Philadelphia: William B. Saunders, pp. 12, 69–70.

Myrenburg K. and Myrenburg M. (1982). *Water-gymnastics*, Stockholm: Spänstituets Gymnastik-förening.

Reid M.J. (1975). *Handling the Disabled Child in Water – an Introduction*, London: Association of Chartered Paediatric Physiotherapists.

Reid Campion M. (1985). *Hydrotherapy in Paediatrics*, Oxford: Heinemann Medical Books.

Slade C. and Simmons-Grab D. (1987). Therapeutic Swimming as a community based programme. *Cognitive Rehabilitation*, March/April: 18–20.

Skinner A.T. and Thomson A.M. (eds) (1983). *Duffield's Exercises in Water*, 3rd edn, London: Baillière Tindall.

Neurosurgical and neurological conditions

Margaret Reid Campion

Overview to Chapters 9 and 10

The question is often asked 'how appropriate is hydrotherapy for patients with neurological conditions?'

Lower motor neurone lesions, such as Guillain–Barré–Landry syndrome or peripheral nerve lesions have long been treated satisfactorily in water. However, the debate ranges around whether or not head injuries, cerebral vascular accidents and other upper motor neurone lesions should be rehabilitated in water.

Only through clinical experience is it possible to suggest that hydrotherapy is a valuable and effective means of rehabilitation for those suffering neurosurgical and neurological conditions as research has not been undertaken.

Opinions vary worldwide and often reflect the philosophy and treatment approach of the physiotherapists working in the field of neurology. In Europe, mainly in Switzerland and Holland, physiotherapists treat both upper and lower motor neurone lesions in water, their approach based largely on the principles of the Halliwick method. In Australia various points of view are held. Carr and Shepherd (1982) tend not to favour rehabilitation in water as, through their motor relearning programme, they aim to retrain muscles to perform precise actions as would be used in everyday normal functions. Since the pool is not a normal environment and muscle activity is different from land one can argue that water is not an ideal medium. The other side of the argument is that if functional activity is not possible on land but can be facilitated in water so that the 'idea' of the movement is implanted and commenced early it may carry over to land.

In a recent paper Carr, Shepherd and Ada (1995) indicate the need for early, active rehabilitation in environments that provide a challenge; water is such an environment, demanding activity to its movement, particularly in relation to balance and may assist the person in regaining functional activity.

Views in Britain may be coloured by the recommendation of Davis and Harrison (1988) not to treat upper motor neurone lesions in water because of the difficulty of acquiring stability which may in turn cause associated reactions to occur thus hindering movement re-education.

Bobath-trained physiotherapists will be familiar with the use of reflex inhibiting patterns, stretchings, normalizing tone and facilitating righting and equilibrium reactions. Those physiotherapists who have also made a study of the Halliwick Method can appreciate the similarities between the two techniques. Others who have studied Conductive Education will also appreciate the similarities between it and the Halliwick Method (Chapter 7).

To treat neurologically affected patients effectively physiotherapists need to be fully conversant with the characteristics and properties of water, be able to control their own bodies against any disturbing forces and to be highly skilled in handling their patients physically and psychologically.

Skilled handling is the essence of hydrotherapy especially in this field. Any mishandling will bring about anxiety, tension and inappropriate reactions. Abnormal reactions are invariably the result of poor handling. Unfortunately when this occurs the blame is placed on the water and hydrotherapy condemned.

Rhythmical swaying, swinging and rolling patterns which reduce tone (Sullivan *et al.*, 1982) and aid relaxation (Skinner and Thomson, 1994) form a valuable part of the treatment programme (Smith, 1990). In the hands of an experienced physiotherapist who constantly monitors the patient's reactions these movements extend from very fine to larger ranges as required. Such observation is vital as this determines the range and speed with which the techniques are performed bearing in mind that buoyancy, metacentre and turbulence will also have an effect.

There is a common thread running through the two ensuing chapters. Both authors have wide experience in their field and treat their patients on land and in the water. Both appreciate the critical nature of water, make use of the fine degree of movement possible, utilize rotational patterns and the dynamic environment to develop righting and equilibrium reactions and balance – in many instances using Halliwick techniques. Awareness of the potential risks and the need for care and safety is essential when taking these patients into water.

REFERENCES

Carr J. and Shepherd R. (1982). *A Motor Learning Programme for Stroke*, Oxford: Heinemann Medical.

Carr J., Shepherd R. and Ada L. (1995). Spasticity, research findings and implications for intervention. *Physiotherapy* **81(8)**: 421–429.

Davis B.C. and Harrison R.A. (1988). *Hydrotherapy in Practice*. Edinburgh: Churchill Livingstone.

Skinner A.T. and Thomson A.M. (1994). Hydrotherapy. In *Pain Management by Physiotherapy*, (P.E. Wells, V. Frampton and D. Bowsher, eds), 2nd edn. Oxford: Butterworth Heinemann.

Smith K. (1990). Hydrotherapy in neurological rehabilitation. In *Adult Hydrotherapy – A Practical Approach*, (M. Reid Campion, ed.), Oxford: Heinemann Medical Books.

Sullivan P.E., Markos P.D. and Minor M.A.D. (1982). *An Integrated Approach to Therapeutic Exercise: Theory and Clinical Application*, Reston Va: Reston Pub. Co.

9

The neurosurgical patient and head injuries

G. 'Jega' Jegasothy

This chapter is based on the work done by the physiotherapy team in the neurosurgical unit at Royal Perth Rehabilitation Hospital (RPRH), Western Australia. This unit admits cases of brain trauma from causes such as motor vehicle accidents, motor cycle accidents, industrial and sporting accidents. These patients may or may not have required neurosurgery. Additionally, the unit admits all cases of neurosurgery for vascular complications and space-occupying lesions, such as arterio-venous malformations, aneurysms and tumours.

All cases admitted to the unit require rehabilitation. Due to the extremes in conscious state of the patient case load catered for, from the comatosed patient to the ambulant patient, an individualized treatment programme is drawn up after review by the physiotherapist. The programme offered covers respiratory physiotherapy, orthopaedic physiotherapy, physiotherapy in soft tissue injuries, sensory bombardment, movement rehabilitation and cardiovascular fitness training. The criteria for the choice of hydrotherapy as a treatment modality for the above mentioned cross-section of patients is delineated in the following chapter.

Problems faced by the neurosurgical patient, attempting to regain normal or near normal function, are itemized. Each problem listed is explained and appropriate treatment techniques are provided. It is important to bear in mind that each patient will have multiple problems and these must be addressed simultaneously if a beneficial outcome is to be achieved.

The exercises given in each section are not listed in order of progression, unless otherwise stated. The exercises exemplify the rationale of treatment and often the one exercise can be utilized to achieve a number of goals. Becoming familiar with some of the techniques, the reader should go on to formulate their own list of exercises using the same rationalization of treatment goals.

The chapter is divided into four areas:

- **Indications for hydrotherapy.**
- **Contraindications to hydrotherapy.**
- **Untoward effects.**
- **Hints for success**

The introduction of the patient to water is vitally important. Consideration must be given to the level of functional dependency of the patient, size, weight, shape and density. The neurosurgical patient can pose numerous problems in each of these areas. When a patient is totally dependent, two assistants may be needed to place the patient supine, on the hoist. Keeping this group of patients in mind, we installed a hydraulic bed hoist. This allows us to maintain a patient in the supine position while the bed is swung over and lowered into the water. A physiotherapist or attendant should as far as possible, be in the patient's line of vision or have a reassuring hand on the patient's shoulder. Where an increase in tone has altered the patient's shape, supporting the patient on the hoist safely can be achieved by the physiotherapist sitting alongside the patient on the hoist, being lowered into the water with the patient.

Where a patient has poor or no head control, an inflatable collar is placed around the patient's neck and secured firmly. When the patient is floated off the hoist into the water, his

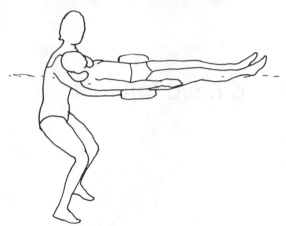

Fig. 9.1 *The physiotherapist's hands should support the patient as low down the trunk as possible, using a backing hold in the horizontal position*

head should rest on the physiotherapist's shoulder. The physiotherapist's hands should support the patient as low down the trunk as possible, using a backing hold in the horizontal position. If the patient is tall, a pelvic float may be required (Fig. 9.1).

INDICATIONS FOR HYDROTHERAPY

Hydrotherapy is indicated for the neuro-surgical patient where the desired goals are to:

- decrease tone
- stimulate movement
- retrain and stimulate righting reactions
- augment and increase the range of weak movements
- retrain centralized, that is rotational, patterns of movement
- retrain reciprocal patterns of movement
- access functional movement patterns
- encourage and develop efficient breath control and voice production
- produce psychological effects
- treat orthopaedic complications
- increase cardiovascular fitness
- offer opportunities for recreation and socialization.

To Decrease Tone

The reduction of tone may occur as a direct result of the warmth of the water. The support

and the uniformity of stimulation provided by this medium help towards a further reduction of tone. The latter effect can be augmented by the use of techniques that utilize the vestibular connections in the central nervous system (CNS).

Research into the physiological effect of heat gives some clues as to the effect of heat on muscle tone. Fisher and Solomon (1965) indicate that the neck exteroceptors in the skin, when stimulated by warmth, show a diminution of gamma-fibre activity, which leads to decreased spindle excitability. Effects of general hyperthermia on the reduction of tone have been documented by Skinner and Thompson (1983). The simplest way to cause general hyperthermia is by immersion in water held at a temperature of 35°C (Franchimont *et al.*, 1983). This pool temperature has proved beneficial in attempts to reduce tone and this is borne out by the experience of the author in treating neurosurgical patients and documented in the work of other physiotherapists (Harris, 1978).

When working with the head-injured patient, in the water or on land, it must be remembered that the patient's thermo-regulatory ability is not as efficient as in the healthy individual. Much research has been done on the reflex increase in the gamma bias in the muscle spindle and an increase in tone can be achieved when core temperature falls by 0.4°C (Blatteis, 1960). It is of utmost importance that due consideration be given to the temperature of the water in the pool if the aim of treatment is the reduction of tone. The best response is obtained when pool temperature is maintained around but not above this temperature when the beneficial effects tend to dissipate (Franchimont *et al.*, 1983).

The support offered by the water and the consequent reduction/elimination of the effects of gravity benefit both the physiotherapist and the patient. On land, the physiotherapist has to contend with the weight of the patient or the weight of the limb, where the patient is dependent. An average male patient may weigh 50–60 kg, which makes considerable demands on the physiotherapist. In any one day, the physiotherapist may treat up to ten patients. This load can be reduced for the physiotherapist if treatment is carried out in the water by the judicious use of buoyancy and flotation, where the changes in position and shape of the patient can be achieved with minimal stress on the physiotherapist.

Activity on land requires the patient to contend with the forces of gravity acting on the affected and unaffected side of the body. In attempting any movement, the patient has to cope with the uneven forces created by the contraction of muscles on two sides of the body, the affected and unaffected side. From this background, patients are not only required to move the weight of their body or limb through space but also to maintain balance. Tone is increased in proportion to the 'perceived effort' – as seen by the patient – being required to achieve the desired movement.

In the water, Archimedes' principle of relative density and Bougier's theorem of metacentre (Reid Campion, 1991) can be utilized effectively to alleviate the above problem. The patient can be led to experience a sense of weightlessness and total support. The physiotherapist is then able to guide the patient through the required movement such that the patient's 'perceived effort' is decreased and tone is thereby reduced.

In attempting to use vestibular stimulation to reduce tone, the physiotherapist must be able to ensure a secure hold on the patient. This is affected by the altered shape of the patient and the distribution of the patient's body weight as a result of this altered shape. Using the principle of buoyancy and flotation, the physiotherapist is able to give the patient the required support only in water while ensuring an effective treatment. Slow rhythmical movements reduce tone while rapid movements increase tone. Slow rhythmical movements comprise all forms of swinging, rocking and rolling movements. Sullivan *et al.* (1983) indicate that rotation around the longitudinal axis of the body aids in the reduction of spasticity.

Exercises to decrease tone

The reduction of tone may be brought about in the following ways:

1. *Starting position*: the patient lies in front of the physiotherapist, who uses a backing hold in the horizontal position.
    Technique: the physiotherapist walks slowly backwards. Initially, the patient is taken backwards through the water in a straight line. Later, the physiotherapist,

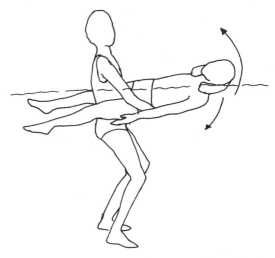

Fig. 9.2   *The physiotherapist moves the patient slowly in an arc. The arc is progressively widened*

by walking in a 'lazy s' shaped path, allows lateral trunk flexion to occur.
Patient appreciation: the patient appreciates the sensory stimulation provided by the warmth and the pressure of the water, and the movement of hips and lower limbs on the trunk

2. *Starting position*: as above.
    Technique: as the physiotherapist walks backwards and sways the patient from side to side, the physiotherapist raises the hip first on one side and then the other at the end of the swing, thereby incorporating some rotation.
    Patient appreciation: the patient feels the sensory stimulation provided by the water, the warmth and pressure, as well as the movement of the hip and lower limbs on the trunk, coupled with rotation.

3. *Starting position*: the patient is in supine lying facing the physiotherapist, who has the patient's legs on either side of the physiotherapist's waist and her hands under the patient's hips. The patient's head is supported by an inflatable neck collar.
    Technique: the physiotherapist moves the patient slowly in an arc. The arc is progressively widened (Fig. 9.2).
    Patient appreciation: the patient appreciates the sensory stimulation of the

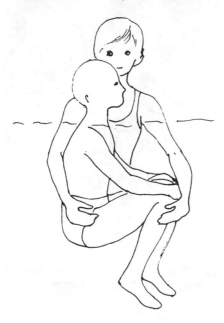

Fig. 9.3   *The patient is held curled up in a ball sideways on to the physiotherapist*

warmth and pressure of the water, the movement of the head and trunk on the hips and stimulation of the vestibular-ocular system (Herman, 1982).

4. *Starting position*: the patient is held curled up in a ball sideways on to the physiotherapist. The patient's knees are flexed up against the chest, with the patient's hands around the knees, where possible (Fig. 9.3). The physiotherapist holds the patient with one arm placed around the back at waist level, the other hand holds the patient's legs in flexion. The depth at which the activity takes place should be such that the greater part of the patient's weight is supported by the water.

Technique: the physiotherapist, by rhythmically and slowly moving her body laterally in a rocking motion, causes a forward and backward movement of the patient's body. Initially, a small amplitude displacement of the patient's head is aimed for.

Patient appreciation: the patient appreciates the movement of the head and neck on the trunk and the vestibular system is stimulated.

To Stimulate Movement

It is necessary to stimulate the return of movement in the severely disabled patient who invariably has very little in the way of voluntary movement. At this stage of the patient's recovery, there is considerable sensory deprivation and the patient thus has very little desire to move. The patient may not know how to move.

It is known that thermal information is carried via collateral pathways from the spinothalamic and lemniscal tracts to the mid-brain and the reticular formation in the brainstem. This information is then carried along neural pathways from the latter areas to the hypothalamic and pre-optic areas (Lee and Warren, 1978). The function of the reticular formation is to stimulate the cortex to wakefulness. Therefore, heat, by stimulating the neural receptors in the skin (Wadsworth and Chanmugam, 1983) and its connections to the reticular formation along with vestibular information, which also has connections in the reticular formation, may help to stimulate and maintain a state of alertness in the patient.

Any movement of the head in space will cause varying degrees of vestibular stimulation. The vestibular system has connections with the reticular formation and the cerebellum. The latter is an important centre, together with the thalamus and mid-brain, in the control of muscle tone and movement. Herman (1982) in his research postulates that the prerequisite of peripheral movement is mid-line structure stability and visual stability, in particular the vestibular-ocular reflex. The latter reflex is brought into operation when the head is moved in space in relation to a stationary object. The above explanation is the basis for the formulation of exercises that will result in the stimulation and establishment of tone and movement. Where the eyes go, the head follows and so the body. Where movement is already present, however little, further movement may be produced as a result of stimulation overflow and recruitment of motor neurones. The latter is the basis for some of the proprioceptive neuromuscular facilitation (PNF) techniques.

5. *Starting position*: the patient is in the horizontal supine float position with his lower limbs on either side of the physiotherapist's waist. The physiotherapist's hands

support the patient as high up the back as possible (Fig. 9.2).

Technique: the patient is rotated to allow the cheek on that side to touch the water, whilst being given instruction to turn the head away. In the initial stages, the whole pattern can be done passively by the physiotherapist. At first, displacement is small, but is progressively allowed to get larger.

Patient appreciation: the patient appreciates vestibular stimulation and head on body rotation.

Techniques 1 to 5 could be introductory lessons before attempting techniques 6, 7 and 8.

6. *Starting position*: the physiotherapist holds the patient as in the previous technique, except that the hands holding the patient support the hips.

   Technique: this technique is a progression from the previous one. The physiotherapist displaces the patient's hips from side to side with an anterior/posterior movement. The patient is instructed not to allow any movement to occur initially. As the range of displacement is increased, the patient is instructed to return head and trunk to midline.

   Patient appreciation: the patient appreciates head on trunk and trunk on trunk displacement. There is static work for the neck and trunk musculature, which is progressed to active contraction.

7. *Starting position*: the patient is held in the horizontal supine float position with the lower limbs astride the physiotherapist's waist (Fig. 9.2). If the patient is tall or heavy, pelvic floats may also be required.

   Technique: the patient is moved in an arc in one direction only. When the appropriate momentum has been gained, the physiotherapist stops the movement abruptly. The patient's trunk will be carried on passively in the line of movement till all momentum is dissipated.

   Patient appreciation: the patient appreciates vestibular stimulation, as well as lateral trunk flexion.

8. *Starting position*: the starting position is the same as that in technique 7 (Fig. 9.2).

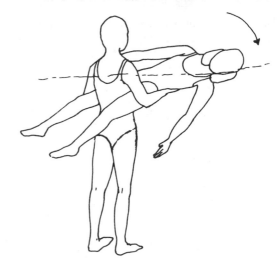

Fig. 9.4   *The patient is moved in an arc to the affected side*

Technique: the patient is instructed to touch the ipsilateral knee with the hand on the side of the direction of movement. For example, if the patient is being moved to the right, the instruction is to touch the right knee with the right hand. This technique is first performed to the stronger side.

Patient appreciation: the patient appreciates vestibular stimulation and lateral flexion of the trunk, which is voluntary assisted. The patient has had to work from the area of turbulence or drag effect and against bow wave, both of which impede the movement.

9. *Starting position*: the patient is held in the horizontal supine float position with the lower limbs astride the physiotherapist's waist (Fig. 9.2).

   Techniques: the patient is moved in an arc to the affected side (Fig. 9.4). When the physiotherapist stops the movement of the patient's body through the water, the patient is instructed not to let the water cause lateral flexion of the body. This will bring about contraction of the trunk flexors of the unaffected side. When the patient has learnt the sequence, the movement can be taken on the unaffected side.

   Patient appreciation: the patient appreciates the static muscle work of the trunk side flexors.

10. *Starting position*: the patient is supported by neck and pelvic floats and is in the horizontal supine float position facing away from the physiotherapist. The unaffected or least affected leg is placed in a ring float with the appropriate amount of air in it, so that the leg is just floated to the surface. The affected leg is allowed to sink in the water. The physiotherapist supports the patient as required.

Technique: the patient is instructed to push the ankle float under the water.

Patient appreciation: the patient appreciates the 'movement' of the affected leg to the surface. The patient is subsequently instructed to augment the movement of the affected limb so that it moves to the surface quickly.

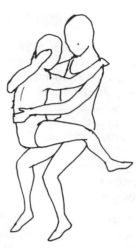

Fig. 9.5   *The patient is facing the physiotherapist in a stride sitting position on the latter's lap*

Retrain and Stimulate Righting Reactions

The ability of the body to right itself is seemingly dependent on tone. When hypotonus is present, for example when there is damage to the cerebellum, few, if any, righting reactions persist. The presence of hypertonus, on the other hand, dampens the body's ability to utilize stepping, propping and righting reactions. These protective mechanisms are difficult to retrain on land as they are the means by which the unsupported body gains stability. It can be extremely difficult to give adult patients enough support to enable them to have the confidence to relearn these antigravity reactions.

In the correct depth of water, with adequate support from the physiotherapist and the appropriate treatment technique, the patient can be given the required feeling of support and security. This is the base from which the patient can be taught the destabilizing effects of limb movements on the body and the appropriate counter-measures to regain stability. The techniques described from 1 to 9 above utilize head and trunk righting and can be used to retrain and stimulate righting reactions.

11. *Starting position*: the patient is facing the physiotherapist in a stride sitting position on the latter's lap. The physiotherapist maintains a stable 'sitting position', one hand being taken under the patient's arm and placed in the thoraco-lumbar area,

whilst the other hand is placed in the occipital and neck area. The patient's upper limbs are placed on the physiotherapist's shoulders. This is the ideal position for the patient's arms, but is not always easy to achieve and maintain (Fig. 9.5).

Technique: the patient is instructed to keep the face level with that of the physiotherapist, who shifts her weight from one leg to the other, thereby displacing the patient's hip and trunk laterally.

Patient appreciation: the patient appreciates the head and trunk righting brought about by this technique.

12. *Starting position*: the patient is in horizontal supine float, supported by neck and hip floats and facing away from the physiotherapist, who stands close to the patient's head supporting the patient in the lower thoracic region with both hands (Fig. 9.6).

Technique: the patient is asked to lift one arm slowly out of the water close to the side of the body. Such action will cause the body to roll to the side on which the arm is lifted. As the trunk begins to rotate, the patient is instructed to turn the head away from the side rolling under and drop the shoulder into the water on the side to which the head is turned. Initially, assistance is given as needed, but as the patient masters the technique the physiotherapist's support is slowly withdrawn.

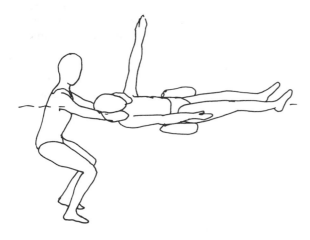

Fig. 9.6   *The patient is in horizontal supine float, supported by neck and hip floats and facing away from the physiotherapist, who stands close to the patient's head supporting the patient in the lower thoracic region with both hands*

Patient appreciation: the patient appreciates the effect of limb movement on the stability of the body. Awareness of the righting reactions required to counter the destabilization of the body and appreciation of static work for the trunk muscles.

13. *Starting position*: the patient assumes a stable sitting position in the water. This position, ideally, requires that there is a right angle at hips, knees and ankle, the feet being hip width apart, the shoulders under the water, the arms stretched forwards and the trunk upright. The physiotherapist adopts a position behind the patient, supporting the patient's hips to stabilize these joints (Fig. 9.7).
Technique: the patient is instructed to stretch the fingers as far as possible. When the physiotherapist feels the patient is about to fall forward, the patient is instructed to sit lower in the water, at the same time the physiotherapist applies pressure downwards on the patient's hips.
Patient appreciation: the patient appreciates the static work of the trunk muscles, the destabilizing effect of limb movement and the activity required to regain balance when the body is falling forward.

14. *Starting position*: the patient is in a stable sitting position as indicated in technique

13, and the physiotherapist maintains the same stable stance.
Technique: the patient is instructed to lower the arms into the water, thus causing the patient to disturb the balanced position. As the physiotherapist feels the patient's balance is disturbed, the patient is instructed to take the head forward and reach as far forward as possible with the fingers. Frequently, it is helpful to have the patient reach towards a visual target, for example the side of the pool.
Patient appreciation: the patient appreciates the contraction of the head and trunk flexors, as well as the destabilizing effect brought about by limb movement and the activity required to regain balance when the body is moved backwards in relation to the base of support.

Once the patient has some knowledge of maintaining the balance of the body against forward and backward displacement, the techniques can be progressed in various ways:

- the patient is instructed to look in various directions, up and down and side to side,
- the patient is instructed to lower one arm and move it forwards and backwards in the water,
- the patient is instructed to move both arms in the water,
- the patient is instructed to flex one leg up.

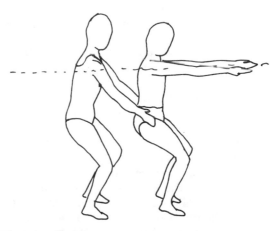

Fig. 9.7   *The patient assumes a stable sitting position in the water. The physiotherapist adopts a position behind the patient's hips to stabilize these joints*

Techniques 12, 13 and 14 utilize the principles of relative density, turbulence and metacentre (Reid Campion, 1991). These techniques are particularly useful for patients who show ataxic signs. It gives the patient a concept of mid-line structure stability while moving peripheral structures. It also allows active relearning of righting reactions while in a stable position.

Augment and Increase the Range of any Weak Movements

With the patient in a stable position, judicious positioning of the limbs or the appropriate angle of movement can augment and increase the range of any weak movement. This can be equally applied to upper motor neuron type paralysis, as well as lower motor neurone type of muscular weakness.

In central nervous system lesions, the increased effort to move the limb against gravity causes further increases in tone. In water, by allowing buoyancy to assist, the weak movement is allowed to move through a greater range than would otherwise have been possible. In doing so, a concomitant increase in tone as a result of co-contraction or associated reactions can be diminished.

15. *Starting position*: the patient assumes a stable sitting position on the physiotherapist's lap, facing away from the physiotherapist who maintains a stabilizing hold on the patient's hips. As an alternative, the patient can be supported by neck and pelvic floats in a horizontal supine float position.
Technique: the affected limb or the more affected limb is pushed passively and rapidly into the water. The upthrust effect of water will ensure that the limb returns to the surface. This action is repeated a number of times. The patient is then instructed to assist in the return of the limb to the surface of the water.
Patient appreciation: the patient becomes aware of the effect of upthrust or buoyancy of the water and once appreciation of the upward movement of the limb has taken place, the patient, when asked to assist the movement, conceptualizes the gradual muscle strength required to move the limb.

16. *Starting position*: the patient is in the horizontal supine float position or in supported side lying, for example on a plinth in the water. Flotation equipment is applied to the limb.
Technique: all the anatomical movements of the limbs can be practised, for example, in the side lying position, upper and lower limb flexion and extension movements can be attempted.
Patient appreciation: the patient appreciates movement practised through as large a range as possible. Such movements are comparable to exercises done in sling suspension on land.

17. *Starting position*: the patient is placed in the standing position in a depth of water that is at the level of the xiphisternum. Depending on the degree of dependence of the patient, one or two physiotherapists may be required to support the patient whose arms are placed around the physiotherapists' shoulders.
Technique: walking practice is encouraged and lateral weight shift is initiated by the physiotherapists.
Patient appreciation: in the water, with minimal effort and the assistance of buoyancy, extensor tone can be overridden and leg flexion is then possible, whereas, on land, the standing position can cause an increase in extensor tone to the extent that the patient is unable to flex the limb against the strength of the extensor tone. Therefore, practising ambulation in the pool will prove beneficial.

Retrain Centralized (Rotational) Pattern of Movement

Lateralizing motor deficits result in abnormal posture. Any peripheral limb or head movement occurring from this central abnormal trunk posture will be inefficient and of poor quality. Control of trunk patterns of movement can be learnt only from a position where the body does not have to work to neutralize the effects of gravity. Water offers this ideal medium.

A common problem encountered in the neurosurgical patient is the lack of shoulder and hip girdle movement and a paucity of trunk rotation. This is often seen in the 'robotic' walking pattern, where the patient has very

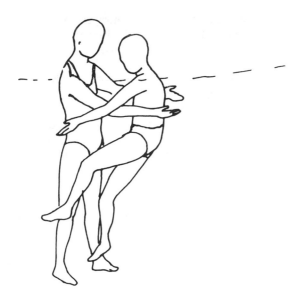

Fig. 9.8 *To create a roll through 360°*

little arm swing, head turning, trunk rotation and 'ambles' along with a 'waddling' gait. Exercise numbers 5, 6, 7, 8, 9, 11, 12, 13 and 14 can be used for this purpose also. The physiotherapist has to choose the exercise appropriate to the patient's level of motor recovery.

18. *Starting position*: the patient is in supine lying at a right angle and to one side of the physiotherapist, who supports the patient on the arm on the side to which the patient is lying. The physiotherapist's arm is at the level of the inferior angle of the scapula.

    Technique: to create a roll through 360° in front of the physiotherapist, the patient is instructed to turn the head towards the physiotherapist and to bring the outer arm and leg across the body. The physiotherapist's free arm acts as a guide and support for the patient's arm as it comes across and may facilitate the rolling action. At the completion of the roll, the patient will be in the same starting position, but on the opposite side of the physiotherapist (Reid Campion, 1991) (Fig. 9.8).

    Patient appreciation: the patient will appreciate marked vestibular stimulation along with head control, trunk rotation and body righting.

19. *Starting position*: the patient is in the horizontal supine float lying position with the physiotherapist standing between the legs at the level of the patient's knees and supporting the patient with the hands placed as high up the patient's back as possible (Fig. 9.2).

    Technique: the patient is instructed to come up to sitting, initiating the movement with the head and reaching forward with the hands, which are placed on the physiotherapist's shoulders. To facilitate the forward movement, the physiotherapist must 'sit' down in the water as the patient comes up to the sitting position astride the physiotherapist's knees (Fig. 9.5). As the patient returns to the starting position, the head must control the movement of the body back into the lying position.

    Patient appreciation: the patient becomes aware of the need for head control in initiating and controlling movement. Additionally, trunk flexion and the achievement of a functional movement from lying to sitting will be appreciated.

Retrain Reciprocal Pattern of Movement

Midline structure stability provides the basis of limb movement as reciprocal patterns of movement provide the basis of functional patterns of locomotion. Reciprocal limb movements are affected by minimal changes in tone. If the patient is well supported and the limbs allowed to move freely, the patient is able to concentrate solely on coordinating the movement and not on the effort of moving. Rhythm contributes to the smoothness in the execution of any movement pattern. This is an important concept to teach the patient when reciprocal movements are being practised.

20. *Starting position*: the patient is in the horizontal supine float position supported by neck and pelvic floats. The physiotherapist assumes a position where the patient can be assisted maximally. This may be at the patient's head to steady the patient, if necessary, but the head itself should never be held, since this destroys the patient's last opportunity to control the body and lower limbs (Reid Campion, 1991). The physiotherapist may find it an advantage

to stand by the patient's feet and guide the movement from that position.

Technique: the patient is instructed to flex and extend each of the lower limbs in turn. To ensure that the limb remains in contact with the water, the movement is done with external rotation of the hip. The patient is encouraged to maintain a smooth movement pattern by counting to four for each cycle of movement.

Patient appreciation: the patient becomes aware of coordination of the limbs, learns control of speed of movement and rhythm, so vital in neurological conditions.

21. *Starting position*: the patient is in the supine floating position as in technique 20. The physiotherapist stands behind the patient's head supporting the patient underneath the back at the level of the patient's waist.

    Technique: the patient is instructed to flex the leg in abduction and external rotation while taking the ipsilateral arm down to the knee, that is, for example, right hand to right knee. The patient will not roll if the contralateral arm and leg are held in extension.

    Patient appreciation: the patient will appreciate the movement of side flexion combined with coordination of the head, trunk and limbs. Body image and awareness of body parts will be enhanced.

22. *Starting position*: as in technique 20. The physiotherapist may stand at either the patient's head or feet. If standing at the head, support is provided underneath the patient's waist. However, if standing at the patient's feet the hold is on the lateral side of the patient's ankles.

    Technique: the patient is instructed by the physiotherapist to abduct and then adduct the legs. It may be necessary to guide the movements of abduction and adduction in which case the physiotherapist should be at the patient's feet.

    A rhythmic counting is essential in the early stages, until the patient has mastered the movement and can take over the counting. Once the movements of the legs have been mastered, abduction and adduction of the arms should be incorporated. Initially, the arms should move in the same direction as the legs. Later, the patient should be encouraged to move the upper and lower limbs in opposite directions. Rhythmical movement must be obtained at all times. In this manner, the patient can learn to propel the body through the water.

    Patient appreciation: the patient appreciates coordination of all four limbs, concentration, movement disassociation and independent mobility in the water.

23. *Starting position*: the patient is placed in the prone horizontal float position supported by a pelvic float and with the hands on the physiotherapist's shoulders. Alternatively, the hands may be placed on an air ring.

    Technique: the patient is instructed to maintain extension at the knees and perform 'straight kicks'.

    Patient appreciation: the patient becomes aware of increasing strength in the neck, trunk and limb extensor muscle groups and lower limb coordination.

Access Functional Movement Patterns

All head-injured patients have problems with new learning, to a greater or lesser extent. This problem is augmented in those patients with perceptual deficits, such as dyspraxia, decreased spatial awareness and decreased body image.

The dyspraxic patient will have great difficulty in planning and sequencing a set of exercises, but may produce the desired movement when the exercise is practised as a functional movement pattern. This is exemplified by the patient who has great difficulty in coordination arm swing while walking, but is able to coordinate all four limbs when swimming. This is especially evident in those patients who enjoyed swimming prior to the hospitalization. It is advisable to provide a float initially, so that the patient is not faced with failure at the first attempt.

24. *Starting position*: the patient is placed in the horizontal supine position facing away from the physiotherapist, who supports the patient's body underneath the back at waist level with the patient's head resting on the physiotherapist's shoulder or close to the shoulder (Fig. 9.9a).

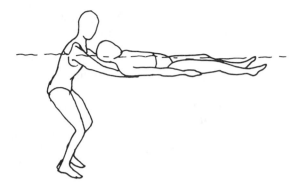

Fig. 9.9a *The patient is placed in the horizontal supine position facing away from the physiotherapist*

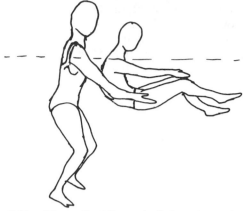

Fig. 9.9b *The patient flexes both legs towards the chest, to bring the head, shoulders and arms forward and come to the sitting position*

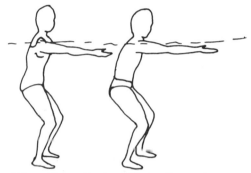

Fig. 9.9c *The patient maintains the sitting position using the head and keeping the arms forward just below the suface of the water*

Technique: the patient is instructed to flex both legs towards the chest, to bring the head, shoulders and arms forward and come to the sitting position. The patient is also instructed to blow out strongly as the head comes forward. Such action assists the forward movement of the head (Fig. 9.9b and c). To return to the starting position, the patient is instructed to bring the legs towards the chest, place the head and shoulders back slowly and then straighten the legs. The physiotherapist initially assists the patient to gain the sitting position. Gradually, such assistance is withdrawn so that the patient is finally able to accomplish the movement independently.

Balancing in the sitting position requires fine adjustments of the head, arms and hands with precise balance of the head of the spine. Turbulence judiciously and appropriately placed around the patient develops balance coordination to a greater degree once the patient is able to perform the lying to sitting action correctly and stabilize the body in the sitting position.

Patient appreciation: the patient becomes aware of how to achieve the functional movement pattern of getting from lying to sitting in water. This may carry over onto land, however, it must be realized that the pattern for land will differ in some ways from that in water. The strengthening of the trunk flexors brought about by this exercise will carry over onto all activities.

There is increasing awareness of a developing range of movements of head, trunk and lower limb flexion, which are involved in vertical rotation control (Reid Campion, 1991).

Due to the support afforded by the water, walking practice is made easier for the physiotherapist and the patient. This support, the relaxation of tone, the assistance provided to movement by buoyancy and the decreased effort required to move limbs, will often allow a patient hampered by a strong positive supporting reaction on land to achieve movement in the water. It is usually inadvisable to take a confused, restless and mobile patient into the water. Where a patient is restless and dependent, the restlessness can be directed to produce movement in the water with the use of appropriate flotation equipment and under the strict supervision of a physiotherapist, on a one-to-one basis with the patient. For the patient who is confused, but compliant and has enjoyed swimming prior to the accident, hydrotherapy is an ideal situation to start the introduction of a structured programme. The patient is allowed to move or swim by whatever means possible. The physiotherapist would be quick to observe the effect of altered body shape and provide appropriate support. Due to residual hemiparesis, a patient attempting to swim may find the affected side lagging in the water and thereby causing his body to roll. Providing the patient with a limb or trunk float or encouraging the patient to use an inflated rubber ring, may give the stability he/she needs. Encouraged by the success of his/her effort, the patient will then persist with this exercise.

Pacing the patient while the latter is 'swimming' allows the physiotherapist slowly to encourage the patient to concentrate on one activity. Aerobic activity is aided and this in turn helps the patient to concentrate. An exercise programme such as mat exercises will have no meaning to a confused patient, and their insistence will only encourage increasing levels of frustration for the patient. The sedative effects of heat and hydrotherapy on the restless patient has been documented by Wilson and Kasch (1963) and Kraus (1973).

Encourage and Develop Efficient Breath Control and Voice Production

Voice production is dependent on good breathing patterns. Many patients who are 'mute' or have poor phonation because of their head injury, have benefited from hydrotherapy conducted in collaboration with the speech pathologist (this is the term used in Australia for a speech therapist).

Briefly, efficient breath control and phonation is hampered by the increase in tone in the muscles of the neck and abdomen. This tone can effectively splint the expansion of the rib cage and diaphragmatic excursion required to produce effective breath control. In the water, emphasis is placed on total relaxation. This is obtained, in the horizontal supine float position, by the use of floats which provide total support to the arms, legs, trunk and head. The relaxation achieved can be utilized to teach the patient proper use of the abdominal musculature to produce and control the rate and

length of inspiration and expiration. The speech pathologist's participation is vital, preferably in the pool alongside the physiotherapist, to ensure that normal phonatory patterns and speech are successfully re-established.

Hydrotherapy encourages movement and play. Both can be used to facilitate and guide patients to produce voice and speech as part of their exercise programme. The speech pathologist should be encouraged to participate and contribute to this activity in the water.

The strength of oral musculature has bearing on both speech and effective feeding. To strengthen these muscles, blowing activities should be encouraged. Such activities include blowing bubbles in the water and also blowing lightweight plastic objects across the surface of the water.

Produce Psychological Effects

Whatever the style and however many floats it takes, the disabled patient gets enjoyment from moving through the water under his or her own volition. This allows the patient a sense of achievement and freedom and helps reinforce a positive attitude necessary for any long-term rehabilitation.

Hydrotherapy is a welcome break from routine for those patients who enjoy the water. When improvement is measured in months, patients enjoy the change of medium. Most people associate the pool with recreation, relaxation and enjoyment and therefore readily accept working in the water.

Treat any Orthopaedic Complications

The treatment of orthopaedic complications by hydrotherapy is covered in another chapter. The force of trauma that produces a head injury may also produce fractured limbs and or spine.

When a patient is initially out of a plaster cast, joint stiffness causes pain and thus a reluctance to move the affected limb. This, in turn leads to increased joint stiffness and further pain. The warmth of the water relieves joint stiffness (Wadsworth and Chanmugam, 1983) and may decrease the pain. In the case of a patient who has suffered a fracture of the tibia and fibula, when the plaster of paris cast is removed the attention is centred on the stiff joint – the knee and ankle. This will cause a stronger perception of pain, largely as a result of the expectation of pain and stiffness. Instead of focusing on knee flexion exercises, the physiotherapist should choose movement patterns that will involve knee flexion, such as technique 24, which provides a means of obtaining the desired increase in the range of the knee movement combined with total trunk patterns of movement (vertical rotation).

Head injured-patients who are expected to grade the degree of weight-bearing on the affected joint, especially when they have associated paralysis, can be helped by practising ambulation in the water. Depending on the depth of water chosen, the weight on the limb can be accurately monitored in terms of weight bearing of total body weight (Harrison and Bulstrode, 1987).

For patients with oedematous limbs, exercising in the deeper end of the pool will help decrease the swelling in the limbs in accordance with Pascal's Law (Reid Campion, 1991).

To Increase Cardiovascular Fitness

A return to the demands of the patient's previous employment is unlikely where the patient has undergone neurosurgery, as the patient's medical condition compromises fitness. All head-injured patients, who have required hospitalization for a length of time have compromised fitness. Therefore, all patients expecting to return to work should be given a programme of cardiovascular fitness training. Energy requirement to move in water is far greater than on land, according to the work of Froud and Zahm (Reid Campion, 1991). Supervising a cardiovascular fitness programme, in the hydrotherapy pool, is less time-consuming than on land. The patient entering the pool for cardiovascular fitness training will find a pool temperature of 35°C very exhausting. A venue with a lower pool temperature will have to be considered for this type of programme.

Opportunities for Recreation and Socialization

The severely disabled patient who finds independent movement difficult on land may achieve such mobility in the water. The properties of water provide a medium where freedom of movement can be obtained.

By providing appropriate flotation equipment, the physiotherapist can teach the patient to utilize whatever mobility has been regained to move through the water. The patient's shape and/or density will have been affected by the injury and this must be carefully assessed prior to using flotation equipment. Wherever possible, such equipment should be kept to a minimum, and the ideal is that the patient should be able to move through the water without any support, if total independence is to be gained. A patient confined to a wheelchair, due to involuntary movements, will demonstrate a considerable diminution of the ataxic or choreoathetoid movements once in the water, provided the strokes are adapted to keep the limb under water. One such patient, despite the presence of severe choreoathetoid, ataxic and occasional ballistic movement as a result of a head injury, was taught to swim. He was initially taught relaxation, breath control and coordination. Selective strengthening of the extensor muscles was then implemented. This was followed by the retraining of rotational movement patterns. The patient was then taught swimming strokes. He now enjoys swimming, totally submerged. The breast-stroke action used is totally coordinated while under the water, but any work on the surface is noticeably less coordinated. Recreational activities on land require modification of equipment and able-bodied helpers. In the water, an efficient assessment of the patient's ability and quality of movement by the physiotherapist is all that is needed to implement a similar programme.

Recreational programmes can be developed to cater for group activities. Neurosurgical patients, especially the head injured, are often socially isolated by a motor, perceptual or behavioural problem. Working in a group helps the patient learn social skills necessary for integration into the mainstream of society.

CONTRAINDICATIONS

Some problems experienced by the neurosurgical patient contraindicate hydrotherapy as a treatment modality.

1. When a diagnosis of fractured base of skull is made, it is important to seek medical clearance prior to instituting a hydrotherapy programme. A fracture in

the base of the skull points to possible communication into the meninges. If the patient inhales water, it is possible for water borne infection to communicate with the brain, giving rise to meningitis.

2. Patients incontinent of bowel and bladder are not taken into the pool. The latter problem in male patients is easily overcome. Most dependent patients establish a routine of bladder and bowel continence spontaneously. This allows a hydrotherapy programme to be undertaken during the patient's 'dry' period.

3. The effect of the heat of the hydrotherapy pool on a patient with high blood pressure, especially if the latter is a result of a head injury, and on unclipped aneurysm, is unknown. These patients are not taken into the pool for a hydrotherapy programme.

4. Royal Perth Infection Control (Microbiology Department) recommends that the following patients should not use the hydrotherapy pool:

   - Patients with Methicillan Resistant Staphylococcus Aureus or Multiple Resistant Gram Negative Bacteria who have not been cleared
   - Patient's with vesicular skin conditions
   - Patient's with open/weeping lesions that cannot be sealed with waterproof dressing
   - Patients with diarrhoea/enteric infection who are incontinent of faeces and those with urinary tract infection who are incontinent
   - Patients with indwelling catheters
   - Patients with short-term CVP line
   - Patients with blood borne infections – HIV, HBV and HCV that have open lesions or lesions which produce exudate/blood. Otherwise, this group need not be excluded.

As part of the hydrotherapy chemical maintenance regime at RPRH, the Physiotherapy Department uses Bromine as the active agent. This was done to reduce cost and for the comfort of staff working in the area for extended periods. Some patients can be sensitive to bromine, hydrotherapy is offered to these patients on advice.

Patients with percutaneous enteral gastrostomy (peg) can be taken into the pool if there is no infection at the site of insertion and the peg is securely capped and sealed. It has been found that the most successful way of sealing the site is to cover the peg with a large sheet of Op-site dressing.

UNTOWARD EFFECTS

Some patients may have adverse reactions after hydrotherapy sessions, and it is important to take note of these:

- Patients may exhibit an increase in tone. If this tone increase is a consistent feature after the second or third session, hydrotherapy should cease and may be reintroduced at a later date.
- Some patients take on a 'hot flushed' look, this usually points to a physiological inability to cope with the heat and hydrotherapy is discontinued for a while.
- Patients on sedative drugs to control restlessness may appear extremely lethargic and tired after a pool session.
- Patients with low blood pressure should be monitored closely. Their blood pressure before and after sessions should be taken.
- Due to the nature of the patient's dependence, they are unable to communicate simple problems, like water being retained in the ear. Due to their debilitation, these patients are prone to persistent ear infections.

HINTS FOR SUCCESS

To be successful in treating a neurosurgical patient in water, a few guidelines should be followed:

- Where hydrotherapy is being used as a treatment modality and not as a recreational facility, treatment should always be on a one-to-one basis. Where group activity is involved in the treatment programme, the one-to-one basis operates within the group.
- Treatment should be goal oriented. Having assessed the patient and analysed the

main problems, the physiotherapist should develop an exercise programme that will achieve specific results.

- Hydrotherapy should not be abandoned as a treatment modality if no success is initially forthcoming. The programme can be reintroduced at a later date for such a patient.
- Where availability of trained assistants is a problem, family members can be trained to assist. This gives the family a sense of participation in the patient's recovery process. Being a part of the patient's programme is important to family members, as it helps in their effort to come to terms with the tragedy that has occurred.
- Introduce games towards the end of each session and allow group participation when possible.

REFERENCES

Blatteis C.M. (1960). Afferent stimulation of shivering. *American Journal of Physiology*, **199**: 698.

Fisher E. and Solomon S. (1965). Physiological response to heat and cold. In *Therapeutic Heat and Cold*, (S. Licht and H.L. Kamenetz, eds), Baltimore: Waverly Press, pp. 126–169.

Franchimont P., Juchmes J. and Lecomte J. (1983). Hydrotherapy – mechamisms and indications. *Pharmacology Therapeutics*, **20**: 79–93.

Harris S.R. (1978). Neurodevelopmental treatment approach for teaching swimming to cerebral palsied children. *Physical Therapy*, **58**: 979–983.

Harrison R. and Bulstrode S. (1987). Percentage weight bearing during partial immersion in the hydrotherapy pool. *Physiotherapy Practice*, **3**: 60–63.

Herman R. (1982). Functional recovery in the visual and vestibular pathways. *Int. Rehab. Med.*, **4**: 173–176.

Kraus R. (1973). *Therapeutic Recreation Services – Principles and Practices*, Philadelphia: W.B. Saunders.

Lee J.M. and Warren M.P. (1978). *Cold Therapy in Rehabilitation*, London: Bell & Hyman.

Reid Campion M. (1991). *Hydrotherapy in Paediatrics*, Oxford: Heinemann Medical Books.

Skinner A.T. and Thompson A.M. (1983). *Duffield's Exercise in Water*, 3rd edn, London: Baillière Tindall.

Sullivan P.E., Markos, P.D. and Minor M.A.D. (1982). *An Integrated Approach to Therapeutic Exercise: Theory and Clinical Application*, Reston, Va: Reston Pub. Co.

Wadsworth J. and Chanmugam A.P.P. (1983). *Electrophysical Agents in Physiotherapy*, 2nd edn, Marrickville, NSW: Science Press.

Wilson I.H. and Kasch F.W. (1983). Medical aspects of swimming. In *Medical Hydrology* (S. Licht, ed.), Newhaven: Elizabeth Licht.

RECOMMENDED READING

Euler C.V. and Soderberg U. (1956). The relation between gamma motor activity and the electroencephalogram. *Experientia*, **12**: 278–279.

Harrison R. and Bulstrode S. (1987). Percentage weight bearing during partial immersion in the hydrotherapy pool. *Physiotherapy Practice*, **3**: 60–63.

Herman R. (1982). A therapeutic approach based on theories of motor control. *Int. Rehab. Med.*, **4**: 185–189.

Herman R. (1982). Functional recovery in the visual and vestibular pathways. *Int. Rehab. Med.*, **4**: 170–173.

Ito Masae (1972). Neural design of the cerebellar motor control system. *Brain Research*, **40**: 81–84.

Reid Campion (1991). *Hydrotherapy in Paediatrics*, 2nd edn, Oxford: Butterworth-Heinemann.

Sullivan P.E., Markos P.D. and Minor M.A.D. (1982). *An Integrated Approach to Therapeutic Exercise: Theory and Clinical Application*, Reston Va.: Reston Pub. Co.

Wadsworth H. and Chanmugam A.P.P. (1983) *Electrophysical Agents in Physiotherapy*, 2nd edn, Marrickville, NSW: Science Press.

ACKNOWLEDGEMENTS

Margaret Reid Campion – whose training and guidance has formed the basis of the treatment of neurosurgical patients in hydrotherapy. My thanks to Margaret for allowing the liberal use of exercises and drawings from her book.

Serena Pearce and other physiotherapy colleagues for helping me in the formulation and practice of the hydrotherapy techniques.

Margaret Davies-Slate, Librarian, RPRH, for title search and reference.

Royal Perth Hospital, Microbiology Department, and J. Buchanan, Superintendent Physiotherapist, RPRH for release of infection control policy and information on pool maintenance.

10

Neurological rehabilitation

Sue Gray

INTRODUCTION

Normal control of our bodies is the outcome of complex interplay between genetics, motivation, training and sensory factors.

Shepherd, 1988

Hydrotherapy, as part of the rehabilitation process for people with neurological conditions, is more widely recognized for those with lower motor neurone lesions than for those who have suffered cortical neurone damage – previously upper motor neurone (Portisky, 1992). It is becoming more accepted though not well understood or routinely used for such conditions. There is a wide spectrum of opinions but limited research or information on the effects or outcomes of treatment of adult neurologically damaged people in water. Rehabilitation aims to restore a person to a life that is as independent as possible. A wide variety of treatment methods are available, hydrotherapy having a definite place in the treatment of neurologically damaged people.

This chapter comprises:

- **A brief outline of current thinking in neurological rehabitation.**
- **Neuromuscular effects of immersion, related to the hydrodynamic principles.**
- **Discussion of potential problem areas and contraindications.**
- **Guidelines for treatment planning.**
- **Indicators for treatment of a variety of specific conditions appropriate for hydrotherapy.**
- **Illustrated practical techniques for use in the treatment of neurologically damaged people.**

BACKGROUND TO NEUROLOGICAL TREATMENTS

The central nervous system (CNS) is constantly receiving information from the environment, processing it and acting on relevant information while disregarding or storing the non-relevant information (Kidd *et al.*, 1992). The normal CNS has a great ability to adapt and change. The term neuroplasticity is used to describe this phenomenon.

Movement occurs because of our ability to stabilize certain parts of our bodies and move others (Bobath, 1990). Many of the abnormalities in movement that occur result as the neurologically damaged patient attempts to move up against gravity (Musa, 1986). The increase in tone that is required often creates a chaotic result due to lack of inhibition. When CNS is damaged, the organizational and monitoring ability of the brain is affected. The recovery potential of the CNS is more diverse than previously thought (Kaplan, 1988; Stevenson, 1993). This provides an even greater incentive to physiotherapists working with these patients to access and exploit this potential. To be therapeutic the physiotherapist has to learn how to aid the patient to access and redirect the remaining available resources to achieve maximum recovery. To be effective treatment needs to produce changes in the neuro-anatomy of the CNS by influencing dendrite construction and neurotransmitters. Therapeutic treatment is that which stimulates a reaction without overstressing the damaged system and minimizes abnormal responses.

Anatomical changes strengthen synaptic connections, guide axonal sprouting and facilitate the unmasking of alternative or subsequent pathways (Goldberger and Murray, 1988). The CNS learns by demand. Left to its own devices, the damaged CNS will adapt to the stimulus created by the environment and gravity, developing stereotypic patterns and compensatory strategies leading to contractures and limited function (Musa, 1986).

Treatment involves physiotherapists in using their handling skills and their own intact CNS to fill in the gaps in the patient's damaged system. This allows patients to experience normal movement and to achieve their intended goal. In practice this means that initially the physiotherapist encourages the patient to perform as much of the intended movement as possible. The physiotherapist then provides the additional control and muscle activity to assist the patient to achieve the chosen goal. Great sensitivity in handling is required by the physiotherapist. Too much support prevents learning, too little allows the movement quality to deteriorate and limits long-term change. *During treatment of a neurologically damaged person in water, the water takes over part of the work of the physiotherapist.* For example, in order to facilitate stabilizing activity around a joint the effects of the negative pressures created by turbulence can be used to create facilitatory resistance (see Facilitation of movement (No. 8, p. 221) in the Practical techniques section.) Verbal commands can be kept to a minimum and direct handling by the physiotherapist is not required allowing greater access to an automatic responses at spinal level. The physiotherapist is manipulating the water environment to assist or resist and facilitate automatic movement. It is therefore essential to understand the properties of water and the effects that can occur. Once verbal commands are used the information is assimilated at a much higher level in the CNS (Dietz, 1992). Treatment that accesses more automatic movements improves carryover of treatment into normal function even after formal treatment has finished.

To summarize, in the course of treating a neurologically damaged person, whatever the medium, the physiotherapist's handling has to provide just enough facilitation to allow achievement of the chosen goal but not so much that the stimulus to change the anatomy of the CNS is absent. Neuro-anatomical change at axonal level is needed to support long-term improvement.

When treating the patient the physiotherapist needs to be on the 'cutting edge', just breaking new ground, but should not be over-challenging or over-supportive. The aim is function not compensation.

NEUROMUSCULAR EFFECTS OF IMMERSION

The neuromuscular effect of placing a human body in water is very variable. A sound understanding of the hydrodynamic principles is essential for effective treatment (Skinner and Thomson, 1989). Hydrodynamic principles are dealt with in Chapter 3, p. 14.

The neuromuscular effects of immersion are:

- changed points of reference for balance
- tonal adaptations
- access to the components of movement.

Changed Points of Reference for Balance

Balance is a state where the body is in stable equilibrium. On dry land, balance is preserved by keeping the Centre of Gravity (COG) within the Base of Support (BOS). In water the COG interacts with the Centre of Buoyancy (COB). A different point of reference is created causing a rotational effect, the relationship between the COB and COG, being termed the metacentric effect. The changed body shape caused by deformity and the changed density which can be caused by increased or decreased muscle tone may affect where the COB is located within the body and therefore the metacentric effect on the floating body.

The stability of the body in water depends on the ability of the person to control these rotational effects at will. The patient has to learn to appreciate where and when stability is lost and to be able to correct it.

The metacentric effect is a very useful tool in the treatment of the neurological patient (p. 14).

For example, with a patient in supine, very small changes in the relationship of the COB and COG create a need to sustain balance. Initially the treatment involves making the patient aware of the changes in balance and then facilitating self-correction. It is possible to help the patient to access the automatic balance reactions (equilibrium and saving and righting reactions). The key point of stability on dry land is the trunk (Bobath, 1990). In water, very fine grading of balance within the trunk can be practised in floating supine, where rotation can occur around the longitudinal or vertical axis. Longitudinal rotation occurs around an axis running head to toe and vertical rotation around an axis running at right angles to this. Working with the patient in water provides increased opportunity to raise the patient's awareness of his trunk control both voluntarily and automatically. A large amount of the muscle activity in the trunk is automatic; it occurs without conscious thought.

The effects of the base of support are different in water from the effects on dry land. The base of support in water is dynamic and moving. The centre of buoyancy is also dynamic and moves as the body posture changes, therefore instability alters balance. Even with a large base of support, i.e. floating in supine, there is a greater potential for instability than with a patient lying supine on a bed. This can again be exploited to enhance the patient's awareness and to facilitate movement and control.

In summary, water creates a change in the points of reference for balance in all postural sets or starting positions. The body is more easily destabilized but within a supportive low gravity environment. Destabilizing effects can be more easily seen and felt by the patient, and therefore re-educated. For example the effect of a slight increase in tone on one side (as in hemiplegia) of a supine patient has a magnified destabilizing effect in water, which may be easier for the patient to appreciate and learn to correct when assisted by skilled handling.

Tonal Adaptations

Several factors affect the tonal changes that are often detectable in the immersed patient. In water, minimal gravity acts on the person because the up-thrust is equal to the weight of the body of water displaced. If this were the only factor then muscle tone would be expected

to fall. On dry land, tone is recruited as the body comes up against gravity. However, the dynamic nature of the base of support and the potential for instability may provide a stimulus to recruit tone and have to be controlled and directed to allow them to be useful in treatment. Another factor that tends to decrease tone is buoyancy. Movement is easier if the buoyancy effect is used to assist and therefore tone recruitment is reduced. The CNS controls distribution of tone very economically; tone reduces when it is not demanded by the environment; for example, a normal person will have less muscle tone when lying than when standing. The afferent input is changed during immersion (Clements, 1984) as there are reduced afferent signals to the tactile and joint receptors. This may lead to gravity functions such as walking being more difficult in water due to the reduced afferent feedback. Assessment of gait in water, however, is always required since experimenting with the patient in different depths may allow a balance between the *advantages* of the assistance of water and the *disadvantages* of lack of afferent feedback. The low toned patient requires stimulus to raise tone and is therefore likely to be better when walking in water up to the waist since gravity will have a greater impact.

The properties of turbulence and drag can also be utilized to recruit more tone and therefore more normal movement in a patient whose tone is abnormally low. If the patient has increased muscle tone the increase of tone recruited by using turbulence and drag will tend to push the movement quality into abnormality. Care must be taken that the recruited tone is functional and not compensatory, i.e. abnormal head and neck fixation often occurring as a compensation for an unstable pelvis.

There is decreased information to the vestibular apparatus in normal people when subjected to a micro-gravity environment (Gabriel, 1968; Homick, 1977). This may offer another explanation as to why tone is reduced as an effect of immersion. After brain trauma there is a loss of inhibition which can lead to 'overreaction' in the CNS. The effect of reduced afferent information reaching the brain results in less chaotic reaction to gravity stimuli, allowing the patient a greater chance to control his or her movements more normally.

Kozlovskya (1983) indicated that a decrease in the gravitational load (microgravity) initiates a significant shift in the motor control system. He detected an increased excitability of the central integrative mechanisms at spinal level. This is very relevant to physiotherapists. It provides another way into the CNS, at a more automatic level. Normal movement facilitated automatically has the best outcome and carryover.

Heat has been shown to affect muscle tone by inhibiting tonic activity. This response occurring quickly after immersion assists the physiotherapist in the release and lengthening of soft tissues and helps the prevention of contractures occurring due to stereotyped patterning and limited movement.

Psychological effects of enjoyment, relaxation on the one hand or fear and apprehension on the other will affect muscle tone. Preparation and good information gathering, either from the patient or from a close relative or friend, will equip the physiotherapist for most problems and allow alteration in the approach accordingly.

The effect of immersion on the sympathetic nervous system due to the depression of noradrenaline production (O'Hare, 1985) may partially account for the feeling of well-being that patients often report after hydrotherapy treatment. The experience of suffering from neurological damage is very traumatic and disruptive on every level, and the psychological effects of immersion should not be overlooked. A boost to the patient's motivation can greatly improve the overall effectiveness of treatment.

Access to Components of Movements

A patient floating in supine can rotate through vertical or longitudinal axis (Reid Campion, 1991). The ability to rotate around a longitudinal axis is more primitive in developmental terms (Golani, 1981). This concept has been further explored in a study completed in rats (Szechtman, 1985). After hypothalamic lesions, the rats were completely akinetic but slowly recovered. Initially they learned to rotate around a longitudinal axis and then when near recovery they learned to rotate around a vertical axis. In treating patients the theory can be explored by working on longitudinal rolling initially on the basis that it is the forerunner of more complex activity (Cools, 1992). Normal child development occurs in this order also. The patient is first helped to feel the roll in the

longitudinal plane and then facilitated actively to correct it.

Progression is then made to the vertical roll. It is important to ensure that the patient is facilitated to use his or her trunk as much as possible to initiate and control the roll rather than the limbs and head. This allows the most normal carryover.

The effects of immersion also allow for the finer breakdown of movement goals or finer breakdown of progressions, by using the effects of buoyancy, turbulence and the metacentric effect. For example, in order to facilitate movement in an upper limb with abnormal movement, initially the effect of buoyancy can be used to float the arm away from the body resulting in a 'letting go' of unwanted muscle tone, specific turbulence can then be used to assist and facilitate movement. The metacentric effect can be used to facilitate automatic saving reactions. This introduces a much more graduated movement progression than is possible on dry land.

PROBLEM AREAS

Many neurological physiotherapists are wary of treating their patients in water, reserving hydrotherapy for the later stages when 'not too much harm can be done and the patient enjoys doing something a bit different'. In the light of this the following is a discussion of some areas that may prove contentious (all treatment techniques mentioned here are described in the illustrated section at the end of the chapter.)

Unwanted Tonal Changes

Although the evidence is overwhelming that immersion should reduce tone, this is often not the experience of the physiotherapist taking her patient into the pool. The causes of unwanted tonal change are many. The pool environment is often noisy and strange and may make the patient tense and apprehensive. The effort required to undress may have an adverse effect and possible variations of temperature can recruit tone that the patient may not be able to control.

Once in the water, apprehension about lack of stability and unfamiliar reactions may overshadow the beneficial effects and cause unwanted tonal abnormality. Any lack of knowledge or of confidence in the medium on the part of the physiotherapist can lead to increased anxiety in the patient; poor handling frequently results in increased tone. The physiotherapist can compensate for all of the above difficulties by careful preparation and skilled handling. Firstly, mental adjustment of the patient (p. 21) both prior to entering the water and on immersion can alleviate anxiety and help avoid an increase in tone. Patients must be given time to acclimatize to the water; those with a damaged CNS may need a longer time to adjust than others. Secondly, it is important not to react to any anxiety and tension by holding the patient too closely or providing support with floats. Thirdly, avoid over-stimulating the patient; even small amounts may provide huge CNS stimulation which might or might not be wanted. Reactions are often slower in water than on dry land and it is tempting to superimpose one activity upon another without waiting to see the initial effect.

The physiotherapist also needs to remember that there is a huge level of hidden activity. Visual assessment of the patient can be inaccurate, and there is also constant equilibrium work within the trunk that is difficult to see. This can be likened to working with a patient on a gym ball where very little input from the physiotherapist can make the patient work hard.

Control and Stability of the Patient in Water

Water is a moving and dynamic environment that makes the acquisition of control and stability essential for everyone entering the medium. Careful choice of starting position is important. Water has properties that are not available on land and these unique features should be used fully if the value of water for hydrotherapy is to be realized.

The physiotherapist needs to acquire the skills of stabilization and control if the patient's treatment is to be adequately facilitated. By its nature water is supportive and it allows the physiotherapist to lift and move the patient easily and to avoid the necessity of supporting the patient too much or too high out of the water.

When working with a patient in water, consideration should be given as to whether a second person may be needed to assist rather than relying on flotation equipment; this may be particularly so where a patient is non-communicating, may inhale water, or be unsafe in taking oral fluids.

Working slowly and letting water assist activities and movements increases control. Every programme should include adjustment of the patient to water and the teaching of breath control (Association of Swimming Therapy, 1992) which when acquired removes one of the main sources of anxiety for both the patient and the physiotherapist.

Any task requiring accurate visual assessment of the part of the body under water, for example early gait re-education, is more difficult in the pool. The advantages of assisted and slower movements need to be utilized and sometimes combined with dry-land assessment and treatment. The components of the movement, for example, in gait, pelvic stability and knee control, can be worked on in water and combined into the functional activity on land during the early stages and in the pool again later.

The pool is an excellent environment for working to improve the patient's saving and equilibrium reactions. The fact that loss of balance occurs more slowly because of the higher density of the water and 'drag' effect allows the patient more time to react, so that there is a feeling of safety and better control is achieved. Unwanted reactions may still occur, however, if the degree of instability allowed is not carefully matched to the patient's level of ability.

The use of the head as the initiator of movement in the pool is crucial to the teaching of rotational control in water. This often raises concern particularly among Bobath trained therapists. Where a patient is fixing or compensating hugely with the head on dry land, work in the pool can be modified to reduce this. If overuse of the head occurs the patient will probably have also recruited excessive tone around the neck and shoulders. This in turn restricts normal movement of the head on the body which is a requirement of normal balance reactions in any medium. A very successful technique is to use the supportive effect of the water to teach the patient to 'let-go' of tone and thus allow more free and normal movement. (Practical techniques 1, using neck collar.) The programme advances to enabling the patient to perceive normal movement of the head on the trunk. Working in supine, the increased instability in water magnifies the trunk and head movements, enabling the patient more easily to perceive, understand and re-learn control.

Lack of Ability to Observe Directly the Quality of Movement under Water

Direct observation of under-water activity is not easy in the pool, the physiotherapist who knows the patient well can get useful and effective feedback by touch. There are a variety of other indicators of the quality of movement being performed, for example head position, body posture, arm movements, facial expression and so on.

Problems of Impaired Sensation

Gross sensory loss has in the past been considered a contraindication to hydrotherapy. Often patients with severe sensory difficulties find working in the water rather disorientating because they cannot see what is happening under water which reduces visual feedback substantially. Usually with careful introduction to the water, skilled handling and well-planned treatment goals, these patients can gain great benefit from hydrotherapy, both physically and psychologically. Care should be taken with the choice of starting positions; walking in water is often more difficult for these patients. Work in supine with longitudinal and vertical rolling offers a 'way in', i.e. access to the Central Postural Control Mechanism, that is not available to the physiotherapist on dry land. The trunk movements that occur are therefore easier for the sensorily damaged patient to perceive as they trigger a higher level of activity in the CNS.

Non-verbal facilitation of automatic movement in water, occurring mainly at spinal level, is an important tool in treating sensorily deprived patients.

Level of Breath Control and Airway Protection

Patients who have been assessed as having unsafe swallowing can be treated in the pool if the airway can be adequately protected. The physiotherapist has to ensure that no water accidentally enters the mouth. On occasion this may mean having a second person in the water to assist with treatment. Even patients who appear to have no deficits in speech or oral function can find that their breath control is not as automatic as before their incident. This is often the root of fear and refusal to continue with hydrotherapy. Careful assessment is required at the beginning of the treatment session. Breath control is carefully monitored as new activities are introduced.

The physiotherapist needs to check breath control both in isolation, and combined with another activity. If the patient's attention is distracted by a physical activity breath control often becomes unsafe and may give rise to anxiety. For example, during · the more advanced stages of the longitudinal roll (Practical techniques 5), the patient needs to control his or her breathing and initiate and control the roll at the same time. It is important that the patient learns to blow out whenever their mouth comes near the water. Breath control does not mean breath holding but blowing out gently on expiration (Association of Swimming Therapy, 1992). Ideally the patient's physical activities should be matched by progressively improving levels of breath control. In the neurologically damaged patient, however, levels of control are sometimes variable, due for example to fatigue and distraction. The physiotherapist needs therefore to be constantly vigilant.

Helping the patient feel confident to have water on their face and control breathing reliably will greatly increase their confidence and ability to make the most of the hydrotherapy session. The effect of hydrostatic pressure increasing with depth provides facilitation to breath control if the patient is upright in the box position (Practical techniques 6) or standing in deep water. For those patients with voice and breath control problems, working alongside a speech and language therapist (SLT) in the pool is very beneficial. The effect of immersion in normalizing the tone in the abdominal muscles is a significant contribution to improved breath control. For those patients who have a problem with associated reactions while attempting to vocalize, working in the pool is useful. The reduction of muscle tone that is achievable improves control and the general effect on body position of the unwanted movements is less dramatic, being slower and easier to control in the water. For example, a patient who experiences increased flexor tone in the upper limbs when making the effort of vocalization or deep breathing will experience a dampening effect on muscle tone due to the increased density of the water, the warmth of the water and the reduced effects of gravity. Maintaining as normal a tone as possible throughout the body improves function and carry-over of improvement.

The patient who is struggling with lip closure and nasal breathing in land-based SLT treatment sessions may well benefit from hydrotherapy. The automatic survival stimulus for lip closure, preventing water entering the mouth, often enables successful lip closure and improved breathing in the water. Patients who have difficulty with air escaping out of the nose when it should not do so benefit from working in water with their speech therapists.

Patients with Limited Communication

Many neurologically damaged people have restricted communication. The effect of the extra noise in a pool, water in the ears and the physiotherapist behind or above the patient may compromise communication. Special care has therefore to be taken. It is much easier if the pool physiotherapist also treats the patient on dry land and is already familiar with any difficulties. Special consideration must also be given to patients with hearing problems; even patients with normal hearing will be compromised in water.

The pool environment distorts noise and this, combined with the effects of having the ears under water, may compromise some patients severely, and they may require additional consideration.

The Visually Impaired Patient

Physiotherapists treating visually impaired patients need to have a working knowledge of their patient's level of vision. Vision may be distorted, reduced in acuity, or both. Water tends to reflect and distort light, which some patients find very disconcerting. If patients wear glasses, consideration may be given to keeping them on in the initial sessions until the patient is well orientated.

Epilepsy

Patients who have had brain trauma have an increased incidence of epilepsy. This need not affect their hydrotherapy treatment (p. 155). All staff must be fully conversant with the emergency procedure and there should always be a member of staff, pool-side. Even in the throes of a highly mobile fit, the patient may be restrained safely in the water until quiet and then lifted or hoisted from the pool and treated appropriately.

Cognitive and Behavioural Disorders

Some patients who suffer a neurological incident also have cognitive or behavioural problems. Care should be taken when assessing these patients for treatment as the benefits to the patient of hydrotherapy need to outweigh the difficulties they present. Assessment needs to take this into account as well as the possible hazards of the pool area and the risks attendant on any activity in water and the possibility that extra staff may be required. Hydrotherapy can be used as a reward in a behavioural programme but liaison with the full rehabilitation team is necessary on a regular basis.

The Staffing Implications of Treating Neurological Patients in Hydrotherapy

Neuro-hydrotherapy may require a higher staff to patient ratio than dry-land therapy. All but some of the most severely disabled patients can be successfully treated for the whole of their treatment, once in the pool, by only one physiotherapist, but more support staff may be needed to assist with showering, dressing and emergency procedure. There may also be a need for training and education of staff as treatment of the neurologically damaged patient in water may have only been covered minimally in undergraduate training and older staff may have received no input at all.

Local variation and staff availability may determine the relative merits of whether patients are better treated by pool-based physiotherapists or neurological physiotherapists trained in hydrotherapy skills. If neurological physiotherapists are also able to treat their patients on land and in the water they gain greatly from the experience and offer continuity to their patient's rehabilitation.

Floats: To Use or Not to Use?

Careful consideration of the use of floats is required; is their use for the benefit of the patient or the physiotherapist? For the treatment of the neurologically damaged person in water the properties that are particularly useful are the dynamic support of the water and the easy access to smooth free movement that is achievable with very little effort.

The use of floats can inhibit this. They give a false image of the body posture in water and this may delay or inhibit learning about independent control. Floats do not compensate for asymmetry, and they compound the problems of learning to control unwanted movement. If floats are thought to be needed for safety, careful assessment is needed. The ideal solution is for the physiotherapist to modify the intended programme to allow for special emphasis on teaching the patient to keep safe. If this is not possible due to the severity of the patient's problem then another technique or a helper should be used to obtain the best outcome from the treatment. Floats are not as adaptable as a helper, who can alter the support as and when required. The involvement of willing relatives or friends of the patient, actually in the water, can often be appropriate and very beneficial both to patients and relatives. In some neurological conditions the use of the modified PNF (Adler *et al.*, 1993), called Bad Ragaz techniques, is appropriate. Floats are then essential.

Some of the techniques in the illustrated section of the chapter use floats. As a general rule those techniques that are aiming to re-educate balance and control do not use floats but those stretching soft tissue or utilizing the drag of the water do.

Occasionally a patient enjoys being totally floated and left to have some time alone, with supervision but without handling. Severely affected patients rarely experience such freedom on dry land. This can also be used to provide relaxation.

Continence Difficulties

Catheterization or urinary incontinence/poor control is not a contraindication to hydrotherapy. Faecal incontinence is a contraindication to hydrotherapy unless a routine has been established that is reliable.

TREATMENT PLANNING FOR NEUROLOGICALLY DAMAGED PEOPLE

Treating a neurological patient in water offers a wide variety of options in a highly dynamic environment. The following are guidelines for assessing the benefits of hydrotherapy and planning the treatment. In each of the three treatment sections there is far more than would be included in one session. For example a whole treatment session might be devoted to only one or two activities in perhaps two starting positions.

Special Considerations for Hydrotherapy

Patients often have quite strong feelings about swimming and possibly bad experiences which colour their perceptions when they are offered hydrotherapy treatment. These need to be discussed and taken into consideration. Each patient needs to be carefully assessed and any potential contraindications to hydrotherapy investigated. Treatment planning is important: definite aims and objectives must be set. This has the added bonus of providing data to support the validity of the service required. Hydrotherapy affects the level of resources required to carry out the treatment and, as it is potentially a dangerous environment, a well thought-out rationale for treatment is essential.

Integration of hydrotherapy into the overall multi-disciplinary treatment of the patient is important and this should include the timing of the course of treatment in the rehabilitation process. Finally, the involvement of relatives and friends where appropriate adds a useful dimension to treatment and enhances the integration of relearned skills into the patient's everyday life after formal treatment has finished.

NEUROLOGICAL CONDITIONS

The following comprises information about specific abnormalities and special considerations for the treatment of some common damaged cortico-neural conditions (Poritsky, 1992): hemiplegia, Parkinson's disease, multiple sclerosis, ataxia and hypotonia perceptual problems, oral and breath control, and the

Table 10.1 Aims and techniques of levels of hydrotherapy treatment

	Primary	*Intermediate*	*Advanced*
Aims	Acclimatization to the pool environment and the water	Continuing adjustment to the pool environment	Total adjustment to the pool environment
	Improved breath control	Continuing breath control	Consistently reliable breath control with no prompting
	Appreciation of longitudinal roll and stability	Self-stability in supine	Safe self-entry into the pool
	Understanding the principles of buoyancy and roll if appropriate	Initiation of longitudinal roll alone	High level balance work
	Evaluation of the potential for normalization of tone during treatment	Independent vertical roll with good breath control	Possible work on gait
	Introduction to vertical and longitudinal roll	Facilitation of normal movement, voluntary and automatic	Cardiovascular fitness work
			Swimming
			Ability to go along to local pool alone or with a relative or friend and enjoy a recreational swim
Techniques	Seaweeding and 'letting go' with a short lever (Practical techniques 1)	Seaweeding with a longer lever (Practical techniques 1)	Underwater work with eyes open if possible (Practical techniques 6)
	Head rotation in supine (Practical techniques 5)	Trunk control work, rhythmic stabilizations, the use of the metacentric effect and turbulence in supine (Practical techniques 2, 8, 9, 10)	Over side entry, off wall or down steps (consider the amenities of their local pool)
	Trunk-sway and release (Practical techniques 1, 3)	Balance in the box position (Practical techniques 8, 5)	Combine vertical and longitudinal rotation initially between two (Practical techniques 5)
	Breath control in the 'box' position (Practical techniques 6)	Breath control with vertical rolling, with two helpers initially (Practical techniques 5)	Elementary propulsion and basic strokes – see p. 130
	Releases and stretches as appropriate (Practical techniques 3, 4, 7)	Facilitation of normal movement by using buoyancy, turbulence and drag (Practical techniques 8, 10)	Prone to supine to prone swimming (Practical techniques 12)
	Longitudinal rocking, balancing and rolling (Practical techniques 2, 10)	In supine, facilitation of normal movement using turbulence and buoyancy (Practical techniques 8)	Turbulence and buoyancy work in standing (Practical techniques 8)

Primary	Intermediate	Advanced
Vertical roll with breath control (Practical techniques 5)	Use of the facilitatory aspects of Bad Ragaz – minimal resistance where appropriate	Rhythmic stabilization and trunk stability work with a longer lever, checking for abnormal mass contraction and compensatory movements (Practical techniques 9)
	Box position facilitation of normal reactions using the metacentric effect, turbulence and buoyancy (Practical techniques 8)	Gait work especially if low tone is a problem (Practical techniques 10)
	Patient initiated longitudinal rolling with good breath control (Practical techniques 5)	Carefully constructed cardiovascular work
		Bad Ragaz (low resistance)

Guillain–Barré–Landry syndrome, a lower motor neurone condition.

Hemiplegia

The patient who has suffered a cerebral vascular accident resulting in one side of the body being affected will have altered shape and density which allows the metacentric/disability effect to be utilized in treatment. Associated reactions and overcompensation on the non-affected side need to be monitored and controlled. The patient's CNS is less able to inhibit unwanted activity so over-stimulation by tasks that are too difficult needs to be avoided otherwise unwanted tonal activity through the whole body becomes a problem.

Abnormal muscle tone with a disrupted central postural control mechanism will be present. There is great potential even in the early stages to use the properties of water to gain maximum rehabilitation once the patient is medically stable. As some cases have altered breath control special care will be needed to protect the patient's airway.

Any tendency to over-stress the CNS needs to be avoided. Treatment sessions should be individually planned and the fine grading of movements in water understood. Due to the body's asymmetry, attaining and maintaining stability in all positions needs considerable attention (p. 170).

Buoyancy and turbulence can be used to facilitate early function especially in the upper limb. Those patients who have a painful shoulder benefit from release work because movement becomes relatively more pain free in the pool. Other problems that may present and require special consideration are those of sensory and proprioceptive impairment, compensation and dyspraxia.

Gait re-education in the initial stages of hydrotherapy treatment is probably best omitted, but active functional work such as swimming can actually reduce muscle tone most unexpectedly. Individual treatments are most beneficial throughout the hydrotherapy programme although in the later stages there may be aspects of the programme that the patient can do alone. The psychological effect of hydrotherapy on the patient's mood and motivation is very significant.

Parkinson's Disease

Parkinson's disease and the Parkinsonian syndrome comprise a group of disorders characterized by tremor and disturbance of voluntary movement, posture and balance.

Disorder of posture usually presents with slight flexion in standing at all joints. Correction of posture often requires effort and concentration. Other common features are bradykinesia, rigidity, especially in the trunk, paucity of movement, weakness of extensor groups of limb and trunk muscles, reduced thoracic expansion and loss of postural and normal equilibrium responses. Akinesia and bradykinesia are often lessened in the water, possibly due to the abnormal stimulus of the water pressure and turbulence on the body giving an increased feedback to the brain (Reid Campion, 1991). In water these patients have an altered shape and density to normal. Rotational movements are limited and balance reactions from within the trunk are reduced. In treatment this disability/metacentric effect can be exploited to give them greater movement experience. Use of longitudinal and vertical rolling is very beneficial. Water tends to initiate freer movement to counteract the inertia problems. They have a tendency to develop flexion contractures so working to improve active extension counteracts this. Cardiovascular fitness work is an important objective of treatment and is safer and more interesting in the pool. Difficulties with communication may be encountered due to the mask-like face, a tendency not to socialize and increased levels of anxiety. It is important to keep the pool area relatively quiet during early visits and to allow them to acclimatize gradually. The drugs used to treat Parkinson's disease have a tendency to induce a degree of hypotension so care should be taken when the patient leaves the pool. If the patient has any degree of altered breath control extra care may be needed to protect the airway.

Occasionally hydrotherapy increases the effects of rigidity. Cooler water may be more beneficial.

Guillian–Barré–Landry syndrome

This syndrome can affect both sexes at any age. It is most commonly seen between the ages of 20 and 50. At present the cause is unknown. In around 50% of cases the onset is preceded by a mild gastro-intestinal or respiratory infection.

The patient experiences symmetrical muscle weakness. The motor symptoms usually start distally and move proximally with lower limb involvement preceding that of the upper limb. The disease can proceed to involve the trunk and cranial nerves. Pain is a variable and often overlooked symptom. Parasthesiae are often present. Autonomic functions are sometimes affected, e.g. involvement of cardiac muscle may lead to sinus arhythmias and variable blood pressure. The symptoms progress over a period of weeks, then plateau out and gradually function returns in reverse order. Patients recover in 3 months to 2 years.

Hydrotherapy becomes appropriate when there is some motor recovery occurring. The patient does not usually suffer cortical neurone damage therefore the problems of tone abnormality are that of weakness due to reduced velocity of nerve impulses. The brain is unaffected and cerebral function is unimpaired. Spasticity is not one of the problems. These patients do often have reduced respiratory function and this needs to be taken into account in hydrotherapy. Treating them in supine will reduce the effect of hydrostatic pressure at this stage. Where pain is a problem the pain relieving properties of hydrotherapy will be helpful. Treatment should be directed at carefully building up muscle power, coordination and balance. Fatigue is often a problem so programmes must be carefully constructed. If patients have been left with any degree of soft tissue shortening, stretches can be interspersed with more active work to allow the patient to rest. Care is required to protect very flaccid joints. The pool environment is an excellent medium in which to work on trunk rotational control and balance mechanism re-education both in the early stages and much later. If sensory loss has occurred, careful protection of the skin is required. The patient may need to wear socks. In the later stages patients may work on more functional activities such as walking and step ups. Cardiovascular fitness is an important part of the programme. These patients often have long admissions and hydrotherapy offers a variation in treatment which improves motivation and enhances cooperation with treatment.

Multiple Sclerosis

Multiple sclerosis (MS) is a degenerative and progressive disease of the CNS, although a high proportion of patients are still leading independent lives 20 years after diagnosis. There is markedly variable symptomatology. Fatigue can be a great problem: patients need to be helped to pace activities, learning their own limitations and accepting that they need to rest when they reach them. Fatigue may also be due to sensitivity to heat, but a pool temperature that is thermo-neutral should not cause a rise in body temperature and therefore produce fatigue. Each patient should be assessed on an individual basis.

Occasionally patients experience a loss of tone after treatment. This may be because the patient needs to be taught how to pace their activity and to be allowed to rest after treatment if necessary. Hydrotherapy is effective for people with MS if they enjoy it and feel it is beneficial. There are potential psychological and physiological gains to be enjoyed. Treatment needs to be adapted to cope with abnormal increases and decreases in muscle tone.

The patients may also have changes of body shape and density. Balance reactions may have become abnormal, and rotational movements difficult. Impaired sensation sometimes occurs, contributing to dyspraxia. Feet may require protection with socks. Patients with MS sometimes have memory, cognitive and behavioural difficulties or mood changes which require consideration if they occur. Hydrotherapy can provide much needed social contact but care needs to be taken that they do not become too reliant on treatment and lose their independence. Treatment contracts for a certain number of treatments are useful. Urinary problems are a common feature of MS which may lead to problems with incontinence and need monitoring. Altered breath control may require increased awareness to protect the airway.

Ataxia and Hypotonia

A patient with hypotonia inevitably shows a form of ataxia. Ataxia means that movements are uncoordinated and ill-timed. Team work between the muscles is lost giving a jerky appearance to the movement. Stopping and starting are difficult and overshooting occurs (Downie, 1992). There is great tendency to overcompensation distally, causing for example increased tone in the upper limbs which inhibits recovery proximally. Release work is first required to facilitate a 'letting go' of the overcompensation. Treatment then needs to facilitate recruitment of tone dynamically without overcompensation. Patients often experience a disruption of their breathing pattern; care and attention to breathing control to protect the airway is required in the water. It may be beneficial to work alongside the speech and language therapist. Fatigue can be a problem,

since it is very hard work for the patient to maintain any form of control. Treatment goals must be realistic and well paced.

Tremor can be a problem but may be 'damped' down in water. These patients have less asymmetry but still require work in supine to centralize control and to re-educate central posture control. Metacentric work in the 'box' position is very beneficial. Problems are encountered in initiating and controlling rotation, therefore work on longitudinal and vertical rolling is important. Special care is needed when combining the need for breath control with a roll, if their breath control is not fully automatic. Treatment should progress slowly enough to allow them to adjust.

Tone is reduced, therefore buoyancy, drag and turbulence should be used extensively to facilitate activity.

Standing and gait re-education are often beneficial because the water assists in supporting the patient. Some effects of gravity are required though to recruit tone. The patient receives a tremendous boost to morale on achieving activities not possible on dry land.

Disrupted sensation and proprioception can present increased difficulties in the water due to reduction of sensory inputs usually provided by normal weight bearing in gravity. Bad Ragaz techniques can be helpful, but care is required so that they do not reinforce compensation, which can be avoided by alternating these with 'let go' techniques.

Deficient Oral Function and Breath Control

Many neurological conditions leave patients with impaired oral and facial function, impaired sensation and altered breathing patterns. Hydrotherapy can be beneficial in providing alternative methods to encourage re-education of the breathing pattern; for example hydrostatic pressure assists the recoil of the chest wall on expiration. The normal automatic recoil assisted by the abdominal muscles can be impaired in a patient with abnormal increased muscle tone both intercostally and abdominally and can therefore create voicing difficulties. The pressure of the water assists in the expiration phase when voice is produced. Close liaison with the patient's speech and language therapist is essential for work in this area.

It is helpful to explore different starting positions in order to achieve the maximum effect. Some patients who have recruited increased muscle tone around the shoulders, and are breathing largely with their accessory muscles of respiration as a result, may respond best to lying supine with a neck ring, with the physiotherapist standing between the patient's knees (Practical techniques 1, p. 217). This aids the reduction of compensatory tone in the upper chest and allows the experience of diaphragmatic breathing to develop more easily.

Breathing exercises can be made fun and different in the pool; for example blowing objects along the surface as a game and underwater blowing through mouth and nose.

Cardiovascular exercise and swimming can all be used appropriately to normalize breath control.

It should be remembered that the increased effort of controlling breathing may increase tone and reduce normal movement. Constant monitoring and guidance by the physiotherapist is required.

Perceptual/Cognitive and Behavioural Problems

Perceptual, cognitive and behavioural problems can all be features of neurological trauma and disease. They may lead to difficulties with all functional activities and usually become more noticeable as activities become more complex and demanding. The patient may appear clumsy, careless or unintelligent when in fact they are struggling to assimilate the incoming information and act on it. Patients can also be overexcitable or have no sense of danger. Particular care is therefore required in the pool area with its potential dangers. Patients' awareness of how they are failing may lead to angry outbursts or withdrawn behaviour. It is important to liaise with the clinical psychologist and occupational therapist to gain the fullest picture of the patient's difficulties and how best to treat them.

Hydrotherapy can sometimes be used as part of the patient's treatment programme or there may be physical problems that respond to hydrotherapy alongside the behavioural ones. When working with these patients it is desirable to keep the pool are as quiet as possible, to keep

Key to drawings

⊙	Front facing
♀	Side view
W	Wall fixation
∼∼∼	Water surface
♀	Person with feet on the bottom of the pool
♀	Person without feet on the bottom of the pool
⟩	Turbulence
→←	Direction of movement or pressure
⌒	Rotational/diagonal movement or pressure
↔↕	Movement in all directions
⊘	Float
⟨⟩	Float may be required

instructions simple and to use structured repetitive programmes initially. Inclusion of cardiovascular aspects to the programme is helpful in dissipating emotion and promoting natural sleep. Where possible the patient should remain with the same physiotherapist.

SUMMARY

Normal control of our bodies is highly complex. Rehabilitation after neurological damage requires resourceful and varied approaches. Hydrotherapy has a definite role to play in the rehabilitation of the neurologically damaged person.

Water is a wonderfully dynamic environment that can recreate for the person the 'freedom of movement' they have lost, if sensitively guided by the physiotherapist. Water allows a subtle and intuitive approach to treatment.

The skill in treatment is to challenge patients to their limits, where maximum useful stimulus of the CNS occurs, but not beyond. In water it is very much easier to overchallenge the damaged CNS beyond its ability to perform normally. A physiotherapist who is skilled in handling a neurologically damaged person in water can use the water to take over part of the role of facilitator.

Physiotherapists need to remember to take the treatment session slowly and wait for reactions before changing to a new activity. It is also very important and beneficial for the physiotherapist to gain an understanding of hydrodynamic principles by working with *normal* subjects in water. This leads to greater sensitivity of handling, increased skill and enhances the physiotherapist's confidence.

PRACTICAL TECHNIQUES

1 Seaweeding

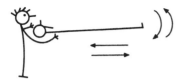

- Keep body moving to keep feet up
- Minimize head support, use the water
- Move forward/backward/snake side to side
- Occasional use of floats on feet if speed needs to be kept slow. Floats are better than a second person as free movement is required

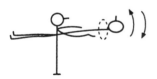

- Selective release using a short lever
- Stand between the patient's legs
- Side-to-side movement
- Incorporate rotation by facilitation with flat hands on the patient's back
- A neck float can be used to encourage 'let go' at the neck and shoulders

2 Appreciation of roll

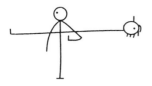

- Find balance point
- Use edge of hand not palm
- Maintain good communication/ explanation
- Allow the patient to roll a little, initially you correct
- Encourage them to play with the movement they felt

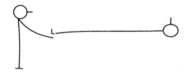

- Working from the feet allows the physiotherapist to alter balance by raising one foot slightly
- Watch for change in limb positions
- *Warning*: beware of compensation/ fixing
- Is the stress or compensation too great?

3 Stretching

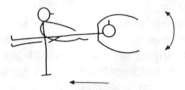

- See Seaweeding. Add prolonged circles with stretch
- Moving forward and back can mobilize shoulders
- Add rotation
- Physiotherapist can stand between legs
- Stretches in the box position. PT on left

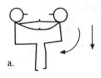

a.

(a)   Use for trunk rotation, flexion and side flexion

b.

(b)   Patient's knees held between physiotherapist's for added localization if required

c.

(c)   Bell, useful for small stretches or movement appreciation

- Trunk sway from the head

4 Prolonged stretches

- Tendo-achilles, soleus and intrinsic muscles of the foot

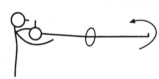

- Shoulders/trunk on pelvis
- Aids selective flexion/extension

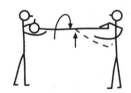

- Total body stretch with extension and rotation

Combine with passive mobilization techniques for specific joints

5 Rotation

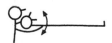

- Head on body
- Use eyes 'look at me'

Longitudinal rotation

- Initially totally controlled by physiotherapist with no submersion
- Take care when including submersion that the patient has adequate automatic breath control
- Teach to blow or hum as they roll
- Ensure the movement is in both directions

Vertical rotation

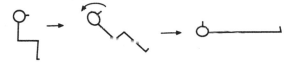

- Come forward again with the command 'lift head, reach forward and bend in the middle'
- Teach the patient to allow the movement to happen
- Not to be rushed
- Disallow use of the limbs, use trunk and head
- Teach to hum or blow, as they go just below the surface

Combination rotation

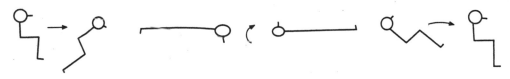

This is started between two people on either side of the patient holding under the arms. *Beware* of patient overusing the helper

6 Breath control

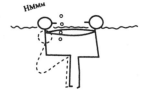

- Use box position at start of breath control
- Aid selective flexion/extension
- Beware of the patient pulling on the physiotherapist
- Patient can be stabilized between physiotherapist's knees or with feet on the bottom. One leg may require more stabilization than the other

- For a patient with memory problems this may need repeating at the start of every session
- Beware of patients with speech/ swallowing problems
- Involve speech and language therapist

7 Buoyancy

- Trunk rotation

- Lateral flexion

- Hip extension

- Extension

- Thoracic rotation

8 Facilitation of movement using metacentric effect, turbulence and buoyancy

Examples

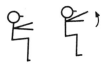

- Box position, lifting all limbs individually

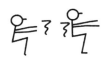

- Isometric holding using specific turbulence

- Shoulder protraction. Using specific turbulence for both assistance and resistance

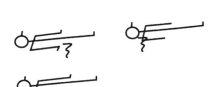

- Elbow extension

- Hip extension and protraction. Using specific turbulence for both assistance and resistance

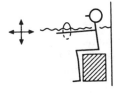

- Use of a stool for upper limb work

9   Rhythmic stabilizations

Beware of unwanted fixing and compensation. Reduce the resistance to regain more selective movement. Swop during treatment between rhythmic stabilizations and release/stretch work to ensure the patient retains the ability to 'let go' of the increased tone facilitated.

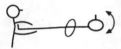

- Rotation. Ask patient to 'keep nose in line with toes'
- Flexion and extension

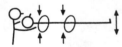

- Physiotherapist applies gentle displacement pressure around the trunk and asks the patient to 'hold their position'

10   Balance and saving reactions

Sensory input – movement awareness. Very subtle handling and careful instructions to the patient are required.

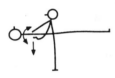

- Longitudinal rocking
- Also the 'bell' and the appreciation of roll section (sections 2 and 3)

More active

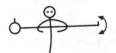

- Standing between patient's legs

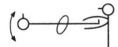

- Gentle trunk resistance using a combination of rotation and side flexion to disturb balance

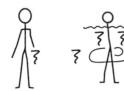

- Using turbulence to disturb balance and facilitate reaction

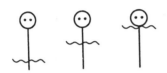

- Progress using change of depth and increased turbulence in late stages where a high level of selective reactions are available to the patient

- Beware of overstimulation leading to overcompensation and fixation

Warning: during treatment swop between this activity and release/stretch work to ensure the patient retains the ability to 'let go' of the increased tone facilitated.

11 Swimming

Patients who are very disabled on land can learn to swim independently. They need to be able to do combined rotations with good breath control and have the ability to maintain stability in supine when using their arms for propulsion.

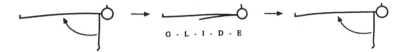

- Simple propulsion
- Arm out at 90°, pull to side and glide
- Stroke suitable for uni- or bilateral swimming
- Front crawl or breast stroke leg kicks

12 Combined rotation swimming

Two stokes supine, two strokes prone.
A high level of breath control is required.

13 Gait work

Walking in all directions at varying speeds and depths utilizing turbulence and drag.

REFERENCES

Alder S.S., Beckers D. and Buck M. (1993). *PNF in Practice*, Berlin, Heidelberg: Springer Verlag.

Association of Swimming Therapy (1992). *Swimming for People with Disabilities*, London: A&C Black.

Bobath B. (1990). *Adult Hemiplegia: Evaluation and treatment*, 3rd edn, London: William Heinemann.

Clements G. (1984). Adaptation of postural control in weightlessness. *Experimental Brain Research*, 57: 61–72.

Cools A. (1992). Brain plasticity and central planning of movement. *AOG Nijega Januer*, 1: 3–72.

Dietz V. (1992) Human neuronal control of automatic functional movements: interaction between central programs and afferent input. *Physiological Reviews*, 72(1): 33–69.

Downie P.A. (ed.) (1992). *Cash's Textbook of Neurology for Physiotherapists*, 4th edn, London: Mosby-Year Book Europe Ltd.

Gabriel A. (1968). Contribution of space programme to our knowledge of motion sickness. Third Symposium on basic environmental problems of man in space. Geneva. European Space Agency, 8–10 rue Mario-Nikis, 75738 PARIS CEDEX 15, France.

Golani I. (1981). 'Warm up' along directions of movement in the ontogeny of exploration in rats and other infants animals *Proc, Natl. Acad. Sci.*, 78(11): 7226–7229.

Golderberger M. and Murray M. (1988). Patterns of sprouting and implications for recovery of function. *Advances in Neurology, 47: Functional Recovery in Neurological Disease* (S.C. Waxman, ed.), New York: Raven Press.

Homick J.L. (1977). The effects of prolonged exposure to weightlessness on postural equilibrium (R. Johnson Dictlin, ed.) Biomechanical results from Skylab, NSA SP3–377: 104–112.

Kaplan M.S. (1988). Plasticity after lesions of the brain: Contemporary concepts. *Archives of Medical Rehabilitation*, 69: 984–991.

Kidd G., Lawes N. and Musa I. (1992). *Understanding Neuromuscular Plasticity*, London: Edward Arnold.

Kovlovskya I.B., Aslanova I.F., Barmin V.A., Grigorieva L.S., Gevlich G.I., Kirenskaya A.V. and Sirota M.G. (1983). The nature and characteristics of gravitational ataxia. *The Physiologist*, 26: 108–109.

Musa I. (1986). The role of afferent input in the reduction of spasticity: a hypothesis. *Physiotherapy*, 72: 531–536.

O'Hare J.P. (1985). Observations on the effects of immersion. *British Medical Journal*, 12: 21–28.

Poritsky R. (1992). *Neuroanatomy*. Philadelphia, USA: Hanley and Belfus Inc.

Reid Campion M. (ed.) (1991). *Adult Hydrotherapy: A Practical Approach*, London: Heinemann Medical Books.

Shepherd G. (1988). *Neurobiology*, Oxford: Oxford University Press.

Skinner A. and Thompson A. (1983). *Duffield's Exercise in Water*, London: Ballière Tindall.

Stevenson P. (1993). A review of neuroplasticity: some indications for physiotherapy in the treatment of lesions of the brain. *Physiotherapy*, 79(10): 699–702.

Szechtman H. (1985). The morphogenesis of stereotyped behaviour induced by the dopamine receptor agonist apomorphine in the laboratory rat. *Neuroscience*, 14(3): 783–789.

ACKNOWLEDGEMENTS

With special thanks to Wendy Adamson, Charles Dean, Jane Golden, Jeremy Gray, Bridget Peace, Kate Saville, Bernice Statton, Sheila Watters and Helen Whitelock.

The pictorial method of representing techniques was devised by Helen Whitelock.

Spinal mobilizations, spinal cord injuries

Margaret Reid Campion

Overview to Chapters 11 and 12

The field of spinal mobilization in water is a comparatively recent development in hydrotherapy techniques. It is growing vigorously in various countries such as Britain and Australia. Physiotherapists with an interest and/or training in manipulative techniques who are also aware of the properties, characteristics and advantages of water are forging ahead evolving these techniques. There are several ways in which these can be carried out and the reader is referred to the ensuing chapter and to hydrodynamic exercises (p. 179).

Hydrotherapy has long proved an exceptionally useful modality in the rehabilitation of spinal injuries not only as an addition to the formal rehabilitative programme but as a sound basis for future recreational skills.

Rehabilitation programmes comprise specific exercises and re-education of movement. The buoyancy and resistance or impedance provided by water allows attempts at activities impossible on land; the skills of stroking learned during the hydrotherapy programme help increase the patient's confidence and safety, thus participation in many aquatic sports adapted for the disabled becomes possible.

11

Spinal mobilizations

Jan Hill

INTRODUCTION

This chapter details two treatment approaches for the hydrotherapy management of spinal mobility problems. These are passive manual mobilization (PMM) and passive mobilization using turbulent drag (PMTD). Other techniques such as hydrodynamically progressed exercise, Bad Ragaz and Halliwick techniques, stretching and relaxation, all of which could also be used to mobilize the spine, have been previously outlined and therefore will only be mentioned with reference to other texts.

Additionally this chapter will cover the incidence of spinal dysfunction, research of passive mobilization and the benefits, disadvantages and special considerations in using passive mobilization techniques in water. Indications and contraindications appropriate for passive mobilization in water will be outlined only, as these are similar to the land-based approach. Assessment and types of equipment will be mentioned and techniques of PMM and PMTD will be detailed including self-management. As with land-based management of spinal mobility problems, passive mobilization adds to the range of hydrotherapy treatment. Other presenting signs and symptoms of spinal dysfunction must be also managed in the total treatment plan. However these will not be mentioned in this chapter.

INCIDENCE OF SPINAL PAIN

Spinal pain and particularly low back pain is one of the major public health problems facing industrial societies today and it usually occurs in individuals during their most productive years (Mayer *et al.*, 1984). It constitutes 60% of consultations in any physiotherapy department) (Bogduk and Twomey, 1991). Although the figures have not been reported hydrotherapy services are in demand for the treatment of spinal dysfunction and various texts advocate specific treatment approaches for spinal pain (Davis and Harrison, 1988; Langridge and Phillips, 1988; Reid Campion, 1990; Smit and Harrison, 1991; Whitelock, 1992). The incidence of spinal pain is similar throughout the western world where 80% of the population experience low back pain at some stage in their life. The costs relating to injury are extremely high, financially, socially and psychologically and 10% will have prolonged disability. Acute lower back pain is self limiting and most recover in two months, however there is a high recurrence rate. Detailed statistics are well documented (Mayer *et al.*, 1986; Langridge and Phillips, 1988; Maher and Adams, 1994). Spinal pain is a major medical and social problem.

RESEARCH IN PASSIVE MOBILIZATION

The incidence of spinal pain has facilitated extensive research to increase the understanding of spinal pain and its management. In hydrotherapy treatment for spinal dysfunction, Langridge and Phillips (1988) studied group hydrotherapy for chronic lower back and Smit and Harrison (1991) studied effects of individual hydrotherapy treatment demonstrating reduction of pain levels of spinal dysfunction, with improved thoracic lumbar mobility. Neither studied the effects of passive mobilization in hydrotherapy. Other research evaluates land-based passive mobilization techniques, specifically of the lumbar spine. However the efficacy of only a few techniques has been supported by research. Some of these studies are relevant to the application of passive mobilization in water. Lee and Evans (1994), in assessing the effect of posteroanterior (PA) mobilization of the fourth lumbar vertebra found that preconditioning (resistance of viscoelastic properties of the lumbar spine) and creep (deformation under load) decrease with each loading of PA mobilization, finally reaching a steady rate. Therefore if PA mobilization is to be effective it will be evident in the initial phase of the application. The physiotherapist should consider increasing the PA force so that preconditioning or creep can occur to produce further improvement (Lee and Evans, 1994). This is dependent however on logical and gradual progression and must not result in irreparable damage. Normal tissues have only a temporary response to preconditioning and creep after PA mobilization and quickly return to the original state. Clinical improvement with this technique may be explained by the fact that in scar or abnormal tissue the preconditioning or creep effect may not be temporary (Lee and Evans, 1994).

Land PA mobilization provides a bending or sagging resulting in movement of the mobilized vertebrae relevant to the supporting ends, that is the pelvis and the thorax, this is much greater than the true intervertebral motion (Lee and Evans, 1994). Posteroanterior mobilization of the lumbar spine does not produce a single glide of one vertebra on another but a complex motion in both extension and translatory (every point of the vertebrae moves in the same direction) movement and thus an increase in the lordosis of the lumbar spine (Lee and Evans, 1994). This would tend to support the PA mobilization of the spine in water which is usually one of general mobilization.

Important knowledge for the clinical application of passive mobilization techniques is that coupling (motion in which rotation or translation of the body about or along one axis is constantly associated with simultaneous rotation or translation about another axis) (White and Punjabi, 1978; Brown, 1990) movements

occur in the cervical and lumbar spines. Therefore the physiotherapist cannot expect to mobilize either rotation or lateral flexion in isolation. Between C2 → C7 lateral flexion and rotation is a coupled movement. The C2 → C4 facet joints translate to either side and the movements of lateral flexion and rotation are three dimensional. Translation is an integral part of the motion (Schneider and Pardoe, 1985). Rotation and lateral flexion are a coupled movement in with the lumbar spine. Coupling varies with intra-vertebral level and with flexion and extension of the lumbar spine (White and Punjabi, 1978; Pearcy and Tibrewal, 1984; Punjabi *et al.*, 1989; Yamamoto *et al.*, 1989; Vicenzio and Twomey, 1993; Brown, 1990). The exact coupling patterns to expect at various levels of the lumbar spine are yet to be determined (Punjabi *et al.*, 1989; Bogduk and Twomey, 1991). Abnormal coupling patterns in the lumbar spine may be an indicator of low back pain disturbing the expected normal coupling response. There may be alterations in the muscles to compensate for the loss of stability (Punjabi *et al.*, 1989). In hydrotherapy, where movement is freer, coupling can be observed when mobilizing either rotation or lateral flexion of the cervical and lumbar spine.

Twomey and Taylor (1982), when testing for creep and hysteresis (the amount of energy lost when the structure was initially stressed and occurring with the removal of a load) with loading of the lumbar spine, found that advancing age results in decreased range of flexion movement of the lumbar spine but an increased amount of flexion creep deformation. Age changes reflect increased lumbar stiffness, together with decreased stability near the end of range of movement. Hysteresis recovery is prolonged and less complete in older than younger spines (Twomey and Taylor, 1982). On land the magnitude of the force of PA mobilization is larger at the vertebral joints below the mobilized vertebrae than above (Lee and Evans, 1994). In water this force may be increased by buoyancy and density of body parts.

Flor and Turk (1984) suggest that, although patients show some immediate pain relief, the value of manipulation is questionable, supporting the need for more research in all techniques used for the management of spinal pain. The major problem in much of the medical research of chronic low back pain is that it tends to disregard the psychological and learning factors that may have taken place when pain existed for a long time (Flor and Turk, 1984).

PASSIVE MOBILIZATION IN WATER

The water provides a unique environment for passive mobilization. The rotating torque of buoyancy/altered metacentre and/or relative density of the body/body part can assist mobilization and vary the amplitude of passive movement. Dynamic properties of water provide additional forces to assist the physiotherapist with mobilizing techniques.

Benefits of Passive Mobilization in Water

The water provides for passive mobilization a medium which is supportive, friction-free/and, if warm, relaxing and hypnotic (Whitelock, 1992). It assists the patient's and physiotherapist's movements creating ideal conditions for passive mobilization of the spine. The success of passive mobilization depends on a water-confident patient, suitable depth for the physiotherapist, patient comfort in flotation equipment, non-slip pool floor and pool design features for fixation. The benefits of using warm water for treatment of physical and psychological conditions are numerous and have been well documented (Skinner and Thomson, 1983; Davis and Harrison, 1988; Reid Campion, 1990).

Disadvantages of Passive Mobilization in Water

Passive mobilization may be compromised by the patient's condition such as acute spinal pain, especially when it is aggravated by movement, fear of water or an unwillingness to be placed in the starting position. Highly turbulent water and inadequate pool design can make application of the techniques difficult. Disadvantages associated with applying passive manual mobilization to the spine in water include: difficulty in gaining fixation of the patient with the flotation equipment or pool features, and fixation of the physiotherapist in relation to pool design and water depth. Localization of treatment to a specific joint, the line of force to the spinal level, and controlling the amplitude of the mobilization is also difficult. Therefore the application of small amplitude oscillations may not be effectual.

Special Conditions for Passive Mobilization Techniques in Water

In water passive mobilization of the spine has specific requirements; these include patient comfort and water confidence, physiotherapist stability and control of application of mobilization. Therefore it may not be directed to all patients with spinal problems. If the patient is a non-swimmer and is frightened of the water, the technique cannot be introduced until the patient is mentally adjusted to the water and confident in the position required for the technique. The Halliwick Method (Skinner and Thomson, 1983; Reid Campion, 1991; Association of Swimming Therapy, 1992) would be implemented to gain water confidence prior to application of a passive mobilization technique. Patient comfort will be individual and gained using a variety of flotation equipment to support the neck and/or pelvis and/or other body parts. In every case the patient must be able to relax fully. The physiotherapist needs to stand with a wide base of support on a non-slip pool floor, preferably working at a water depth no greater than the eleventh thoracic spine (TII) (McMillian, 1984), to treat effectively and to obtain maximal stability when applying the technique. The physiotherapist directs the force by utilizing the buoyancy effect on their own body. The position must capitalize on buoyancy but at the same time there must be control of its unwanted effects.

Aims of Passive Mobilization in Water

The hydrotherapy programme for the management of patients with spinal mobility problems includes the aim to increase range of motion. The techniques utilize the properties of water such as its buoyancy, skin friction and turbulent drag, temperature, depth and behaviour in the static and dynamic situation (Bolton and Goodwin, 1974; Horsfield *et al.*, 1982; Skinner and Thomson, 1983; Davis and Harrison, 1988; Reid Campion, 1990; Whitelock, 1992). These properties can be used to gain increased range of motion of the spine through exercise, relaxation, Bad Ragaz techniques (Skinner and Thomson, 1983; Davis and Harrison, 1988;

Reid Campion, 1990), Halliwick Method (Association of Swimming Therapy, 1992; Horsfield *et al.*, 1982; Skinner and Thomson, 1983; Reid Campion, 1985), stretching (Whitelock, 1992) or passive mobilization.

The specific aims of passive mobilization in water are to:

1. Reduce local muscle spasm. Mobilization is thought to reduce gamma gain by producing a barrage of spindle output which convinces the central nervous system (CNS) to reduce the contraction of intrafusal fibres and muscle spasms (Korr, 1975). This activates better muscular activity especially post mobilization. Also oscillations may inhibit reflex muscle contraction and produce a temporary sense of relief in certain individuals by breaking the pain–fear cycle. This may allow the individual to realize that activity does not necessarily result in increased pain (Zusman, 1986).

2. Reduce muscle tone by warming the affected part to reduce the gamma firing, and relax the neuromuscular stretch receptors and thereby decrease the striated muscle tone (Franchimont *et al.*, 1983), and reduce pain perception. Unlike land treatment, hydrotherapy warms the body throughout the treatment period. Mobilization reduces muscle tone not only in those muscles passing over the joints being mobilized but also in more remote muscles by stimulation of mechanoreceptive afferent fibres which project synaptically to neurones in the motor neurone pools within the CNS (Wyke, 1985; Guyton, 1991).

3. Relieve pain and effusion of a joint by reducing joint pressure, periarticular tension and increasing circulation and movement (Giovanelli *et al.*, 1985). The warmth of the water and hydrostatic pressure will also have a similar effect. Oscillations or stretching techniques stimulate the joint mechanoreceptors to produce inhibition of nociceptive activity and therefore CNS perception of pain (Wyke, 1985; Wall and Melzack, 1994). According to Corrigan and Maitland (1983) short-term bombardment followed by rapid stretch of articular and myofacial nerve endings by passive mobilization

may disrupt the pain and spasm cycle. In water such a stretch can be achieved by adding flotation equipment to body parts to change specific gravity/relative density, and manual techniques such as contract/hold relax or prolonged stretch.

4. Assist over time in the optimal repair and extensibility of soft tissue by improving metabolic functioning of joint tissue with oscillations (Zusman, 1986).

5. Increase the range of motion of the spinal movements.

6. Gain weight reduction on the spine in buoyancy supported flotation to enable rehydration of the disc by osmotic pressure as occurs in rest periods or traction on land. According to Bogduk and Twomey (1991) the therapeutic effects of traction on land occur only during the period of traction. In hydrotherapy, the treatment time is more prolonged and the patient may concurrently perform various gradations of exercise in the vertical or other postures where weight reduction on the spine is maintained.

7. Gain general relaxation (Skinner and Thomson, 1983) and facilitate the reduction of pain and stress,

8. Use the water for post-mobilization activity to achieve other aims of the treatment. Water provides a medium for fine graduation of exercise in a weight-reduced environment to maintain the effect of mobilization and to enable muscle strength/coordination work to be trained with improved spinal alignment.

Indications for Spinal Mobilization

The indications for spinal mobilization are clearly outlined (Maitland, 1973; Corrigan and Maitland, 1983; Grieve, 1984) for land-based mobilization and are also applied to spinal mobilization in water. Chronic spine problems with the predominant feature of stiffness are the most appropriate group for passive mobilization in water, although selected sub-acute conditions may be indicated. The signs and symptoms most suitable for the technique are those where pain and resistance are of equal importance, where resistance not pain is dominant or where pain is not aggravated by minor movement. The condition is not irritable (Maitland, 1973).

Contraindications for Passive Mobilization in Water

1. Acute spinal problems where pain is a major problem, where there is significant functional limitation because of pain and there are many specific aggravating factors. The condition is irritable (Maitland, 1973).
2. Conditions requiring small amplitude grade mobilizations.
3. Patients with significant fear of water, or reluctance to move into the starting positions required for mobilization.

Assessment for Passive Mobilization in Water

Assessment of the patient for passive mobilization of the spine in water includes land-based assessment, screenings for precautions and possible contraindications for hydrotherapy (Skinner and Thomson, 1983; Davis and Harrison, 1988; Reid Campion, 1990; Australian Physiotherapy Association, 1990), a water confidence assessment (Reid Campion, 1991) and assessment of the patient's ability to accommodate and be comfortable in the starting position for the application of the technique.

Passive mobilization of the spine in water is reliant on a thorough subjective and objective land-based assessment (Maitland, 1973; Caillet, 1981; Corrigan and Maitland, 1983; Grieve, 1984; Butler, 1991). The assessment should include a 24-hour pattern of symptoms, aggravating and easing factors, posture, functional movement analysis, range of motion (active and passive), muscle imbalance, neural and special tests and palpation. The research of assessment procedures is important for hydrotherapy. Maher and Adams (1994) found that stiffness assessment is not reliable. Matyas and Bach (1985) found that tests of pain are more reliable than passive mobilization tests, such as Passive Accessory Intervertebral Movement (PAIM), Passive Physiological Intervertebral Movement (PPIM), Straight Leg Raise (SLR) and forward flexion. Tests of pain and patient feedback should be used in combination with manual assessment initially during and following hydrotherapy treatment. The water assessment determines if the patient is at ease with water on the face and in the eyes and ears and

can protect the nose and mouth if submerged. Assessment must also determine if the patient is able to move through vertical and lateral rotation (Reid Campion, 1991). It is important that the physiotherapist understands the spinal movements required for these activities and how a patient's spinal symptoms could be aggravated while moving through planes of rotation to accommodate treatment positions for spinal mobilization.

Equipment

Equipment required for passive mobilization of the spine includes: cervical and pelvic flotation, rings, armband floaties, swimming rope (a rubberized rope that is attached to the handrail and to a strap wrapped around the patient's waist. It is usually used to provide stationary swimming), hydroplinth and tyre.

PASSIVE MANUAL MOBILIZATION (PMM) IN WATER

PMM techniques do not necessarily replicate those on land. When buoyancy assists, the mobilization should be in harmony with buoyancy. The mobilization is proportionate to the change of the specific gravity/relative density of the body/body part which is altered by the addition of air-filled floats and with the moment of force of buoyancy. When buoyancy supports the mobilization the physiotherapist dictates the speed and amplitude of the mobilization. Water provides freedom from friction and therefore offers little counterforce to PMM as would occur from the treatment surfaces, such as the plinth, in a land-based technique. The technique uses slow, large-amplitude oscillations and greater forces used in this technique are produced by the physiotherapist and buoyancy. Although techniques are directed to joint mobilization and are applied to single joints, a general mobilization of the region is often the result.

The technique is performed with even speed and amplitude to allow for the rebound effect of buoyancy and is much slower than land mobilization. The slower speed is generally more effective and there is less irritation of pain when directing treatment to end of range in a stretching movement by stretch hold, release, stretch hold again technique (Maitland, 1973).

In water this application is easily assisted by the rebound of buoyancy and the physiotherapist or by the patient adding prolonged stretch techniques. The physiotherapist's hold should be close to the area of the spine being mobilized and the mobilizing force may be assisted by flexion and extension of the legs.

Choice of Mobilization Technique

The choice of technique is the same as that recommended by the authors of the land-based techniques (Maitland, 1973; Corrigan and Maitland, 1983; Grieve, 1984; Butler, 1991) providing the water allows a safe breathing position for the patient.

Position of patient and physiotherapist

The position of the patient and physiotherapist is described at the beginning of the section for each level of the spine. Unless otherwise stated refer to this section for the starting position.

Cervical spine

Position: the patient lies supine with pelvic flotation. The physiotherapist stands at the patient's head and holds the head against their chest supporting the occiput with the one hand. A small collar is optional for patient comfort. The patient may be free floating or with the knees bent at 90° and a swimming rope looped around the top of the lower legs and then loosely tied to the pool handrail.

Posteroanterior glide (PA) ↑

The level to be mobilized is palpated with the fingertips on the relevant articular pillar of the vertebra, or spinous process. In the latter case one hand directs the fingers of the other hand on the spinous process and oscillates in a PA direction. The physiotherapist can vary the degree of neck flexion/extension to place the spinal level in the desired position. Special attention is necessary to achieve a PA glide or flexion/extension. The latter should occur however when aiming for physiological movement (Fig. 11.1).

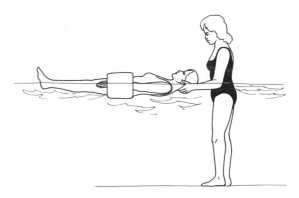

Fig. 11.1 *Cervical spine: posteroanterior glide (PA)*

Variation: The physiotherapist mobilizes unilateral facet joint for unilateral PA glide.

Transverse glide (TG) ← →

The physiotherapist supports the patient's head with a chin hold, as per the land technique. The other hand palpates the transverse process at the level to be mobilized. A transverse force is applied. The head is moved either on the body or the body is moved on the head.

Rotation ↓

The physiotherapist supports the patient's head with a chin hold, the other hand pushes down on the shoulder opposite to the desired rotation and then released to allow rebound. The physiotherapist holds the head still to gain body on head rotation. The amplitude of mobilization varies proportionally to the physiotherapist force.

Variation: The physiotherapist reaches across and above the patient's chest to the shoulder on the same side to the rotation, and pulls shoulder out of water and oscillates (Fig. 11.2).

Variation: Outer range rotation. Position: if the patient is able to lie in side lying in pelvic flotation the physiotherapist supports the patient's head in end outer range rotation and stands in front of the patient. The physiotherapist mobilizes to end outer range rotation by pulling the uppermost shoulder towards him/herself and then oscillates. Care must be given to avoid overmobilization or placing the patient in a precarious breathing position.

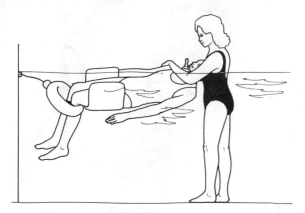

Fig. 11.2   *Cervical spine rotation*

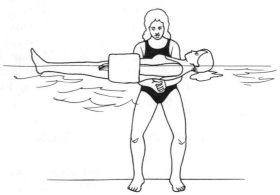

Fig. 11.3   *Posteroanterior glide (PA): lower thoracic spine (T6–T12)*

Longitudinal ⟷

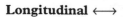

The legs may be fixed at rail with a swimming rope or by another physiotherapist. The physiotherapist flexes the spine to treat the level, i.e. 30° flexion for lower-cervical spine and head in line with body for mid-cervical spine and holds the head with a chin hold. The physiotherapist stands with a wide base of support and then oscillates in a longitudinal direction by leaning backwards. Care must be taken to avoid over-pulling and aggravation of thoracic spinal symptoms.

Traction

The longitudinal technique is sustained not oscillated to obtain traction. The physiotherapist can provide a counterforce with one hand on the dorsal aspect of the upper thoracic spine.

Variation: Position: traction can also be achieved in the vertical with the patient wearing two collars in vertical standing, kneeling, or sitting in the water so that the patient hangs freely by the neck in the water. The physiotherapist can assist the traction by applying controlled downward forces on the shoulder girdle.

Flexion

The physiotherapist moves the neck to achieve flexion/extension instead of a PA glide.

Variation: Position: the physiotherapist holds the occiput with one hand, the other hand is placed on the sternum and oscillates with an anteroposterior (AP) force on the sternum to flex predominantly the lower cervical spine.

Variation: Position: the physiotherapist holds the occiput with one hand. The other hand holds the chin in retraction and then oscillates the head by pushing upward on the occiput to flex predominantly the upper cervical spine.

Thoracic Spine

Position: the patient lies supine with cervical spine and pelvic flotation equipment. The cervical spine support may vary from no flotation equipment to one or more partially or fully inflated neck collar/s. The pelvic support may be adjusted to lie between the thorax and knees to maximize comfort for the individual.

Posteroanterior glide (PA) ↑

Upper Thoracic Spine (T1–T5): Position: the physiotherapist stands at the head of the patient and places fingers, index and middle, on the spinous process and oscillates in a PA direction.

Lower Thoracic Spine (T6–T12): Position: the physiotherapist stands to one side of the patient and palpates the spinous process with the lateral aspect of his/her first metaphalangeal joint of the index finger of one hand. The other hand stabilizes the working hand and oscillates in a PA direction (Fig. 11.3).

Variation: The physiotherapist mobilizes the unilateral facet joint for unilateral PA glide.

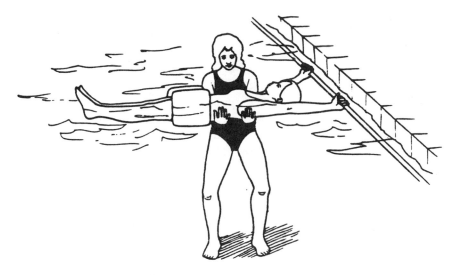

Fig. 11.4   *Thoracic spine: thoracic shunt*

Thoracic shunt

The physiotherapist's position is the same for lower thoracic PA. Both arms are placed under the patient's thorax and holds the opposite lateral thorax with lightly cupped hands. A shunting mobilization is produced by the physiotherapist pushing with one upper arm on the near lateral trunk, pulling with the other hand on the far lateral trunk and oscillating with a 'piston-like' action. This can be applied to levels T5 → T12 of the thoracic spine and include the lumbar spine (Fig. 11.4).

Variation: Fixation of the trunk by one of the physiotherapist's mobilizing arms and oscillation by one arm only. The greater spinal movement occurs distal to the moving arm. Fixation may occur at a lumbar level and mobilization at the thoracic spine or vice versa. This technique can be used to gain relaxation for the trunk musculature prior to using spinal mobilization or other treatment techniques. This technique is contraindicated where there is internal spine fixation or fusion of the spine.

Lumbar Spine

Position: the patient lies supine with cervical spine and pelvic flotation equipment. The pelvic float may be varied to obtain various degrees of flexion and extension of the lumbar spine to assist both the technique and patient comfort.

The techniques to achieve PA glide, Shunting and Unilateral PA glide are mobilized using the same technique as for thoracic spine. The unilateral PA glide will also produce degrees of rotation relative to the force of mobilization.

Transverse glide ← →

Position: the patient lies in side lying on the hydroplinth. The physiotherapist stands in front of the patient and palpates the spinous process at the level to be mobilized. A transverse force is applied. Initially, a float may be placed on the legs proximally and then moved distally using leverage to increase the mobilization.

Rotation ↓ (Fig. 11.5)

Position: the patient in supine lying may be fixed holding along the handrails at the wall or at a corner of the pool. The patient flexes the knees keeping them in the water. Variations of flexion and extension of the lumbar spine will direct mobilization to different levels of spine. The physiotherapist stands on one side of the patient fixing the anterior aspect of the lower thoracic cage on the same side with one hand; the other hand is placed under the patient's body to hold the pelvis on the opposite side. The fixation of the thorax reduces transmission of rotation through the whole spine. The patient is asked to rotate the feet towards the

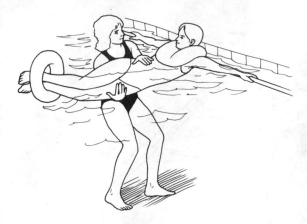

Fig. 11.5   *Lumbar spine rotation*

physiotherapist who oscillates through the patient's pelvis by pulling the opposite side of the pelvis backwards. Alternatively the physiotherapist places the other hand on the near side of the pelvis and oscillates through the pelvis by pushing it forwards. Rotation of the lumbar spine is assisted by the buoyancy effect on the lower limbs moving to one side. Increased mobility is gained by placing flotation equipment on the feet bilaterally.

Variation: To gain greater rotation the flotation equipment is placed on the patient's underneath leg only. Initially, a float may be placed proximally and then moved distally using leverage to increase the rotation.

Longitudinal glide ⟷

Position: supine float with cervical collar and a hydroplinth. The patient is strapped onto a hydroplinth and with counter fixation attached to the handrail. The physiotherapist stands on the side to be mobilized gripping the patient's upper thigh and holding it firmly between their forearm and body, the other hand is placed on the anterior ribcage on the same side to provide counterforce. The physiotherapist stands in step-forward stance with a wide base and transfers their body weight backwards and forwards to oscillate.

Variation: Position: instead of using the hydroplinth, a second physiotherapist stands at the head of the patient holding the lateral thorax bilaterally and pulls backward in a wide stance position to provide counterforce.

Traction

The longitudinal glide is sustained while using either position described in longitudinal glide. *Variation:* Position: the patient is in a vertical sit or kneel posture in an inner tube and hangs free floating in the water. The physiotherapist provides additional lengthening of the spine by prolonged downwards pressure on the pelvis. *Variation:* A weighted belt may be applied to the pelvic region.

Flexion

Position: supine float with cervical and pelvic flotation and handrail hold at poolside or corner. The physiotherapist stands on one side, holds the anterior superior iliac spine bilaterally, pushes down and oscillates in an AP direction. The degree of flexion is proportional to the physiotherapist's force. *Variation:* Position: patient stands back to wall holding handrail and bends knees to chest. The physiotherapist holds the patient's lower legs with knees and hips in full flexion and oscillates by pushing the legs up and down. Further mobilization is gained by adding a small float to the feet (Fig. 11.6).

Extension

Position: the patient is fixed prone on hydroplinth with a cervical collar positioned so that its widest part is placed underneath the patient's chin to obtain a safe breathing position. The physiotherapist palpates the spinous

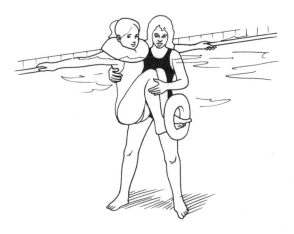

Fig. 11.6   *Lumbar spine flexion*

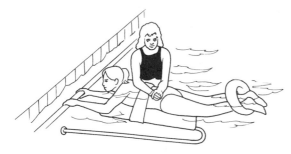

Fig. 11.7 *Lumbar spine extension*

process and oscillates in a PA direction. Further mobilization is gained by adding a small float to the legs using leverage to increase the mobilization force (Fig. 11.7).

Variation: Position: prone with cervical (optional) and pelvic float, the patient grips the handrail and rests their elbows on it, a small float is placed on the feet and the physiotherapist oscillates in a PA direction.

Sacro-iliac Joint (SIJ)

Position: the patient faces the pool wall, grips the handrail with the elbows resting on it and places one knee on the wall in front. On the side to be mobilized the leg hangs below the trunk with the knee flexed.

In lumbar flexion: the physiotherapist stands on the opposite side to be mobilized and stabilizes the patient by holding the handrail diagonally in front of the patient using their body to stabilize the patient posteriorly. The other hand is placed on the opposite side of the pelvis lateral to the SIJ and oscillates diagonally and in a PA direction.

In lumbar extension: the patient is in prone float lying or fixed prone on the hydroplinth. The physiotherapist stands on the opposite side to be mobilized and places one hand on the medial aspect of the opposite SIJ to be mobilized. The physiotherapist holds the anterior aspect of the pelvis with the other hand and oscillates diagonally in an AP direction.

Straight Leg Raise (SLR)

Position: the patient stands with their back to the corner/wall and holds the handrail with both hands. The physiotherapist holds the pelvis against corner/wall and assists the patient to raise one leg in hip flexion with knee extension.

The force can be increased by adding a float on the foot.

Variation: The physiotherapist can add the movement of internal rotation by holding the femoral condyle and rotating in an internal direction.

Neuromeningeal

Position: the patient stands parallel to the wall holding the handrail with the hand opposite to the test/treatment side lifting the leg with hip flexion and knee extension. The physiotherapist stands on the test/treatment side and with one hand on the patient's occiput to vary neck and trunk flexion. The other hand is free to vary dorsiflexion of the foot. A float on the leg can be added to increase the mobilization and progressed using the principle of leverage (Fig. 11.8).

PASSIVE MOBILIZATION USING TURBULENT DRAG (PMTD)

PMTD uses the theorem of Bernoulli (Reid Campion, 1990). The patient is positioned comfortably in flotation equipment placed on the neck and pelvis and is asked to relax fully. The physiotherapist moves the patient away from the direction of the movement to be mobilized. A negative drag is thus produced on the surface of the body near the direction of the

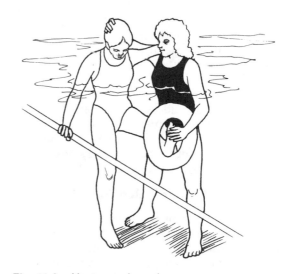

Fig. 11.8 *Neuromeningeal*

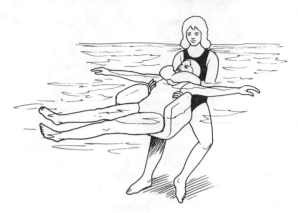

Fig. 11.9   *Spinal lateral flexion*

movement required. When the patient is relaxed the drag will produce a gross mobilization of the spine towards the negative pressure of the water. The drag effect can be graded with speed and controlled change of direction. As well as mobilizing the spine these movements can enhance relaxation, via their hypnotic effect (Whitelock, 1992).

Spinal Lateral Flexion

Position: the patient lies supine in sufficient flotation equipment for comfort. The physiotherapist stands either between the patient's legs or to one side of the lower limbs holding the lateral aspect of both thighs bilaterally and moves the patient to the opposite side of the lateral flexion required.
Variation: Position: the physiotherapist stands at the head of the patient holding either side of the thorax and moves the patient to the opposite side of the lateral flexion to be mobilized (Fig. 11.9).
Variation: Position: the patient is free floating in the vertical kneel or sit position in a tyre or holding the shoulders of the physiotherapist who is facing the patient. The physiotherapist holds the tyre or the patient's lateral chest and moves the patient to the opposite side of lateral flexion to be mobilized (Figs. 11.10a, b).

Spinal Flexion/Extension/Rotation

Position: the patient and the physiotherapist are face to face in the water with the patient's legs astride those of the physiotherapist. The physiotherapist holds the patient's lower trunk moving the patient in the opposite direction to the

mobilization required. In the case of flexion/extension the physiotherapist moves forwards or backwards but in the case of rotation moves in an arc or circle.
Variation: Position: the patient is positioned in a tyre facing the physiotherapist or holding the physiotherapist's shoulders in a sitting or kneeling position and free floating. The physiotherapist moves in the direction opposite to that of the required mobilization.

SELF-MANAGEMENT

Patients who have been treated by hydrotherapy for spinal problems should be provided with a self-management programme to control spinal symptoms and to prevent relapse of the condition. This programme could include a water-based and land-based programme to be carried out in their own time at an appropriate community pool and home/office (Smit and Harrison, 1991). The pool programme will require flotation equipment including a cervical collar and pelvic float, either commercial or hand made (tubigrip, sailcloth filled with polystyrene blocks or balls), and armband floaties or rings available at standard swim shops. The programme should be individualized and may include exercises to maintain or improve range of spinal motion, particularly for patients whose hydrotherapy programme includes any form of passive mobilization. A complete self-management programme would include posture, range of motion, muscle strength, both concentric/eccentric work with coordination of

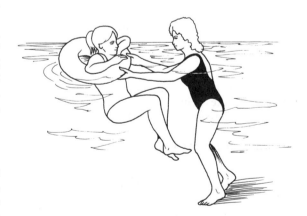

Fig. 11.10a   *Spinal flexion/extension*

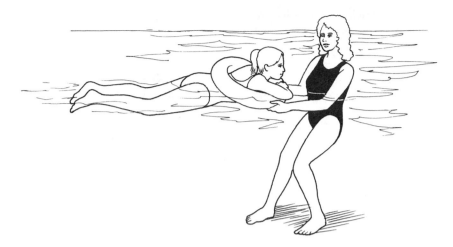

Fig. 11.10b   Spinal flexion/extension

trunk (Miller and Medeiros, 1987) and peripheral limbs, endurance, power and fitness. Swimming strokes must be modified for the individual so that the spinal symptoms are not aggravated. The mobility section of the self-management programme aims to maintain or improve the range of movements gained by passive mobilization techniques used in the hydrotherapy treatment.

Self-management spinal mobility exercises in the water may include some of the following:

Position 1

Lie in supine with flotation equipment under the neck and pelvis. The number and position of flotation equipment is individual to the patient's comfort.

1.1 Feet hooked under handrail

Exercise 1: Push the back of head down against the neck float with chin tucked in. Hold the float down for 5 counts and slowly release.

Exercise 2: Rotate the head to right hold against the neck float for 5 counts slowly return to middle. Repeat to the other side.

Exercise 3: Place a small float or kickboard under the back between the shoulder blades. Push back down against float or kickboard for 5 counts, hold and slowly release.

Exercise 4: Keep the body flat on top of the water and bend sideways from the waist to reach hand down to the foot. Repeat on other side. (Neck collar is optional.)

1.2 Rest head/shoulders on handrail and grip with hands

Exercise 1: Bend knees so that feet are directed to the pool floor, keeping the knees in the water, take both feet to the one side, return to the middle and repeat to the other side. A small ring float can be added under the arches of the feet to increase the stretch.

Position 2

Lie in prone with flotation equipment on neck (optional) and feet. Grip the handrail resting elbows on it. A hydroplinth can be used for this exercise.

Exercise 1: Push feet down against the float with knees straight and relax very slowly to allow feet to rise to the top of the water.

Position 3

Stand facing the pool wall, shoulders underwater, grip the handrail with both hands and rest elbows on it. Hang the body down in the water with knees together and bent. Keep the lower legs parallel to the pool floor and the body close to the wall.

Exercise 1: Keeping the knees pointing directly down to the bottom of the pool twist the feet together to one side allowing the spine to rotate. Return the feet to the middle and repeat to the other side.

Exercise 2: Swing both legs like a pendulum to one side allowing the spine to bend but keep the body close to the wall, return the legs to the middle and repeat to the other side. Add a ring float to both legs close to the knees to increase the stretch.

Exercise 3: Using two neck collars and keeping the chin tucked in, lightly hold hand rail, hang in a kneel or sit position and allow the neck to stretch gently.

Position 4

Place a tyre around the body under armpits. Lightly hold the handrail and hang in a kneel or sit position.

Exercise 1: Allow the spine to stretch gently.

Position 5

Sit down in a chair position (a 'sitting' like position with hips flexed and abducted slightly wider than the body's width with the knees flexed to 90° and feet flat on the pool floor. Shoulders are flexed and abducted slightly with the rest of the arms extended) facing and holding the handrail at arms length from the wall.

Exercise 1: Stretch one hand across in front of body and as far to the side as possible. Keeping the feet still during the movement.

Position 6

Stand or sit with the back to the wall hold along the rails with both hands keeping the shoulders under the water. The depth of the water is dependent on spinal comfort.

Exercise 1: Push the chin forwards along the top of the water and return to tuck the chin in and stretch the back of the neck. Keep looking straight ahead throughout the movement.

Exercise 2: Keeping the back against the wall bend both knees to the chest. A small ring float can be placed under the arches of the feet to increase the stretch.

Exercise 3: Keep leg straight, lift it up in front as high as possible. Add a small ring float to the ankle to increase the stretch.

Position 7

Stand facing the wall and hold the handrails at arms length from the wall.

Exercise 1: Keeping the feet on the floor, look upwards and bend backwards to extend the spine and return to the standing position.

Position 8

Stand parallel to the wall holding the handrail with one hand at arms length from the wall.

Exercise 1: Keep leg straight lifting up in front as high as possible, bend head and body forward. Add a small ring float to the ankle to increase the stretch.

Position 9

Hold a dumb-bell/kickboard in each hand with arms straight, shoulders abducted and keeping clear of pool wall. Squat down so that the shoulders are underwater and the body's position is in a free floating kneel position.

Exercise 1: Tuck both knees to the chest slowly, tip the head back, straighten the legs and lie flat in supine on top of the water. Tuck both knees to the chest, bring the head forward to return to the squat position.

Exercise 2: Tuck both knees to the chest and then tip the head forward and lie flat in prone on the top of the water. Tuck both knees to the chest and return to the squat position. Exercises 1 and 2 can be combined into one exercise.

Exercise 3: Swing both legs like a pendulum to one side, return to the midline and then repeat to the other side.

SUMMARY

Mobilization, passive or active, of the spine in water is only one aspect of physical treatment and management of spinal problems. The physiotherapist must select passive mobilization as a treatment technique based on a knowledge of the patient's presenting signs and symptoms. The type of technique selected is based on current knowledge of effectiveness and outcome. At all stages the physiotherapist must critically analyse and evaluate these treatment techniques to deliver the highest level of care. Research also supports muscle strengthening, particularly abdominus transversus and obliquus for stability problems of the spine (Tesh *et al.*, 1987; Miller and Mederios, 1987; Richardson *et al.*, 1990; Jull *et al.*, 1993), and fitness for ongoing management (Cady *et al.*, 1979; Mayer *et al.*, 1986). Posture, balance and coordination, correct lifting techniques, as well as general or specific advice on back protection for all activities of daily living including occupation must also be advocated.

ACKNOWLEDGEMENTS

Bronwyn McIveen: Physiotherapy colleague with hydrotherapy and manipulative therapy qualifications, who has helped me enormously in hydrotherapy development. Her critical analysis, knowledge and enthusiasm are admirable.

Ann Hallum: Hydrotherapy assistant, whose constant support and devotion to hydrotherapy is much appreciated.

Veronica Delafosse: Librarian, for title search and support.

Siang Jeffries: Typist, my sincere thanks for her patience.

Anthony Rigby: Dear friend, my special thanks for proof reading.

REFERENCES

Association of Swimming Therapy (1992). *Swimming for People with Disabilities*, 2nd edn, London: A&C Black.

Australian Physiotherapy Association (1990). Clinical standards for hydrotherapy. *The Australian Journal of Physiotherapy*, 36(3): 207–210.

Bogduk N. and Twomey L.T. (1991). *Clinical Anatomy of the Lumbar Spine*, 2nd edn, Melbourne: Churchill Livingstone.

Bolton E. and Goodwin D. (1974). *Introduction to Pool Exercises*, Edinburgh: Churchill Livingstone.

Brown L. (1990). Treatment and examination of the spine by combined movements – 2. *Physiotherapy*, 76(2): 66–74.

Butler D.S. (1991). *Mobilisation of Nervous System*, Melbourne: Churchill Livingstone.

Cady L.D., Bischoff D.P., O'Connell E.R., Thomas P. and Allen J. (1979). Strength and fitness and subsequent back injuries in firefighters. *Journal of Occupational Medicine*, 21: 269–272.

Caillet R. (1981). *Low Back Pain Syndrome*, Philadelphia: FA Davis Co.

Corrigan B. and Maitland G.D. (1983). *Practical Orthopaedic Medicine*, Sydney: Butterworth and Co.

Davis B.A. and Harrison R.A. (1988). *Hydrotherapy in Practice*, Edinburgh: Churchill Livingstone.

Flor H. and Turk D.C. (1984). Etiological theories and treatments for chronic back pain, 1: Somatic models and interventions. *Pain*, 19: 105–121.

Franchimont P., Juchmes J. and Lecomte J. (1983). Hydrotherapy – mechanisms and indications. *Pharmac. Ther.*, 20: 79–93.

Giovanelli B., Thompson E. and Elvey R. (1985). Measurements of variations in lumbar zygapophyseal joint intracapsular pressure: A pilot study. *Australian Journal of Physiotherapy*, 31(3): 115–121.

Grieve G.P. (1984). *Mobilization of the Spine, Notes on Examination, Assessment and Clinical Method*, 4th edn, London: Churchill Livingstone.

Guyton A.C. (1991). *The Textbook of Medical Physiology*, 8th edn, Sydney: W.B. Saunders Co.

Horsfield R., Solomons S. and Ward A. (1982). *Physics and Chemistry for the Health Sciences*, Marrickville, New South Wales: Science Press Australia.

Jull G., Richardson C., Toppenberg R. and Bang B. (1993). Towards a measurement of active muscle control for lumbar stabilisation. *The Australian Journal of Physiotherapy*, 39(3): 187–193.

Korr I.M. (1975). Proprioception and somatic dysfunction. *Journal of American Osteopathic Association*, 74: 638–650.

Langridge J.C. and Phillips D. (1988). Group hydrotherapy exercises for chronic back pain sufferers – Introduction and monitoring. *Physiotherapy*, 74(6): 269–273.

Lee R. and Evans J. (1994). Towards a better understanding of spinal posteroanterior mobilization. *Physiotherapy*, 80(2): 68–73.

McMillian J. (1984). Unpublished lecture material. Halliwick Aquatics instructions training course, supervised by James McMillian, conducted by VicSwim in conjunction with the Australian Physiotherapy Association, March 1984.

Maher C. and Adams R. (1994). Reliability of pain and stiffness assessment in clinical manual lumbar spine examination. *Physical Therapy*, 24(9): 801–811.

Maitland G.D. (1973). *Vertebral Manipulation*, 3rd edn, London: Butterworths & Co.

Matyas T.A. and Bach T.M. (1985). The reliability of selected techniques in clinical arthrometrics. *The Australian Journal of Physiotherapy*, 31(5): 175–199.

Mayer T.G., Gatchel R.J., Kishino N., Keeley J., Mayer H., Capra G. and Mooney V. (1986). A prospective short-term study of chronic low back pain patients utilising novel objective functional measurement. *Pain* **2S**: 53–68.

Mayer T.G., Tencer A.F., Kristofferson S. and Mooney V. (1984). Use of noninvasive techniques for quantification of spinal range-of-motion in normal subjects and chronic low-back dysfunction patients. *Spine*, **9(6)**: 588–595.

Miller M.I. and Mederios J.M. (1987). Recruitment of internal oblique and transversus abdominus muscles during the eccentric phase of curl-up exercise. *Physical Therapy*, **67(8)**: 1213–1217.

Pearcy M.J. and Tibrewal S.B. (1984). Axial rotation and lateral bending in the normal lumbar spine measured by three-dimensional radiography. *Spine*, **9**: 582–587.

Punjabi M., Yamamoto I., Oxland T. and Crisco J. (1989). How does posture affect coupling in the lumbar spine. *Spine*, **14(9)**: 1002–1011.

Reid Campion M. (1990). *Adult Hydrotherapy: A Practical Approach*, Oxford: Heinemann Medical Books.

Reid Campion M. (1991). *Hydrotherapy in Paediatrics*, 2nd edn, London: William Heinemann Medical Books.

Richardson C., Toppenberg R. and Jull G. (1990). An initial evaluation of eight abdominal exercises for their ability to provide stabilisation of the lumbar spine. *The Australian Journal of Physiotherapy*, **36(1)**: 6–11.

Schneider G. and Pardoe M. (1985). Translation of the facts during coupled motion in the cervical spine: A pilot study. *The Australian Journal of Physiotherapy*, **31(2)**: 39–44.

Skinner A.T. and Thomson A.M. (1983). *Duffield's Exercise in Water*, 3rd edn, London: Ballière Tindall.

Smit T.E. and Harrison R. (1991). Hydrotherapy and chronic lower back pain: A pilot study. *The Australian Journal of Physiotherapy*, **37(4)**: 229–234.

Tesh K.M., Shaw Dunn J. and Evans J.H. (1987). The abdominal muscles and vertebral stability. *Spine*, **12(5)**: 501–508.

Twomey L. and Taylor J. (1982). Flexion creep deformation and hysteresis in the lumbar vertebral columns. *Spine*, **7(2)**: 116–122.

Vincenzio G. and Twomey L. (1993). Side flexion induced lumbar spine conjunct rotation and its influencing factors. *The Australian Journal of Physiotherapy*, **39(4)**: 299–306.

Wall P.D. and Melzack R. (1994). *Textbook of Pain*, 3rd edn, Edinburgh: Churchill Livingstone.

White A.A. and Punjabi M.M. (1978). *Clinical Biomechanics of the Spine*, Philadelphia: Lippincott Co.

Whitelock H. (1992). *Water Exercise for Better Health*, Melbourne: Lothian Publishing Co. Pty Ltd.

Wyke B.D. (1985). Articular neurology and manipulative therapy. In *Aspects of Manipulative Therapy*, 2nd edn, E.F. Glasgow, L.T. Twomey, E.R. Scull, A.M. Kleynhaus and R.M. Ideyak (eds), Melbourne: Churchill Livingstone, pp. 72–77.

Yamamoto I., Punjabi M.M., Crisco T. and Oxland T. (1989). Three-dimensional movements of the whole lumbar spine and lumbarsacral joint. *Spine*, **14(11)**: 1256–1260.

Zusman M. (1986). Spinal manipulative therapy: Review of some proposed mechanisms, and a new hypothesis. *The Australian Journal of Physiotherapy*, **32(2)**: 89–99.

ADDITIONAL READING

Battié M., Bigos S.J., Fisher L.D., Spengler D.M., Hansson T.H., Nachemson A.L. and Wortley M.D. (1990). The role of spinal flexibility in back pain complaints within industry – A prospective study. *Spine*, **15(18)**: 768–773.

Biering-Sorensen F. (1984). Physical measurements as risk indicators for low-back trouble over a one-year period. *Spine*, **9(2)**: 106–119.

Blomberg S., Hallin G., Grann K., Berg E. and Sennerby U. (1994). Manual therapy with steroid injections – A new approach to treatment of lower back pain – A controlled multicenter trial with an evaluation by orthopaedic surgeons. *Spine*, **19(5)**: 569–577.

Dalton P.A. and Jull G.A. (1989). The distribution and characteristic of neck–arm pain in patients with and without a neurological deficit. *The Australian Journal of Physiotherapy*, **35(1)**: 3–8.

Elvey R.L. (1986). Treatment of arm pain associated with abnormal brachial plexus tension. *The Australian Journal of Physiotherapy*, **32(4)**: 225–230.

Güeken L.N. and Hof A.L. (1994). Instrumental straight leg-raising: Results in patients. *Arch. Phys. Med. Rehabil.* **75**: 470–477.

Hall J., Bisson D. and O'Hare P. (1990). The physiology of immersion. *Physiotherapy*, **76(9)**: 517–521.

Herzog W., Conway P.J., Kawchuk G.N., Zhang Y. and Hasler E.M. (1993). Forces exerted during spinal manipulative therapy. *Spine*, **18(9)**: 1206–1212.

Maitland G.D. (1985). Passive movement techniques for intra-articular and periarticular disorders. *The Australian Journal of Physiotherapy*, **31(1)**: 3–8.

Maitland G.D. (1985). The Slump Test: examination and treatment. *The Australian Journal of Physiotherapy*, **31(6)**: 215–219.

Marras W.S. and Wongsam P.E. (1986). Flexibility and velocity of the normal and impaired lumbar spine. *Arch. Phys. Med. Rehabil.*, **67**: 213–217.

Philip K., Lew P. and Matyas T.A. (1989). The inter-therapist reliability of the Slump Test. *The Australian Journal of Physiotherapy*, **35(2)**: 89–94.

Tibrewal S.B., Pearcy M.J., Portek J. and Spivey J. (1985). A prospectus study of lumbar spine movements before and after discetomy using biplanar radiography. *Spine*, **10**: 455–460.

Von Korff M. (1994). Studying the natural history of back pain. *Spine*, **19(185)**: 20415–20465.

12

Spinal cord injuries

Aliçon Bennie

The physiotherapist may encounter a patient with spinal cord injury (SCI) either during the initial stage of rehabilitation or, later, as part of an ongoing fitness programme or as a result of a complication of their injury, e.g. contracture. It is widely accepted that hydrotherapy can augment SCI rehabilitation (Guttman, 1976; Nixon, 1985; Bromley, 1991). The physiological effects of warm water, the principles of turbulence as a form of impedance, and the use of buoyancy to assist weak muscles can all be utilized effectively when treating a person with SCI in water.

Spinal cord injury can affect anyone at any stage of their life. Paralysis may occur through trauma or disease. An injury to the spinal cord will affect motor power, sensation and control of the bladder, bowel and sexual function. High thoracic and cervical lesions will also have disturbances of the autonomic nervous system.

Lesions may be (a) complete, i.e having no innervation below the level of injury or (b) incomplete, i.e having some sparing of muscle power or sensation below the damaged segment. The degree of incompleteness can be classified using the American Spinal Injury Association (ASIA) Impairment Scale (Ditunno, 1992) (Table 12.1). For the purpose of this chapter, incomplete lesions will refer to those who have some motor sparing, i.e. ASIA grade C, D, E.

Paraplegia is the term describing someone who has acquired loss of movement and sensation to the legs or legs and trunk. A person exhibiting paralysis in their arms, in addition to their legs and trunk, is described as having tetraplegia.

Many newly acquired SCI people will be admitted to specialist centres solely treating SCI or other neurological conditions. Others may remain in an orthopaedic or general hospital.

The physiotherapist should take into account the stage of rehabilitation the patient is at when devising a hydrotherapy programme. The person with a newly acquired SCI will normally be referred for hydrotherapy as part of a comprehensive and extensive rehabilitation programme. Hydrotherapy should complement the dry-land programme, supplementing rather than duplicating activities which are already being undertaken, perhaps more effectively, on dry land. Frequently the hydrotherapist and the dry-land physiotherapist are one and the same person. Water has unique properties and, as previously emphasized in other chapters, these should be used to maximum effect. In no other medium can a paralysed person be totally independent without the use of artificial aids. The ease with which a severely disabled person can be handled in water should also be utilized.

People with a long standing paraplegia or tetraplegia may be referred for hydrotherapy with a specific problem, e.g. contracture, spasticity. Treatment sessions should reflect these needs.

Initial treatment sessions need to be on a one-to-one basis. This will help the patient to build confidence and assist the physiotherapist in providing adequate support for exercises and swimming. Fatigue may be a problem for high lesions and treatment sessions should be kept short initially. Adequate rest periods should follow pool treatment to allow the impaired autonomic nervous system to recover.

Table 12.1 ASIA Impairment Scale (Ditunno, 1992)

The following scale is used in grading the degree of impairment in spinal cord injuries

A = Complete. No sensory or motor function is preserved in the sacral segments S4–S5.

B = Incomplete. Sensory but not motor function is preserved below the neurological level and extends through the sacral segments S4–S5.

C = Incomplete. Motor function is preserved below the neurological level, and the majority of key muscles below the neurological level have a muscle grade less than 3.

D = Incomplete. Motor function is preserved below the neurological level, and the majority of key muscles below the neurological level have a muscle grade greater than or equal to 3.

E = Normal. Sensory and motor function is normal.

INDICATIONS FOR HYDROTHERAPY

Patients should be orthopaedically and physiologically stable prior to hydrotherapy treatment. Different methods are utilized to stabilize the spine of the person with an acute traumatic SCI. Postural reduction, surgical fixation or reduction are all commonly used. The method chosen will determine the time when a patient is able to commence hydrotherapy. Consultation should be made with the medical team about restrictions imposed on trunk or neck movements when in the pool.

CONSIDERATIONS, PRECAUTIONS AND CONTRAINDICATIONS

Physiological Changes

Changes in the autonomic nervous system need to be considered during hydrotherapy treatment of lesions above T6.

Temperature control

Temperature control may be affected in lesions above T6 (Guttman *et al.*, 1958; Johnson, 1992).

The inability of the blood vessels to constrict quickly, due to a lack of sympathetic control, can lead to a rapid drop in core temperature. There is much debate regarding pool temperatures. In general, the pool temperature should reflect the level of activity of the patients. Swimming or aerobic training sessions will require a pool with a temperature lower than one where the emphasis is on pain relief and reduction of tone. Temperatures between 32–35°C are acceptable for sessions where there is a low level of activity. Lack of temperature control may lead to difficulties for the person with high tetraplegia, who cannot move sufficiently to stay warm, if they wish to continue swimming in a public swimming pool, where the temperature is considerably lower.

Postural hypotension

Postural hypotension is common in the early stages of SCI (Mathias and Frankel, 1992). This is caused by a drop in blood pressure during changes in position. Baroreceptor reflexes control short-term changes in blood pressure (Barron and Blair, 1993). The patient with tetraplegia may experience postural hypotension when coming out of the pool. This usually occurs when the patient is lifted with the hoist. The physiotherapist should be aware of this to allow time for the autonomic nervous system to react during changes in position.

Considerations for Hydrotherapy Treatment

Incontinence

Many people with paraplegia and tetraplegia will be incontinent of urine and faeces. Most will develop a regular bowel routine but should ensure they have emptied their bowels prior to entering the pool. Catheters may be spigotted if the bladder capacity can accommodate this. An over extended bladder may instigate autonomic dysreflexia. This may lead to raised blood pressure and a throbbing headache (Mathias *et al.*, 1992). Otherwise, a clean urinary leg bag should be used. Small volume collection bags are available and can be worn discreetly tucked into the swimming costume. People with no collection devices should empty their bladder prior to entering the pool. All pools should have a wheelchair accessible toilet.

Open wounds

Patients with extensive open wounds should not be allowed in the hydrotherapy pool. The risk of infection to that person may result in several months of bed rest to allow the wound to heal. There is also the risk of infecting others. Small wounds may be covered with an occlusive dressing, although prolonged submersion may be detrimental to healing.

Lack of sensation

SCI affects sensation below the level of the lesion. Care should be applied when assisting the patient into the pool. Rough tiling around the pool may cause grazing of delicate skin.

The physiotherapist should also consider the lack of sensation when choosing hand positions for support. This is particularly relevant when teaching a person with tetraplegia to swim as they may not realize that they are being supported. This can lead to a lack of confidence.

Decreased vital capacity

Vital capacity will be decreased in the person with SCI whose intercostal and abdominal muscles are denervated. Carter (1992) states that there is a 26% mean reduction of total lung capacity in people with tetraplegia and that the vital capacity (VC) is 55% of the predicted value. It is also noted that VC will alter according to position, e.g. supine and sitting. This should not be a contraindication to pool treatment, however, the physiotherapist must be aware of reduced reserve capacities particularly in prone swimming.

ENTRY TO THE POOL

Many patients will enter the pool with the help of a hoist. Patients who suffer from postural hypotension may benefit from using a stretcher attachment, although most find a chair attachment sufficient.

In later stages, people with paraplegia may be able to transfer from their wheelchair to the floor, then lower themselves into the pool. Precautions need to be taken to avoid damage to the skin over bony prominences when getting out of the pool. A towel or mat can be put on the polished surfaces to avoid grazes.

TREATMENT

The main aims of treatment are:

1. Reduction of spasticity.
2. Relief of pain.
3. Increase range of movement.
4. Improve muscle power.
5. Increase aerobic capacity.
6. Re-educate gait.
7. Re-educate swimming.

When devising any treatment programme a problem solving approach should be taken. Treatment will consist of many techniques previously described in this book and others (Skinner and Thomson, 1983; Davis and Harrison, 1988). Adaptations of these techniques and specific exercises suitable for the treatment of SCI in the pool are outlined in this chapter.

Reduction of Spasticity

Most people with SCI above the level of T12 will have some degree of spasticity (Edgar, 1992; Illis, 1992). This may interfere with sitting posture or with activities of daily living. Physiotherapy techniques which include inhibition of reflex activity are often used to reduce spasticity (Illis, 1992). The pool provides a useful medium for facilitating a reduction in tone.

Spasticity may mask underlying muscle power. Buoyancy can facilitate voluntary movement when tone has been reduced. Conversely, excessive demand on weak muscles may result in a further increase in tone due to associated reactions.

Warm water can produce temporary relaxation of muscle tone (Skinner and Thomson, 1983). Specific exercises, particularly those with a rotation component, may enhance this further. Passive movements can also help to decrease tone (Lammertse, 1992).

Passive exercises

1. *Using turbulence*:
   (a) the patient lies supine wearing neck and body floats. The physiotherapist stands between the patient's thighs. The patient is then swayed from side to side in an arc. Turbulence will help to side flex the trunk. The physiotherapist accelerates

through the arc thus increasing the turbulence. If deceleration, towards the end of the arc, occurs it will help to prevent the patient from spasming, as the turbulence will dissipate before changing the direction of movement.

The physiotherapist can also push down on one hip to add a rotation component to the exercise.

(b) The patient lies supine with neck, body and, if necessary, leg floats. The physiotherapist is at the head end of the patient and sways the patient from side to side. The physiotherapist can facilitate selective segmental movement by placing her hands either at the top of the trunk or at the waist. This exercise is not usually suitable for someone with excessive extensor spasticity.

2. Two physiotherapists are required to rotate the patient in opposite directions. One stands at the head end rotating the shoulders in one direction, while the second stands between the patient's thighs and rotates in the opposite direction. The physiotherapist who is between the patient's thighs should feel an immediate reduction in adductor spasticity. Water is an ideal medium for this stretch as it allows the shoulder to be pushed down into the water while the pelvis is raised, thus getting a true rotation around the axis of the spinal column. On land, the supporting surface would prevent the last few degrees of rotation.

Active exercises for the person with an incomplete lesion

1. The patient holds on to the corner of the pool whilst having their hips and knees bent to 90°. The knees are rotated in one direction and the shoulders in the opposite (Fig. 12.1). The knees must stay on the same horizontal plane throughout the exercise. This position is held, then the knees and shoulders are rotated to the other side.

2. *Cycling*:
   (a) The patient is upright in deep water and cycles. This position can be achieved by holding on to the corner of the pool while facing outward or while supported

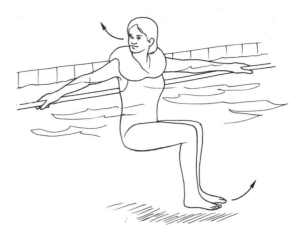

Fig. 12.1 *Patient rotating trunk to decrease spasticity*

with a float-belt or 'Wet-vest'. This reciprocal exercise helps to decrease tone in the lower limbs. It should, however, only be performed within a range which the patient can control. The knees should not be extended to the point where extensor spasticity is initiated.

(b) The patient sits on the stool in the water and cycles. The maintenance of flexion at the hips should help to avoid an extensor thrust.

Relief of Pain

Pain sometimes occurs in the acute SCI. This may be in the back or neck as a result of the weakness induced by prolonged bed rest or fixation. The shoulders may also be affected due to spasticity or a decreased range of movement.

Warm water can have a sedative effect on pain and therefore allow more effective exercising (Skinner and Thomson, 1983).

Neurogenic or root pain may be temporarily relieved in some patients.

Increasing Range of Movement

The reduction in range of movement of a single joint can be severely debilitating to a person whose independence is already compromised by a lack of muscle innervation. For example, a shortened biceps tendon in a person without an innervated triceps can prevent independent transfers.

Warm water may help to relieve pain which will make stretching more comfortable. General exercises can maintain range of movement in all joints although specific attention will be required to affected joints.

Lower limbs

Passive movements to maintain range of movement to the lower limbs may be facilitated by the reduction in tone which warm water may produce. Patients can be in float lying or strapped or held on to submerged inclined plinth. However, adequate fixation of the physiotherapist's body may be difficult to achieve full range of movement in stiff joints. In this instance, passive movements may be achieved more effectively on dry land.

Shoulders

Many people with tetraplegia have painful shoulders with a resultant decrease in range of movement. Passive stretches are more effective and comfortable when utilizing the pain relief and reduction in spasticity which warm water promotes.

Passive stretching can be performed in float lying. The physiotherapist can fixate either the arm while the trunk moves away or the trunk while the arm moves away. Some patients find it more comfortable when the trunk is moved away from the arm. The pool offers the ideal method of doing this.

Stretching can also be done as active assisted or resisted exercises. Momentum gained during resisted movement can stretch contracted muscles. Care should be taken if using this technique in the presence of acute inflammation.

Elbows

A complication for some C5 lesions is contracted elbows. This is due to the unopposed contraction of biceps. Range of movement can be gained using hold/relax techniques while in float lying. The warmth of the water will reinforce relaxation of the biceps.

Trunk

The acute SCI person often has a stiff trunk due to the postural reduction or surgical fixation that has been performed. Consultation regarding trunk exercises should be made with the medical staff prior to the initial hydrotherapy session. The patient may need to wear a brace while in the pool. There may also be restrictions in the amount of trunk movement allowed. Once trunk mobilization is allowed, exercises as described in 'Reduction of spasticity' may be performed.

Improving Muscle Power

Exercising in water can prove invaluable for strengthening weak muscles. Buoyancy assisted exercises will produce movement in joints where muscle power is only grade 1 or 2 of the Oxford Scale (Hollis, 1981).

Incomplete lesions or those with fully innervated muscles weakened by prolonged bed rest will benefit from a strengthening programme in the hydrotherapy pool. It is not so beneficial for direct strengthening of muscles which are already Oxford grade 5. When hydrotherapy is used as part of a complete rehabilitation programme, further strengthening exercises can be performed using multi-gym or weight-training equipment on dry land. Time in the pool would be more effectively spent, as described later in this chapter, increasing aerobic capacity.

Upper limbs

Bad Ragaz techniques, increasing leverage, e.g. with table tennis bats or floats, exercises involving the body or limbs in an unstreamlined position or exercises where turbulence is increased can all be used to strengthen the upper limbs (Skinner and Thomson, 1983; Davis and Harrison, 1988).

Adaptation of Bad Ragaz techniques can be particularly effective for people with C6 lesions. They can perform the abduction, lateral rotation pattern well but usually find difficulty performing the adduction, medial rotation pattern, due to the lack of full innervation of latissimus dorsi, pectoralis major, teres major and triceps.

1. Pectoralis major can be facilitated by using maximal fixation to medial rotation and keeping the elbow extended when adducting the arm from a starting position of 90° abduction.
   Starting position: Supine float lying with right arm at 90° abduction. The physiotherapist's right hand is placed over the

patient's wrist to fixate the arm in lateral rotation. The physiotherapist's left hand is placed under the elbow to maintain extension.

Action: The patient then pulls their trunk towards their arm.

Note: This technique will not be successful if full elbow extension cannot be maintained. The strong biceps muscle will produce elbow flexion rather than allowing the weak pectoralis major to adduct the shoulder.

2. Triceps can be facilitated using the abduction, lateral rotation pattern.

   Starting position: Supine float lying with the elbow flexed across the trunk, the shoulder in adduction.

   Action: When maximal fixation is given to the shoulder abduction component while minimal fixation is given to the elbow extension component, irradiation to the triceps muscle will occur as the arm straightens and the trunk moves away from the arm.

Trunk

Bad Ragaz techniques with stabilization from the shoulders, while useful for some people with incomplete lesions, are extremely difficult for those without muscle power in the legs. Techniques with stabilization at the pelvis or thigh are more useful for the person with a complete paraplegia. Rhythmic stabilizations can be used to strengthen muscles where movement is prohibited. Other exercises which are also useful for the person with paraplegia who has weak trunk flexors are described here.

1. *Starting position*: Patient in supine lying with neck float and the physiotherapist between the patient's thighs.

   Action: Patient comes up to touch the physiotherapist's shoulders with their hands. The physiotherapist can allow the hips of a patient with poor trunk innervation to sink or can push the hips up for those with more trunk control. This exercise is not suitable to strengthen fully innervated trunk muscles because the physiotherapist will have difficulty maintaining a stable position.

2. *Starting position*: as before.

Action: Patient comes up with the right hand to touch the physiotherapist's right shoulder. The exercise can be repeated to the opposite side. This produces flexion with rotation.

3. *Starting position*: as before.

   Action: The physiotherapist starts to swing, in an arc, towards the patient's right. The patient is then told to pull the right hand down towards the right knee. This produces side flexion. Turbulence will provide impedance to the movement. The exercise is then repeated to the opposite side.

   Note: The body must remain on a horizontal plane. No rotation should occur.

Lower limbs

Care needs to be taken when treating patients with increased tone. Exercises should be performed in a range which the patient can fully control. As further control is gained, the range of movement can be increased. There is nothing to be gained from extension exercises which are achieved through facilitating extensor spasms.

A variety of starting positions can maximize the effect of lower limb strengthening, e.g. sitting, supine float lying, submerged plinth, upright floating, standing. The pool is particularly useful for patients who have Oxford grade 1 or 2 muscle power (Hollis, 1981). Standing exercises should be performed only when balance and trunk control are sufficient.

Bad Ragaz techniques, floats, manual resistance and turbulence can all be used to add impedance to lower limb exercises.

Flaccid low lesions may have weak or no innervation of hamstrings, gluteii, plantar and dorsi flexors, while having strong hip flexors and quadriceps. Appropriate use of buoyancy assisted exercise can facilitate these weak muscles. Care needs to be taken when using flippers as a means of resistance. Overstretching of weak dorsiflexors may occur if flippers are worn on the flaccid foot.

Increasing Aerobic Capacity

Swimming is an ideal way of improving aerobic capacity. It does not put the same stress on the shoulder joints as other wheelchair sports, e.g. wheelchair basketball, but will achieve the same goal. Gerhart *et al.* (1993) stated that shoulder pain was noted as one of the main causes for a decrease in independence of long-standing SCI.

Many people with a high tetraplegia who cannot push a manual wheelchair find it extremely difficult to exercise aerobically. They may also not be able to swim independently. Good aerobic exercise can be achieved in supine lying while progressing up and down the pool by lifting the arms out of the water, abducting and vigorously pulling in. Neck and hip floats may be required to prevent sinking. It should be noted that this is not a progression to independent swimming and other techniques (p. 130) should be employed if this is the aim. It does, however, enable a person with a high tetraplegia to exercise vigorously enough to raise his heart and respiratory rates. This type of exercise may help to prevent the drop in core temperature, described earlier, when immersed in a cooler pool. Likewise, care should be taken to prevent overheating when in pools heated to around body temperature.

Re-educating Gait

The pool may be the ideal medium for gait re-education of the person with a flaccid paraplegia but may not be so suitable for the person with a spastic incomplete lesion. Spasticity may be increased during this activity and, if so, it would, perhaps, be more appropriate to leave walking to dry land where normal movement techniques can be more effectively applied. Assessment in different depths of water and evaluation of spasticity, following initial sessions, are the key factors when selecting future treatment programmes. Exercises in standing may not produce an increase in tone.

Standing and walking may be facilitated by using buoyancy to support the weight of the weak flaccid lesion. Weight-bearing can be reduced by increasing the depth of water (Harrison and Bulstrode, 1987, p. 26). This may allow some people with insufficient muscle power to stand on dry land to commence gait training or pre-gait training exercises earlier.

SWIMMING

Swimming is an extremely valuable form of exercise for almost everyone. The person with an SCI is no exception. They can gain independence in water, free from any form of aid or appliance, that cannot be achieved on land. It is an activity which may start as a therapeutic exercise, i.e. increasing strength and endurance, go on to be a recreational activity and then, for some, offer an opportunity for competition, be it at club or international level.

Density

Prior to teaching a person with SCI to swim, the physiotherapist should consider changes which may have occurred to that person's density. The body is at its most dense between 18 and 36 years of age approximately. Many spinal injuries happen during this time, therefore the physiotherapist will be handling someone who is, physiologically, at the most dense period of their life. Muscle atrophy will alter the ratio of the major body components with a specific gravity less than one, i.e. fat, cancellous bone and those which are greater than one, i.e. muscle, compact bone. This could have the effect of decreasing the overall density, thus assisting the person to float.

Bone may become osteoporotic after the acute stage of SCI (Bergman *et al.*, 1977; Cole, 1988). This would further decrease the overall density.

Spasticity, particularly when present in the lower limbs, may increase the overall density. This is reasonable to assume as muscle contraction will decrease volume while maintaining mass.

Upthrust Effect

The effect of upthrust may be disturbed in the patient who has either more muscle power or greater spasticity on one side of the body. This may shorten the trunk, therefore decreasing the effect of upthrust on that side. This change in shape would cause the patient to rotate to that side (p. 15). This may be corrected by turning the head to the opposite side or by lifting the opposite arm higher out of the water when sculling.

Many adults who sustain SCI will have been able to swim prior to their injuries. This experience should be utilized when re-educating their swimming technique. However, many able-bodied people are not confident and water-safe swimmers. Hydrotherapy sessions are the ideal safe environment for the person with an SCI to improve their confidence in water. Learning to submerge the face and exhale into the water may be a new experience for the swimmer who, for the last 20 years, swam with their head above water. Conversely, a previously confident swimmer will be able to use prior experience to adapt the strokes quickly to allow for changes in body position and lack of leg propulsion.

It should also be remembered that most people learn to swim when they are confident about the way their body works on land. The person with a newly acquired paraplegia or tetraplegia may not fully appreciate the lack of balance or sensation which their injury has produced. It is therefore important to spend time in the initial stages teaching the patient to roll vertically and horizontally and to be able to adopt safe positions in the water.

It is not proposed to detail all methods used in teaching a person with SCI to swim. It is relevant, however, to bring the reader's attention to some problems which may occur.

Back Sculling

This is usually the first choice of stroke. The head should be placed well back into the water. This should help to keep the legs afloat. However, if the head is extended too far, the body will arch over the centre of buoyancy and may start to sink from the feet.

Manual assistance from the physiotherapist may be required to support the body. Floats around the hips or ankles can be helpful if manual assistance is insufficient.

Both arms should be kept under the water during both the propulsive and the recovery phases. Some people with tetraplegia, whose triceps are not innervated, may find insufficient power using this stroke.

Back Stroke

A progression of the back scull is the bilateral over water recovery or 'Old English' back-stroke. This stroke allows a more powerful propulsive phase. However, the body may start to sink as the arms are lifted over the water to recover. This occurs as there is no momentum from a following leg kick and due to the meta-centric effect of taking the arms higher over the water. This can be minimized by modifying the position of the arms as they start the propulsive phase.

Unilateral back crawl alleviates the drop in momentum as one arm starts its propulsive phase as the other one finishes. Patients who have high lesions without trunk control usually find difficulty maintaining their balance and may feel their body rolling from side to side. This rolling can be reduced by losing the 'catch' on the water just below 90° abduction and sculling the remainder of the propulsive phase. The head can also be rotated away from the side to which the body is rolling.

Breast Stroke

Physiotherapists should ensure the person with paraplegia has good breathing control and has the ability to roll vertically and horizontally before considering any prone swimming. Many find it disconcerting when their bottom rises quickly to the surface thereby forcing their head into the water. Those with innervated back extensors should easily learn to raise their head to breathe. People with higher lesions may find it easier, initially, to roll onto the back to breathe until the technique of pushing down during the later part of the propulsive phase is learned. It is usually more efficient to do two or more strokes between each breath. The legs drop when the head is raised therefore increasing the frontal resistance. This in turn slows the momentum gained from the stroke.

People with tetraplegia, particularly those without innervated triceps, may find it extremely difficult to lift their head out to breathe or indeed to roll. Careful consideration should be given to each individual prior to allowing them to swim prone. Extra time may be needed to teach rolling.

People who have lesions causing extreme extensor spasticity may find it difficult to raise the head to breathe. They should roll onto the back or may find front crawl a more efficient stroke to use.

Front Crawl

For many people with SCI, front crawl is a difficult stroke to master. People with low lesions or those with extensor spasticity should have good horizontal body positions and therefore find it an efficient and effective stroke to perform.

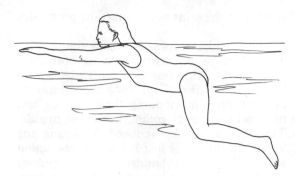

Fig. 12.2 *Body position of a person who has flexor spasticity when swimming prone*

Those whose body position is flexed when prone (Fig. 12.2) may find it difficult. The legs will act as a pendulum and will swing from side to side during unilateral propulsion. This should diminish as the person becomes more proficient at the stroke. More turbulence will be created by a strong pull. This in turn will assist the legs to extend therefore reducing the pendulum motion, thus making it easier to raise the arm out of the water to produce a more efficient pull.

Butterfly

A few people with tetraplegia find butterfly an easier stroke than front crawl. As the body does not rotate during bilateral strokes, this will allow them to concentrate on the propulsive phase of the stroke.

It should be remembered that this type of butterfly will not have the undulating movement of a swimmer who has a leg kick.

Incomplete Tetraplegia

Most people with an incomplete tetraplegia will have a degree of spasticity. Extensor spasticity may be accentuated when swimming in the supine position and therefore it may be easier to swim in the prone position.

The physiotherapist should consider the benefits of teaching people with this type of lesion to swim in the early stages of rehabilitation. Those with weak muscle power, i.e. less than Oxford grade 3, may increase their spasticity greatly due to the effort involved in trying to keep their bodies afloat and produce a coordinated movement. It may be more beneficial to use the short hydrotherapy session learning to control small ranges of movement or using techniques to reduce their increased tone. Swimming may be introduced at a later stage.

Cardiovascular Benefits

As previously stated swimming is an excellent form of aerobic exercise. Many people with a newly acquired SCI will have spent a considerable period on bed rest. They will have lost a lot of their previous stamina. They may also have used their legs as a major form of exercise prior to their disability, e.g. jogging, football. Swimming is a tremendous way to increase endurance, therefore making activities of daily living (ADL) easier.

Many hydrotherapy pools are small and therefore unsuitable for long-distance swimming. While efforts should be made to gain access to a larger swimming pool, resisted or tethered swimming may be a useful compromise. The swimmer can be attached to one end of the pool by an elastic cord, e.g. Theratubing or 'bungee' which is tied around the waist. They then swim, either to the other end of the pool or to a predetermined distance where they then remain for a set time. As the person improves more tension can be added by shortening the rope or the time at the predetermined spot can be increased. Care should be taken not to cause overheating in a hot hydrotherapy pool.

OTHER WATER ACTIVITIES

Many water activities are available to the SCI person who can swim. Scuba diving, water polo, sailing and water skiing are a few of these activities. These activities should be undertaken in the supervision of specially trained instructors.

Gerner *et al.* (1992) report that dry sauna bathing is a safe procedure for people with paraplegia and tetraplegia. This may help to reduce spasticity in some people with an SCI.

Hydrotherapy and swimming can be fun, exciting and, of course, beneficial to people with SCI at any stage of their injury. There is an opportunity to create a social environment with family and friends. Learning to swim following an SCI can facilitate a healthy lifestyle and can help avoid complications.

REFERENCES

Barron K.W. and Blair R.W. (1993). The autonomic nervous system. In *Neuroscience for Rehabilitation*, (H. Cohen, ed.), Philadelphia: J.B. Lippincott Company, pp. 218–244.

Bergman P., Hellporn A., Schoutens A., *et al.* (1977). Longitudinal study of calcium and bone metabolism in paraplegic patients. *Paraplegia*, **15**: 147–159.

Bromley I. (1991). *Tetraplegia and Paraplegia. A Guide for Physiotherapists*, 4th edn, Edinburgh: Churchill Livingstone.

Carter R.E. (1992). Respiratory management, including ventilator care in tetraplegia and diaphramatic pacing. In *Handbook of Clinical Neurology*, Vol. 17 (61). *Spinal Cord Trauma* (P.J. Vinken, G.W. Bruyn, H.L. Klawans and H.L. Frankel, eds), Amsterdam: Elsevier Science Publishers BV, pp. 261–274.

Cole J.D. (1988). The pathophysiology of the autonomic nervous system in spinal cord injury. In *Spinal Cord Dysfunction: Assessment* (L.S. Illis, ed.), Oxford: Oxford University Press, pp. 201–235.

Davis B. and Harrison R. (1988). *Hydrotherapy in Practice*, Edinburgh: Churchill Livingstone.

Ditunno J.F. (1992). *Standards for Neurological and Functional Classification of Spinal Cord Injury*, American Spinal Injury Association. Illinois.

Edgar R.E. (1992). Post-traumatic spinal spasticity. In *Handbook of Clinical Neurology*, Vol. 17 (61): *Spinal Cord Trauma* (P.J. Vinken, G.W. Bruyn, H.L. Klawans and H.L. Frankel, eds), Amsterdam: Elsevier Science Publishers BV, pp. 367–373.

Gerhart K.A., Bergström E., Charlifue S.W., *et al.* (1993). Long-term spinal cord injury: functional changes over time. *Archives of Physical Medicine and Rehabilitation*, **74(10)**: 1030–1034.

Gerner H.J., Engel, P., Gass, G.C., *et al.* (1992). The effects of sauna on tetraplegic and paraplegic subjects. *Paraplegia*, **30**: 410–419.

Guttman, L. (1976). *Textbook of Sport for the Disabled*, Aylesbury: H.M. & M. Publishers.

Guttman, L., Silver, J. and Wyndham, C.H. (1958). Thermoregulation in spinal man. *Journal of Physiology*, **142**: 406–419.

Harrison R. and Bulstrode S. (1987). Percentage weight-bearing during partial immersion in the hydrotherapy pool. *Physiotherapy Practice*, **3**: 60–63.

Hollis M. (1981). *Practical Exercise Therapy*, 2nd edn, Oxford: Blackwell Scientific Publishers.

Illis L.S. (1992). Spasticity 1: Clinical aspects. In *Spinal Cord Dysfunction*, Vol. II, *Intervention and Treatment* (L.S. Illis, ed.), Oxford: Oxford University Press, pp. 81–93.

Johnson R.H. (1992). Temperature regulation in spinal cord injuries. In *Handbook of Clinical Neurology*, Vol. 17 (61): *Spinal Cord Trauma* (P.J. Vinken, G.W. Bruyn, H.L. Klawans and H.L. Frankel, eds), Amsterdam: Elsevier Science Publishers BV, pp. 275–289.

Lammertse D.P. (1992). Managing spasticity. In *Management of Spinal Cord Injury*, 2nd edn (C.P. Zejdlik, ed.), Boston: Jones and Bartlett, pp. 583–591.

Mathias C.J. and Frankel H.L. (1992). The cardiovascular system in tetraplegia and paraplegia. In *Handbook of Clinical Neurology*, Vol. 17 (61): *Spinal Cord Trauma* (P.J. Vinken, G.W. Bruyn, H.L. Klawans and H.L. Frankel, eds), Amsterdam: Elsevier Science Publishers BV, pp. 435–456.

Mathias C.J., Frankel H.L. and Cole J.D. (1992). Management of cardio-vascular abnormalities caused by autonomic dysfunction in spinal cord injury. In *Spinal Cord Dysfunction*, Vol. II, *Intervention and Treatment* (L.S. Illis, ed.), Oxford: Oxford University Press, pp. 101–120.

Nixon V. (1985). *Spinal Cord Injury: A Guide to Functional Outcomes in Physical Therapy Management*, London: William Heinemann Medical Books.

Skinner A.T. and Thomson A.M. (1983). *Duffield's Exercise in Water*, 3rd edn, London: Baillière Tindall.

Rheumatic, orthopaedic conditions and sports injuries

Margaret Reid Campion

Overview to Chapters 13, 14 and 15

The use of hydrotherapy in the treatment of rheumatic and orthopaedic conditions is widely recognized. The particular values come about because of the warmth of the water which decreases pain and muscle spasm and the buoyancy of the water which relieves the stresses on all joints especially the weight-bearing joints.

Buoyancy is a vital factor in the fine grading of progressions of exercise and in increasing range of movement and muscle strength and allowing early re-education of walking.

Sports injuries respond well to hydrotherapy, a modality that has been used for centuries largely by means of hot springs and and whirlpool baths (Hopper, 1990). Currently the swimming pool is in demand for exercise whether this is for recreation, pleasure, rehabilitation or fitness and the maintenance of general health. The pool can be utilized by professional and amateur athletes to train in the early stages following injury. The injured athlete is always in a great hurry to recover and return to the favoured sport!

Hydrotherapy for sports injuries, sadly neglected till fairly recently, is benefiting from increased exposure and success rate in rehabilitation and hopefully will become an 'integrated treatment regimen' (Hopper, 1990: 177). Physiotherapists working in the field are usually aware of the benefits of the modality but fail to use water specifically, allowing patients to pursue exercise in the medium that have come straight from the gymnasium. This means that the unique advantages of water are not used to enhance the speedy recovery of these injuries. There is a marked tendency to allow the patient to exercise in the water with minimal instruction and supervision; the particular advantages of water cannot be employed from the bathside!

Water running has been and is the subject of research (Hamer *et al.*, 1984; Hamer 1985; Bishop *et al.*, 1989; Gleim and Nicholas, 1989) and physiotherapists are optimizing its potential in rehabilitating sports injuries (Hopper, 1990).

13

Rheumatic diseases

Lynette M. Tinsley

INTRODUCTION

In this chapter, consideration will be given to a variety of rheumatic conditions under the following headings:

- **Inflammatory arthritis.**
- **Degenerative arthritis.**
- **Spondyloarthropathies.**

ADVANTAGES OF HYDROTHERAPY

The advantages of hydrotherapy for rheumatic conditions are similar to those for all conditions. Of particular value are the warmth of the water, which decreases pain and muscle spasm, and buoyancy, which relieves the stresses on joints especially those involved in weight bearing.

Assessment and Planning of Treatment

For each of the categories given above, the person should be individually assessed both subjectively and objectively (p. 24). The assessment will help to establish the patient's needs, aims of treatment, realistic goals of treatment and treatment priorities (Harrison, 1980). In rheumatic diseases alterations in shape and density are as relevant to a water activity programme as in any other condition (p 17).

Clinical signs and symptoms in rheumatic disorders

Common clinical signs and symptoms in the rheumatic disorders are pain occurring in and around affected joints, creating tension and muscle spasm; decreased range of motion and increased stiffness of joints; muscle weakness; deformities in some conditions and diminished functional ability.

Contraindications

The contraindications of hydrotherapy for the rheumatic disorders are common to all pool users: cardiac or respiratory failure, infective skin conditions including tinea pedis, excessively low, high or uncontrolled blood pressure, active TB, urinary infections, urinary or faecal incontinence and morbid hydrophobia (Atkinson and Harrison, 1981; Golland, 1981).

There are no contraindications peculiar to the rheumatic diseases patient, except for those people in the early stages of recovery from a generalized flare of rheumatoid arthritis, when overactivity or exertion could cause a recurrence of the symptoms of pain and swelling. Abnormal physiological measurements, for example altered blood pressure or diminished vital capacity, should form no barrier to the person participating in hydrotherapy, providing the condition is recognized and monitored (Harrison, 1980; Harrison, 1981). Occasionally a patient will complain of hypersensitive skin in response to pool chemicals, chlorine or bromine, the reactions to both varying from mild irritation to severe itching and rashes. This may be a drug-induced reaction. A person with a single inflamed joint need not be excluded from the pool provided the affected joint is adequately restrained by a splint. Plastazote thermoplastic splinting material can be used but, for the very frail, an alternative material or weighting of the splint may be necessary due to the increased buoyancy created by the splint. Similarly, a cervical collar of moulded Plastazote can be used for those people with cervical spine involvement, this can be individually moulded or commercially manufactured.

Whilst not being a contraindication to hydrotherapy, a person with *osteoporosis* should be treated with caution, bearing in mind that even a slight degree of overexertion or sudden movement can lead to fractures.

As well as hydrotherapy, the patient should be encouraged to participate in weight-bearing exercises to stimulate the bone, as there seems to be little evidence from scientific studies on the effect of exercising in water and the effect of other non-weight-bearing exercises on bone density. Recent research indicates that bone density is increased by swimming (Orwoll *et al.*, 1987). Water provides a safe environment for exercising and, for the severely osteoporotic, may be the only safe exercise medium.

Primary aims of treatment

The primary aims of treatment for most rheumatic conditions are:

- relief of pain, swelling and stiffness
- promotion of relaxation
- joint mobilization
- muscle strengthening
- correction/prevention of contractures
- improvement of coordination and functional ability
- improvement of morale.

INFLAMMATORY ARTHRITIS

Rheumatoid arthritis is a systemic, inflammatory disorder characteristically involving peripheral joints, often symmetrically. It can also manifest itself in other tissues and organs, for example the heart, lungs, eyes or nervous system. Weight loss, fever, depression, altered functional abilities and body shape and frequently, poor self esteem are common features.

Aims of Treatment

The aims of treatment for inflammatory disorders are:

- relief of pain and muscle spasm
- maintenance or restoration of muscle strength
- reduction of deformities and increased range of motion of all affected joints; the stretching of contractures, maintenance of range of motion and muscle power around unaffected joints
- promotion of relaxation
- re-education of correct walking patterns
- improvement of functional abilities and morale (Golland, 1981; Reid Campion, 1985).

Water temperature

In the author's experience, a water temperature of 35°C is that of choice (see also p. 7). Patients immersed in warm water should be carefully observed for adverse reactions and where these occur appropriate action should be taken.

Procedure Prior to an Exercise Programme

Following the initial assessment on land, and the decision to provide a water activity programme, the patient should be prepared for the procedure. The physiotherapist should describe the pool, the mode of transport from the ward to the pool, the method of entry into the water, an outline of what is expected of the patient and the type of activity to be carried out. If the analysis of the patient's shape and/or density has shown alteration which may produce rotational effects of the body when in the water these can also be explained to the patient who can be given instructions as to how to control these patterns when they occur. Thus the person is prepared for hydrotherapy and any apprehension diminished.

Safety

Safety procedures are not different for the rheumatic disease patient. The same principles apply as for all patients undertaking hydrotherapy treatment (Martin, 1981; Campion 1983; Reid Campion, 1985). The initial assessment will determine the person's capabilities and suitability for either individual or group treatment.

Individual programme

It is advisable, whenever possible, to conduct the earliest treatments on an individual basis for a short duration of time. Five to ten minutes to begin with gradually increasing the length of time. The emphasis of the treatment should be on relaxation, gentle movements and controlled stretching.

Technique

Method of entry and introduction to water

The technique of entry into the pool at this early stage is in most cases by mechanical hoist to diminish activity and stress on affected joints if recovering from a recent flare. Once in the water, the person is either positioned on a plinth in support lying, held in head support lying by the physiotherapist or in float support lying for the exercises. An apprehensive person may well be less concerned if allowed to stand in the deeper water holding onto the grab rail, with the physiotherapist nearby, for a period of time, until they are confident in water; or they may sit on a weighted chair, strapped in and instructed to keep the head forward to maintain the upright sitting position. Mentally adjusting the patient to the element of water and teaching balance restoration will help to overcome any problems of apprehension (p. 21). Early exercise can begin with relaxation using gentle active, sweeping movements within a pain-free range, the patient limiting the movement, and breathing exercises, until the person feels relaxed and confident in the water. Once confidence is gained, more formalized exercises can be introduced for mobilizing the strengthening. Again, the Halliwick means of blowing to keep the nose and mouth clear of water should be taught.

Mobilization

The movement of acute or very painful joints should be avoided and care should be taken not to overstretch peri-articular structures during joint mobilization. This can easily occur in a pool due to the difficulty with fixation and isolation of movement of a specific joint. The physiotherapist must therefore control the amount of activity during the exercise, or ensure isolation of movement by the use of appropriate floats. Techniques which can be employed for joint mobilization are *Bad Ragaz patterns* which use mass movement of the limbs and the trunk, isotonically, or isometrically, (Davis, 1967; Davis, 1971; Skinner and Thomson, 1983). Uncontrolled stretchings should be avoided to prevent damage to peri-articular structures and an increase of the inflammatory process, therefore modification of the techniques, either by alteration of grip or limitation of range of motion, may be necessary (Harrison, 1980).

Hold–relax techniques – in some instances hold–relax techniques can be used to improve range of motion of a joint where muscle spasm is the limiting factor. In water the position of the patient is important so that buoyancy assists movement in the required direction. They are valuable techniques useful in the treatment of ankylosing spondylitis (Barefoot – Lecture Notes, 1988).

Strengthening

Muscle strengthening around a painful joint

Muscle strengthening requires care. A method of achieving this is by the use of stabilizations or isometric contractions, whereby the physiotherapist puts the joint into a pain-free position and holds distally to the joint. The patient 'holds' the position whilst the physiotherapist moves the patient in different directions, causing different muscle groups to contract. Range of movement is gradually reduced and the direction of movement changed more quickly, giving rise to co-contraction of muscles around the joint. This method prevents stress on the joint, but allows for an increase of resistance.

Muscle strengthening can be achieved by the use of finely graded exercises using buoyancy as assistance, support or resistance; turbulence whereby resistance can be given either by increasing the speed of movement, altering the length of the lever arm or by using equipment such as floats or bats, which can be used to streamline or unstreamline and thus alter the resistance to movement. A narrow surface offers little resistance, a flat surface increases the resistance. Bad Ragaz techniques of mass patterns of movement using those patterns which counteract deformity and move pain-free joints can also be used for muscle strengthening.

When using floats as a resistance to a movement, the amount of resistance represented should be known. To prevent further damage to a joint, the person should have sufficient control over the active elements of the exercises (buoyancy resistance and assistance) and the return to the starting positions.

As a guideline to the amount of resistance provided by a float, a 3 in (8 cm) cube of polystyrene requires 1 lb (0.5 kg) of pressure to submerge it (Harrison, 1980). At all times, care must be taken to prevent stress on an already compromised joint, for example the lever arm may need to be shortened in the exercise abduction of the hip and the resistance may need to be given over the knee joint rather than at the ankle (Skinner and Thomson, 1983).

Group treatments

It may be necessary, due to large patient numbers and restricted staff levels in many departments and hospitals, to conduct treatments as a group rather than individually. As soon as practical after the initial introductory treatment, the patient should be included into a group activity.

A general programme of exercises is given as a toning workout incorporating warm-up, mobility, strengthening exercises, an aerobic component (if participants are confident and capable in water), cool down, relaxation, breathing exercises, posture awareness and patient education.

Time is allowed at the end of the session for attention to the specific needs of the individual. To participate in a group activity, patients should be confident in the water and at least semi-independent. Ideally, the group should be made up of those with similar disabilities, but as this is rarely the case, the physiotherapist must be prepared to conduct a session in which participants may be in the starting positions of lying, sitting or standing, so the exercises will need to be modified according to the restrictions placed on the individual by the apparatus.

Advantages

The advantages of group activity are encouragement, stimulation, motivation and social interaction, which occur while working with people with similar disabilities.

Disadvantages

Certain disadvantages can be experienced when working in groups. These are related to the size of the group, the positioning of group members and the physiotherapist, the size, shape and depth of the pool and the ability of the physiotherapist to provide safely adequate control and supervision of the exercises. Too large a group may make positioning the group members in the appropriate depths difficult, in that the group may become too widely spread for adequate control of safety and accurate supervision of exercise performance. This is particularly so where the pool is larger. However, the smaller pool, especially one where the depth is the same, poses the problem of positioning group members in appropriate depths.

Further difficulties arise within a group situation where visual and auditory problems exist amongst the participants. Distractions within the group itself and movements around the pool area can add to the difficulty of the physiotherapist's task. The number of participants should be limited, preferably to 8–10, provided most people are able to maintain their balance and feel reasonably confident in water. Positioning within the pool should enable the physiotherapist to be within easy reach of each person for correction of the exercises or in the event of patients experiencing difficulties.

The role of education

The treatment time spent in the pool can be utilized as an important education period, creating body awareness and promoting the principles of joint preservation and work simplification. For example, during exercises for the hands, the physiotherapist can emphasize the stresses placed on wrist and meta-carpophalangeal joints during activities of daily living, such as dusting, turning taps and opening of jars. Alternative ways to perform these tasks can be suggested to prevent ulnar drift and strain on the joint. While performing an exercise, explanation of the specific joint movement involved can highlight the importance of the activity, for example internal rotation and adduction of the shoulder, to put the hands behind the back, is an important movement required for toileting. A further example is the importance of strong quadriceps muscles to maintain stability of the knee and to facilitate walking, getting in and out of chairs, or walking up and down stairs. The importance of correct postural habits can be related to their effect on body mechanics. Explaining simply the functional activity of an exercise and the muscles involved in the performance of the action can give a greater understanding of the importance of the exercises.

As part of the education process it is useful to ask the patient to select an exercise and for them to explain the reason for the exercise, which muscles are working and thus the functional activity of the movement involved in, for example, opening doors, hanging up clothes and walking. Performance of the exercises should be slow, gentle and non stressful. Gentle exercise is emphasized as opposed to vigorous. Many people tend to believe that the harder they work the more beneficial it is, whereas if practised, there is a greater likelihood of further damage.

Exercise Programmes for Patients with Inflammatory Arthritis

In the case of the person with inflammatory arthritis, the exercises will be modified according to the individual's abilities and disabilities. There will also be variation between the programmes selected for individual treatments and group treatments.

Individual treatments

Individual treatments are usually given for the sub-acute and immediate post-acute phases. The initial sessions can be from 5–10 minutes, gradually progressing in time according to the patient's tolerance. Exercises are commenced as non-weight-bearing exercises, concentrating on relaxation techniques and large functional movements.

Relaxation

Relaxation can be practised with the person floating, using the effect of buoyancy. Support can be given by the use of floats around the neck and hips and possibly the ankles. In the supine floating position, the person can be encouraged to breathe deeply, to tense muscles

and relax them and consciously to allow the body to be supported by the buoyancy of the water. Imagery, such as imagining oneself floating in a peaceful environment, may be used. To promote relaxation, the physiotherapist can sweep the lower limbs and trunk from side to side slowly and rhythmically through the water. The hold should be at the centre of balance of the body, approximately waist level, thus giving the physiotherapist maximum control and the person a feeling of security.

Modification of this hold may be necessary where a large or tall person presents a problem. The physiotherapist will need to take the hands nearer the hips to achieve the swinging movement easily. To achieve this hold the person's neck should rest on one of the physiotherapist's shoulders which has been lowered slightly to allow the head to pass over the shoulder.

Individual Treatment Relaxation

In some cases, e.g. the more severely disabled, those who have been bed ridden for long periods or isolated from caring touch, a modified version of Watsu (Dull, 1993) can be employed. This is a method whereby the person is cradled in the physiotherapist's arms, the neck being well supported in the crook of the elbow and gently rocked, stretched and carefully rotated in a series of relaxing movements. Gentle mobilization of the vertebrae can be specifically performed in this position.

Based on Eastern philosophers, derived from Zen Shiatsu, Watsu affects the body on all levels, emotional, psychological and physical, and requires the patient to be completely trusting of the skill of the physiotherapist. In turn, the physiotherapist must be mindful of the pathology of the disorder.

The benefits derived from Watsu are decreased muscle tension and pain, stretching of soft tissue contractures, decreased anxiety levels, improved body awareness, increased joint range of movement, release of emotional stress, improved circulation, improved breathing pattern, less fatigue/increased energy.

Mobilizing and Strengthening Exercises

Mobilizing and strengthening exercises can be carried out in flotation on a one-to-one basis but care must be taken to prevent overstretching of peri-articular structures. The physiotherapist must be able to control the amount of activity, to isolate the movements with adequate fixation and to be aware of the amount of resistance by the floats when used. The patient should be able to control the active element of the exercise and the return to the starting position (Harrison, 1980).

Mobilizing exercises – can be active assisted movements, hold–relax techniques, active sweeping movements or pattern movements, e.g. for the shoulder joint the flexion–abduction lateral rotation pattern; for the knee single or double knee flexions patterns.

Strenthening exercises – around a painful joint can be achieved by isometric contractions or stabilizations. With a pain-free joint the techniques of choice are graded exercise using buoyancy, altered speed of movement or length of weight arm turbulence and patterns of movement.

Group treatments

Once the inflammatory processes have subsided and the person enters the immediate post-acute phase or is in the chronic phase of the disorder, they can be included in a group situation. In such a group generalized exercises are given, followed by specific individual exercises according to the needs of the individual. The starting positions for the exercises can be variable, either lying, sitting or standing, with the exercises modified according to the position. Selected starting positions will be governed by the patient's physical condition.

General Mobility Programme

A general mobility programme along the following lines could be used and include mobility and strengthening exercises, postural awareness, gait retraining and relaxation techniques.

The person should be encouraged to begin with a suggested maximum of ten repetitions for each exercise gradually increasing the number of repetitions as their tolerance permits, and also to work within the limits of pain. Stretching should be encouraged, but a warning against stressing already compromised tissues should be given.

The exercise programme should have a *warm-up* phase, a *specific exercise* phase and a *cool down* phase. For the more able the warm-up phase of three to four minutes in a depth of water at xiphisternum level may consist of rhythmical walking through the water, in changing directions, with exaggerated arm and trunk movements. For the less able the warming phase may be in a depth of water at xiphisternum level with alternate leg and arm movements in different directions followed by trunk rotations and side flexion movements. The period of time can be set at 3–4 minutes with 10–15 repetitions of each movement. With the emphasis on gentle rhythmic movement there should be minimal stress on joints and peri-articular structures. The cool down phase can include swimming, walking, relaxed trunk and arm movements at a gradually decreasing rate of activity.

At the end of the warm-up phase, group members are positioned for the specific exercises. For those who are unable to stand for long periods or by virtue of disability, or for those who are fearful of deep water, most lower limb exercises can be done in the lying position, but in this instance for ease of description, all exercises will be described as for the standing patient; alternative positions being given where appropriate.

Legs

Starting position: the person stands in the water, preferably in the depth in which buoyancy is neutral. Ideally this means the water should be at the level of the xiphisternum. Some people may need to exercise with the water at waist level where there is a greater degree of gravity acting on the body, providing a feeling of greater security to the nervous or anxious person. If the patient has been taught the skills of mental adjustment and balance restoration such action may be obviated (p. 21).

Exercises that form the basis of the 'conventional' method, that is buoyancy assisted, neutral or resisted exercise (Davis and Harrison, 1988), and utilize all movements of the hips, knees and feet, may be used. Care must be taken with the application of those exercises that take the legs into adduction, across midline. Smaller joints such as the ankle are less effectively exercised in the water, as a rule, but movements that are aimed at flexibility of the feet and ankles should not be ignored.

Approaching these exercises using the principles of hydrodynamic exercise (p. 179) are of value. The warmth of the water, the support and buoyancy, producing relaxation, allow greater mobility without the stresses of a gravity-dominated situation and thus there is merit in including exercises that develop flexibility in the ankle and foot in any programme.

Posture

The posture of some patients suffering from rheumatic disorders is altered and exercises and activities that will improve this altered posture should be included in the programme. Taking patients with a forward flexed posture into deeper water, while in the vertical position, will often bring about a more upright stance. Since buoyancy has taken the stress off the weight-bearing joints and spine and with the patient's natural desire to keep the face and mouth clear of the water, a more erect posture results. Specific exercises involving the quadriceps, gluteal, abdominal, shoulder retractors and neck muscles are carried out to improve trunk control along with exercises for the trunk muscles. While these exercises are frequently carried out in standing they may also be performed sitting on a chair with the shoulders immersed.

Back mobility

Flexion, extension, lateral flexion and rotation of the trunk can be developed in both the sitting and standing positions. The choice of depth is important as it is inadvisable to allow the head to go under the water when performing forward flexion and lateral flexion. A wide base, in either standing or sitting, is important for balance, and this is achieved by having the patient stand with the feet wide apart sideways, or in sitting placing the feet apart and keeping the head forward. Once again depth is important.

Arms and shoulders

These exercises should be carried out in the sitting or standing starting positions with the depth of water at shoulder level. Movements that involve flexion, extension, abduction, adduction, internal and external rotation can be used for the shoulders. All these movements should be carried out as rhythmical swinging actions and various components can be combined. The shoulder girdle may be exercised by movements involving elevation, depression, retraction and protraction.

Hands

There is no specific advantage of doing hand exercises in water other than that the warmth of the water promotes ease of movement, and relaxation and that all joints are thus included in the programme. All movements of the fingers, thumbs and wrists should be included, care being taken not to stress the metacarpophalangeal joints or spread into ulnar deviation.

Thought should be given to exercises that combine a variety of movements in functional patterns. As the movements considered above have been discussed in relation to group work the physiotherapist is not able to carry out Bad Ragaz patterns which require a one-to-one relationship between the patient and the physiotherapist. Yet these patterns incorporate all the movements both anatomical and physiological of joints and muscles. It is possible there is a place for the appropriate timetabling of group sessions to permit individual work with the patients so that more functional patterns involving all joints of the limbs may be utilized (Reid Campion, 1988).

Neck

Neck movements can be made more effective if techniques carried out on a one-to-one basis are used (p. 180).

To exercise the neck effectively in water is not easy and requires the patient to be immersed as fully as possible if the patient's neck is to benefit from the warmth of the water, so a stable position is essential. This may be achieved if the patient is seated securely on a chair or leaning with the back against a wall, the hips, knees and ankles flexed and the feet placed flat on the floor of the pool, well forward of the body and wide apart. The movements of the neck and head of flexion, extension, side flexion and rotation can be performed, but should not be continued if they cause dizziness or nausea. The physiotherapist should be aware of any bony destruction or instability of the cervical spine and proceed with care.

Functional activities

Functional activities can be promoted in water although differences occur to similar activities on land due to buoyancy. The advantages of the support of water, warmth, weight relief and relaxation encourage and motivate the patient to carry out such activities early, thus facilitating their use on land. There is a psychological benefit for the patient in being able to achieve movement and perform activities with greater care than without the benefits of water. Functional activities include:

- sitting to standing
- standing balance on both legs or either leg
- walking forwards, sideways and backwards
- stepping up and down.

Balance is a vital factor in all functional activities and can be increased in a variety of ways. Both static and dynamic balance may be developed by means of hydrodynamic exercise (p. 160) and with the use of turbulence.

Relaxation

Relaxation is brought about by the support and warmth of the water. It is important that, apart from the body, the neck, shoulders and arms are relaxed. Rhythmical, relaxed sweeping movements of the arms may also involve the trunk but the emphasis is on the release of tension from the neck and shoulder areas. Increased range of motion can be achieved by encouraging the patient to gently 'stretch' into the movements.

Swimming

Patients who have swum in the past may find swimming a useful means of activity, maintaining mobility and fitness and providing social and psychological benefits. Care should be taken in choosing the stroke or strokes for a patient.

Generally floating on the back and sculling is suitable for most patients and this can be extended to a back stroke action. Side stroke may prove suitable for some patients, but careful consideration must be given to the selection of breast stroke. Cervical, thoracic and lumbar extension may be compounded in breast stroke and the kick into abduction and extension with rotation of the lower limbs may stress the lumbar spine, hip and knee joints. Swimming skills should be taught to the non-swimmer and adaptations made for physical disabilities and limited mobility. General teaching techniques for strokes (Elkington, 1978) and modifications for disabilities (Reid Campion, 1985) may be employed.

SAFETY AND CARE IN THE HANDLING OF THE RHEUMATOID ARTHRITIS PATIENT

The handling and holding of the rheumatoid arthritis patient is of utmost importance to prevent an increase of pain and damage to compromised and painful joints, soft tissues and osteoporotic bones. When lifting or transferring patients from a chair to the hoist, commode, chair or wheelchair, care should be exercised by holding the patient around the chest wall, using the length of the lifter's arms. The lift should *not* be done by lifting under the shoulders, *nor* by grasping the patient's forearms or wrists (as is commonly done with a through-arm lift). Support for the legs should be given under the *thighs* and the *lower legs*.

When employing a standing transfer to the hoist, support from the helper should be given around the body, not grasping the upper arm and dragging on the shoulder(s). Support, while lifting the legs, should be given under the thighs and lower legs, so there is no strain on the knee joints. As the patient is lowered on the hoist into the water, the physiotherapist, already standing in the water, should place one hand or arm over the legs to prevent the legs floating up due to buoyancy and also to reassure the patient against the sensation of floating away (Fig. 13.1).

When transferring from the hoist, the patient should be requested to keep their arms folded over their chest to prevent pulling on the patient's shoulders and to prevent the patient grasping around the physiotherapist's neck due to panic, or should an emergency arise whereby the physiotherapist would be needed to move quickly and unhindered. The person should be held firmly around the body and close to the physiotherapist with one arm while the physiotherapist's other arm supports under the person's thighs. In this manner, the patient feels

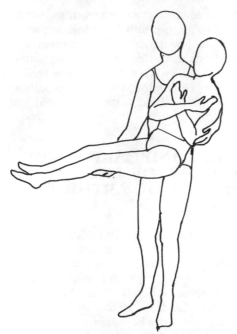

Fig. 13.1   *When employing a standing transfer to hoist, support should be given under the thighs and lower legs*

secure, can be floated across the pool and positioned appropriately into the standing position or either lying, sitting or standing.

If the patient is supported on a plinth, a restraining band may be secured firmly across the hips and abdomen and a neck support placed beneath the cervical spine. In this position the patient can perform arm, leg and trunk side flexion and rotation exercises. If the patient is seated on a chair, a restraining band may be placed over the hips and abdomen and firmly secured. Many patients, if fearful of tipping over, may need the chair to be placed near the wall of the pool. The patient should be instructed to keep their head forward in order to maintain the upright position.

When standing a severely disabled rheumatoid arthritis patient from the supine float position, often the most comfortable and secure method is for the physiotherapist to have one arm around the body supporting behind the shoulders and in some cases the head as well. The other hand and forearm is placed over the front of the patient's thighs. An upward pressure is applied to the body by the arm supporting behind the shoulders at the same time that a downward pressure is applied by the arm

across the front of the thighs, equally, until the patient is brought to an upright position with the feet on the bottom of the pool. As the legs go down and the centre of equilibrium is established, the arm pushing on the legs should be moved to support the body at waist level or on the rib cage. If possible, the patient should be encouraged to tuck the chin in, bringing the head forward at the beginning of the movement; blowing out strongly will further facilitate this action of the head. This method is used successfully and comfortably for most persons with severely limiting rheumatoid arthritis, who are unable to employ the self-righting method of forward rotation used in the Halliwick Method (Fig. 13.2).

To walk the severely disabled or fragile patient, the physiotherapist should stand in front of and facing the patient. The physiotherapist's hands should hold and support preferably at waist level or over the lower rib cage. The patient rests their hands and forearms along the physiotherapist's forearms, distributing the weight away from the patient's wrists. In this way facial expression can be observed and gait can be analysed and corrected. A feeling of security is provided by the support to the trunk and the patient can bear weight along the

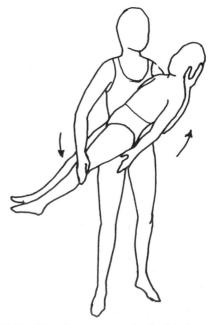

Fig. 13.2   *Standing a severely disabled rheumatoid arthritis patient from line supine float position*

forearms without stressing the wrists and hands.

To transfer the patient onto the hoist, the reverse procedure to that of transferring into the pool is used. The physiotherapist should maintain a restraining hold over the front of the legs until the hoist is raised from the water. If the neck or back are painful during the transfer, either into or out of the water, consideration should be given to providing some support by means of rubber cushions or neck supports. The patient's comfort is of paramount importance at all times.

Safety Points

While acknowledging the following points are applicable to all patients the author feels it is essential to emphasize them here in relation to the handling of rheumatoid arthritis patients. A number of points for safety should be remembered. Buoyancy can override equilibrium of the elderly or debilitated patient, so the righting position should be taught (Martin, 1981; Campion, 1983; Reid Campion, 1985).

Poor eyesight, hearing, fear of the water, reflection of the light on the water, turbulence of the water, noise and echo and lack of understanding of body mechanisms can all lead to confusion and stress for many patients, particularly the elderly, frail or severely disabled. Awareness of the over-enthusiastic person must also be considered. This person, on finding himself in a warm and welcoming medium, can lean to overactivity and a subsequent increase of pain and swelling.

The use of ladders and steep stairs for entry or exit into or out of the pool should be discouraged because of the degree of stress placed on affected joints and weakened muscle groups. Entry and exit for the rheumatoid arthritis person should, in preference, be either by hoist, ramp or wide shallow steps and the method of entry is determined by the degree of disability.

New or nervous patients should be oriented to the pool beforehand, either by explanation, or better still, by a tour of the pool site itself. Mental adjustment and balance restoration skills should also be taught (p. 21).

Pool therapy is tiring, thus following a pool session the patient should shower, be adequately rested and warmly wrapped or clothed. A minimum of 15 minutes and preferably up to 45 minutes should be allowed for heart rate, respiration, blood pressure and skin temperature to return to normal. Patients should take some fluid refreshment to replace body fluid loss (Atkinson and Harrison, 1981; Golland, 1981).

Treatment times are variable according to the patient's tolerance. For some severely disabled patients, 5 minutes may be enough initially, while others may work for 20 minutes without adverse side effects. A full exercise programme can be achieved in 20 minutes, but many patients, particularly the fitter osteoarthritic or ankylosing spondylitic, will tolerate a session of up to 45 minutes or more, but no longer than one hour, depending on the water temperature and the severity of the condition and exercise. Patients with respiratory or cardiovascular problems generally tolerate only a short period of treatment (Harrison, 1980; Atkinson and Harrison, 1981; Golland, 1981; Skinner and Thomson, 1983).

DEGENERATIVE ARTHRITIS

The conditions treated under this heading include osteoarthrosis, a common disorder of central and peripheral diarthrodeal joints; disc degeneration, also a common disorder frequently co-existing with osteoarthrosis; and osteoporosis of the spine. The most common signs and symptoms will be pain, muscle spasm and weakness and loss of range of motion.

Treatment of Osteoarthrosis (OA)

The aims of treatment for OA are similar to those for inflammatory arthritis. They include relief of pain; relief of muscle spasm; strengthening of the muscles around the affected joints; increased range of motion of the affected joints; improved walking pattern where the lower limbs are involved and encouraging and teaching swimming skills.

Techniques

The techniques employed include relaxation, mobilizations using hold–relax methods, strengthening using Bad Ragaz patterns, stabilizations and repeated contractions, reeducation in walking and the teaching or promotion of swimming skills (Elkington, 1978;

Reid Campion, 1985). In most cases of OA especially where the hips and knees are involved there is an associated low level of general fitness and mobility and one aim of treatment should be to improve strength and mobility of the trunk muscles.

'Free' exercise programme for osteoarthritis

As in all exercise programmes there should be a 'warm-up' session. Warm-up activities should take place in an appropriate depth which means that the water should be at xiphisternum level if the patient is safe exercising at that level. Such activities include exercises for the legs, arms and trunk using the 'conventional' method (Davis and Harrison, 1988) and walking in various directions.

Specific exercises for the affected joints would aim to increase the range of motion in all directions of movement at the joint(s) as well as strengthening the muscles around those joint(s). Progression for strengthening can be achieved by attaching floats to the limbs, or increasing the speed of the exercises. The starting positions for the exercises may include standing, sitting, kneeling and support lying both supine and prone. Special consideration of the osteoarthritic spine, back pain and the osteoporotic spine is provided below.

Walking

The physiotherapist should observe and correct abnormal patterns of gait. Instruction should begin with a discussion on posture, correction of the patient's posture, analysis and demonstration of the normal walking pattern. The walking pattern on land is not the same as that for walking in the water. Different muscle work is involved due to the effect of buoyancy assisting and resisting movements of the lower limbs and to the effects of turbulence around the body (Reid Campion, 1985; Davis and Harrison, 1988). The patterns of movement for walking which demand balance and coordination described on p. 185 may be used. These patterns can be modified, either by the physiotherapist instructing the patient to make, for example, smaller ranges of movement, smaller steps, depending on the mobility and ability of the patient to balance.

Functional activities

Functional activities particularly those involving the lower limbs are most important for the osteoarthritic patient. These would follow similar activities to those already described (p. 261) but emphasis would be placed on ascending and descending the 'stairs'; the latter being stools of various heights. It is important that the physiotherapist ensures correct functioning especially of the quadriceps muscle using buoyancy assisted (concentric) and buoyancy resisted (eccentric) exercises.

Swimming

All swimming strokes may be utilized but the physiotherapist must assess the patient's mobility, at the same time being aware of the movements involved in all the strokes, and must ensure that no movement aggravates any joints and produces pain.

Osteoarthrosis Spine, Back Pain, Osteoporotic Spine

The back conditions most commonly seen amongst the arthritic disorders result from inflammatory and degenerative conditions, for example spondylosis, spondylolisthesis and osteoporosis. Many patients may be overweight, underfit, immobile and have poor posture, all brought about by pain, muscle spasm and weakness. The whole person needs treating, but care must be taken to treat within the point of aggravation of signs and symptoms.

Aims of treatment

The aims of treatment are to relieve pain and muscle spasm; to mobilize, specifically the spine and generally the whole body; to strengthen the abdominal, back extensor, hip and leg muscles; to correct the posture; to improve general fitness; to create body awareness and to educate in and promote back care. Selection of appropriate exercises will depend on the findings of the individual's assessment.

It is important that extra care is given with the choice of exercises for the osteoporotic spine, particularly with extension and rotation exercises. The emphasis should be on gentle mobility exercises with a gradual progression of strengthening exercises. The leg muscles must be exercised as well as the trunk muscles.

The physical properties of water can allow for the gradual progression of exercise in terms of weight relief since the effects of buoyancy increase with depth. In the horizontal position, exercises can be totally non-weight-bearing, whilst in the vertical position weight-bearing can be gradually increased by decreasing the depth of water.

Techniques

The techniques of choice would be those for relaxation which as stated earlier (p. 260) may be commenced in flotation. Mobilization can be obtained through the Bad Ragaz patterns specifically designed for the trunk.

Free exercise programme

Free exercises should be performed within the point of aggravation of any symptoms. The exercise routine commences with a general warm-up session which would include relaxed neck and shoulder exercises so that tension in those areas is relieved. The starting positions may be those of standing, sitting or lying. Whichever position is used the patient should be immersed as deeply as possible.

Free exercises involve movements of the upper and lower limbs, the trunk, head and neck. When neck exercises are performed specifically for cervical mobility they follow the movements and guidelines provided on p. 180. The usual progressions of exercise, such as increasing the speed, the range of motion and the repetitions, can be utilized.

Isometric exercises can be included for muscle strengthening, for example standing with the back against the wall, pressing the arms against the wall, holding then relaxing. Posture correction should be included by getting the patient to practise tightening the quadriceps, the gluteals and the abdominals at the same time as retracting the scapulae and elongating the cervical spine by stretching the crown of the head towards the ceiling.

Balance, posture and walking skills must be maintained. Balance control not only involves control in standing on both feet but includes the ability to counteract the effects of buoyancy and turbulence. Ways in which balance can be maintained and improved are given in Chapter 8. In all these exercises an upright posture is desirable and the patient requires careful instruction about posture correction and maintenance. Walking should be practised in all directions with the resistance being varied by increasing the speed of motion and therefore the turbulence around the moving body.

Swimming

Patients are encouraged to swim using any stroke which is comfortable; generally the stroke of preference is back stroke to prevent hyperextension. For the osteoporotic patient, back stroke again would be the choice as it involves most work for the posterior shoulder girdle muscles and thoracic spine movements. Breast stroke may be used, but only if there is no discomfort due to hyperextension of the spine, especially the cervical spine.

SPONDYLOARTHROPATHIES

The conditions grouped under this heading are also known under the heading of 'sero-negative spondarthritis' and include such conditions as ankylosing spondylitis, psoriatic arthritis, Reiter's disease, ulcerative colitis or Crohn's disease (Moll, 1980). A similar exercise routine can be applied for all conditions. The example used is for ankylosing spondylitis.

Ankylosing Spondylitis

Ankylosing spondylitis is a sero-negative inflammatory arthropathy affecting mainly the axial skeleton, but it may involve some peripheral joints such as the hips, shoulders, knees or feet. It is characterized in the early stages by low back pain, stiffness and impaired chest mobility; in the later stages by permanent stiffness, intermittent episodes of pain, loss of range of motion of the spine and possibly of the hips and shoulders, the latter often due to soft tissue contractures.

Aims of treatment

In the early or *acute stages* of the condition where pain is the predominant feature, the aims of treatment are to relieve pain and muscle spasm; to increase respiratory expansion, function and vital capacity; to maintain mobility of the spine, hips and shoulders; to create body awareness and to establish postural habits.

In the later stages of the condition when pain and muscle spasm are reduced and on into the *chronic stage* of the disorder, the aims of treatment are as stated for the early stage, but attention is paid also to increasing muscle strength to counteract deformities; to improving mobility and to teaching or improving swimming ability.

It is of interest to note that the Chartered Physiotherapists Policy Statement (*Physiotherapy*, January 1979) gives as a contraindication to hydrotherapy, chest conditions where the vital capacity is below 1500 cc; a statement which would exempt some people with ankylosing spondylitis and a low vital capacity from participating in hydrotherapy. However, Harrison (1981) disputes this figure and it has been the experience of this author that a low vital capacity and/or restricted chest mobility in the person with ankylosing spondylitis is no reason to preclude the person from an active hydrotherapy programme.

Technique

In the early or acute stages individual treatment is preferable, particularly if pain and muscle spasm are the predominant features. On a one-to-one basis it is easier to gain relaxation of muscle spasm by having the person supported in floats with the physiotherapist passively moving their body from side to side in large movements, inducing relaxation. Once relaxation is achieved the person is encouraged to assist the movement actively.

Breathing exercises can also be introduced with the person actively trying to expand the ribcage laterally or by the physiotherapist assisting by passively moving the trunk into side flexion to gain unilateral chest expansion. Mobilization of the trunk and limbs can also follow once relaxation has been achieved using the Bad Ragaz patterns of movement involving the trunk and upper and lower limbs (Bolton, 1971; Boyle, 1981). Swimming can be introduced at the early stage with the person choosing the stroke they find most comfortable and which does not aggravate the pain or muscle spasm. In the case of non or poor swimmers, water safety should be taught using the Halliwick principles (Martin, 1981; Campion, 1983; Reid Campion, 1985).

Modification of Watsu movements to relax, stretch and increase range of joint movement may also be of use in the acute stage, working carefully within pain tolerance. A more vigorous approach may be used in the more chronic stages when stiffness and soft tissue shortening are the main features.

Free exercise programme

Free exercises for the patient with ankylosing spondylitis can be divided into early and later rehabilitation programmes.

From the beginning, the programmes are active ones which place great emphasis on chest mobility, neck movements, posture, trunk, hip and shoulder mobility. Relaxation can be practised either by floating with supports or freely using large sweeping movements of the limbs and trunk. As with any exercise programme a warm-up session is important. Emphasis should be on lateral costal movement rather than diaphragmatic breathing. Some patients may find the pressure of the water on the chest wall uncomfortable, in which case the exercises can be carried out in supine lying on a plinth with part of the chest clear of the water. As the patient is able to tolerate the pressure so the starting position is changed to standing. Trunk movements may be combined with the breathing patterns to increase mobility and flexibility in the spine.

Neck exercises can be carried out in the 'more usual' manner in a free exercise programme but it is suggested that a more effective method of working the neck muscles is for the physiotherapist to work individually with the patient using both the flexed position and rolling techniques previously provided (p. 180). Good posture is vital for the patient with ankylosing spondylitis and in treatment this should be emphasized. Arm movements, with the importance of scapulae retraction and shoulder extension being stressed, assist in good postural control. Breast stroke arm action for example can achieve this type of movement.

Trunk mobility is developed through the 'conventional' trunk exercises emphasizing the extreme ranges of movement with over pressure to increase the range. Combining arm and trunk actions assists trunk mobility. Trunk movements may be carried out lying on a plinth in various positions, and when leg movements are incorporated they prove helpful in mobilizing the trunk and hip joints.

All exercises should be governed by the amount of pain and modifications to an exercise should be determined by individual needs. In the later stages of rehabilitation the exercise programme is expanded and the workload added to by increasing the speed, which ensures there is greater turbulence effect and therefore requires more effort and a greater range of movement is developed.

Flotation equipment may be used for some exercises to increase the workload. For example, an exercise for the trunk and shoulders could be progressed by the use of a flotation ring. With the arms in the 'reach' position and grasping the ring with the hands the patient swings the arms from side to side at the same time rotating the trunk. At the end of the range of movement to each side the patient pauses and attempts to push the ring under the water at the same time extending the trunk.

The various arm movements for the swimming strokes of overarm, breast stroke and back stroke can be incorporated in the programme and combined with body movements. The speed of the arm movement can be varied and breath control included by encouraging the patient in breathing techniques used for individual swimming strokes (Elkington, 1978; Reid Campion, 1985).

Stretching techniques (in a group)

A number of techniques can be used effectively to stretch tightened structures particularly of the hips, hamstring muscles, trunk and shoulders by the use of floats and buoyancy assistance. The method of contract–relax then employs passive stretching. Adequate fixation is necessary to localize the movement. The stretches should be done three times to maximize the effect before changing to the opposite side or limb (Barefoot – Lecture Notes, 1988).

The physiotherapist's imagination and ingenuity can devise a wide variety of exercises and activities for these patients in a free programme. Such programmes should be interesting and varied regularly as these patients will require a considerable amount of treatment over the years. Provided the aims of treatment are incorporated there are no limits to the activities than can be developed.

Hydrodynamic exercises may be used to strengthen muscles, particularly those of the trunk, and to increase the range of motion. These may be incorporated in free programmes provided they have been taught carefully and frequent checks are made to observe that the patient is carrying out the exercises correctly.

Swimming

All the swimming strokes can be attempted with modification according to the needs of the individual and the problems associated with stiffness. It may be necessary for some people to have a neck ring and hip float to enable them to perform back stroke. Others may be unable to perform breast stroke due to spinal rigidity. Underwater swimming can be included, not only to improve breath control, but as a competitive incentive. Some swimmers employ the use of a snorkel to overcome the problems due to stiffness. As there is some medical concern over breath holding in underwater swimming, controlled blowing out should be encouraged, whereby the air is gradually expelled from the lungs (Strauss 1982; Reid Campion, 1985).

Posture check

Before leaving the water, a posture check can be carried out as a reminder to maintain an upright stance and correct head position. Standing with the feet slightly apart, the knees are braced into extension by tightening the quadriceps, the gluteals and abdominals are tightened to control pelvic tilt (an integral part of posture correction and awareness), the shoulders are drawn back by adducting the scapulae and the head position corrected by extension and retraction of the lower cervical spine attempting to glide the neck back at the cervical, thoracic level. This movement is followed by cervical elongation by stretching upwards from the crown of the head.

REFERENCES

Atkinson G.P. and Harrison R.A. (1981). Implications of the health and safety at workout in relation to hydrotherapy departments. *Physiotherapy*, **67**(9): 263–265.

Barefoot J. (1988). Unpublished lecture notes.

Bishop P.A., Frazier S., Smith J. *et al.* (1989). Physiological responses to treadmill and water running. *The Physician and Sports Medicine*, **17**(2): 87–94.

Bolton E. (1971). A technique of resistive exercise adapted for a small pool. *Physiotherapy*, **57(10)**: 481–482.

Boyle A.M. (1981). The Bad Ragaz method. *Physiotherapy*, **67(9)**: 265–268.

Campion M. (1983). Water activity based on the Halliwick Method. In *Duffield's Exercise in Water* (A.T. Skinner, A.M. Thomson, eds), London, Baillière Tindall.

Davis B.C. (1967). A technique of re-education in the treatment pool. *Physiotherapy*, **63(2)**: 57–59.

Davis B.C. (1971). A technique of resistive exercise in the treatment pool. *Physiotherapy*, **57(10)**: 480–481.

Davis B.C. and Harrison R.A. (1988). *Hydrotherapy in Practice*, Edinburgh: Churchill Livingstone.

Dull, H. (1993). Watsu: *Freeing the Body in Water*, Harbin Springs Publishing.

Elkington H.J. (1978). *Swimming: A Handbook for Teachers*, Cambridge: Cambridge University Press.

Gleim G.W., Nicholas J.A. (1989). Metabolic costs and heart rate responses to treadmill walking in water at different depths and temperatures. *American Journal of Sports Medicine*, **17(2)**: 248–252.

Golland, A. (1981). Basic hydrotherapy. *Physiotherapy*, **67(9)**: 258–262.

Hamer P., Writtingham D., Spittles M. *et al.* (1984). Cinematographical comparison of water running to treadmill running. (Unpublished paper.)

Hamer P. (1985). Water-running: training effects on aerobic, anaerobic muscle parameters following an eight week interval exercise programme. Unpublished honours degree thesis at the University of Western Australia.

Harrison R.A. (1980). Hydrotherapy in rheumatic conditions. In *Physiotherapy in Rheumatology*, (Hyde, S. ed.), Oxford: Blackwell Scientific Publications.

Harrison R.A. (1981). Tolerance of pool therapy by ankylosing spondylitis patients with low vital capacities. *Physiotherapy*, **67(10)**: 296–297.

Hopper, D. (1990). Hydrotherapy for sports injuries, In *Adult Hydrotherapy – a Practical Approach*, (Reid Campion, M. ed.), Oxford: Heinemann Medical Books.

Martin J. (1981). The Halliwick method. *Physiotherapy*, **67(10)**, 288–291.

Moll J.M.H. (1980). *Ankylosing Spondylitis*, Edinburgh: Churchill Livingstone.

Orwoll E.S., Ferar J.L. and Oriatt S.K. (1987). The effect of swimming exercise and bone mineral content. *Abstracted Clin. Res.* **35(1)**, 194A.

Reid Campion M. (1985). *Hydrotherapy in Paediatrics*, Oxford: Heinemann Medical.

Reid Campion M. (1988). Unpublished lecture.

Strauss R.H. (1982). Concerns in underwater sports, *Pediatric Clinics of North America*, **29(6)**: 1431.

ADDITIONAL READING

Berson D. and Ray S. (1979). *Painfree Arthritis (Exercises in Water)*, Boston: G.K. Hull.

Cadogan D.R. (1971). Handling the handicapped. *Physiotherapy*, **57(10)**: 467–470.

Dick W.C. (1972). *An Introduction to Clinical Rheumatology*, Edinburgh and London: Churchill Livingstone.

Elkington H.J. (1971). The effective use of the pool. *Physiotherapy*, **57(10)**: 452–460.

Fries J.F. (1979). *Arthritis: A Comprehensive Guide*, Massachusetts: Addison-Wesley Publishing Co.

Gardiner M.D. (1963). *Principles of Exercise Therapy*, 3rd edn, London: G. Bell and Sons.

Harris S.J. (1971). Bathside management, pool hygiene and resuscitation. *Physiotherapy*, **57(10)**: 471–475.

Harrison R.A. (1980). A quantitative approach to strengthening exercises in the hydrotherapy pool. *Physiotherapy*, **66(2)**: 60.

Hart F.D. (1981). *Overcoming Arthritis*, Sydney: Methuen Australia Pty. Ltd.

Jagger M. and Smood D. (1984). Hydrotherapy by physiotherapists in a community health clinic. *Australian Family Physician*, **13(12)**: 878–881.

Jetter J. and Kadlec N. (1985). *The Arthritis Book of Water Exercise*, London: Granada Publishing Co.

Kacavas J., Morrison D. and Thurley M. (1977). The use of aqua therapy with geriatric patients. *American Corrective Therapy Journal*, **31(2)**: 52–59.

Reed B. and Rose M. (1985) *Water Workout*, Melbourne: MacMillan Sun Books.

Roth A. (1975). Therapeutic water exercise: A treatment modality in orthopaedic management. *Journal of Western Pacific Orthopaedic Association*, **XII(1)**: 15–20.

Scott J.T. (1980). *Arthritis and Rheumatism*, Oxford: Oxford University Press.

Tinsley L.M. (1983). Ankylosing spondylitis programme, *Australian Physiotherapy Newsletter* (W.A.), 9–12.

Williams L. (1987). Get wet, get moving. *Western Australian Arthritis & Rheumatism Foundation Newsletter*, No. 73.

Wynn Parry C.B. and Deary J. (1980). Physical measures in rehabilitation. In *Ankylosing Spondylitis* (J.M.H. Moll, ed.), Edinburgh: Churchill Livingstone.

14

Orthopaedics

Christine Lee

Hydrotherapy is utilized as a form of treatment in a wide variety of orthopaedic conditions. Physiological effects of immersion combined with the warmth of the water and buoyancy make the hydrotherapy pool an ideal place to initiate management of the orthopaedic patient. As the patient progresses, properties of water such as turbulence and moving against buoyancy can exercise all patients to their full potential.

AIM

The aim of this chapter is to give an overview of the hydrotherapy treatment of several orthopaedic conditions seen regularly in the hospital setting. The list is by no means exhaustive and the information should be utilized to apply the main principles to the ever expanding field of orthopaedic medicine.

INDICATIONS

Common characteristics of the orthopaedic patient may include the following:

Pain and Muscle Spasm

On immersion in a heated pool the circumferential warmth will relax muscles by initiating a peripheral vasodilatation. Buoyancy will decrease the loading onto weight-bearing joints which should help to reduce pain. The sympathetic nervous system is suppressed by immersion and will thus decrease the perception of pain (Mano *et al.*, 1985). To achieve

these responses the exercising limb needs to be fully immersed in water throughout the treatment session.

Oedema

Hydrostatic pressure increases with depth (Pascal's law). This pressure can result in several physiological changes occurring which may assist in reducing swelling:

1. The gradient pressure difference in the upright position will precipitate a body fluid movement from distal to proximal, thus reducing peripheral swelling.
2. During immersion a diuretic response will occur due to central volume expansion which will suppress anti-diuretic hormone (Hall *et al.*, 1990). This diuretic effect may help decrease swelling.
3. A combination of hydrostatic pressure and exercising the appropriate limb will enhance circulation and thus help reduce swelling.

To achieve the above effects the oedematous body part needs to be fully immersed and exercised as deep as possible in the water.

Decreased range of movement

This may be due to pain or swelling, as listed above, or stiffness. Stiffness may be eased by the warmth of the water causing a vasodilatation and increasing the skin temperature (Ring *et al.*, 1989). The buoyancy of the water will help move the stiff joint into further range with minimal increase in pain.

Using floats to obtain a good stretch with hold–relax followed by passive physiological or passive accessory movements will gain extra range of movement. An example could be a hold–relax technique to improve knee flexion. This can be followed by buoyancy assisted passive physiological knee flexion to take the range of movement further into flexion.

Muscle Weakness

Buoyancy acts differently to gravity. There is no value in using a land-based exercise which works the muscle at grade 3 or 4 (Oxford muscle scale) and doing that same exercise in the water environment as a strengthening exercise. For example, on land, hip abduction when standing is gravity resisted, when done in the water in the same standing position the exercise is now buoyancy assisted and not exercising the muscle to its full potential. In this situation, the position of the patient needs to be changed into a buoyancy resisted position to be comparable to the land-based exercise.

When addressing the problem of muscle weakness, make sure the position of the patient makes the muscles work to their optimal level to gain the strengthening effect required.

A useful progression of exercises to consider is the modified Oxford scale in water. The scale which helps to determine when to progress to a harder form of the exercise can be used as a means of objectively assessing and progressing a patient's exercise regime.

Poor Balance

Patients who have been on extended bed rest or non-weight-bearing through a limb will have balance problems. Support given by the water due to hydrostatic pressure will give patients longer reaction times before losing their balance. This allows for re-education of balance and also improves the patient's confidence in their ability to maintain their balance. Reaction times were shown to improve in a study on a group of patients doing a regular water exercise programme (Lord *et al.*, 1993).

Poor Posture

After sustained bed rest, poor mobility on land, or prolonged sitting, the hydrotherapy pool becomes an ideal environment for postural education. While the water provides support in the upright position the physiotherapist can give verbal instructions to correct poor postural habits.

Turbulence can be used to work the trunk muscle groups. By creating turbulence in front of a patient in the upright position near their centre of buoyancy there will be a tendency for the patient to fall forward. To counteract this movement the patient must use their back extensor muscles. Similarly turbulence created behind a standing patient will draw the patient backwards. The patient must work their abdominal muscles to maintain a static position.

Decreased Cardiovascular Fitness

Whether a problem is spinal, upper limb, or lower limb, the patient can be supported appropriately to enable them to exercise aerobically in the hydrotherapy pool. This can be in support standing doing upper limb work with bats, supine support float doing patterkick or modified swimming strokes. Whenever possible an aerobic component should be included in a patient's treatment programme.

On immersion in water there is a rise in cardiac output which can lead to an initial decrease in heart rate. The heart rate will then rise proportionally to the level of physical exertion and the temperature of the water. This needs to be considered when checking the heart rates of patients after their aerobic session.

PROGRESSION OF EXERCISES

The water environment allows for numerous progressions of exercise using the conventional method. An exercise can be progressed by working through the stages of buoyancy assisted, neutral, and resisted.

In each of these positions the following can be used:

1. *Speed of the movement.* In a buoyancy assisted situation the limb is moved slower than buoyancy to make the exercise harder. For a buoyancy resisted position the limb is moved quicker through the water to increase difficulty.
2. *Lever length.* In a buoyancy assisted situation the shorter the lever length the harder the exercise, while in a buoyancy

resisted situation, the longer the lever the more difficult the exercise.

3. *Turbulence*. This can be created by the moving limb, the patient or the physiotherapist. Turbulence can be used to assist the movement into the low pressure area or resist the movement by working against turbulence.
4. *Floats*. These can be used to assist a movement when it is buoyancy assisted or can increase the exertion required when utilized against buoyancy. Harrison (1980) suggests polystyrene 8 cm cubes which are equivalent to 0.5 kg to be used when trying to increase the exertion required by the patient.
5. *Streamlining*. A body part is easier to move through water if it is streamlined. To make a body part unstreamlined you can increase the surface area exposed to the water during movement by changing the position of the hand or foot or using bats and flippers.

Each of the progressions above can be used individually or combined together to give a fine grading system for the progression of exercise.

GAIT RE-EDUCATION

Patients suffering from spinal pain and lower limb complaints will require some form of gait re-education. The warmth of the water and the support given in the upright position allows the patient a longer reaction time to correct their gait pattern. This is ideal in patients who can progress from non-weight-bearing through to full weight-bearing by altering the depth of the water in which they are standing. A patient who is touch weight-bearing (10%) with crutches on land is able to immerse to C7 level (8% weight-bearing) and practise a proper heel strike/push off in the water. This is extremely difficult for the patient to do on land. Harrison and Bulstrode (1987) and Harrison *et al.* (1992) determined the weight-bearing at different depths of immersion with the patient stationary and walking.

Ideally re-education is done on a flat surface in the pool. On a sloped-bottomed pool consideration must be given to the effect on the gait pattern especially if there is a leg length discrepancy.

TREATMENT PLANNING

A thorough land-based assessment needs to be conducted to determine the aims and objectives of hydrotherapy. In addition, all patients need to be checked for contraindications to pool treatment. Ideally the physiotherapist doing the land-based assessment is also the person conducting the pool treatment. This allows for further assessment of body shape and density, and how water will affect the patient's balance on immersion. It also enables the physiotherapist to update land-based exercises in keeping with the patient's progress.

It is important to be able to reassess objectively the effectiveness of hydrotherapy intervention. This can be done with goniometry measures, assessing functional activities, noting changes in gait pattern, or the amount of flotation used during a specific exercise.

The length of treatment will vary greatly from one patient to the next. Variables to consider include the type of injury, whether the problem is acute or chronic, any associated medical problems, the duration of bed rest prior to mobilization, the age of the patient, the general fitness of the patient and the pain level. Initial treatment time in most cases commences at 20 minutes building up to 45 minutes for rehabilitation patients.

As far as possible the treatment plan should contain the following stages:

1. *Warm up* – General range of movement exercises for the affected limb and body.
2. *Stretches* – Specific to the affected limb.
3. *Strengthening* – Specific to the condition.
4. *Aerobic* – To improve cardiovascular fitness.
5. *Functional activity* – Attempt an activity that the patient cannot do on land in the water. If this is not possible then break down the activity and practise components of it. Examples would be gait re-education, attempting the action of putting shoes on or kicking a ball.
6. *Cool down* – Range of movement exercises.
7. *Relaxation* – Performed by the patients themselves or with the assistance of the physiotherapist. The patient must be in a completely relaxed position and submerged as much as possible to gain benefits from the warmth and buoyancy of

the water. Supine floating and support lean sitting are two possible positions.

The length of the treatment session and priority of aims of treatment will dictate the time spent on each treatment component and how many stages are used.

COMMENCEMENT OF TREATMENT

Post surgical patients can commence treatment as soon as they are medically stable and do not have evidence of contraindications such as wound infection or leakage from the suture line. Sutures can be covered with 'Op-site' or a sprayed plastic dressing.

ORTHOPAEDIC CONDITIONS

In the following section the most frequently seen orthopaedic conditions in the hydrotherapy pool will be discussed and progression of exercises suggested. This is by no means a recipe list of exercises and should only be seen as a possible progression for the presenting conditions. The ability to progress exercise programmes in water must come from a sound knowledge of the properties of water and the physiological effects of the body being immersed. The physiotherapist with this knowledge base will be able to advance or alter programmes to work the patient to their full capability.

Shoulder Girdle

Fractured scapula

The most common form of fracture involves the body or neck of the scapula. The injury is usually caused by a direct blow to the area such that bruising, swelling and severe pain are evident. Treatment consists of wearing a sling for comfort but range of movement exercises are begun immediately.

Aims: To encourage active use of the affected side and to improve scapulothoracic rhythm.
Exercises: The shoulder should be immersed throughout the treatment session to provide it with warmth and support by the buoyancy of the water. Buoyancy assisted flexion, extension and abduction are commenced in the standing

or sitting position. When the patient can achieve 90° flexion in the water, horizontal abduction and adduction can be incorporated. These patients usually progress rapidly and only require a few weeks treatment in the pool before being able to be maintained on a full home programme.

Glenohumeral Joint

Fractured neck of humerus

This fracture is seen mainly in elderly, osteoporotic women (Apley and Solomon, 1988) who fall onto an outstretched hand. The fracture is often impacted due to the method of fall, so mobilization can be commenced early.

Aims: To improve range of movement and decrease pain.

Considerations:

1. It is possible that the patient has never been in a hydrotherapy pool and the fall may have been caused by gait or balance problems, thus they will feel unsteady in water. Mental adjustment to the water environment is vital and the patient must develop the ability to restore their balance both vertically and longitudinally. This will help to decrease the patient's anxiety during the treatment session.
2. These fractures can be very painful with the patient unwilling to initiate movement or using 'trick' movements instead of scapulo-thoracic rhythm.

At the initial hydrotherapy sessions these patients need close supervision.

Early exercises:

Standing/sitting

1. Buoyancy assisted shoulder flexion, extension and abduction with emphasis of movement occurring at the glenohumeral joint.
2. Hold–relax buoyancy assisted flexion, extension and abduction.
3. Horizontal abduction/adduction using a float to support the arm.
4. Shoulder protraction/retraction by punching the arm gently forward (flotation as required).

5. Sliding the hand up the side of the body and pushing down again progressing to using floats to increase difficulty.
6. Active range of movement of the elbow, wrist and finger joints.

Supine float

7. Bad Ragaz techniques utilizing isometric holds while the body is moved through the water.
8. Relaxation in the sitting or supine float position so that the patient will relax the shoulder girdle musculature.

Later exercises:

1. Walking through the water with an arm swing pattern. This will increase turbulence and make the arm movement more difficult through the water.
2. Push-ups against the wall in the lean standing position.
3. Bad Ragaz upper limb isotonic patterns incorporating rotation.
4. If shoulder joint stiffness has become a problem then passive mobilizations both accessory and physiological should be used whilst the patient is in the water. Caudad glides in abduction stabilizing the arm and moving the body caudally through the water will improve shoulder abduction. By moving the body through the water while the arm is at the patient's end of range abduction combined with the caudad glide will use turbulence to provide an end of range stretch.

The same principle can be applied to the other ranges of movement. It is vitally important that these patients start mobilizing early and that their water-based and land-based exercise programmes are kept up to date with each other.

Arthroplasty

These patients can commence hydrotherapy 10–14 days post-operatively, with emphasis initially on buoyancy assisted exercises, until three weeks post surgery when full range of movement can be encouraged.

Aims: To improve range of movement and strength.
Exercises: Buoyancy resisted exercises are utilized but Bad Ragaz isotonic techniques should be used only when pain allows. Early exercises listed under fractured neck of humerus may be used.

Fractured shaft of humerus

This can result from a fall onto the hand with a rotation force (spiral fracture), a fall onto the elbow with the arm in abduction, or a direct blow to the arm (transverse fracture). In most fractures a collar and cuff sling is used to immobilize the arm for six weeks at which time range of movement exercises of the elbow and shoulder can be commenced. If there is marked displacement a U slab of plaster may be required for immobilization or internal fixation may be necessary, especially if there is a case of pathological fracture from a metastatic tumour.

Aims: To regain movement at the shoulder and elbow joint and strengthen muscles.
Exercises: The exercises used for fractured neck of humerus can be utilized, with the exception of shoulder abduction which should be avoided until the fracture has shown signs of uniting.

Elbow joint

Injuries around the elbow joint can include fractures to the supracondyles, epicondyles and condyles of the humerus. Special care needs to be taken with these fractures due to potential risk to the brachial artery. Treatment consists of three to six weeks in plaster of paris following an undisplaced fracture while manipulative reduction is required for displaced fractures.

Aim: To regain range of movement at the elbow joint.
Exercises: No resisted work should be carried out until the X-rays show good union. Once this is achieved Bad Ragaz techniques can be utilized to take the joint through its full range of movement. The use of bats and floats will help strengthen the muscles around the elbow after union has been achieved. This can be in the form of isometric or isotonic exercises.

Swimming should be encouraged with emphasis on breast stroke to help with triceps and biceps strengthening. The stroke may have to be modified if there are associated shoulder problems.

Wrist and Hand Joints

Even though fractures and injuries are common in the wrist and hand, hydrotherapy is rarely used as a form of management.

These patients can immerse their forearm and hand in warm water at home to carry out their range of movement exercises if pain or stiffness is limiting their ability to mobilize.

Pelvis

Fractures of the pelvis are usually caused by direct injury or by violence transmitted longitudinally through the femur. After bed rest to allow for commencement of union of the fracture, as well as relief of pain, the patient can begin to ambulate as pain allows. Hydrotherapy becomes an ideal medium to encourage the patient to move.

Aims: To increase weight-bearing, improve lower limb muscle strength and maintain range of movement of the hip joint.
Considerations: If there has been disruption of the pelvic ring the use of hip abduction should be restricted.

Early exercises:

Standing

1. Walking in the most comfortable depth of water. This will probably be at 10% weight-bearing at the beginning. Support is given by the physiotherapist as required. Maximum support is given with the patient's hands on the physiotherapist's shoulders, the patient walking forwards as the physiotherapist moves backwards. As the patient improves, this can be progressed from a short arm hold to a long arm hold and then to no support.
2. Buoyancy assisted hip flexion and extension.

Side lying

3. Lumbar extension and flexion buoyancy neutral.

Supine

4. Patterkick with the legs in float support supine lying.

Later exercises:

If pain allows:

Standing

1. Walking sideways across the pool. Commencing with small steps and progressing to larger steps. Walk the patient at a depth where their pain is comfortable.
2. Balance work. Examples – one leg standing, one leg standing working against turbulence created by the physiotherapist or forward hopping, stopping between each hop. The patient should commence at a depth which is comfortable painwise and progress to shallower water as tolerated.

Supine float

3. Swimming freestyle or back stroke. It may be several months before the patient finds breast stroke kick comfortable.
4. Isometric Bad Ragaz techniques can be used initially and then progressed to isotonic techniques.

Hip Joint

Total hip replacement

There are numerous forms of prothesis used to carry out total hip replacements. The majority of procedures are carried out on elderly patients following a fall or those with severe osteoarthritis of the hip. Hydrotherapy can be used effectively on patients with osteoarthritis of the hip (Sylvester, 1989) to improve functional ability and this can also apply to post total hip replacement patients.

Aims: To improve joint mobility, strengthen hip musculature and commence gait re-education if the patient is allowed to weight-bear.

Considerations:

1. Those patients having elective total hip replacements could have had periods of decreased mobility as well as several joints affected with osteoarthritis. This will

affect their ability to mobilize post-operatively. Commencing these patients on a pre-operative hydrotherapy programme will improve muscle strength and familiarise the patient with the post-operative regime. Exercises from the early and later exercise lists would be appropriate.

2. Cemented or uncemented procedure. Usually cemented total hip replacements can commence partial weight-bearing the day after the operation whilst uncemented procedures commence touch weight-bearing through the limb. This will determine the depth of the water in which the patient should exercise when exercising in the upright position.

3. The surgical approach. With any patient post arthroplasty there is the possibility of dislocation.

   Where an anterior incision has been used it is essential to limit extension and external rotation. With a posterior incision flexion should be limited, whilst when a postero-lateral incision has been employed adduction, internal rotation and flexion must all be limited.

4. Limiting rotation movements. The exercise regime should contain minimal rotation exercises during early post-operative treatment due to the possibility of dislocation. Bad Ragaz techniques should be modified to limit the rotation component.

Early exercises:

Standing

1. Buoyancy assisted hip flexion, extension and abduction.
2. Hold–relax stretches of any tight muscle group. Consideration must be given to the type of surgical approach and which movements must be limited.
3. Knee flexion and extension in standing.

Supine float

4. Supine plinth lying bicycling action unilateral or bilateral.
5. Bad Ragaz isometric hip abduction.

Later exercises:

Standing

1. Decrease the depth of water the patient walks in as increased weight-bearing is allowed.
2. Balance work in a depth which is dictated by the degree of weight-bearing allowed.
3. Functional activities such as lifting the leg to touch the toes with the knee flexed. This will improve the ability to put socks and shoes on. It is important to limit the degree of hip flexion early post operatively.

Supine float

4. Hip extension with a float on the ankle.
5. Progress to buoyancy resisted work as able. This will depend on the strength of each particular muscle group.
6. All Bad Ragaz isometric leg patterns.

Fractured neck of femur

These fractures are seen in the elderly patient who has had a fall directly onto the hip. Most will require surgery with a pin and plate.

Aims: To regain confidence in walking, improve joint mobility and strengthen hip musculature.

Considerations:

1. These patients may have balance problems which caused their initial fall.
2. Pain will lead to an unwillingness to mobilize so considerable encouragement will be required.

Exercises: Those listed under total hip replacement can be utilized.

Fractured shaft of femur

This type of fracture is usually seen in the younger adult following road traffic accidents, falls from a height, and crushing injuries. Conservative treatment is with traction to overcome the displacement of the fracture and the shortening of the quadricep and hamstring muscles due to the fracture and muscle spasm. Surgical intervention can incorporate intramedullary nailing or pin and plating. This type of management and the severity of the fracture will determine when hydrotherapy can commence.

Aims: To regain hip and knee range of movement, gait re-education, strengthening hip and knee musculature.

Considerations: These patients will often have marked wasting of the quadriceps and shortening following traction, therefore they will be lacking knee stability and flexion. Post-surgical repair patients could have marked soft tissue injury following their accident which requires appropriate land-based intervention as well as hydrotherapy.

Early exercises:

Standing

1. Buoyancy assisted hip flexion, extension and abduction.
2. Buoyancy resisted knee extension. Progress by increasing the speed of the movement.
3. Buoyancy assisted knee flexion with the hip in the neutral position.
4. Buoyancy resisted knee flexion with the hip flexed to 90° flexion.
5. Stretches for quadriceps, hamstrings and hip adductors by using a hold–relax technique. The hold component can be given by the physiotherapist or by the use of floats. The stretch should always be taken to a feeling of muscle pull rather than pain.
6. Gait re-education with weight-bearing as allowed. Commence the patient in deeper water and progress to shallower water dependent on pain, percentage of weight bearing allowed and gait progression.

Supine float

7. Bicycling action unilateral or bilateral.

Later exercises:

Once there is good union at the fracture site, these patients can be worked harder in the pool.

Standing

1. Balance work using turbulence created by the physiotherapist or the patient themselves.
2. Hold–relax stretches for any range that has not been regained.
3. Physiological and accessory mobilizations used in the pool as required. For example knee flexion may be limited by poor patella mobility, when the use of medial and cephalic glides of the patella may be helpful. Physiological knee extension with buoyancy assisting will also improve limitations of knee extension.

Supine float

4. All Bad Ragaz isotonic, isometric patterns unilateral and bilateral.
5. Swimming with or without flippers mainly using back stroke and freestyle to improve quadriceps and hamstring muscle strength.

Knee Joint

Total knee replacement

This type of surgery is usually carried out on older patients with osteoarthritis of the knee joint.

Aims: To increase knee flexion, improve quadriceps and hamstring muscle strength and mobility.

Considerations:

1. Pre-operatively mobility could have been greatly restricted leading to muscle weakness and a poor gait pattern. If possible these patients should be commenced on a pre-operative programme consisting of exercises from the suggested early and later exercise sections. This will improve muscle strength and familiarize the patient to the post-operative hydrotherapy regime.
2. Other weight-bearing joints may also be affected by osteoarthritis which will affect the post-operative outcome.
3. The surgical procedure may be cemented or uncemented. Patients with cemented replacements will be allowed to weight-

bear as tolerated post surgery but uncemented replacements will be partially weight-bearing only.

Early exercises:

Standing

1. Buoyancy assisted knee flexion and extension.
2. Hold–relax techniques to increase knee flexion. The hold can be given by the physiotherapist or by the use of floats. Buoyancy is used to give the stretch into the new range of movement.
3. Gait re-education. The depth of the water will be determined by the degree of weight-bearing allowed with emphasis given to the heel strike and toe push off.

Supine float

4. Supine plinth lying performing bilateral bicycle action.
5. Bad Ragaz isometric patterns through varying ranges of knee flexion. The physiotherapist can apply the movement through the water by holding distally to the knee or the patient can be moved through the water from their shoulders while holding knee flexion.
6. Repeated contractions to the knee.

Later exercises:

Standing

1. Progression of weight-bearing by decreasing the depth of the water in which the patient is standing and decreasing the support given by the physiotherapist.
2. Balance exercises such as maintaining balance against turbulence created by the patient or the physiotherapist. This can then be progressed to one leg standing while turbulence is created.

Supine float

3. Bad Ragaz lower limb patterns incorporating the hip and knee.

Knee reconstruction

This type of surgery is usually seen in young sportspeople following ligamentous ruptures of one or more of the anterior cruciate, post cruciate or collateral ligaments.

Post-operative regimes vary greatly from surgeon to surgeon. It may include wearing a brace limiting range from 30° to 60° knee flexion for six weeks or immediate gentle mobilization of the knee joint. Contact sports are limited for 9–12 months.

Aims: To strengthen the muscles around the knee joint, gait re-education, improve range of movement and proprioception.

Early exercises:

Once the patient is allowed to mobilize the knee joint, exercises are used to improve range of movement but the knee should not be forced into extension.

Standing

1. Buoyancy assisted knee flexion and extension.
2. Buoyancy resisted knee flexion taking care not to allow the knee into forced extension if floats are being used.
3. Gait re-education commencing in deeper water and progressing to shallower water.

Supine float

4. Rhythmic stabilizations through varying degrees of knee flexion.
5. Bad Ragaz isometric techniques for the lower limb avoiding forced knee extension.

Later exercises:

Standing

1. Functional activities related to the sport to which the sportsperson wishes to return. Examples are practising the action of kicking a ball or hopping and landing on one leg, using appropriate depths.
2. Metacentric exercises to improve balance.
3. Water running (deep or shallow). This is performed using some form of buoyancy

vest. Emphasis is given to technique to maintain the sportsperson's style of running. Aerobically it can push the athlete significantly.

Supine/prone float

4. Swimming to improve cardiovascular fitness.

Fractured patella

This can be caused by falls against a hard surface or by heavy objects falling across the knee. Treatment can consist of placing the patient in plaster for six weeks in full extension, wiring the fractures or excising the patella; whichever procedure is undertaken there will be trauma to the quadriceps tendon and an inability to flex the knee.

Aims: To increase knee flexion and improve hamstring and quadriceps strength.

Early exercises:

Standing

1. Buoyancy assisted knee flexion and extension.
2. Hold-relax knee flexion. The hold component can be given by the physiotherapist or by the use of floats.
3. Squats.
4. Marching on the spot with the emphasis on the knee flexion.

Supine float

5. Bad Ragaz isometric knee patterns.
6. Patterkick. In supine, knee flexion will be encouraged while in prone the emphasis will be more on knee extension.

Later exercises:

1. Metacentric exercises in the squat sitting position (p. 182).

Fractured tibial plateau

These fractures generally result from a severe valgus stress to the knee joint. Treatment can be by traction or open reduction and internal fixation.

Aims: To regain knee joint range of movement and improve muscle strength of the quadriceps and hamstrings.

Exercises: The progress of the patient will usually be rapid with this type of fracture. Exercises listed under fractured patella can be utilized and progressed quickly since there will be less limitation of knee flexion.

Fractured tibia/fibula

This type of fracture can result from torsional stresses as may happen in sporting injuries, falling from a height landing onto the feet or from direct blows.

Treatment usually consists of a full leg plaster on which a walking heel is applied three to six weeks post injury. The plaster is retained till union is achieved, up to 12 weeks approximately. After such prolonged immobilization muscle wasting could be marked with stiffness affecting the hip, knee and ankle joint.

Other forms of management may include intramedullary nail or pin and plating and these patients can commence mobilization earlier than those whose open fractures have been treated with external fixation. Patients with external fixators are not allowed to commence hydrotherapy until the fixators have been removed and the wounds have healed.

Aims: To improve range of movement of the knee and ankle joint plus regain muscle strength.

Early exercises:

Standing

1. Emphasis on weight-bearing with a good gait pattern. Encourage knee flexion during the swing phase and good heel strike and push off.
2. Bilateral heel raising in standing, using appropriate depths.
3. Buoyancy assisted and resisted knee flexion and extension.

Supine float

4. Bad Ragaz ankle dorsiflexion/plantarflexion.
5. Bad Ragaz knee flexion/extension.

Later exercises:

Standing

1. Metacentric exercises in the squat sitting position (p. 182).
2. Balance exercises that involve maintaining balance against turbulence created by the patient or the physiotherapist. Progress to one leg standing and then one leg standing in the heel raised position.

Supine float

3. Flipper work incorporating knee extension with ankle dorsiflexion and knee flexion with ankle plantarflexion.

Ankle Joint

Fractures affecting the ankle joint may include the medial and lateral malleolus, talus or the anterior and posterior tibial margins. Fractures with little displacement will be treated with plaster while those affecting the talus tibial alignment will be pinned.

Aims: To regain ankle and forefoot range of movement, progress weight bearing and improve muscle strength especially of the calf muscles.

Early exercises:

Standing

1. Hold-relax stretches to the calf muscles.
2. Bilateral heel raising in varying depths of water as pain allows.
3. Balance exercises including two-legged stance, one leg standing and in the heel raised position. Turbulence and the depth of the water can be varied to progress the activity.
4. Graduated weight-bearing as pain allows. Maintain the patient at a depth that achieves the best gait pattern.

Sitting

5. In the sitting position, knee flexion and extension with ankle dorsiflexion and plantarflexion. Progress by increasing the speed of the movement.

Supine float

6. Bad Ragaz dorsiflexion/plantarflexion pattern.

Later exercises:

Standing

1. Jogging in water commencing in deep water and progressing to shallower water as pain and technique allow.
2. Deep water running to encourage the patient to return to activities like jogging and to improve/maintain aerobic fitness.

Supine float

3. Bad Ragaz techniques incorporating dorsiflexion and plantarflexion with inversion and eversion.

Cervical Spine

Treatment for neck pain in the pool can only be effective if the neck is submerged during treatment. In the early stages of rehabilitation muscle spasm may be the main limiting factor. The patient may find cervical float collars extremely uncomfortable so the patient must inform the physiotherapist of any increase in pain. Initially it will be more comfortable to give exercises which move the body on the head rather than the head on the body.

Aims: Whether the patient is post whiplash injury or post laminectomy the aim of treatment is to decrease muscle spasm and improve range of movement.

Early exercises:

Standing or squat sitting with the neck submerged as much as possible.

1. Horizontal abduction and adduction with the upper limbs to stretch the trapezius muscle gently.
2. Arms at 90° shoulder abduction. Stretch one arm to the side to encourage cervical side flexion one way and then reach to the other side to gain side flexion in the opposite direction.
3. Arms at 90° shoulder flexion with palms together. Moving the arms side to side to

encourage cervical rotation by moving the body on the head.

4. Arms at 90° shoulder flexion. Stretch forward with one arm at a time, encouraging cervical rotation by moving the body on the head.
5. Active range of movement of the cervical spine into flexion, extension, side flexion and rotation.
6. Practise moving from sitting to the standing position. The head will have to initiate the movement.
7. Relaxation in squat sitting encouraging the patient to relax the cervical musculature as much as possible.
8. Walking sideways across the pool with emphasis of leaning into the movement, thus involving side flexion of the head and trunk.

Supine floating

9. 'Seaweeding' (p. 101), swaying the patient from side to side while in supine float, can help relaxation. If the patient is also encouraged to look at the physiotherapist – 'Hallo' (p. 102) – as the movement occurs cervical rotation will result.
10. The physiotherapist supporting the patient in supine float, laterally rotates the patient's body while the patient maintains their head position. This will encourage cervical rotation.

Bells hold (p. 51)

11. The patient is rocked backward and forward to initiate cervical flexion and extension.
12. The patient is rocked side to side to initiate cervical side flexion.

Later exercises:

1. The patient performs resisted bat work to improve strength of the upper limbs and cervical musculature.
2. Swimming is encouraged. For those patients with restriction of rotation, freestyle is encouraged, while for limitation of flexion and extension, breast stroke is used. Side stroke will improve cervical side flexion, if attempted in both side lying positions.

3. Hold relax stretches for stiff ranges of movement. It is important to isolate the stretch to the cervical movement and not allow shoulder movements to occur. The hold can be given by the physiotherapist or by the patient. The cervical musculature should be submerged as much as possible to allow the warmth of the water to aid the stretch.

Thoracic Spine

Thoracic stiffness can be effectively treated with stretches, active range of movement exercises, strengthening work and mobilizations in the hydrotherapy pool. Most of the exercises listed use movements of the upper limbs to work the musculature of the thoracic spine.

Aims: To improve joint mobility and strengthen thoracic musculature.

Exercises:

Standing

1. Horizontal abduction/adduction with the upper limbs going through full range of movement.
2. Shoulder flexion/extension through full range of movement in combination with thoracic rotation.
3. Breast stroke arm action taking the action to full thoracic extension.

Sitting

4. Place palms together at 90° shoulder flexion and move the arms side to side under the surface of the water.

These exercises can be progressed by increasing the speed of the movement, walking while doing the activity or using bats in the hands to increase the resistance and lever length.

Forward lean position

5. Hold the rail with one hand. Pass the other hand underneath as far as possible

and stretch. A float may be required to gain a full stretch.

6. Facing the wall, hold onto the rail with one hand and stabilize the anterior shin of both legs against the wall. This will stabilize the pelvis. The free hand moves in a horizontal abduction movement to full end of range thoracic extension.

Lumbar Spine

Hydrotherapy is used extensively in the treatment of lumbar pain for a variety of causes including post surgery, soft tissue injury, arthritis, fractures and disc pathology. It is vital that a full land-based assessment determines the cause of the lumbar pain so appropriate treatment can be given.

Hydrotherapy can be very effective in decreasing lumbar stiffness and improving range of movement. Special care needs to be taken with acute back pain patients that they do not overstretch in the pool or do sudden unprotected movements. These patients enjoy the support and the warmth of the water but can easily overdo their exercises if not closely monitored.

The following exercise regimes assume that the patient has no neurological involvement and is being referred for hydrotherapy for treatment of low back pain or stiffness.

Spinal surgery

This may include discectomy, laminectomy or spinal fusion of one or several levels. Patients may commence hydrotherapy as soon as they are medically stable, the suture line closed and no infection evident. This can be as early as four days post surgery in laminectomies but will be later in spinal fusions.

Aims: To allow the patient to gain confidence in walking, encourage movement of the lumbar spine, gain relaxation of the back extensor muscles and decrease pain.

All exercise regimes should take into account the specific instructions of the orthopaedic surgeons especially if an emphasis towards lumbar flexion or extension is preferred. If a generalized programme is required the following exercises can be utilized.

Early exercises:

Supine float

1. The physiotherapist moves the patient slowly around the pool to encourage muscle relaxation. The patient may be supported by the physiotherapist (p. 48) or by neck, pelvic, knee and/or ankle floats.
2. Gentle isometric contractions of the back extensor muscles can be encouraged by the physiotherapist applying light pressure and asking the patient to hold the position in the water.
3. Trunk side flexion with the legs moving side to side. Support is given by the physiotherapist initially at the pelvis and can be progressed to giving support under the shoulders, which will increase the lever length and the difficulty of the exercise.

Standing

4. Hip flexion, extension and abduction buoyancy assisted encouraging good posture throughout.
5. Unilateral hip and knee flexion.
6. Walking sideways, backwards, forwards across the pool with support as required. This progresses from physiotherapist support, to holding a large tube, to no support.

Supine plinth lying

7. Back extension work. Progression:

   - one leg hip extension
   - one leg hip extension while the other leg holds an isometric contraction just beneath the surface of the water
   - bilateral hip extension
   - bilateral hip extension with a small float around the feet.

8. Bilateral knee flexion to the chest followed by the knees coming to one side then the other to work the oblique abdominal muscles.

Later exercises:

Vertical hanging, back to the wall, holding the rail with outstretched arms

1. Bring both knees to the chest and then up diagonally.
2. Bicycle riding action with the legs, then reverse bicycle riding action to increase lower abdominal strength.

Vertical hanging, facing the wall

3. Anterior thighs against the wall with the knees flexed. Trunk side flexion ensuring that the patient controls the movement.
4. Same starting position as 3, but rotate the legs side to side to gain lumbar rotation.
5. As above, but holding the rail with extended arms, flex at the hips to bring the knees towards the chest. This will cause lumbar flexion with rotation.

Standing

6. Hamstring stretches with appropriate flotation for the stretch.
7. Stretches to full range of trunk rotators, side flexors, extensors and flexors using the hold–relax technique. Buoyancy is to give the stretch. For example, to stretch the trunk side flexors the patient faces the wall resting both forearms on the edge of the pool. A float is placed around both feet. The patient keeps the anterior thigh in contact with the wall as they raise both legs to the right to gain the stretch for the left trunk side flexors. They then press down against the float to gain contraction of the left side flexors, relax and allow a higher movement of the legs to the right.
8. Forward lean push ups against the wall.
9. Walking across the pool changing direction so that the patient is working against turbulence.

Supine float

10. All the Bad Ragaz trunk techniques can be utilized as pain allows. Work the patient within their limits of comfort if pain is the restricting factor. With a stiffness problem push the patient physically into a muscle stretch.

The upper limb and lower limb patterns can also be used if pain and muscle spasm are limiting the use of the trunk patterns.

Prone lying

11. Holding onto the wall with both hands bring both knees towards the chest then extend the legs again. Flotation may be required depending on the floating ability of the patient. Prone floating may be assisted by placing one hand against the wall below the other which is holding the rail.
12. Holding onto two large floats, one under each arm, slowly roll from prone lying to supine lying and return to prone.

An aerobic component should be encouraged in the programme such as swimming or sculling in supine float with a patterkick action. Posture correction and gait re-education instruction are vital throughout all treatment sessions.

Spinal fractures

These patients will have a period of bed rest prior to commencing hydrotherapy. The period of rest will vary greatly depending on the location and level of the fracture and the degree of displacement. In some cases the patients will wear their body brace in the pool during treatment. Pain is a common factor and the progression of rehabilitation is determined by pain levels and the degree of fracture union.

The exercises utilized for spinal surgery can be used with these patients. Rotation movements especially in combination with extension should be restricted in the early days.

Disc pathology

Land-based treatment such as electrotherapy, mobilizations and exercises can be augmented with hydrotherapy if pain and muscle spasm are major limiting factors to movement. Range of movements that are being used on land to help the patient should be the same as those that are encouraged in the water. An example would be if a patient's home programme is directed towards lumbar extension then the hydrotherapy treatment should do the same. In later rehabilitation, joint stiffness can become a major problem, so lumbar mobilizations in the water can be incorporated (p. 233).

SUMMARY

The exercises listed in this chapter are only examples of regimes that may be utilized in the treatment programmes. The scope and progression of exercises in the hydrotherapy pool are vast especially with the orthopaedic patient who can progress rapidly with the correct intervention.

ACKNOWLEDGEMENTS

1. Mr and Mrs Rathmann for their support.
2. Trish Starling for her comments regarding the chapter content.

REFERENCES

Apley A. and Solomon L. (1988). *Concise System of Orthopaedics and Fractures*, London: Butterworth.

Hall J., Bisson D. and O'Hare P. (1990). The physiology of immersion. *Physiotherapy*, **76(9)**: 517–521.

Harrison R. (1980). A quantitative approach to strengthening exercises in the hydrotherapy pool. *Physiotherapy*, **66(2)**: 60.

Harrison R. and Bulstrode S. (1987). Percentage weight-bearing during partial immersion in the hydrotherapy pool. *Physiotherapy Practice*, **3**: 60–63.

Harrison R., Hillman M. and Bulstrode S. (1992). Loading of the lower limb when walking partially immersed: implications for clinical practice. *Physiotherapy*, **78(3)**: 164–166.

Lord S., Mitchell D. and Williams P. (1993). Effect of water exercise on balance and related factors in older people. *Australian Journal of Physiotherapy*, **39**: 217–222.

Mano T., Iwase S., Yamazaki Y. and Saito M. (1985). Sympathetic nervous adjustments in man to simulated weightlessness induced by water immersion. *Journal of UOEH*, **7**: 215–227.

Ring E., Barker J. and Harrison R. (1989). Thermal effects of pool therapy on the lower limbs. *Thermology*, **3**: 127–131.

Sylvester K. (1989). Investigation of the effect of hydrotherapy in the treatment of osteoarthritic hips. *Clinical Rehabilitation*, **4**: 223–228.

RECOMMENDED READING

Crawford Adams J. and Hamblen D. (1990). *Outline of Orthopaedics*, 11th edn, London: Churchill Livingstone.

Crawford Adams J. and Hamblen D. (1992). *Outline of Fractures*, 10th edn, London: Churchill Livingstone.

McRae R. (1990). *Clinical Orthopaedic Examination*, 3rd edn, London: Churchill Livingstone.

McRae R. (1994). *Practical Fracture Treatment*, 3rd edn, London: Churchill Livingstone.

15

Management of sports injuries

David FitzGerald and Margaret Reid Campion

INTRODUCTION

This discussion will outline the role of hydrotherapy in the rehabilitation of sports injuries. It will attempt to describe rational therapeutic intervention, graded according to the nature of injury and stage in the healing process. It is not intended to be an exhaustive account of aetiology, structural pathology or the physiotherapeutic procedures which may be employed in the treatment of sports injuries, but rather an overview of the principles of hydrotherapy relevant to patient management.

Treatment of pain resulting from sporting injuries requires a systematic search for the structures at fault. Unlike visceral or systemic disease where a collection of signs and symptoms are usually attributable to specific pathological processes, the symptoms resulting from soft tissue injury are often multifaceted in origin.

'Functional analysis' (as opposed to diagnostic, structural labelling) is more relevant to the physiotherapist because it represents the integrated assessment of multiple elements of the musculoskeletal system. While one structure may be primarily implicated, it is rarely affected in isolation. Function will be the recurring theme of this discussion. Physiotherapists treating musculoskeletal conditions need to seek *optimal solutions* to clinical problems. Optimization requires the manipulation of a number of factors to provide the most efficient combination (Crosbie, 1993). Optimization of variables is necessary because traumatic insult or a new set of external constraints placed upon the body (altered training intensity) provide a new set of variables to which the body must adapt. These adaptations or compensations are not always optimal and may create further problems.

The format of the chapter is as follows:

- classification of injury
- aspects of tissue response to injury
- aspects of healing and influential variables
- formulation of rehabilitation principles based on tissue properties
- regional injury and hydrotherapy rehabilitation overview.

TISSUE RESPONSE TO INJURY

Any injury to the soft tissues will initiate an inflammatory response. Because rehabilitation of sports injuries involves minimizing the inflammatory reaction and progressively rehabilitating damage structures to full capacity, it is necessary to have a thorough understanding of the associated biological events. Categorization of injury in relation to the stage of inflammation is a valuable scale on which to gauge progression.

These stages are generally referred to as:

1. Acute.
2. Sub-acute.
3. Chronic.

These categories are often loosely applied by referring to the time since onset of symptoms. While this may be generally true, it is important to note that the timescale relates to the cellular and biochemical processes which occur in the inflammatory process. Three phases can be identified (modified from Oakes, 1982).

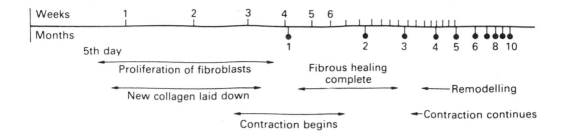

Fig. 15.1 *Collagen timescale.*

1. *Acute inflammatory phase* (up to 72 hours): vascular rupture and cellular infiltration, scar tissue very fragile, weak and unstable type 3 collagen.
2. *Repair phase* (72 hours up to 8 weeks): 72 hr–21 days – High collagen synthesis/degradation, increased scarring.
   21–60 days – Consolidation, predominantly fibrous, increasing strength, reduced capacity to respond to treatment
3. *Remodelling phase* (3/6 months–1 year): Type 1 collagen, minimal cellular composition, hypertrophic response to progressive stretching.

The concept of the 'collagen time-scale' (Evans, 1980, Fig. 15.1) is particularly relevant because good functional recovery is governed by the time constraints of normal physiology and does not necessarily relate to the level of pain. From a rehabilitation perspective the relevance of this lies in the fact that the mechanical properties (maximum failure load, energy absorption capacity, stiffness and compliance) of a tissue are directly related to its collagen content (Noyes *et al.*, 1974).

Tissue healing and remodelling

An extensive review of this topic has been undertaken by Cummings and Tillman (1992) and a summary is presented below. The purpose of this discussion is to provide a basis for planning hydrotherapy regimes commensurate with the degree of pathology and stage in the healing process.

1. Immobilization of non-traumatized tissues:

– significant loss of dense connective tissue strength
   80% in muscle after 4 weeks
   50% in MCL (knee) after 8 weeks
   39% ACL (knee) after 8 weeks
– slower loss of length and flexibility than strength (> 7 weeks for contracture)
– trauma prior to immobilization accelerates contracture (4 weeks).

2. Prevention of dense connective tissue shortening:

   – immobilization in lengthened position
   – inducing stress by isometric contractions
   – inducing stress by protected motion during healing
   – prevention of accelerated remodelling by reducing acute inflammatory reactions, and preventing chronic irritation
   – early protected mobilization promotes healing, minimizes scar tissue and increases strength of union.

3. Overuse injuries and stress fractures:

   – may be prevented by a controlled, phased build up to increased sports activities.

The great advantage of hydrotherapy is that the properties of water allow *controlled* loading of tissues which cannot be achieved on land. Secondly, and most importantly, it allows *functional* patterns of load to be utilized which have been shown to be effective (Vasey and Crozier, 1980; Oakes, 1982; Ihara and Nakayama,

1986) and is the ultimate aim of *all* rehabilitation.

CLASSIFICATION OF SOFT TISSUE INJURY

Soft tissue injuries may be classified in terms of (1), aetiology or (2), severity (Oakes, 1982).

1. Aetiology

(a) Direct injuries due to trauma, e.g. contusions, lacerations.
(b) Indirect injuries which may be further subdivided into:
   (i) acute – occurs with sudden overloading such as muscle tears or ligament ruptures
   (ii) chronic – due to repeated overload, e.g. tendonitis
   (iii) acute on chronic – due to sudden rupture of a persistent lesion, e.g. rupture of Achilles tendonitis.

2. Severity

(a) Grade 1 – Mild pain at the time of injury or within 24 hours of injury, especially when stress is applied to the injury: local tenderness may or may not be present.
(b) Grade 2 – Pain during activity, usually requiring cessation of activity; pain and local tenderness when the injury is stressed.
(c) Grade 3 – Complete, or near complete rupture of a portion of ligament or tendon with severe pain and loss of function; a palpable defect may be present but stressing the structure may be paradoxically painless, due to loss of continuity of the tissue.

Treatment of Acute Injury

If the severity of the injury is such that the activity must cease then the well-described first aid measures of **rest, ice, compression** and **elevation** (RICE) are appropriate. The specifics of these components are well described in the literature but of particular interest in relation to hydrotherapy is the rest component.

The role of rest

It is the exception rather than the rule that absolute rest (no movement) is indicated in sports injury management. The 'rest' component should strictly be considered as 'relative rest'. A large body of scientific evidence has now accumulated documenting the physiological, biomechanical and functional benefits of early controlled tissue mobilization as opposed to absolute rest by splinting immobilization (Tipton *et al.*, 1970; Vailas *et al.*, 1981; Leach, 1982; Zairns, 1982; Frank *et al.*, 1983; Salter *et al.*, 1975, 1989). It has been shown that the use of continuous passive motion assists the nutritional support of synovial joint components, especially articular cartilage, ligaments and synovium (Woo and Akeson, 1987). It has also been shown to have a significant effect on the clearance of haemarthrosis (O'Driscoll, 1983). Whether these effects can be achieved with hydrotherapy is not certain but clinical experience suggests that motion of any description, as opposed to immobilization, is more likely to produce the desired physiological effect. Controlled movement of the tissues within the region of trauma can be imparted by movement of structures proximal or distal to the affected area. For example, hamstring pain which is increased by neck flexion – a movement which increases tension in the nervous system (Brieg, 1978) but has no direct effect on muscle length, indicates a neural component to the symptomatology (Worth, 1969; Kornberg and Lew, 1989). Clinically, such neural involvement is commonly seen in association with primary muscle tears in that region (Fig. 15.2) illustrates this example.

Selective motion of neural structures can be achieved by moving proximal or distal to the site of symptoms but maintaining the pathological structures in an unloaded position. This imparts relative motion between the neural structures and the interfacing tissue.

Clinical evidence suggests that functional movement, modified as required, should be incorporated as early as possible (Vasey and Crozier, 1980; Oakes, 1982; Ihara and Nakayama, 1986). This is required to facilitate optimal recovery of proprioception and return to normal movement patterns. Of particular

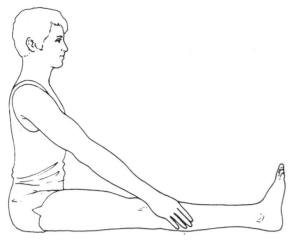

a

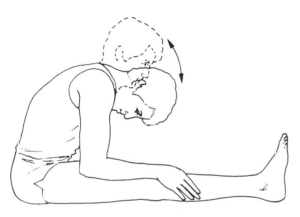

b

Fig. 15.2 *a. Symptoms are noted in long sitting prior to 'slump', b. Long sitting slump, approximating the shoulders towards the hips to increase the length of the spinal canal. Cervical flexion is added, then subtracted, monitoring the effect on hamstring pain*

importance in the axial skeleton and lower limbs is the degree of weight-bearing involved in the functional activity. If structures normally function under load of body weight then the closest approximation to this should be instituted as early as possible in rehabilitation. For example, immersion to the level of C7 is equivalent to approximately 8% weight-bearing (Harrison and Bulstrode, 1987) and could be used as a baseline loading level. The progression can then be made from relatively static loads to more dynamic weight-bearing activity using body weight, and finally through to

explosive jump or sprint work depending on the rate of progression.

Clinical Foundations prior to Hydrotherapy Rehabilitation

The subjective history and clinical features differentiate acute lesions from those resulting from an inflammatory response at a site of previous pathology, indicating a failure of the tissues to withstand the applied stress. Frequently, there may be some suspicion of dysfunction indicated by increased tightness, fatiguability, or subtle un-coordination and such symptoms may be indicators of imminent failure. Conversely, examination of an apparently 'acute onset' injury often reveals evidence of previous sub-clinical trauma such as tissue thickening, adaptive shortening, or restriction of joint range. Therefore the significant difference between this patient group and the 'initial acute onset' injury is that there may be residual soft tissue changes or functional disturbance from previous episodes. In the evaluation of pain related to chronic injuries the critical question to ask is 'Why has this problem occurred?' Is it related to extrinsic factors, such as running surface, footwear, racket size or equipment? If the source of the problem relates to intrinsic factors, can these be treated or modified to allow continuation?

Extrinsic factors

The extrinsic contributory factors in recurrent overuse injuries relate to those factors external to the body but which can exert a direct influence on the way in which it functions. These may include general environmental factors such as temperature or playing surface, or relate more specifically to the type of equipment used such as the style of running shoe, the length of cleat/stud (Cook *et al.*, 1990) or the size of racket in racket sports. If it is considered that extrinsic factors are contributing to the injury than they should be adjusted as appropriate. The level or grade of participation is an important consideration in all age groups and particularly so in contact sports. In adolescence it is mandatory to participate on an equal basis in terms of age or size because the unnecessary risk of injury to immature growing tissue during development is unacceptable. Likewise, it is important to match the intensity, frequency and duration of training, and the type of equipment used, to the stage of skeletal maturity. Abnormal or excessive force applied to an immature skeleton may not only produce pain at the time of insult but also induce structural alterations which may be pain provoking in later life, e.g. asymmetrical activities such as rowing or tennis).

Intrinsic factors

The intrinsic factors which may precipitate sports injuries are closely related to general anthropometrical considerations. While there is a certain 'self-selection' process in relation to chosen activity there is always the individual who decides to 'take up' a sport for which they are neither physically nor mechanically suited (i.e. episodic fun runner, social squash or tennis player). The physical attributes which facilitate safe participation in sport relate not only to size and strength but also to the individual's coordination and the degree of muscular control. Detection of the muscular imbalances which may produce pain or functional alteration may not be evident on routine static muscle tests (Kendall and McCreary, 1983). More specific evaluation of functional movement in terms of patterns of muscle recruitment is necessary to detect pathomechanics (Janda, 1983a,b). Such imbalances may manifest themselves as muscle or tendon damage due to hyperactivity/overuse of a particular muscle group, or as damage to articular structures due to abnormal stress transmission through joint surfaces and peri-articular tissues.

Another important component of muscle function, together with strength and coordination is the flexibility of the musculo-tendinous unit. Safran *et al.* (1988) have shown that greater force and increase in length are needed to tear an isometrically preconditioned (warmed) muscle. In the case of chronic Achilles tendonitis it is considered that lack of flexibility is a significant aetiological factor (Reynolds and Worrell, 1991) in the development of this condition.

In determining whether there is a significant intrinsic aetiological component, two aspects should be considered:

1. Structural anomalies.
2. Functional compensations.

Structural factors refer to osseous anomalies such as genu valgum, patella alta or scoliosis. Acquired factors refer to the connective tissue changes which may develop secondary to abnormal biomechanics (i.e. shortening of hyperactive muscle such as hamstrings, psoas) or tightening of fascial structures (iliotibial band).

Evaluation and treatment of structural anomalies

The range of structural anomalies which may occur is extensive and the existence of an anomaly does not in itself dictate that dysfunction will follow. In relation to the effects of asymmetries during running it has been demonstrated in asymptomatic individuals that the lower limbs of distance runners possess a multifaceted asymmetry for touchdown and foot contact as well as for the entire phase of foot support of the running stride (Vagenas and Hoshizaki, 1992). Thus deciding on the significance of asymmetries is a complex decision which depends on addressing the most evident abnormalities first, but may ultimately depend on hard-earned clinical experience! The body's adaptability may be extremely variable and the mechanisms of compensation for structural faults is not fully understood.

Obviously, conservative treatment cannot hope to alter structure but it can provide adequate functional compensation to allow pain-free motion. An example of the patello–femoral joint will serve to illustrate. Historically, pain in the anterior knee region has proved to be particularly resistant to physiotherapy. Most anterior knee pain in adolescence was diagnosed as chondromalacia patella (Goodfellow *et al.*, 1976) and when conservative treatment of rest and physiotherapy failed various surgical procedures were undertaken (Install *et al.*, 1976; Install, 1979; Bentley and Dowd, 1984). However, the success rate of surgical intervention was not consistent and an alternative conservative approach was pioneered by McConnell (1986) addressing some of the many variables known to influence patello–femoral joint mechanics (Laurin *et al.*, 1978; Marks and Bentley, 1978; Sikorski *et al.*, 1979; Gerrard, 1987). The result of this approach has been a significant improvement in treatment of anterior knee pain and a reduction in surgical intervention.

In situations where no amount of joint and soft tissue mobilization or muscle strengthening can provide adequate, pain-free function then external compensation for structural faults should be considered. In the lower limb this may involve a shoe raise to compensate for leg length discrepancy or a more sophisticated form of orthotic appliance to modify foot function.

Treatment of functional compensations

Changes in joint and soft tissue develop secondarily to the functional demands placed upon them. That this is so is verified by the well-documented, deleterious effects of immobilization (Tipton *et al.*, 1970; Salter *et al.*, 1975, 1989; Vailas *et al.*, 1981; Leach, 1982; Zarins, 1982; Frank *et al.*, 1983). Indeed, there is ample evidence documenting structural adaptations to imposed functional demands (Poss, 1984; Marks, 1991; Cameron *et al.*, 1992). Patterns of functional use and disuse, both in athletic activity and routine daily living, are commonly observed clinically. This habitual use may not only place the inert structures under constant, repetitive load but initiates a tendency for dominant muscles groups to become overused, or hypertonic (Jull and Janda, 1987; Janda, 1988). The result of this is a tendency for the hyperactive muscle groups to become shortened, in association with a lengthening of the antagonistic muscle groups due to reciprocal inhibition. The implications on movement are such that the normal synergies of muscle activation may become disturbed. These alterations should not be viewed as due to an isolated muscle weakness which must be strengthened, but in terms of a disturbance in the complex mechanisms of neuromuscular control (Janda, 1978). Poor motor regulation will subject other elements of the musculoskeletal system to potentially harmful stresses which may result in repeated microtrauma and eventually pain. Therefore effective treatment must address cause as well as symptoms.

GENERAL PRINCIPLES OF REHABILITATION

Rehabilitation is commonly classified in a somewhat arbitrary three-stage system, early, middle and late, but is in fact a continuum, graded according to the applied workload. The vast spectrum of potential rehabilitation procedures is beyond the scope of this discussion but in general terms progression can be made by manipulation of the following variables with attention to quality of task execution and the associated pain response prior to further progression:

1. Degree of weight-bearing.
2. Range of joint motion.
3. Type of muscle contraction.
4. Force of muscle contraction.
5. Speed of contraction.
6. Level of static/dynamic load.

Careful monitoring of the tissue response following each progression should be undertaken on an ongoing basis and any signs of increased irritation dictate caution, if not a reduction in the rate of progression.

The rehabilitation programme must attempt to stimulate collagen synthesis in an organized manner in order to improve the tensile strength of the tendon. To this end an 'eccentric training programme' has been devised by Curwin and Stanish (1984) and this has proved to be effective in the rehabilitation of many chronic tendonoses including the Achilles tendon.

There are three parameters on which the eccentric exercise programme is based:

- Length
- Load
- Speed.

Normalization of musculo-tendinous length reduces the strains which occur with joint motion. Progressive increase in load causes adaptive changes in collagen synthesis and mechanics with a subsequent increase in tensile strength. Changing the speed of contraction also increases the tensile stress on the tendon. An example of an eccentric programme based on a 'calf-raising' exercise is outlined in Fig. 15.3.

Primary muscle damage may occur at virtually any anatomical site and may be due to either intrinsic or extrinsic factors. Injuries to muscle have been graded in a similar fashion to ligament – based on a four-tier system according to the degree of anatomical disruption and percentage of fibres torn (Muckle, 1982;

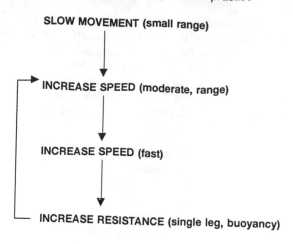

SLOW MOVEMENT (small range)

↓

INCREASE SPEED (moderate, range)

↓

INCREASE SPEED (fast)

↓

INCREASE RESISTANCE (single leg, buoyancy)

Fig. 15.3

Hamer, 1991). In association with early passive mobilization, active, or active-assisted movement must also start as soon as pain allows. In the case of primary muscle injury this may commence from 48 hours (Herring, 1990) but sub-maximal isometric contractions, incremented through range, may be acceptable earlier. The progression is then made to low intensity, small range motion, paying particular attention both to the eccentric and concentric phases of muscle activity (Belka, 1968; Costill et al., 1971; Steadman, 1979; Hakkinen and Komi, 1981).

The obvious potential of hydrotherapy to facilitate these requirements dictates an important role in the rehabilitation process. As active movement imparts motion to both the contractile and inert structures these principles can be employed in the treatment of both muscle and tendon.

Subsequently, re-establishment of normal movement patterns then requires conscious activation of normal synergies with further progression to increasingly demanding, spontaneous activities. Frequently, an apparent lack of strength in a particular muscle group improves immediately following appropriate stimulation in a functional pattern. Examples of typical hydrotherapy rehabilitation programmes incorporating these principles are outlined below.

The advantages of hydrotherapy for injuries with primary muscle damage are:

- decreased stress on joints, especially weight-bearing

- reduction of pain and muscle spasm
- improved circulation leading to the dispersal of haematoma and oedema
- decreased swelling.

The depth at which exercise takes place is dictated by the degree of weight-bearing allowed, or carried out in the horizontal position.

Active and buoyancy assisted small-range movements using the 'conventional method, together with modified isometric Bad Ragaz patterns and hydrodynamic exercise (p. 179) using minimal alterations in shape to facilitate movement of the affected part, would commence the treatment. The physiotherapist needs to monitor the movements carefully to avoid an excess of range of movement due to buoyancy and/or turbulence.

Progressions would be to buoyancy neutral 'conventional' exercises, the movements being slow and streamlined with changes in the length of the lever arm as appropriate. These exercises can be further progressed to quicker, unstreamlined movements, increasing the speed and range as appropriate. Controlled isotonic Bad Ragaz patterns may be commenced but no resistance given and alterations in shape may be increased gradually in the hydrodynamic exercises. Repeated contractions may be introduced and, where appropriate, rhythmic stabilizations.

All techniques would progress to the advanced stages as the condition improves. 'Conventional' exercises would become buoyancy resisted, performed with increasing speed and range. Further resistance may be provided manually or by increasing the size and number of floats. Bad Ragaz patterns to strengthen muscles and increase the range of movement would be employed and the changes in shape in hydrodynamic exercise would be larger, demanding greater muscle work, balance and coordination.

Gait re-education and other functional activities are begun immediately, the choice of depth being vital. The usual and hydrodynamic approaches of gait re-education can be used, progression being by decreasing the depth in the former, but in the latter too shallow a depth is of little value. A buoyancy neutral depth, that is with the water level at the xiphisternum, is optimal.

Hydrotherapy in the Rehabilitation of Musculo-tendinous Injuries

The spectrum of tendon injuries ranges from an acute tendonitis (inflammation of the tendon and surrounding paratenon), through to degenerative changes within the substance of the tendon (tendonosis) and potential tendon disruption (partial or complete). The pathophysiology is usually related to an intrinsic mechanism of injury – gradual, sustained overload, or sudden, severe overload. Less frequently tendons are subjected to direct trauma – extrinsic mechanisms, except in the case of the rotator cuff of the shoulder where impingement is common. The commonly involved tendons in sports injuries are: Achilles, peroneal, hamstring, iliotibial band, rotator cuff, common extensor origin and wrist extensors. The principles of rehabilitation are similar whether one is addressing a post-surgical repair or a chronic tendonosis. The application of the principles varies according to the initial level of loading (reduced load tolerance of a surgical repair relative to a tendonitis) and the duration of each phase of rehabilitation.

Once the inflammatory responses have settled in acute trauma, hydrotherapy is an ideal means of rehabilitation. Athletic fitness can be maintained by swimming and deep water running supported by a buoyancy aid (Hopper, 1990). Specific techniques would include the 'conventional' method, Bad Ragaz patterns and hydrodynamic exercise, all being progressed as described above.

The chronic conditions where the need for strength and muscle control is essential, the use of distal holds in the Bad Ragaz patterns, especially if pain has decreased, allow for an increased range of movement and stronger muscle work.

Exercising the smaller joints of the body – the ankle and wrist joints – is considered by some authorities to be difficult in water. However, the use of Bad Ragaz patterns and hydrodynamic exercise negates this argument, and where the ankle tendons are involved, activity taking place in a buoyancy neutral situation will not only help disperse swelling (Pascal's law), but at this depth activities may include standing on the affected leg and balancing against turbulence applied around the athlete by the physiotherapist – a technique similar to the wobble board on land, but having the supportive factor of hydrostatic pressure to assist the athlete in the early stages. Hold–relax, stabilizations and progression from buoyancy dominated to gravity dominated situations assist recovery.

Hydrotherapy in the Rehabilitation of Lower Limb Stress Fractures

Stress fractures occur anywhere but predominate in the lower limb and particularly involve the tibia (Kues, 1990; Taube and Wadsworth, 1993). Other anatomical sites include the fibula, ischium, metatarsals, navicular, calcaneus, femur, patella, pars intra-articularis, ribs and olecranon. The precise pathophysiology has not been clearly defined but appears related to mechanical overload. If the applied stress stimulates excessive bone resorbtion in relation to formation, microfactures may result. Such altered stresses may result from repetitive compression, torsion, ligament tension, muscle hyperactivity or muscle fatigue impairing force attenuation. There may also be intrinsic contributory factors previously discussed. The fundamental principle of rehabilitation is progressive, pain-free activity. The therapeutic exercises relating to hydrotherapy involve the following:

- 'Conventional' method and Bad Ragaz patterns for joints above and below the fracture site and hydrodynamic exercise.
- Progressions from buoyancy assisted to buoyancy resisted exercise with alterations of lever length.
- Bad Ragaz patterns, from isometric to isotonic, and increasing amounts of turbulence appropriately placed round the athlete in 'sitting' and standing will stimulate muscle activity as well as balance mechanisms.

(Reid Campion and Hamer, 1995)

Hydrotherapy in the Treatment of the Lumbopelvic Complex

Injury and loss of function in this region is extremely common and may be due to intrinsic or extrinsic mechanisms. Confirmed structural diagnosis is the exception rather than the rule in this region. Radiological evaluation in the form of CT, MRI or bone scan confirm pathology at the severe end of the spectrum (fracture, pars defect or disc protrusion) but are less helpful for more minor pathology; 66%–78%

of all low back pain does not have a specific diagnosis! (Loeser, 1977). It is likely that the pathological entities established by radiography represent 'end-stage pathology' which is likely to have resulted from functional disturbances which existed prior to the development of pathology (Nyberg, 1993). There are a number of reasons for caution in interpreting radiographic abnormalities as significant in relation to functional disturbance. Studies using CT scans interpreted positive findings in 50% of asymptomatic subjects over 40 on the basis of degenerative findings (Weisel *et al.*, 1984). X-ray studies demonstrate no significant difference in the incidence of spondylosis and disc degeneration between patients with and without low back pain (Witt *et al.*, 1984).

There is substantial evidence accumulating (Jull and Richardson, 1994) which implicates a highly specific muscular control system in this region and this information must be incorporated into hydrotherapy regimes. Briefly stated the concepts of dysfunction are based on the following tenets:

1. Although all trunk muscles contribute to lumbopelvic control the obliques and transversus abdominis have key roles (Kendall and McCreary, 1983; Gracovetsky *et al.*, 1985; Tesh *et al.*, 1987; Richardson *et al.*, 1990).
2. The above muscles appear to be particularly vulnerable to disuse and loss of supporting role (Caix *et al.*, 1984; Nouwen *et al.*, 1987).
3. The gluteus maximus, gluteus medius and iliopsoas muscles also commonly show signs of dysfunction relative to their synergist partners (Janda, 1978; Janda and Smith, 1980; Sahrmann, 1987).
4. Dysfunction of these stabilizing systems may predispose to overload of spinal structures.
5. Rehabilitation of the lumbopelvic complex should address automatic coordination of muscle activity to control posture as well as addressing torque producing capability (Jull and Richardson, 1994).

Armed with this knowledge a hydrotherapy regime for the lumbopelvic complex would include the following:

1. Bad Ragaz patterns commencing with static trunk patterns progressing to isotonic patterns without rotation and later to those with rotation.
2. 'Conventional' exercises from buoyancy assisted to buoyancy resisted, added resistance being provided by flotation equipment. Rotation is introduced gradually.
3. Hydrodynamic exercise commenced in a semi-sit/stand position immersed to C7 using small changes of shape within the pain-free range. Static and dynamic activity as well as balance mechanisms are developed.
4. Small range rapid movements of the upper and lower limbs performed on a stable trunk, allowing no trunk movement to occur, whilst normal respiration continues, maintains and improves the strength of the lumbopelvic complex. An upper limb movement may comprise flexion/extension of the shoulder, the arms kept close to the body, combined with pronation and supination of the forearm. For the lower limbs flexion of the hip and knee, followed by extension of the whole leg to just beyond the vertical, avoiding extension of the lumbar region.
5. Spinal mobilizations (p. 233) may be of value in some instances.

Hydrotherapy in the Treatment of the Neck/Shoulder Complex

Serious neck injury in the form of fracture or instability is a medical emergency and will not be considered further here. The two regions are considered together because functionally they are interdependent – much like the lumbar spine–pelvis–hip complex. The mechanisms of injury may be extrinsic or intrinsic. Because much of the suspensory mechanism of the shoulder girdle attaches to the cervical and thoracic spine good stability function of the postural muscles in these regions is necessary to ensure that shoulder girdle motion does not exert excessive stress on spinal structures. Conversely, impaired range of shoulder motion may force compensatory motion in the spine – the concept of relative flexibility (Kendall and McCreary, 1993).

The concept of relative flexibility (i.e. the proportional contribution of individual components to a total movement pattern) is essential to understanding pathomechanics of the scapulohumeral complex. The proportional motion between glenohumeral–scapulothoracic joints is approximately 2:1. This proportion is not constant throughout the range and varies as follows:

- First 30° variable greater glenohumeral motion
- Last 60° equal contribution of glenohumeral/scapulothoracic joints
- Mid-range variable.

These movements also require the sternoclavicular and acromioclavicular complex to undergo upward rotation, A/P rotation and axial rotation. These movements require the integrated action of almost 30 muscle groups! From a biomechanical perspective external rotation of the humerus is essential during elevation in order to achieve clearance of the coraco-acromial arch. This is achieved by a combination of upward scapular rotation on the thorax, derotation of the retroverted humerus by the rotator cuff muscles and the resultant slackening of the inferior GH ligaments. The high incidence of impingement syndromes in athletes performing overhead activities (swimmers, racket sports and throwers) commonly involves a failure of one or more of these mechanisms. It should be noted that in impingement syndromes, regardless of the symptomatic structures (rotator cuff, biceps tendon, sub-acromial bursa, coraco-acromial ligament or brachial plexus) two divergent mechanisms can lead to symptoms. The supraspinatus outlet is approximately 9–10 mm in area (influenced by acromial shape). Impingement due to capsular restriction can effectively wedge the humerus into the sub-acromial space causing irritation of the structures within. Conversely, capsular/muscular laxity may allow excessive translational motion of the humerus resulting in impingement. The centrode of motion in glenohumeral rotation is a 6–8 mm radius in geometric head of humerus. In instability this centrode becomes larger indicating excessive, aberrant motion. Important muscles to address in rehabilitation are:

- upper trapezius	
- levator scapulae	upper force component
- upper serratus anterior	
- lower trapezius, lower serratus anterior	lower force component, increasingly active through elevation
- lower trapezius	more active component of lower force couple during abduction
- lower serratus anterior	more active component of lower force couple during flexion
- middle trapezius	abduction to 90° maximal activity; flexion reduced in early range, building
- rhomboids	as middle trapezius
- teres major	resisted adduction, medial rotation, extension
- latissimus dorsi	active movements recruit

These principles must then be incorporated into the hydrotherapy programme. Specific attention to technique may also be required in chronic overuse injuries. Relaxation may need to be obtained prior to introducing other techniques.

Relaxation in the pool can be acquired in a fully supported float lying position, with the body being swayed gently from side to side. Turbulence will draw the arm away from the body thus facilitating movement.

Buoyancy assisted, followed by buoyancy neutral, movements are introduced. Repeated contractions, isometric Bad Ragaz arm patterns and carefully monitored and controlled isotonic patterns using proximal holds are used as the condition improves.

As pain decreases, and in chronic conditions, the aim is to increase muscle strength and range of movement. Resistance would be added to the Bad Ragaz patterns. Slow reversals, successive induction, stabilizations and repeated contractions may also be introduced.

Where injury has involved the cervical region and pain is paramount, inhibiting movement of the head and cervical spine, vertical suspension in deep water by means of one or two neck collars arranged to provide optimal comfort and support of the chin and occiput, with one or more ankle rings placed around each shoulder, can bring about pain reduction. The athlete must be carefully supervised and the time spent 'hanging' is dictated by the athlete's tolerance and the effectiveness of this stretching for pain relief.

REFERENCES

Belka D. (1968). Comparison of dynamic, static and combination training on dominant wrist flexor muscles. *Research Quarterly*, **39**: 244.

Bentley G. and Dowd G. (1984). Current concepts of etiology and treatment of chondromalacia patellae. *Clinical Orthopaedics and Related Research*, **189**, 209–227.

Breig A. (1978). *Adverse mechanical tension in the central nervous system*, Stockholm: Almqvist and Wiksell.

Caix M., Outrequin G., Descotes B., *et al.* (1984). The muscles of the abdominal wall: a new functional approach with anatomical deductions. *Anatomy Clinics*, **6**: 101.

Cameron K.R., Wark J.D. and Telford R.D. (1992). Stress fracture and bone loss – the skeletal cost of intense athleticism. *Excel*, **8**: 39–55.

Cook S.D., Brinker M.R. and Poche M. (1990). Running shoes – their relationship to running injuries. *Sports Medicine*, **10(1)**: 1–8.

Costill D.L., Fink W.J. and Habansky A.J. (1971). Muscle rehabilitation after knee surgery. *Physician and Sports Medicine*, **5**: 71.

Crosbie J. (1993). Optimisation and musculoskeletal physiotherapy. In *Key Issues in Musculoskeletal Physiotherapy* (J. Crosbie and J. McConnell, eds), Oxford: Butterworth-Heinemann, pp. 1–16.

Cummings G.S. and Tillman L.J. (1992). Remodelling of dense connective tissue in normal adult tissues. In *Dynamics of Human Biologic Tissues* (D.P. Currier and R.M. Nelson, eds), Philadelphia: F.A. Davis Company, pp. 45–47.

Curwin S. and Stanish W.D. (1984). *Tendinitis: Its etiology and treatment*. Lexington, Ma.: Collamore Press, D.C. Health and Co.

Evans P. (1980). The healing process at cellular level: A review. *Physiotherapy*, **66(8)**: 256–259.

Frank G., Woo S.L.-Y., Amiel O., Harwood F., Gomez M. and Akeson W. (1983). Medial collateral ligament healing. A multi-disciplinary assessment in rabbits. *American Journal of Sports Medicine*, **11**: 379–389.

Gerrard B. (1987). The McConnell technique – applied science or applied persuasion. In *Manipulative Therapists Association of Australia – Fifth Biennial Conference*, Melbourne, Australia: Manipulative Therapists Association of Australia.

Goodfellow J., Hungerford D.S. and Zindel M. (1976a). Patello-femoral joint mechanics and pathology: 1. Functional anatomy of the patello-femoral joint. *Journal of Bone and Joint Surgery*, **58B(3)**: 287–290.

Goodfellow J., Hungerford D.S. and Zindel M. (1976b) Patello-femoral joint mechanics and pathology: 2. Chondromalacia patellae. *Journal of Bone and Joint Surgery*, **58B(3)**: 291–299.

Gracovetsky S., Farfan H. and Helleur C. (1985). The abdominal mechanism. *Spine*, **10(4)**: 317–324.

Hageman P.A. and Sorensen T.A. (1991). Eccentric isokinetics. In *Eccentric Muscle Training* (M. Albert, ed.), New York: Churchill Livingstone, pp. 99–105.

Hakkinen K. and Komi P.V. (1981). Effect of different combined concentric and eccentric muscle work regimes on maximal strength development. *Journal of Human Movement Studies*, **7**: 33.

Hamer P. (1991). Classification of injuries. In *Postgraduate Sports Physiotherapy Resource Manual* (D. Hopper, ed.), Perth: Curtin University, pp. 2–11.

Harrison R. and Bulstrode S. (1987). Percentage weight bearing during partial immersion in the hydrotherapy pool. *Physiotherapy Practice*, **3(2)**: 60–63.

Herring S.A. (1990). Rehabilitation of muscle injuries. *Medicine and Science in Sport and Exercise*, **22(4)**: 453–456.

Hopper D. (1990). Hydrotherapy for sports injuries. In *Adult Hydrotherapy* (Reid Campion M., ed.), Oxford: Heinemann Medical.

Ihara H. and Nakayama A. (1986). Dynamic joint control training for knee ligament injuries. *American Journal of Sports Medicine*, **14(4)**: 309–314.

Install J. (1979). 'Chondromalacia patellae': Patellar malalignment syndrome. *Orthopaedic Clinics of North America*, **10(1)**: 117–127.

Install J., Falvo K.A. and Wise D. (1976). Chondromalacia patellae. *Journal of Bone and Joint Surgery*, **58A**: 1–8.

Janda V. (1978). *Muscles: Motor Regulation and Back Problems*. New York: Plenum.

Janda V. (1983a). *Muscle Function Testing*, London: Butterworths.

Janda V. (1983b). On the concept of postural muscles and posture in man. *The Australian Journal of Physiotherapy*, **29(3)**: 83–84.

Janda V. (1988). Muscles and cervicogenic pain syndromes. In *Physical Therapy of the Cervical and Thoracic Spine*, (R. Grant, ed.), New York: Churchill Livingstone.

Jull G.A. and Janda V. (1987). Muscles and motor control in low back pain: Assessment and management. In *Physical Therapy of the Low Back* (J.R.

Taylor and L.T. Twomey, (eds), New York: Churchill Livingstone, pp. 253–278.

Jull G.A. and Richardson C.A. (1994). *Rehabilitation of Active Stabilisation of the Lumbar Spine*, 2nd edn.), New York: Churchill Livingstone.

Kendall, F.P. and McCreary E.K. (1983). *Muscles: Testing and Function*, 3rd edn, Baltimore: Williams and Wilkins.

Kornberg C. and Lew P. (1989). The effect of stretching neural structures on grade one hamstring injuries. *Journal of Orthopaedic and Sports Physical Therapy* **(June)**: 481–487.

Kues J. (1990). The pathology of shin splints. *Journal of Orthopaedic and Sports Physical Therapy*, **12(3)**, 115–121.

Laurin C.A., Levesque H.P., Desalt R., Labelle H. and Peides J.P. (1978). The abnormal lateral patello-femoral angle. *Journal of Bone and Joint Surgery*, **60A(1)**, 55–60.

Leach R.E. (1982). The prevention and rehabilitation of soft tissue injuries. *International Journal of Sports Medicine, (Suppl.)*: **3** 18–20.

Loeser J.D. (1977). Low back pain. In *Low Back Pain* (J.J. Bonica, ed.), New York: Raven Press, pp. 155–162.

Marks K.E. and Bentley G. (1978). Patella alta and chondromalacia. *Journal of Bone and Joint Surgery*, **60B(1)**: 71–73.

Marks R. (1991). Effect of altered functional demand on the structural and functional properties of articular cartilage. *New Zealand Journal of Physiotherapy* **(April)**: 31–34.

McConnell J. (1986). The management of chondromalacia patellae: A long term solution. *Australian Journal of Physiotherapy*, **32(4)**: 215–223.

Muckle D.S. (1982). Injuries in sport. *Royal Society Health Journal*, **102**: 93–94.

Nouwen A., Van Akkerveeken P.F. and Versloot J.M. (1987). Patterns of muscular activity during movement in patients with low back pain. *Spine*, **12**: 777.

Noyes F.R. Torvik P.J., Hyde W.B. and DeLucal J.L. (1974). Biomechanics of ligament failure. *Journal of Bone and Joint Surgery*, **56–A(7)**: 1406–1417.

Nyberg R. (1993). Clinical assessment of the low back: History and structural evaluation. In *Rational Manual Therapies* (B.J.V. and R. Nyberg, eds), Baltimore: Williams and Wilkins, pp. 71–95.

Oakes B.W. (1982). Acute soft tissue injuries: nature and management. *Australian Family Physician* (suppl.), **10**: 3–16.

O'Driscoll S.W., Kumar A. and Salter R.B. (1983). The effect of continuous passive motion on the clearance of a haemarthrosis. *Clinical Orthopaedics and Related Research*, **176**: 305–311.

Poss R. (1984). Functional adaptation of the locomotor system to normal and abnormal loading patterns. *Calcified Tissue International* (suppl.) **36**: 155–161.

Reid Campion M. and Hamer P. (1995). Hydrotherapy; In *Sports Physiotherapy*, (Zulnaga *et al.*, eds), Melbourne: Churchill Livingstone.

Reynolds N.L. and Worrell T.W. (1991). Chronic Achilles peritentinitis: etiology, pathophysiology and treatment. *Journal of Orthopaedic and Sports Physical Therapy*, **14(4)**: 171–176.

Richardson C., Toppenberg R. and Jull G. (1990). An initial evaluation of eight abdominal exercises for their ability to provide stabilisation for the lumbar spine. *The Australian Journal of Physiotherapy*, **36(1)**: 6–11.

Safran M.R., Garrett W.E., Seaber A.V., Glisson R.R. and Ribbeck B.M. (1988). The role of warm up in muscular injury prevention. *American Journal of Sports Medicine*, **16(2)**: 123–128.

Sahrmann S.A. (1987). Muscle imbalances in the orthopaedic and neurological patient. In *10th International Congress of the World Confederation of Physical Therapy*, Sydney, Australia.

Salter R.B. (1989). The biologic concept of continuous passive motion of synovial joints: The first 18 years of basic research and its clinical application. *Clinical Orthopaedics*, **242**: 12–25.

Salter R.B., Simmond D.F., Makolm E.J., Rumble E.J. and MacMichael D. (1975). The effect of continuous passive motion on the healing of articular cartilage defects. *Journal of Bone and Joint Surgery*, **57–A**: 570–571.

Sikorski J.M., Peters J. and Watt I. (1979). The importance of femoral rotation in chondromalacia patellae as shown by serial radiograph. *Journal of Bone and Joint Surgery*, **61 B(4)**: 435–442.

Steadman J.R. (1979). Rehabilitation of athletic injury. *American Journal of Sports Medicine*: **147**.

Taube R.R. and Wadsworth L.T. (1993). Managing tibial stress fractures. *The Physician and Sports Medicine*, **21(4)**: 123.

Tesh K.M., Dunn J.S. and Evans J.H. (1987). The abdominal muscles and vertebral stability. *Spine*, **12**: 501.

Tipton C.M., James, S.L., Mergner W. and Tcheng T. (1970). Influence of exercise on strength of medial collateral knee ligaments of dogs. *American Journal of Physiology*, **218**: 894–902.

Vagenas G. and Hoshizaki B. (1992). A multivariate analysis of lower extremity kinematic asymmetry in running. *International Journal of Sports Biomechanics*, **8**: 11–29.

Vailas A.C., Tipton C.M., Matthews, R.D. and Gart M. (1981). Influence of physical activity on the repair process of medial collateral ligaments in rats. *Connective Tissue Research*: 25–31.

Vasey J.R. and Crozier L.W. (1980). A neuromuscular approach to knee joint problems. *Physiotherapy*, **66(6)**: 193–194.

Weisel S.W., Tsourmas N. and Feffer H.L. (1984). A study of computer-assisted tomography: 1. Incidence of positive CT scans in an asymptomatic group of patients. *Spine*, **9**: 459–551.

Witt I., Vestergaard A. and Rosenklint A. (1984). A comparative analysis of X-ray findings in the lumbar spine in patients with and without lumbar pain. *Spine*, **9**: 298–300.

Woo S.L.-Y. and Akeson W.H. (1987). Response of tendons and ligaments to joint loading and movements. In *Joint Loading* (H.J. Helminen, I. Kiviranta, M. Tammi, A.-M. Saamanen, K. Paukkonen and J. Jurvelin, eds), Bristol: Wright, pp. 40.

Worth D.H. (1969). The hamstring injury in Australian rules football. *Australian Journal of Physiotherapy*, **15(3)**: 111–113.

Zarins B. (1982). Soft tissue injury and repair – biochemical aspects. *International Journal of Sports Medicine* (suppl. 1), **3**: 9–11.

Section IV

Health Promotion

Margaret Reid Campion

Overview to Chapters 16, 17 and 18

This section of the book is concerned with promoting health for individuals and in the community. It is the role of the physiotherapist to help in the restoration and maintenance of health and increasingly the psychosocial model is emerging. As Collins (1987) argues the physiotherapist may prove more effective in this role if he or she acts more as a partner than a prescriber in health care. This means that the physiotherapist must appreciate the definition of health and have an understanding of both the psychological and sociological dimensions of health. Collins (1987) quotes several definitions of health such as that of the World Health Organization (1978); that of Herzlich and Graham (1974) and a more simplistic definition – 'the absence of disease'.

All definitions see physical, mental and social well-being as important and interrelated and that these must be acceptable to the individual. Values, beliefs, attitudes and the environment will influence the individual and the community and it is vital in a psychosocial approach that the physiotherapist understands and is able to modify treatment and education programmes to allow for the psychological and social influences on the individual.

BENEFITS OF EXERCISE IN WATER

The benefits of exercise in general terms are widely known, but some physiotherapists may be less familiar with the benefits of exercise in water.

It is fun, refreshing, exhilarating and relaxing to participate in water activity. All degrees of exercise can be undertaken without weight-bearing. There is no need to assume the upright position unless required. Muscular strength, physical fitness, and range of movement may be maintained and increased. Balance and coordination can be improved; pain decreased, swimming and safety skills acquired. The psychological and social benefits are numerous, especially when activity takes place in a group.

The following chapters relate strongly to the psychosocial approach with an emphasis on maintaining and improving health and physical and mental well-being for all ages from the young to the frail elderly. How effective such activity can be is epitomized in the pages of Meme Macdonald's book *Put Your Whole Self In*.

REFERENCES

Collins M. (1987). *Women's Health through Life-stages*, Sydney: Australian Physiotherapy Association.

Herzlich C. and Graham D. (1974). *Health and Illness*, New York: Academic Press.

Macdonald M. (1992). *Put Your Whole Self In*, Sydney: Penguin Books Australia Ltd.

16

Aquanatal exercise

Georgina Evans

One of the most striking aspects of antenatal and postnatal care in recent years has been the growth in popularity of aquanatal classes, exercise classes in water designed specifically for women who are pregnant or are in the first few months after delivery. In the development of these classes Britain is to some extent following the lead of other countries. The French *Association Nationale Natation et Maternité* (ANNM) for example was founded in 1977 (Vleminckx, 1988) and now runs biannual five-day courses to train midwives and swimming instructors to lead aquanatal classes. The *Fédération Internationale d'Hydrothérapie Périnatale*, which has headquarters in Brussels, was established in 1989 to foster links between the ANNM and various other countries. There was also significant progress in the theory and practice of aquanatal exercise in Australia, where physiotherapists took a prominent role.

In Britain aquanatal classes were rare in the 1980s (Collins, 1988) but their number is now rising in response to a rapidly expanding demand, and here too physiotherapists have played an important part. The Association of Chartered Physiotherapists in Women's Health (until 1994 the Association of Chartered Physiotherapists in Obstetrics and Gynaecology) published preliminary guidelines for aquanatal classes in 1990, replaced by fuller guidelines in 1995 (ACPWH, 1995). A few training courses for aquanatal instructors are now available in Britain, though there is not the central direction characteristic of France. The ideal team to lead an aquanatal class is a physiotherapist with special training in obstetrics working alongside a midwife. The combined skills and expertise of these two professions can offer mothers thorough screening, safe exercise and informed advice.

THE MAIN BENEFITS OF EXERCISE IN WATER DURING PREGNANCY

Weightlessness

Buoyancy gives a feeling of weightlessness in water, which is accentuated by hydrostatic pressure. Because the hydrostatic pressure of water exerts a force proportional to the depth of immersion (Pascal's law) the swelling of feet and ankles will be reduced more easily if the exercises are performed well below the surface of the water. There is less jarring of the joints in water than on land. It is suggested that a woman submerged to the level of the xiphisternum will experience only 28% of her body weight (Harrison and Bulstrode, 1987). The women feel lighter and more graceful, which bolsters their self-esteem.

Body Temperature

The body's ability to eliminate heat is increased in water. The thermoconductivity of water, which is twenty-five times greater than that of air, may reduce the risk of hyperthermia. Maternal core temperature is unlikely to reach a critical level (Katz *et al.*, 1991; McMurray *et al.*, 1993).

Circulation

By the twenty-fifth week of pregnancy the blood volume increases by 40%. The heart increases in size and accommodates more blood; thus the stroke volume rises and the cardiac output increases by 30–50%. The physiotherapist must appreciate that the same amount of exercise increases cardiac output more in a pregnant than in a non-pregnant woman. The increased blood volume is accompanied by increased dilatation of veins from the lower abdomen downwards, and this may give rise to varicose veins, haemorrhoids and swelling of the legs (Vleminckx, 1988). The leg movements of swimming and exercise aid venous return, while contact with water below body temperature narrows the blood vessels in the skin in order to maintain body temperature; all this is said to reduce varicosities and oedema. Exercise during pregnancy trains the heart, as muscle activity generates a demand for oxygen which increases the flow of blood to the heart. A small drop in the heart rate after immersion has been observed (McMurray *et al.*, 1988). Water-related exercises for pregnant women should not be based on land-derived heart rates, as these may not truly represent the cardiovascular or metabolic demand during immersion. As a general rule the target heart rate for exercise on land should be lowered by approximately 15 beats per minute for pregnant women exercising in water.

Respiration

During pregnancy the diaphragm may be elevated by as much as 4 cm to accommodate the enlarging uterus. The upward pressure of the uterus causes the ribs to flare. The increased levels of progesterone during pregnancy make the respiratory centre more sensitive to carbon dioxide. The resting respiratory rate increases from about 15 to 18 breaths per minute. Consequently pregnant women notice breathlessness on activity. During immersion hydrostatic pressure also causes changes in pulmonary function. Chest mechanics are altered directly by hydrostatic pressure on the chest wall and indirectly by a shift of blood from the extremities into the thorax (Hong *et al.*, 1967). These changes reduce vital capacity and expiratory reserve volume and produce an increase in inspiratory capacity. The inspiratory muscles have to work against the hydrostatic pressure and the higher intra-abdominal pressure caused by the lowering of the diaphragm; therefore exercise in water helps to tone up the respiratory muscles. The effects of pregnancy on pulmonary function and ventilation are not compounded by immersion or exercise while immersed. Thus exercise in water appears to be suitable for the pregnant woman (Berry *et al.*, 1989).

Diuretic Effects

The diuretic and natriuretic effects of exercise in water during pregnancy are profound (Goodlin *et al.*, 1984). The diuretic effect peaks within one hour and after four hours the urine flow has returned to normal. Conversely the natriuretics increase steadily, peaking at about four hours. The diuretic effect of immersion will help a pregnant woman who is troubled by fluid retention, as immersion for 20–40 minutes results in a loss of 300–400 ml of fluid. It is possible that immersion could be used to alleviate symptomatic oedema in some women (Katz *et al.*, 1991).

Reduced Risk of Injury

There is less risk of injury to the joints during exercise in water, as movements are slower and thus more easily controlled than on land and the joints are supported by the water. The abdominal muscles can be toned up without straining them.

Fitness

It is possible for pregnant women to participate regularly in aerobic exercise in water without harm to themselves or their unborn child, and they can therefore maintain their initial level of fitness (Sibley *et al.*, 1981; Katz *et al.*, 1991).

The benefits of exercise in water noticed by pregnant women include weightlessness and the relief of back pain, for hours or days, or in some cases completely. They report that they sleep better the night following the exercise; in addition bowel function is activated because the abdominal wall is massaged by the water. Pregnant women find that they are less self-conscious exercising in the water than on a mat! They often come feeling tired and go home feeling invigorated. The social benefits too are extremely important.

SETTING UP AN AQUANATAL CLASS

Instructors

Two people are needed to run a class. The ideal combination is a physiotherapist with a special interest in and knowledge of obstetrics working alongside a midwife. It is desirable that the two instructors should have attended a specially designed course on the teaching of exercise in water to pregnant women.

Size of Class

The need for the women to be well spaced in the water, to be a good distance from the poolside and to have room for relaxation places practical limits on the total size of a class. For reasons of safety there should be no more than ten women to each instructor. An ideal group would probably have two leaders and up to 15 women.

Time of Sessions

Daytime classes often suit non-working women, although a crèche may be needed. Mothers may have to get older children to and from school, so mid-morning is often a good time. As many mothers now work through many weeks of their pregnancy evening classes are often more popular than daytime classes.

Venue

Aquanatal classes are normally held in a public swimming pool, but it may sometimes be possible to arrange for the use of some other pool, for example in a school or hospital. Before deciding where to hold a class it is advisable to look at all the pools in the area which might be made available. The advantages and disadvantages of each pool should be listed and balanced, as the chances of finding a pool that is absolutely ideal are slim.

Privacy

The peace and tranquillity of a private session in the pool is ideal, but this is not often available. A session during a women-only night helps the women to be less self-conscious and it is usually less noisy. Failing these, the class should be in an area roped off from the other swimmers.

Depth of Water

Ideally a pool should be gently graduated to accommodate the various heights of the women. Preferably the floor of the pool should not descend in steps but should slope, as refraction makes it very difficult for the women to see steps through the water. The ideal level of the water is the xiphisternum. This covers the woman's abdomen without putting any traction on breast tissues, and does not make it difficult for her to maintain an upright position. If the pool is too shallow for this degree of immersion more exercises should be performed in a squatting or kneeling position. On the other hand a shallow pool is often warmer and is not a threat to non-swimmers, so it may have some advantages.

Temperature

A water temperature of 30°C puts the minimum of strain on the pregnant woman. If the water is too cold it will cause an increase in muscle tone in order to maintain core temperature; this would eliminate some of the potential benefits of the class. If the water is too warm (36°C or above) vasodilatation will limit the women's capacity for exercise.

Shower Facilities

There should be enough warm showers to ensure that the women do not have to wait long for a shower after the class, especially if they all have to leave the pool together. If there is likely to be any delay between leaving the water and taking a warm shower the women should be advised to bring their towels to the poolside to keep them warm.

Refreshments

Because the blood sugar level drops in the water it is very important for the participants to remain for a while in the surroundings of the pool to have a drink before they leave. This time can be both very enjoyable and educative.

It is an ideal opportunity to discuss any health issues or worries the women may have. It may in effect be a parent education class, when the expertise of the physiotherapist and midwife may be called upon in the discussion of such topics as the pelvic floor, back pain, breathing exercises, pain relief and water birth. If the instructors are unable to help with an antenatal problem, they should know where to refer the woman for expert advice.

Clothing

Pregnant women may be more comfortable in swimwear with inner support for the breasts, or wearing a bra under their costume. Verruca socks may help to prevent slipping in the pool. An alternative is to cut a section from the cuff of each of a pair of rubber gloves and to wear these over the balls of the feet.

Payment and Charges

The method and rate of payment of the instructors and the charge to the members of the class should be agreed before the classes begin. The arrangements may of course vary from place to place. If the authority which owns the pool is paying the instructors and charging the members of the class directly, the level of each must be negotiated with the managers of the pool. Some health professionals lead a class in their working time and are thus paid by the health authority. Some instructors may wish to hire a pool and recoup the cost from the fees they charge the participants, but this will not normally be a viable economic arrangement.

SAFETY

Safety in the Pool

The pool's health and safety policy should be known and followed. The instructors should make sure that they know the location of the first-aid box and telephone, and that they are familiar with the fire procedure. The members of the class are advised not to jump or dive into the pool. They should not get the tops of their heads wet before the end of the class, as this would make them feel colder.

Lifeguard

A lifeguard is essential if neither of the two instructors has a current life-saving qualification. Even if one of the instructors has such a qualification it is preferable for there to be a separate lifeguard to take full responsibility for life-saving duties. A woman lifeguard is preferable.

Screening and Record-keeping

It is essential that time should be allowed at the first session for the screening of all the women who wish to take part. They must be checked individually for contraindications and for other conditions which may be relevant. Contraindications include heart disease, most kinds of infection (for example bronchitis, influenza, ear, nose and throat, urinary or vaginal infection), some skin diseases or open wounds, active TB, continuing bleeding, leakage of amniotic fluid, gastrointestinal problems or viruses. Epilepsy and diabetes, if well controlled, are not contraindications. Women with certain conditions should only be admitted to an aquanatal class with the explicit approval of their consultant; these include high or low blood pressure, a history of miscarriage or premature labour, cervical suture, bleeding and low-lying placenta. Conditions which are not contraindications but which should be noted and may call for special attention and perhaps some modification of the exercise programme include pains in the back, neck or symphysis pubis and orthopaedic problems.

At this stage the instructors should establish whether a woman is on any medication, whether she is a swimmer or non-swimmer and if she knows her latest recorded blood pressure. It is important for the instructors to be aware of any non-swimmer in the group, as she may need extra guidance and support during the session. If a woman's reported blood pressure is significantly high or low, or if she is unsure of it, one of the instructors should measure it before she enters the pool. If it is found to be high she should not be admitted to the session in the water but should be referred back to her GP or consultant. In fact it is desirable to have a base reading for all participants, as any change in blood pressure may be significant at a later stage. It is helpful to prepare standard summary sheets on which all pertinent details may be recorded; it is then easy for the instructors to check before each session and to decide whether anyone should be given alternative exercises. The women are instructed that in subsequent weeks they should notify the instructors of any change in their health or pregnancy or any problem they have experienced since the preceding session.

A register should be kept of all members of the class; it should record each woman's name, address, telephone number and expected date of delivery and her GP's name and address.

Musculoskeletal Changes in Pregnancy

The physiotherapist must be aware of changes in the musculoskeletal system of the pregnant woman which are caused by the hormones oestrogen, progesterone and relaxin, as they have important implications for the safety and suitability of exercise during pregnancy. These hormonal changes give rise to a general laxity of the joints and an increase in their range. Relaxin is thought to be produced as early as two weeks into gestation (Weiss, 1984). It can take up to six months after the birth to return to the pre-pregnant state. Joint range is increased more in a second pregnancy than in the first, but there is no further increase in subsequent pregnancies (Calguneri *et al.*, 1982). The main joints that are commonly affected are the symphysis pubis (Fry, 1992) and the sacro-iliac joints (Polden and Mantle, 1990: pp. 144–145). Women can feel tenderness, discomfort or pain over these joints and radiating from them. This must be noted before the exercises begin so that the physiotherapist will be in a position to make appropriate modifications. Women experiencing problems with these joints should probably avoid hip abduction (for example, large side-steps through the water) and should replace large backward steps with smaller steps, during which the pelvic tilt should be maintained so as not to increase the lumbar lordosis. Indeed it is probably advisable to make these modifications for aquanatal classes in general. Squatting in the water will be more comfortable for those with painful joints if the knees are kept closer together. All pregnant women should keep their chins in the water when they swim in order to lessen the lumbar lordosis, and the leg movements of the breast stroke should be modified.

The muscles of the rectus abdominis separate as pregnancy advances. If these muscle fibres become overstretched the linea alba may divide. When a gap of two fingers' breadth or more develops the condition is known as diastasis recti, or divarication or separation of the rectus. It is most common in multiple pregnancies or when the baby is large, but it may occur in any pregnancy. It is believed that diastasis recti may be caused by the mother doing unsuitable exercise late in pregnancy. In an aquanatal class care should therefore be taken to avoid hard abdominal exercises which would further stretch the already extended muscles of the abdomen, for example holding onto the edge of the pool and lifting two straightened legs. For similar reasons the women should be given clear instructions as to how they should rise to a standing position from supine lying. They should be sure to draw in their abdominal muscles and then to roll onto their side as they begin to stand.

LEADING AN AQUANATAL CLASS

Supervision of the Class

The acoustics are generally poor in public swimming pools, but the participants must be able to hear and see the physiotherapist clearly, who should speak slowly and distinctly in a voice that will carry to the back of the class. Each exercise should have unambiguous and concise instructions and be demonstrated so the women understand how to perform it correctly. It is normally best for the physiotherapist to lead the class from the poolside, but swimwear is advisable as it will occasionally be helpful to enter the water, for example to help position the women for relaxation. The physiotherapist must be able at any time to establish eye contact with everyone in the pool, partly to maintain constant observation of exercise technique but also to see how the members of the class are coping with the session. Are they too cold, shivering, tense and showing poorly coordinated movements? Are they too warm, flushed, nauseous or dizzy? Are they smiling, laughing and chatting in a way that shows they are enjoying the class? Every member of the class must know that if she feels unwell she must stop exercising and raise her hand so that the midwife in the pool can help her. When the session in the water ends, one of the instructors should leave with the first member of the class and the second instructor should follow the last one out.

Length of the Session

Excessive fatigue and shortness of breath should be avoided. An ideal session would last between 45 and 60 minutes. This would include 5–7 minutes of relaxation at the end of the class; unless the water is very warm a longer period of relaxation will allow the women to get too cold.

Music

A battery-operated cassette or disc player is preferable for use at the pool; if the machine is connected to the mains electricity a circuit breaker must be used. Having the music played over a tannoy system is not ideal as the physiotherapist may need to stop the music to demonstrate an exercise, and she needs immediate control over the music. Instrumental music is more suitable than vocal, and it is helpful if it is familiar to the class. The music should be uplifting with an easy beat. It is important not to expect the women to change direction quickly. Similarly some thought must be given to the speed of the music in relation to the constraints of exercise in water. Remember that during the relaxation most of the women will be on their backs and unable to hear the music. If commercially recorded music is being used the pool must have a current licence from PPL (Phonographic Performance Limited, 14–22 Ganton Street, London W1V 1LB). It is an infringement of copyright to copy tracks from commercial recordings for use in a class.

Use of Water

Water exercises should be considered in their own right and should not simply be borrowed from the gym or an aerobic class. If the classes are run as a course it is easy to make the exercises progressive. At first many of the exercises may be assisted by the water, but later the water may provide resistance; resistance may be increased by the use of floats or table tennis bats and the creation of turbulence.

THE EXERCISE PROGRAMME

The principal aim of the exercise programme of an aquanatal class is to promote exercise that is both beneficial and safe and to encourage good posture.

Components of a Class

An aquanatal session will normally include:

- warm-up and stretching of the relevant major muscle groups
- exercise for muscular strength and endurance
- an aerobic (huff-and-puff) section
- cool-down and stretch
- relaxation.

An antenatal class will also incorporate breathing exercises. Correction of posture and exercise of the pelvic floor muscles are introduced at various times in the course of the session.

Posture

Each class should start and finish with the women adopting a correct posture. They should stand in the water with their feet hip-width apart, the weight falling evenly through the outer border of each foot. The knees should be slightly bent and not locked. They should be shown how to perform a pelvic tilt, drawing in the abdominal muscles and tucking the buttocks under. Then lift the ribs away from the hips, holding the shoulders down and back and the head high, with the chin tucked in a little. If a woman is standing well she should feel the pelvic floor muscles lift.

Pelvic Floor Exercise

The women should be urged to perform the pelvic floor exercise diligently not only throughout pregnancy but for the rest of their lives. Making them aware of the pelvic floor will enable them to release these muscles during the delivery. Continuing with the exercise will help to avoid problems of incontinence later in life. It is very difficult to convey a great deal of information during the class, especially if the acoustics are poor, but this is an ideal topic of discussion over coffee at the end of the class. The physiotherapist can then ensure that the women know exactly where the muscles are, how to exercise them and the problems they may encounter later in life if they are not toned up. It has been shown that pelvic floor muscles are stronger postnatally in women who exercise during pregnancy than in those who do not (Nielsen *et al.*, 1988).

The exercise can be performed in different positions throughout the class. It is important that the exercise should be clearly and correctly explained:

> Close the back passage as if preventing wind escaping; close the front passages as though stopping the flow of urine; lift the passages up and hold as strongly as possible and for as long as possible up to a count of ten, breathing normally throughout the exercise; rest for three seconds and repeat as many times as is possible up to ten.

After doing the exercise according to these instructions the women should try lifting and releasing the pelvic floor muscles quickly up to ten times, so they work both the fast and the slow-twitch muscle fibres.

Warm-up

Warm-up exercises are designed to mobilize the joints, promote the circulation and warm the muscles. These changes increase the range of movement and thus protect the body against injury. The warm-up exercises should work all the main muscle groups. They should raise the heart rate gradually, and the rate at which their intensity increases should be geared to the individual participant. The following are examples of suitable warm-up exercises:

Heel lift

Standing with the feet hip-width apart, lift one heel, pressing through the ball of the foot; lift each heel in turn, swinging the opposite arm; gradually speed up so the action resembles a walking movement; the weight should go through the big toe.

Knee bends

Standing with the feet just over hip-width apart, with the toes pointing slightly outward, bend and then straighten both knees at the same time, keeping a straight back and a pelvic tilt; add movement of the arms, which start outstretched to the side and are brought down as the knees bend, crossing in front of the body before being extended to the side again.

Pelvic tilting

Standing with the feet hip-width apart and the knees bent, pull in the abdominal muscles and tuck the bottom under; hold for a count of four and then slowly let go.

Hip circling

Standing with the feet slightly more than hip-width apart, with both knees bent and hands on hips, circle the hips first to the right and then to the left, keeping the abdominal muscles pulled in as the hips come forward.

Diagonal reaching

Standing with the feet slightly more than hip width apart, bend both knees then straighten them, taking most of the weight on the right leg while stretching onto tiptoes with the left leg; bend both knees again and straighten them, this time transferring the weight to the left leg while stretching to the toes on the right side; add a movement of the arms, reaching towards the ceiling with the arm on the same side as the leg that is taking the weight.

Shoulder circling

As a variant of the preceding exercise, instead of stretching the arms alternately, rotate both shoulders backwards as the legs are straightened.

Knee lifts

Starting with the feet hip-width apart and the arms extended sideways at shoulder height, lift alternate knees while bringing the arms forward at shoulder level and stretching them out to the sides once again.

Arm circling

Standing with the feet hip-width apart, bend and straighten both knees, swinging alternate arms backwards in a circle past the ear.

Arm reaching

Standing with the feet hip-width apart, bend and straighten both knees, extending alternate arms directly above the head as the knees straighten; hold the abdominals tight, and look at the arm as it is lifted.

Pelvic tilting and hip-circling are helpful in maintaining abdominal muscle strength, correcting posture and easing backache. Shoulder movements should concentrate on retraction, as the shoulders are often rounded by the downward traction caused by the weight of the breasts. Several of these exercises help to correct kyphosis, by stretching the upper back and rotating the arms outward. Arm stretches lift the ribs off the baby and ease stiffness.

Stretches

During pregnancy the hormones oestrogen, progesterone and particularly relaxin are responsible for a generalized laxity of the joints. Therefore pregnant women must be aware that they should not overstretch and must not bounce at the end of the stretches. Holding a stretch for eight seconds will achieve the desired effect. Short static stretches are effective in reducing tension and promoting relaxation. The main muscle groups of the legs which need to be stretched are the quadriceps, hamstrings, gastrocnemius, soleus and adductors. The standard stretching exercises for these muscles may normally be performed safely in pregnancy, but any woman who feels discomfort in the symphysis pubis should omit the adductor stretch. When doing shoulder stretches the women must maintain a pelvic tilt so as not to increase the lumbar lordosis. The leg stretches are more fun if performed in pairs and this also helps the class to gel.

Muscle Strength and Endurance

Strong muscles are certainly needed for the daily lifting and carrying which follow the birth of a baby, and to maintain posture and body shape. The following are examples of exercises which may be performed in the water in order to develop muscular strength and endurance.

Prone kicking

Lying prone in the water with the arms outstretched to hold a float, kick alternate legs up and down, keeping the knees straight.

Seated paddling

Sitting on two or three floats with the feet just off the floor of the pool, tighten the abdominal muscles and use the arms to push forward through the water; vary by going backwards.

Bunny hops

Facing each other in pairs and holding hands, bunny-hop round the pool, changing direction on command; this is a good way to practice squatting for the delivery, as it is so much easier in water.

Foot and leg exercises

Form pairs in which one woman lies supine, supported by the other who either allows her partner's head to rest on her shoulder or places two hands under the small of her back; the woman who is lying supine may perform ankle circling, inversion and eversion, dorsiflexion and plantar flexion and bicycling exercises. So as not to put a strain on the rectus abdominis when returning to the standing position, the woman who has been lying supine should pull in her abdominal muscles and roll onto her side with the help of her partner.

Deep knee bends

Facing each other in pairs and holding hands, do a deep knee bend, keeping the back straight and the abdominals tight; relax and remain in the squatting position while doing the pelvic floor exercise, before slowly rising together.

Squatting in pairs

In pairs in the squatting position, arms outstretched and holding hands, pull and push back and forth.

Exercises with table-tennis bats

Table-tennis bats are a convenient means of increasing resistance, as in the following examples. When they take the bats out to the side the women must take care that they do not arch their backs.

1. With the shoulders under the water, the arms stretched out to the side and with a bat in each hand, bring the arms together into the midline, return them to outstretched position, then bring them down to the side of the body.
2. Starting with the arms stretched forward, bend and straighten each elbow alternately, pushing the bats through the water.
3. With the bats held out straight in front, pronate and supinate the forearms.
4. With the right hand pass a bat over the right shoulder, taking it with the left hand which has come behind the back to reach it; repeat from left to right.

Aerobic Section

This section starts gently and gradually increases in intensity before decreasing again. The following are among the many exercises which can be used:

Marching on the spot

Start by marching on the spot, progressing to bringing the knees up higher and taking the hands alternately to the opposite bent knee.

Back kicks

Standing with the feet hip-width apart, kick first one foot then the other backwards towards the buttocks; continue, holding the arms outstretched and bringing them both back towards the body by bending the elbows with each kick.

Punches

Standing with the feet hip-width apart, punch alternate arms forwards; vary with upward or downward punches.

Arm swinging

Standing with the feet hip-width apart, swing both arms in an arc through the water to the right as you bend and then straighten both knees; repeat to the left; swing both arms together through a big circle in front of the body, again bending the knees; repeat the sequence.

Grapevine

Combine small steps forward and backwards through the water with grapevine steps to the side, clapping to the beat of the music.

St Clements

Many sequences can be based on two parallel lines, with those at the bottom of each line moving up between the line together before peeling off and skipping round to the bottom again, either singly or in pairs or even in fours; these routines normally generate great hilarity, especially as they become progressively more intricate, but at the same time they can be the means of introducing some quite strenuous exercises.

Dance routines

Dance routines can work well in the water. The actions of the hokey-cokey, for example, can be adapted to suit an aquanatal class. The conga too can be used in the water, the class copying the different arm movements of the leader as they jog through the water, for example stretching the right arm up and then the left. Country dancing is also a very useful basis for exercise routines in the water.

Breathing Exercises

Mothers today are taught to tune into their own natural breathing pattern during labour, concentrating on the outward breath. This breathing technique can be introduced into the aquanatal classes in various ways, for example:

1. Lying prone and holding a float with outstretched arms, kick with straightened legs, concentrating on the breath out; take a deep breath in when necessary and sigh the air out gently; count how many

breaths are taken in crossing the width of the pool.

2. Form well-spaced groups of three; one woman swims to one of the others in her group while gently blowing a table-tennis ball ahead of her; her breathing should be gentle and not forced; the table-tennis ball makes this exercise amusing as well as useful.

This breathing goes hand in hand with the relaxation and can be practised again during the relaxation session.

Stretch and Cool-down

The main muscle groups that have been used throughout the class need to be stretched again at the end of the session. This can be done separately or incorporated into the cooling-down exercises. The cool-down consists of easy mobilizing exercises, performed slowly and smoothly, with the water providing assistance rather than resistance; music with a slow rhythm is a suitable accompaniment. Examples of exercises that can be used are pelvic tilting, hip circling, arm circling, slow marching and pelvic floor and breathing exercises. It is important to ensure that the women do not become too cold. The cool-down finishes with a final check on posture.

Relaxation

Five to seven minutes of relaxation at the end of the session is usually enjoyed by all the class. Most participants are happy to lie supine in the water. Some are very much at home in the water and float without aids, while others prefer to have support. It is suggested that these women have one float under each forearm and a third under the tops of their thighs to help keep their backs straight; some may like to have a neck float too. All instructions for relaxation need to be given before the women go onto their backs, as once they are in their relaxation position they will be unable to hear what is said. At this stage it is useful for the physiotherapist to get into the water with the class to help with the floats and to stop any collisions! As the women get cold very quickly they are told to relax only for as long as they feel comfortable, and to have a short swim before taking a warm shower. As the women near full term they may be vulnerable to supine hypotension even in the

water, and should not be left to relax on their backs for more than ten minutes. Some may choose to relax lying prone or standing, supported for example by a pair of floats under their forearms.

POSTNATAL EXERCISE CLASSES IN WATER

Women may swim postnatally once the discharge of lochia has ceased; if all is well at their six-week check-up they may join a postnatal class. Aquanatal classes sometimes combine antenatal and postnatal exercise; alternatively separate postnatal classes may be offered. A postnatal class in the water will have the same components as an antenatal class. It must be explained to the women that for four or five months after delivery their bodies' ligaments and collagenous connective tissue will remain soft and more elastic then before pregnancy. In postnatal as in antenatal classes the same care is needed, for example, not to overstretch or work too strenuously. Start gently and gradually build up the intensity. The women's swimming strokes should still be modified if they feel any discomfort in their pubic symphysis or sacro-iliac joints. The abdominal muscles should be checked by the physiotherapist before the first session. If the diastasis is less than two fingers in width the abdominal exercise can be progressive; but if the gap is greater, rotational and side flexion exercises should be omitted until it has been reduced to two fingers or less. The pelvic floor muscles will be much weaker than they were before pregnancy, and a concentrated effort to perform the pelvic floor exercise in many different positions throughout the class is essential. The women will be looking for a more dynamic class once they have delivered. They will be especially keen to work on their vertical and oblique abdominal muscles in order to trim their waists. They will still however enjoy a time for relaxation at the end of the class.

CONCLUSION

Water is a medium in which pregnant women can exercise with both safety and pleasure. Antenatal and postnatal exercise classes in water are provided to promote a feeling of well-being at a time when women can feel heavy, tired and uncomfortable. The classes often help to minimize the minor discomforts of pregnancy and the postnatal period and promote health education. Most important, however, the classes should be sociable and fun. The joy on the faces of the women as they first enter the pool says it all.

REFERENCES

ACPWH (1995). *Aquanatal Guidelines* (available from the leaflet secretary, ACPWH, c/o Chartered Society of Physiotherapy, 14 Bedford Row, London WC1R 4ED).

Berry M.J., McMurray R.G. and Katz V.L. (1989). Pulmonary and ventilatory responses to pregnancy, immersion, and exercise. *Jnl Applied Physiology*, **66**: 857–862.

Calguneri M., Bird H.A. and Wright V. (1982). Changes in joint laxity occurring during pregnancy. *Annals of the Rheumatoid Diseases*, **41**: 126–128.

Collins M. (1988). An innovation: teaching aquanatal exercises. *Jnl Association of Chartered Physiotherapists in Obstetrics and Gynaecology*, **63**: 20–21.

Fry D. (1992). Diastasis symphysis pubis. *Jnl Association of Chartered Physiotherapists in Obstetrics and Gynaecology*, **71**: 10–13.

Goodlin R.C., Engdahl Hoffmann K.L., Williams N.E., Buchan P. (1984). Shoulder-out immersion in pregnant women. *Jnl Perinatal Medicine*, **12**: 173–177.

Harrison R. and Bulstrode F. (1987). Percentage weight bearing during partial emersion in a hydrotherapy pool. *Physiotherapy Practices*, **3(2)**: 60–63.

Hong S.K., Cerretelli P., Cruz J.C. and Rahn H. (1967). Mechanics of respiration during submersion in water. *Jnl Applied Physiology*, **27**: 535–538.

Katz V.L., McMurray R.G. and Cefalo R.C. (1991). Aquatic exercise during pregnancy. In *Exercise in Pregnancy* 2nd edn, (R.A. Mittelmark, R.A. Wiswell and B.L. Drinkwater, eds), Baltimore: Williams & Wilkins, pp. 271–278.

McMurray R.G., Katz V.L., Berry M.J. and Cefalo R.C. (1988). Cardiovascular responses of pregnant women during aerobic exercise in water: a longitudinal study. *International Jnl Sports Medicine*, **9**: 443–447.

McMurray R.G., Katz V.L., Meyer-Goodwin W.E. and Cefalo R.C. (1993). Thermoregulation of pregnant women during aerobic exercise on land and in the water. *American Jnl Perinatology*, **10(2)**: 178–182.

Nielsen C.A., Sigsgaard I., Olsen M., Tolstrup M., Danneskiold-Samsoee B. and Bock J.E. (1988). Trainability of the pelvic-floor. *Acta Obstetricia et Gynecologica Scandinavica*, **67**: 437–440.

Polden M. and Mantle J. (1990). *Physiotherapy in Obstetrics and Gynaecology*, Oxford: Butterworth-Heinemann.

Sibley I., Ruhling R.O., Cameron-Foster J., Christensen C. and Bolen T. (1981). Swimming and physical fitness during pregnancy. *Jnl Nurse-Midwifery*, **26(6)**: 3–12.

Vleminckx M. (1988). Pregnancy and recovery: the aquatic approach. In *Obstetrics and Gynaecology* (J. McKenna, ed.), Edinburgh: Churchill Livingstone, pp. 107–128.

Weiss, G. (1984). Relaxin. *Annual Review of Physiology*, **46**: 42–52.

Aqua relaxation for mothers and babies

Rosalie Mori

The physical and emotional adjustment that a new mother needs to make on the birth of her child continue for many weeks. It places a great strain on a mother's energy levels.

Extra energy and patience are immediately required with the onset of any difficulties that may arise during those first few months of motherhood. It is in such situations that tension levels increase, which may interfere with the dynamics of the family and the establishment of a healthy mother–infant attachment.

The most beneficial aspect of relaxation is in relieving these tensions. Gentle swimming in warm water can promote relaxation. Also early childhood is the optimal time to learn to relax and enjoy water (Madders, 1979).

AIMS

The overall aim of the programme is to reduce tension in both the mother and her child. It has been found that a group situation is beneficial but the group should not be too large. Approximately four to six mothers and their infants is optimal. To some extent the size of the group will also be dependent on the size and shape of the pool.

Primary aims:

Specifically the aims of the relaxation sessions are to:

- promote relaxation in the mother and child
- promote mother and infant attachment
- provide a self-support situation.

Secondary aims:

Certain secondary aims result from the child's activity with the mother in the water. These are:

- the promotion of sensory–motor development
- the promotion of head control
- the promotion of head and truncal righting reactions.

Relaxation

The therapeutic qualities of warm water for relaxation have been well documented. Immersion of a person in warm water aids relaxation as does the support given by buoyancy (Skinner and Thomson, 1983) and the apparent weightlessness that is experienced (Harris and McInnes, 1963). Leboyer (1975) subjectively reported the effectiveness of warm water immersion inducing a calming effect on the newborn. Other authors, Wilson and Kasch (1963) and Kraus (1973) cited by Reid Campion (1985) have noted the sedative effect of warm water, and research by Euler and Soderberg (1956), quoted by Harris (1978), report the reduction in muscle tone brought about by warm water.

Anxiety

In a study of the effect of hydrotherapy on anxiety Levine (1984) found both subjectively and with electromyographic measures (EMG) a reduction in anxiety with only 15 minutes of hydrotherapy. Although no long-term assessment was made this study suggests that immersion in warm water can have a significant short-term effect on anxiety.

Discussions concerning anxiety and its effects on the mother–infant relationship vary, but most agree that anxiety affects the relationship to some degree (Mertin, 1986; Barnett *et al.*, 1987). In so far as 'the mother–infant relationship' is an ongoing developmental process rather than a post-partum event occurring in the first few days after birth (Mertin, 1986), it seems important to reduce anxiety and to ensure every opportunity to maximize the mother–infant relationship.

Reducing the mother's level of anxiety will thus optimize her ability to cope with the adjustment needed with a newborn.

Self-Support

The group situation provides support and comfort from other participants experiencing similar problems. This is important in our society where there has been a decline in the extended family.

Sensory-motor Development

Piaget's (1963) theory of development emphasizes the importance of the development of the sensory-motor system, whereby a motor output requires a sensory input. The brain responds to messages it receives from the environment and the body's relationship to that environment as well as to internal factors such as body parts in relation to another body part and to the state of the muscle tone. Such sensory feedback requires an intact sensory system, which is provided by the various somatic receptors located in the muscles, joints, tendons, ligaments and the skin and the specialized receptors in the eyes and ears, resulting in the appropriate reactions in the motor system (Shepherd, 1980).

In the pool various senses are stimulated to promote sensory-motor integration. The senses stimulated are:

- tactile
- vestibular
- auditory
- proprioception.

The tactile system is stimulated by the water which is all encompassing but also by contact with the mother's body. Movement through water creates turbulence which promotes body awareness especially distally in the limbs. The turbulence created by others moving in the water further aids tactile awareness. The movement in the water stimulates the vestibular system especially by the 'jumping' up and down, the swaying from side to side and moving round in circles in some of the activities.

The songs that are sung in the activities provide stimulation to the auditory system at the same time as developing rhythm which further promotes relaxation in mother and child. The proprioceptive system receives information from muscles, joints and tendons and the resistance and impedance to movement provided by water stimulates proprioception. An intact sensory-motor system will also enable the child to be an active participant in the development of the mother–infant bond.

Head Control

The importance of promoting head control is recognized in this programme, especially with the decline of infants being placed in prone due to 'cot death' fears. The Halliwick approach to head control (Reid Campion, 1985) is used. Activities which facilitate head control are chosen and the appropriate songs and rhymes are employed. The main actions used are:

- jumping
- swaying, i.e. deviating laterally whilst in the vertical position
- moving from the vertical position to supine and returning to the vertical.

Head and Truncal Righting Reactions

Head and truncal righting reactions can be promoted using modified activities as suggested by Reid Campion (1991). Full explanations of these techniques and the appropriate holds are provided by that author, however, some of these holds can be seen in Figs 17.1, 17.2, 17.3, 17.4.

CRITERIA FOR THE AQUA-RELAXATION PROGRAMME

Certain criteria for the programme have been formulated. It has been found valuable to utilize a group situation, but in some instances this has been varied to suit particular situations.

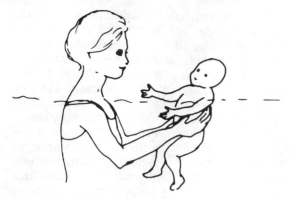

Fig. 17.1   *Child with good head control*

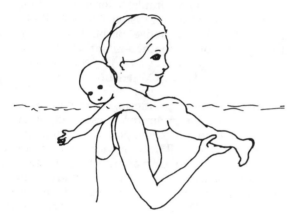

Fig. 17.2

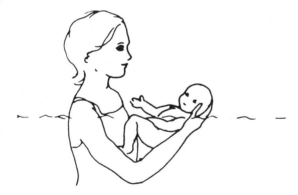

Fig. 17.3   *Full support for the head*

- It is of paramount importance that the mother and her child have had their six weeks post-partum examination by their doctor. There should be no contraindications to hydrotherapy.

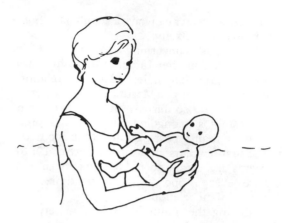

Fig. 17.4   *Cradling used when there is greater head control*

- Mothers suffering from postnatal depression are seen on an individual basis until such time that both the mother and the physiotherapist feel that they are ready to be included into a group.
- The number in the group is largely determined by the size and the shape of the pool, small groups are always advisable. There must be adequate space for the mothers to float; where large numbers are involved the situation may not be sufficiently relaxing.
- In regard to the infants the criteria are that they must wear snugly fitting pants.

Referrals

New or expectant mothers are made aware of the aqua-relaxation programme through antenatal classes (hospital or private based), postnatal exercise classes, or by the maternity ward physiotherapist. The local office of the Physiotherapy Association can also direct the public to centres that offer this service. However, it appears that the majority hear of the programme from friends and relatives. Some mothers are referred by infant health nurses, private physiotherapists and doctors.

The most common reasons for referral are:

- poor sleeping (either amount or pattern)
- 'colic'
- mother not coping
- feeding difficulties
- unsettled baby

- other medical problems, e.g. low birth-weight
- postnatal depression
- mother seeking a water familiarization programme for infant.

Assessment

A subjective history should be taken including the following items:

- details of the pregnancy
- details of the labour
- feeding and sleeping patterns of the infant
- attendance at antenatal classes
- knowledge of relaxation skills and ease of implementation
- the referral source
- the mother's swimming ability.

Also the mother is asked about the frequency that pelvic floor exercises are performed. Objectively, a brief developmental assessment of the child should be carried out. Age appropriate milestones are assessed. In the pool the mother's and infant's reactions to the water are observed and recorded, as well as the mother's confidence in handling the baby.

Procedure

Prior to the first pool session it is advisable to discuss baby massage with the mother, the advantages of the technique and if desired the chance to practise it.

Baby massage in different forms has been used in other cultures for centuries. However, in our society touching comes less easily. A physiotherapist who is trained in massage and with 'permission to touch' is the ideal person to teach mothers how to massage their baby. When used correctly it becomes part of the total handling of the baby and provides the tactile sensation to the skin that is so important in a child's development. Baby massage is a loving and caring way of helping babies and young children to feel that the world is a pleasurable, familiar and safe place. It can prove relaxing for the mother as well. For the baby with special needs baby massage can have beneficial effects (Auckert, 1981).

Similar effects can be brought about by water: the child and its mother appreciate the all encompassing nature of water, the uniform pressure and the warmth all helping to provide tactile sensation and relaxation. The pool sessions involve 15 minutes of total relaxation for the mothers while the babies are cared for by volunteer aides. The mothers are usually supported by neck, pelvic and ankle rings, but they use whatever flotation equipment they find comfortable. Music, to enhance relaxation, is played and the mothers are encouraged to use the relaxation technique with which they are familiar. If they have no particular method, physiological relaxation is taught (Mitchell, 1977).

Following the relaxation period, in approximately 34°C (93.2°F) water temperature, the babies are brought to the pool and join their mothers. Initially, the infants are introduced into the water very slowly, the mother holding her child close to her and attempting to maintain eye contact. It is essential that the child feels secure and this security can be provided by the mother's arms and closeness and from the sensation of the fluid environment which is similar to that experienced prenatally (Reid Campion, 1985).

The time spent in the pool by the infant needs to be carefully monitored as their thermo-regulatory mechanisms are not as well developed as those of adults (Quinn, 1981). For the first visit, the time the child spends in the bath at home is used as a guide. On subsequent sessions this time may be increased, and the activities extended using songs with appropriate actions, e.g. the Halliwick method (Reid Campion, 1991).

The mother is shown various ways of holding her baby in the water. The main positions used are vertical, supine lying and prone lying. In the vertical position support is given by the mother's hands at the upper chest or mid-trunk, depending on the child's head and truncal development (Fig. 17.1). In supine the mother has the child's head on her shoulder and supports the body with the hands. When the prone lying position is used the baby's upper trunk is supported by the mother's shoulder, while her hands support the child's legs (Fig. 17.2).

When the baby requires full support for the head and body he or she is cradled in the mother's arms as shown in Fig. 17.3. The child is facing the mother who supports the child's head with one hand and the body with the other. This cradling can be modified as head control improves (Fig. 17.4).

From the first session onwards action songs can be initiated. These are carried out gently from the beginning but as the baby becomes more confident they become more vigorous. If a baby is not ready to be taken through the songs even when conducted slowly and gently, they are held close as the mother moves through the water. Water toys are often floated on the surface to break up the large expanse of water: this helps to increase the baby's confidence.

Following the programme of activities for the child, the mothers leave the pool one at a time and dress first while the physiotherapist who has been in the water throughout holds the babies individually.

Prior to leaving the department the mother should have the opportunity to feed her baby, particularly as the majority of the babies are either hungry or thirsty after the pool sessions. This is also an opportunity for the mothers to socialize and discuss with each other about their children, and being a mother.

DEVELOPMENTAL FACTORS

Physiotherapists need to be aware of certain developmental facts so that these can be explained to the mothers when questions are raised.

Density

A comment often made is 'my baby feels as if he or she will float'. This phenomenon is quite normal and is due to the infant's specific density of approximately 0.86 when compared to the specific density of water.

Reflex Swimming Action

'Swimming is one of the oldest phylogenetic functions of which there is a residual in the behaviour of the newborn infant' (McGraw, 1969). The neuromuscular organization for such a pattern requires a high level of control over and above that needed for other behaviours such as creeping. McGraw (1969) suggests that when faced with more difficult and dangerous situations the infant uses subcortical centres rather than cortical areas which are less developed, to combine motor actions.

The reflex swimming actions are 'violent' and 'random in nature' (Wielki and Houben, 1983) and occur on presentation of the water. Wielki (1983) described four types of movement occurring at this stage (3–11 months). These are:

- a 'cigarette lighter' movement, manifesting mainly in the vertical position
- alternating reflex leg movements
- simultaneous flexion and extension movements of the legs
- alternating flexion and extension movements of the legs.

According to McGraw (1969) the movements range through reflex swimming, to disorganized actions, to voluntary movements and in the latter phase represent more automatic movements to gain a more secure environment. The acquisition of sufficient head extension above the surface to breathe comes at a later date, thus the infant's head must be supported when placed prone in the water.

This reflex has been noted as early as 11 days of age (Cratty, 1979). After approximately eight months of age movement in the water becomes more deliberate and kicking and cycling motions increasingly vigorous.

The Supine Position

The child who is becoming proficient at sitting may dislike the supine position in the pool. Although this can be seen in older children who are further advanced in their motor development it may be that the child is busily observing the environment. As a stage in development of activity in water disliking the supine position may be expected. This stage may pass quickly, but with some children it may persist for sometime; with ingenuity and distraction the physiotherapist can overcome the difficulty.

There have been no specific studies of the effects of relaxation classes in the hydrotherapy pool for mothers and their infants. Sweeney (1983) found that when premature infants were introduced to water baths, and activity was encouraged, there was improvement in abnormal muscle tone, enhancement of visual and auditory orientation responses, improvement in feeding behaviour and an increase in parent participation.

Similar effects have been noted in the children who participate in the programmes offered as a postnatal service to mothers and their children in Western Australia. Anecdotally mothers have often commented how 'they live for the session'.

This early introduction of the child to water may continue as the child develops as a water familiarization programme and form the basis of learning to swim. Children who have made friends with water at an early age are likely to accept learning to swim more readily (Elkington, 1978). Physical activity has been shown to be vital to both the normal growth of the child and to its psychological well-being (Bailey, 1976). Van Vielt and Howell (1973) state that 'there is perhaps no physical activity that can contribute to more of the combined physical, social and emotional development than swimming and diving: it helps growth, self esteem and confidence and provides a sport that can be used from the cradle to the grave.'

Swimming is a skill that has to be learnt. Early independence in water may occur in the water familiarization programme and depending on the child's physical and mental development the teaching of swimming can be gradually introduced under optimal conditions of trust and safety by a suitably trained instructor who has a sound knowledge and understanding of child development, both physical and emotional, and who values the parents' cooperation and encourages their involvement.

REFERENCES

Auckett D.A. (1981). *Baby Massage*, Melbourne: Hill of Content.

Bailey D.A. (1976). The growing child & the need for physical activity. In *Child in Sport and Physical Activity* (J.G. Albinson, G.M. Andrew, eds), Baltimore: University Park Press.

Barnett B., Blignaut I. and Holmes S., *et al.* (1987). Quality of attachment in a sample of one year old Australian children. *Journal of American Academy of Child and Adolescent Psychiatry*, **26(3)**: 303–307.

Cratty B.J. (1979). *Perceptual and Motor Development in Infants and Children*, 2nd edn, New Jersey: Prentice Hall Inc.

Elkington H. (1978). *Swimming: A Handbook for Teachers*. Cambridge: Cambridge University Press.

Euler C. and Soderberg U. (1956). The relation between gamma motor activity and the electroencephalogram. *Experientia*, **12**: 278.

Harris R. and McInnes M. (1963). Exercises in water. In *Medical Hydrology* (S. Licht, ed.), New Haven: Elizabeth Licht, pp. 207–217.

Harris S.R. (1978). Neurodevelopmental treatment approach for teaching swimming to cerebral palsied children, *Physical Therapy*, **58(8)**: 979–983.

Kraus R. (1973). *Therapeutic Recreation Service Principles and Practices*, Philadelphia: W.B. Saunders Company.

Leboyer F. (1975). *Birth without Violence*, New York: Alfred A. Knopf.

Levine B.A. (1984). Use of hydrotherapy in reduction of anxiety, *Psychological Reports*, **55**: 526.

McGraw M.B. (1969). *The Neuromuscular Maturation of the Human Infant*, New York: Hafner Publishing Company.

Madders J. (1979). *Stress and Relaxation*, Sydney: Collins.

Mertin P.G. (1986). Maternal–infant attachment: a developmental perspective. *Australian and New Zealand Journal of Obstetrics and Gynaecology*, **26**: 196–198.

Mitchell L. (1987). *Simple Relaxation: the Mitchell Method of Physiological Relaxation for Easing Tension*, 2nd edn, London: Murray.

Quinn S. (1981). *Water Babies*, Report from Northern Ireland Sports Council.

Piaget J. (1963). *The Origins of Intelligence in Children*, New York: W.W. Norton and Co. Inc.

Reid Campion M. (1985). *Hydrotherapy in Paediatrics*, Oxford: Heinemann Medical.

Shepherd R. (1991). *Physiotherapy in Paediatrics*, 2nd edn, Oxford: Butterworth–Heinemann.

Skinner A. and Thomson A. (1983). *Duffield's Exercise in Water*, 3rd edn, London: Ballière Tindall.

Sweeney J.K. (1983). Neonatal hydrotherapy adjunct to developmental intervention in an intensive care nursery setting. In *Aquatics: A Revived Approach to Paediatric Management*, (F.H. Dulcy, ed.), City Haworth Press Inc., pp. 39–52.

Van Vliet M.A. and Howell M.L. (1973). *Be Water Wise*, Canada: The Canadian Red Cross Society and the Royal Life Saving Society Canada.

Wielki C. and Houben M. (1983). Descriptions of the leg movements of infants in an aquatic environment. *Biomechanics and Medicine in Swimming*, **14**: 66–71.

Wilson I.H. and Kasch F.W. (1963). Medical aspects of swimming. In *Medical Hydrology*, (S. Licht, ed.), New Haven: Elizabeth Licht.

FURTHER READING

Brazelton T.B. and Heidelise A. (1979). *Psychoanalyst Study of the Child*, **34**: 349–369.

Burke J.P., Clark F., *et al.* Maternal role preparation: A program using sensory integration, infant- -mother attachment and occupational behaviour perspectives. *Occupational Therapy in Health Care*, **4(2)**: 9–21.

Cobb J. (1980). *Babyshock: A Mother's First Five Years*, London: Hutchinson.

Whiteford B. and Polden M. (1984). *Postnatal Exercises*, London: Courtesy Publishing Co. Ltd.

18

Water fitness for the older adult and frail aged

Ann Levin

Society is becoming more aware that health status and a longer life span are dependent on individual behaviours and lifestyle. Lack of disease prevention and health maintenance measures contribute to disease and decreased functional ability in the elderly (Kimble and Longe, 1989). Physiotherapists working with the geriatric population are developing and implementing health promotion initiatives to help people take greater personal responsibility for their health. These initiatives often involve education and self-management skills in addition to exercise programmes.

The major demographic, epidemiologic and economic changes in society during this century cannot be ignored. The elderly (65 years and older) are now the fastest growing segment of the population (Dychtwald, 1986). With the increase in life expectancy, the old-old (85 years and older) component is the fastest growing subgroup. In addition, the mortality rate in the old-old is decreasing. As a result, our health care systems will be increasingly strained (Kimble and Longe, 1989). Social isolation is frequently a problem, as the number of elderly who live alone in the community is increasing.

The elderly are by far the greatest consumers of health care. Many chronic illnesses in this population result in a decreased ability to perform activities of daily living. Most elderly individuals in the community have at least one chronic condition. This does not mean that most of these people are frail. Most elderly are not in this group until after the age of 75. Many are not frail until after the age of 90 (US Dept. of Health, 1986). The frail elderly are likely to have multi-systems problems. They have poor levels of physical and psychosocial functioning and inadequate social support systems. It becomes difficult or impossible for them to continue living independently in the community or to maintain social contacts without ongoing external assistance.

Within the field of health promotion, there are three types of prevention strategies. Primary prevention aims at preventing disease or injury in a healthy population. In the geriatric population, a water fitness programme is an illustration of this category. Secondary prevention aims at reducing the severity of a disease; it can range from interventions at an early stage, to preventing or limiting disability in advanced disease. Two examples are an early intervention programme designed to meet the needs of people with recently diagnosed Parkinson's disease, and a falls prevention programme, for those identified at risk for falling. In tertiary prevention, the goal is to minimize the effects of disease, disability and loss of independence when the condition is chronic and irreversible (Rothman and Levine, 1992). A self-management programme for people with long-standing arthritis is an example of this type of health promotion approach.

Physiotherapists must provide programmes that incorporate the different kinds of strategies for the elderly population. New initiatives should be based on a comprehensive needs assessment that includes consulting with the target group at the initial planning stages. Programme evaluation using valid and reliable outcome measures is necessary to demonstrate the effectiveness of these interventions. Hydrotherapy can form an integral component of many different programmes, either provided by physiotherapy alone or in conjunction with other disciplines. The therapeutic pool can be the focal point for interventions to address both physical and psychosocial needs. This chapter explores some of these specific programmes.

INDICATIONS FOR HYDROTHERAPY HEALTH PROMOTION INITIATIVES

In general, hydrotherapy health promotion initiatives are designed to increase the number of years of good health by reducing illness, disability and premature death. These programmes recognize that health is dynamic and is more than simply the absence of disease.

Hydrotherapy is indicated for the geriatric elderly client where the objectives are to:

- reduce pain
- increase or maintain range of movement (flexibility)
- improve strength
- improve cardiovascular fitness
- control body weight
- increase postural awareness
- promote relaxation
- utilize functional patterns that may be very difficult or impossible to accomplish on land (e.g. ambulation)
- improve equilibrium reactions
- improve vital capacity
- provide opportunities for socialization and recreation.

POOL ENVIRONMENT

A barrier-free environment for the pool and changing rooms is desirable. Non-slip hand rails installed on the walls surrounding the pool area improve client safety. If pool entry is not ramped but stepped, the physiotherapist should be stationed at the stairs to supervise entries and exits. There should be two hand railings at the stairs. As railings are not as easy to hold if wet, clients need to take extra care when exiting the pool, particularly if they have a weak hand grip.

In the changing rooms, wall bars strategically placed on a diagonal next to benches and toilets improve safety. The height of benches is also of concern. Independence in the transitional movement of sit to stand for clients with impaired mobility and/or strength in the lower extremities is facilitated if the bench exceeds standard height. At community pools, the traditional design of the changing area provides one room for each sex. People requiring assistance with dressing must therefore bring a helper of the same sex. This precludes a person's spouse from providing the necessary aid. A small private family changing room meets this need for many couples.

Water temperature is an important consideration. Ageing reduces the sensitivity of the body's homeostatic regulation of heat control. Mechanisms for gaining, conserving and dissipating heat are affected. In the skin, the epidermis and subcutaneous fat become thinner and provide less natural insulation. Cardiac output decreases with ageing, causing reduced blood flow to the skin. This is the reason that many elders complain of cold hands and feet. There is also a significant decrease in the density of sweat glands with ageing, which impairs the body's ability to lose heat when necessary (Kenney, 1989). The water temperature should be maintained in the thermoneutral range of 33–35°C. A thermoneutral temperature is one that does not change the core temperature of the person immersed (O'Hare *et al.*, 1985).

Even at a thermoneutral temperature, clients who are debilitated and are not very active in the water may complain of feeling chilled shortly after immersion. A shivering response may soon follow. This occurs because the thermal conductivity of water is 25 times that of air and the individual is reacting to the loss of heat through the skin. On the other hand, the more active elderly person who may be swimming laps and exercising at a much higher intensity will require a lower water temperature.

There is no physiological benefit gained by raising the water temperature higher than the thermoneutral range. On the contrary, as the temperature climbs, so does the cardiac output, stroke volume and heart rate (Weston *et al.*, 1987). These increases, when combined with the effects of exercise, can overtax the cardiovascular system of the elderly. In addition, the large fall in mean blood pressure and peripheral resistance at higher temperatures could lead to episodes of syncope.

The ambient room temperature is another important factor. It should be a few degrees cooler than the water, depending on the level of humidity. When the humidity is high, it is harder to lose body heat, and a lower room temperature is necessary for comfort. A heated storage unit for linens is a useful piece of equipment to have close by the pool. Clients can be covered in heated towels and flannel sheets to slow the rate of heat loss after they leave the pool.

CONTRAINDICATIONS AND PRECAUTIONS

Age is not a contraindication for hydrotherapy. Ageing is a normal process, not a disease state, and is associated with some decrease in function. Injury, illness and reduced levels of activity will intensify this decline. A decision on the appropriateness of a water intervention programme must be based on the client's medical history and the physiotherapist's assessment. The contraindications are the same as those in the younger population and are reviewed in an earlier chapter. However, there are some additional precautions:

Cognitive Status

People with impaired cognition may be unsuitable for group hydrotherapy programmes but may do well with an individual intervention. Cognitive deficits can affect attention and concentration, orientation, learning, memory and perceptual abilities. Lack of judgement and insight as well as difficulty following commands are concerns, while impulsiveness and aggression can actually be dangerous in water. Clients with severe dementia (e.g. Alzheimer's, multi-infarct) may become very agitated in the foreign environment of water.

Many of these clients have one or more medical problem in addition to the cognitive impairment. The mental status usually precludes them from attending programmes for which they would otherwise be appropriate. There is a growing need for special programmes designed to meet the needs of this population and their caregivers.

Impaired Hearing

Many elders use an assistive device for hearing. If the water programme does not require clients to immerse their ears (e.g. when working in a supine float position), then hearing aids should be permitted. This enhances communication and increases client satisfaction. Participants cannot wear FM transmitters or body-packs in the pool. People with this level of impairment may still participate if they are able to interpret gestures and to copy other people around them.

Impaired Vision

There is reduced visual acuity, depth perception and visual field with ageing. People wearing corrective contact lenses must wear goggles if they wish to immerse their faces. Clients using glasses are encouraged to keep them on in the water when they are not working in the prone position.

Impaired Balance

Balance is mediated through the visual, vestibular and somatosensory systems. Information about muscle length and joint angle is provided by receptors in the muscle spindle (Kandel and Schwartz, 1985). In the water, input for proprioception is reduced (Mitarai *et al.*, 1972). Buoyancy decreases the stretch of the muscle spindles. In addition, the refraction of light rays reflected from the bottom of the pool gives a false perception of the true bottom. Clients need to have as much afferent input as possible to decrease the likelihood of falls in the pool.

Medications

It is not only important for physiotherapists to be aware of the client's medications, but it is vital to know the possible side effects and their implications for water immersion. For example, many elders take beta-blockers. The bradycardia that occurs as a result of taking this antihypertensive, antianginal medication can combine with the cardiovascular effects of immersion to put the person at risk for syncope, lightheadedness and postural hypotension.

As part of a hydrotherapy risk management programme, clients who use nitroglycerine tablets or puffers for respiratory distress must keep their labelled medication at the side of the pool. It is not sufficient to have the medication among their personal effects in the changing room.

Cardiac Pacemaker

Clients must be reminded to self-monitor for any symptoms such as pressure or pain in the chest. Observe for shortness of breath.

MENTAL ADJUSTMENT

Many elderly people may not have been in a pool for many years or may be very afraid of water. This is particularly true if balance is impaired. It is very important that elderly clients regard their first hydrotherapy session as a success, or they may be reluctant to return. Encourage clients to visit and perhaps observe a session from the pool deck. Seeing others working in the pool is often enough to overcome initial doubts.

Take the time to orient the elderly well to the pool area. Allow them enough time to adjust mentally to the water medium. Before entering the pool, explain to clients that they will feel the water pushing them a little and that they will not be left to stand alone until after their water balance has been assessed. This reassurance will improve confidence. Clients should use the physiotherapist for support until they begin to disengage, first by breaking eye contact and then by allowing the physiotherapist to move further away. Lengthening the arm holds or using an appropriate water device to increase stability are two ways to achieve this.

Safety is a major consideration. When working with groups of elderly in the water, trained volunteers or assistants can be positioned strategically around the pool to ensure safety. Many elderly have balance difficulties that can be exacerbated by movements in the water. From Bernoulli's theorem, we know that pressure energy is lower in faster flowing regions of the water. From this, the physiotherapist can anticipate that, for example, horizontal adduction of the shoulders is going to cause the client to move backwards into the area of lower pressure. By mentioning this ahead of time, clients learn to have confidence in, and to trust, the physiotherapist (p. 15).

HEALTH PROMOTION PROGRAMMES FOR THE ELDERLY

Primary Health Promotion: Water Fitness Programmes for the Well Elderly

In working with the elderly, it is necessary to instil in them the importance of regular exercise. Many older people enjoy exercising in water because of the reduced stress on muscles and joints and the ease of movement. The deconditioned sedentary elderly, with or without chronic diseases, will have a limited cardiovascular reserve, which can severely restrict their daily activities (Skinner, 1987). Physiotherapists are aware that a minimum level of daily activity is necessary to prevent the deterioration associated with immobility. In addition, endurance needs to be addressed in this population. An increase in physical fitness can supply the necessary cardiorespiratory power for an extra eight to nine years of self-care in the elderly (Shephard, 1987).

A medical clearance form for a water exercise programme should be completed by each client's physician. The physiotherapist should educate the physician on the physiological effects of immersion.

Programme Format

The class size will be partially a function of the dimensions of the pool. Even if regulations allow a bather load in excess of 20 people, the maximum number of participants should be kept below this number for safety. If the physiotherapist is in the water leading the group, participants may not be able to see the movement of the part of the body that is submerged. The advantage is that the physiotherapist can easily assist participants with positioning and corrections. In this case, it can be helpful to have another person on the deck of the pool to demonstrate proper starting positions and movements. The other option for the physiotherapist is to conduct the class from the ledge of the pool. The exercise programme can include an aerobic component or can be a low intensity class, depending on the medical history and fitness level of the participants.

The programme should include:

- warm-up
- stretching exercises

- aerobic component (if appropriate)
- strengthening exercises
- games to promote better balance and coordination
- cool-down, including slow stretches.

It is important that previously sedentary individuals begin an exercise programme slowly. The tendency is to overdo exercise because the water allows such freedom of movement.

Clients need to learn that they will retain the benefits of exercise only as long as they continue with a regular exercise programme. Physiotherapists have a responsibility to educate the client in this regard.

Warm-up

The purpose of warm-up exercises is gradually to increase the heart rate. A light activity such as submaximal walking is used. Various walking routines can be done: forwards, sideways, backwards, crossovers. Arm movements can be incorporated. The water level should be at the xiphisternum as long as the person is safe at that depth. This is a buoyancy neutral (B±) depth; vertical balance becomes critical so clients should be made aware of this and supervised till safe.

Stretching

By using a float in the water, buoyancy and the technique of contract–relax can be used to gain a passive stretch. This is an excellent method. In the elderly, however, it is most effective when used on an individual basis with a physiotherapist. This technique may not be suitable for use in a group programme for several reasons. Participants sometimes find it difficult to stabilize themselves and to isolate the correct movement. If they do not have sufficient muscle strength, a stretch can become a forced passive movement. In addition, balance is compromised when a flotation aid is placed on an extremity. The centre of buoyancy moves away from midline and the metacentric effect causes a rotational movement to occur. Conventional exercises without a flotation aid can be used to stretch soft tissue around the joints.

Aerobic component

The goal is to increase and maintain the heart rate at a target range for a period of time. Endurance training will increase maximum oxygen uptake in the sedentary elderly just as in younger clients (Niinimaa and Shephard, 1978). A symptom limited stress test is the most accurate way to determine maximum heart rate in the elderly.

Borg's Rate of Perceived Exertion Scale is useful as a guideline to determine ideal exercise intensity. The subjective feeling of exertion is directly related to heart rate. This scale has ratings from 6 to 20, with descriptors ranging from very, very light to very, very hard. Scores of 12 to 13 (somewhat hard) correspond well with 60–75% of maximum oxygen consumption. This is the optimum range at which a conditioning response occurs. Studies have established the scale's validity for different age groups, sex and cultural origin. Beta-blockers do not affect the validity of this instrument (American College of Sports Medicine, 1991).

The Talk Test can be used concurrently. Participants may self-monitor by ensuring that they are working at an intensity level where they can still carry on a conversation. The formula '220 minus age' will not reliably predict exercise intensity in this population (Londeree and Moeschberger, 1984).

As the resistance caused by water is varied by increasing the walking speed and consequently the turbulence around the moving person, water walking is an excellent aerobic activity. Glcim and Nicholas (1989) showed that oxygen consumption is greatest when walking in water at a mid-thigh depth. There is lower oxygen consumption when walking in waist depth water because of the effect of buoyancy on the immersed part of the body. Fit individuals can continue the aerobic activity for 15–20 minutes. Less fit people will have to begin with as low as six minutes and increase and adapt the intensity level over a period of time.

As part of a risk management programme, inform participants about the symptoms of which they need to be aware. These include dizziness or faintness, nausea, palpitations or any irregular heart rate, and pain, pressure or a squeezing sensation in the chest. If any of these symptoms are experienced, clients must stop exercising and notify the physiotherapist immediately. They should be accompanied out of the pool and monitored on land. It may be necessary to refer the person back to the physician.

Strengthening exercises

Strengthening exercises can be easily devised using the principles of hydrostatics, where buoyancy is used to support, assist or resist a movement. Progressions are made by changing the length of the lever, by increasing the size or number of floats, or by increasing the speed and number of repetitions. There is a great selection of aquatic equipment commercially available which will provide impedance to movement. Often, a resourceful physiotherapist can create inexpensive versions of similar devices.

Games for balance and coordination

People can work individually, in pairs, or in groups when playing games in the pool. Books of games are readily available, and can easily be adapted to the water environment. Frisbees, woggles, balls and floating basketball nets can be incorporated into games. Line dance routines can be used.

Cool-down

The heart rate slows down in this segment. Exercises are done slowly at a light activity level. Stretches are repeated to reduce the change of aching or tight muscles.

SECONDARY PREVENTION

Health promotion initiatives at this level focus on early diagnosis and timely treatment in an effort to limit the severity of a disease or to delay the consequences of advanced disease (Rothman and Levine, 1992). In the geriatric population, an early intervention programme for Parkinson's disease and a programme targeting people at risk for falls are examples of secondary health promotion where hydrotherapy may be effective at an early stage.

Parkinson's Disease Early Intervention Programme

Parkinson's disease is a progressive and degenerative disease that affects the central nervous system. Its incidence is greatest between 70 and 79 years of age. The key clinical signs include bradykinesia, tremor, rigidity and postural instability. The impairment least responsive to pharmacologic management is postural instability (Koller *et al.*, 1989).

Clients with Parkinson's disease are often referred to physiotherapy in the more advanced stages, when they are disabled, and are having considerable difficulty with mobility and functional independence. An early intervention programme can focus on reducing the musculoskeletal limitations and postural deformity. This will hopefully increase the individual's ability to function independently for a longer period.

Schenkman (1989a, b) describes a model for evaluation and treatment that differentiates between the impairments which result as a direct effect and as an indirect effect of the pathology. These together lead to composite effects, resulting in the disabilities associated with this disease. Schenkman proposes that physiotherapy aimed at improving or maintaining soft tissue length and flexibility will affect postural control, bradykinesia and cardiopulmonary conditioning by reducing the musculoskeletal contributions to these impairments. The impairments that are a direct result of the pathology, such as tremor and rigidity, have not been shown to be responsive to physiotherapy intervention.

An early intervention hydrotherapy programme can be part of a health promotion initiative. Regular assessments, updated home exercise programmes, education and medical management would be involved within a multidisciplinary approach.

Goals are:

- to promote relaxation
- to increase flexibility
- to improve postural alignment

- to improve balance (this is accomplished by first addressing the musculoskeletal limitations)
- to increase vital capacity and endurance
- to maintain the ability to perform functional activities.

Relaxation

The warm water can be used to promote relaxation of muscle tone in a supine float position. Initially, this has to be done on an individual basis. If a neck float is required, it should contain a minimum amount of air, so that it does not maintain the neck in too much flexion. Progress to no float as soon as possible so that rotational and lateral movements of the neck can be encouraged. Passive relaxation techniques (e.g. seaweeding, incorporating rotation, p. 101) can be used initially, but the client needs to learn as soon as possible to self-relax actively through small amplitude, rhythmic rotational movements. Encourage slow, deep breathing.

Flexibility

When working on increasing flexibility, begin proximally with the trunk. Various techniques of hydrotherapy can be used to improve extension and rotation of the thoracic and lumbar spine. Bad Ragaz patterns incorporating trunk extension, rotation and lateral flexion are useful, but the client also needs to have a water stretching programme that he or she can perform independently. Righting reactions will be limited if the client is unable to elongate on the weight-bearing side because of tight trunk side flexors. Contract–relax techniques combined with a float can work well to improve flexibility. Pelvic mobility in an antero-posterior direction, as well as hip-hiking and scooting activities at various water depths can be practised while in a sitting position. Contract–relax can be used by the client to increase neck mobility and this will encourage increased proprioceptive input for balance. Hip flexors, abductors and rotators, as well as the hamstrings and calf muscles, often require stretching. In the upper extremities, shoulder flexion, abduction and external rotation, along with elbow extension and supination, and wrist and finger extension, need to be emphasized.

Postural alignment

Postural alignment should be practised in an effort to reduce the postural deformity in the sitting and standing positions. Postural impairment will affect the client's ability to do gross motor activities.

Balance

After addressing the underlying musculoskeletal problems, balance activities can be practised in lying, sitting and standing, Weight shifting can be done by moving the centre of gravity first within and later outside the base of support.

Rotation should be incorporated into these movements. As a progression, clients can create turbulence around themselves by moving their arms in the water, or turbulence can be created by others. These are examples of external perturbation in water.

The typical Parkinsonian standing posture is stooped, with a forward head, kyphosis of the trunk, and flexed hips and knees. Mitarai *et al.* (1972) demonstrated that when normal subjects stand immersed in water, buoyancy causes the line of gravity to move posteriorly. This causes the tibialis anterior muscles to contract to prevent the individual from falling backwards. If clients are standing in water with their centre of gravity too far anteriorly over the balls of their feet, there will be a decreased tendency to propulsion. If they are standing with their centre of gravity too far posteriorly, it is logical to predict that retropulsion will be accentuated. In clients with Parkinson's disease, both these extremes are possible.

Vital capacity and endurance

Respiratory problems are the primary cause of death in Parkinson's disease, so it is important to focus on vital capacity early in the disease process. Breathing exercises can be done with the face in or out of the water, and in a variety of positions at various water depths. The hydrostatic pressure on the chest and abdomen will restrict vital capacity and the expiratory reserve volume. Any increase in tidal volume will be achieved by increasing the inspiratory reserve volume. Maintaining thoracic mobility will help to maintain vital capacity. If swimming is an enjoyable pastime, encourage the client to use swimming strokes that emphasize extension and rotation, such as the front or back crawl.

Swimming is also an excellent aerobic activity to improve cardiovascular fitness and endurance.

Functional activities

Clients can perform functional activities in the water. Rolling, emphasizing segmental movement, should be practised. This movement is lost in clients with Parkinson's disease and greatly restricts their ability to perform activities of daily living, such as getting in and out of bed. Turning while sitting, standing up from a seated position and ambulation are performed after the musculoskeletal problems have been addressed. Some movements will be made easier and others will be more difficult. For example, standing up from a bench in the water is easier because of the buoyancy assisting. During ambulation, the acceleration phase of swing will be harder than on land, due to the turbulence and resistance of the water. For these skills to be effective in daily living, they also have to be practised on land.

A Falls Prevention Programme

A secondary prevention programme targets individuals who are at risk of falling. Falls in the elderly can have serious physical and psychosocial consequences. One third to one half of people over the age of 65 fall at least once per year. Falls are the leading cause of accidental death for those over the age of 75 (Holliday *et al.*, 1992). Fear of falling is an associated problem. Early intervention is desirable to prevent the inactivity and dependence that results from lost confidence for walking (Vandervoort *et al.*, 1990). A programme designed to meet the needs of this population must recognize that the problems are multifactorial, and must address both physical functioning and the environment.

The hydrotherapy component can focus on:

- balance activities
- improving range of motion
- increasing strength and endurance
- practise of gait activities.

Balance activities

Many diseases affecting the elderly have a great impact on balance activities. Degenerative joint changes in the cervical spine can cause a decrease in the functioning of the cervical articular mechanoreceptors. This affects proprioception and postural stability.

The rate of falling in water is much slower than on land because of the high impedance ratio of water. The ankle strategy and a stepping response can be practised at various depths, using shallower water as a progression. Arm or leg movements can be done in unipedal stance. This makes use of turbulence and the metacentric effect to challenge balance. Weight shifting, movement within and reaching outside the base of support in various directions, and ambulation at different speeds and directions are encouraged. Other activities include turning in a circle, stepping up and down, practising timed standing with a narrow base of support or in unipedal stance, and timed standing with the eyes closed. Balance work can be incorporated into games.

Improving range of motion

Adequate joint range is important in maintaining balance. Hip and knee flexors often require stretching. These muscles are prone to shortening in the sedentary elderly who sit for extended periods of time.

Increasing strength and endurance

All the anti-gravity muscles should be strengthened. Knee extensors, ankle dorsiflexors and plantarflexors require particular attention. A small improvement in strength will provide increased endurance for activities such as climbing stairs (Vandervoort *et al.*, 1990).

Practise of gait activities

Walking at different speeds and in various directions is practised. Arm movements can be added to challenge balance even more. Gait deviations, such as insufficient step height during swing phase, can be addressed.

Lord *et al.* (1993) demonstrated significant improvement in body sway, and quadriceps and ankle dorsiflexion strength, following a short duration water programme incorporating the above principles in a group of elderly people as compared to a matched group of controls.

The concepts described here can be generalized to diseases where impaired balance is a factor.

TERTIARY PREVENTION

Prevention strategies at this level focus on minimizing existing disabilities and handicaps. A self-management programme for people with a long-standing chronic disease such as arthritis is an example.

Arthritis Self-management Programme

Arthritis is the leading cause of long-term disability and its prevalence increases with age. For example, between 65 and 70 years of age, the prevalence jumps to 40% of the population. Client-identified problems include pain, the inability to perform activities of daily living, and lack of knowledge of the disease and its management. A health promotion initiative can be designed around the hydrotherapy pool to meet the needs of these people. The benefits of using water for clients affected by arthritis have been described in an earlier chapter (p. 253).

A multidisciplinary approach involving physiotherapy, occupational therapy, pharmacy, nutritional services and social work is recommended. Goals of the hydrotherapy component are to:

- decrease pain
- increase range of motion
- increase strength
- maintain the ability to perform functional activities
- improve balance
- improve endurance
- promote relaxation
- demonstrate to clients that proper exercise in water is an enjoyable activity that does not flare or exacerbate symptoms.

Bad Ragaz techniques are not used. Conventional water exercises are preferred in this type of programming, so that clients can work independently and do not have to be dependent on the physiotherapist to increase strength or improve range of movement. This is an important part of giving control of the disease over to the client.

The water is an excellent medium where the weight-bearing can be graded as necessary by varying the level of immersion of the client (p. 26).

The physiotherapist needs to ensure that clients understand that prolonged inactivity causes many of the problems that they associate with arthritis. This includes decreased strength, flexibility and endurance, atrophy, osteoporosis, depression, cardiovascular changes and sleep difficulties. Studies have shown that people with arthritis can do aerobic work without increasing the disease process (Dial and Windsor, 1985; Danneskiold-Samsoe *et al.*, 1987; Minor *et al.*, 1989).

SUMMARY

Long-term goals for a health promotion strategy must include improving quality of life and increasing independence. Hydrotherapy can play an integral part at all levels of the prevention continuum. A sample of possible programmes has been described. Considerations relevant to this population have been discussed.

ACKNOWLEDGEMENTS

I wish to thank:

Helen Whitelock, for her teaching and enthusiasm.

My colleagues at Baycrest Centre for Geriatric Care, especially Maria Huijbregts, Rebecca Gruber and Shayna Alpern, for their support, encouragement and constructive suggestions.

My husband and children, for doing without me so often, and letting me indulge my passion for water.

REFERENCES

American College of Sports Medicine (1991). *Guidelines for Exercise Testing and Prescription*, 4th edn., Philadelphia: Lea & Febiger.

Danneskiold-Samsoe B., Lynberg K., Risum T. and Telling M. (1987). The effect of water exercise therapy given to patients with rheumatoid arthritis. *Scandinavian Journal of Rehabilitation Medicine*, **19**: 31–35.

Dial C. and Windsor R.A. (1985). A formative evaluation of a health education–water exercise program for class II and III adult rheumatoid arthritis patients. *Patients Education and Counseling*, 7: 33–42.

Dychtwald K. (1986). *Wellness and Health Promotion for the Elderly*, Rockville, Maryland: Aspen Publishers.

Gleim G.W. and Nicholas J.A. (1989). Metabolic costs and heart rate responses to treadmill walking in water at different depths and temperatures. *American Journal of Sports Medicine*, 17(2): 248–252.

Harrison R.A. and Bulstrode S. (1987). Percentage weight-bearing during partial immersion in the hydrotherapy pool. *Physiotherapy Practice*, 3(2): 60–63.

Holliday P.J., Cott C.A. and Torresin W.D. (1992). Preventing accidental falls by the elderly. In *Prevention Practice: Strategies for Physical Therapy and Occupational Therapy* (J. Rothman, R. Levine, eds), Philadelphia: W.B. Saunders Company, pp. 234–257.

Kandel E.R. and Schwartz J.H. (1985). *Principles of Neural Science*, 2nd edn, New York: Elsevier Science Publishing Company.

Kenney R.A. (1989). *Physiology of Aging: A Synopsis*, Chicago: Year Book Medical Publishers.

Kimble C.S. and Longe M.E. (1989). *Health Promotion Programs for Older Adults: A Planning and Management Guide*, Chicago: American Hospital Publishing.

Koller W., Glatt S., Vetere Overfield B. and Hassanein R. (1989). Falls and Parkinson's disease. *Clinical Neuropharmacy*, 12: 98–105.

Londeree B.R. and Moeschberger M.L. (1984). Influence of age and other factors on maximal heart rate. *Journal of Cardiac Rehabilitation*, 4: 44. In *Therapeutic Exercise: Foundations and Techniques*, C. Kisner and L.A. Colby (1990).

Lord S., Mitchell D. and Williams P. (1993). Effect of water exercise on balance and related factors in older people. *Australian Physiotherapy*, 39(3): 217–222.

Minor M.A., Hewett J.E., Webel R.R., *et al.* (1989). Efficacy of physical conditioning exercise in patients with rheumatoid arthritis and osteoarthritis. *Arthritis and Rheumatism*, 32: 1396–1405.

Mitarai G., Mano T., Mori S. and Jijiwa H. (1972). Electromyographic study on human standing posture in experimental hypogravic state. *Annual Report of the Research Institute of Environmental Medicine, Nagoya University*, 19: 1–9.

Niinimaa V. and Shephard R.J. (1978). Training and oxygen conductance in the elderly, II: The cardiovascular system. *Journal of Gerontology*, 33: 354–361.

O'Hare J.P., Heywood A., Summerhayes C., Lunn G., Evans J.M., Walters G., Corrall R.J.M. and Dieppe P.A. (1985). Observations on the effects of immersion in Bath Spa water. *British Medical Journal*, 291: 1747–1751.

Rothman J. and Levine R. (ed.) (1992). *Prevention Practice: Strategies for Physical Therapy and Occupational Therapy*, Philadelphia: W.B. Saunders Co.

Schenkman M. and Butler R.B. (1989a). A model for multisystem evaluation treatment of individuals with Parkinson's disease. *Physical Therapy*, 69(11): 932–943.

Schenkman M., Donovan J., Tsubota J., Kluss M., Stebbins P. and Butler R. (1989b). Management of individuals with Parkinson's disease: rationale and case studies. *Physical Therapy*, 69(11): 944–954.

Shephard R.J. (1987). *Physical Activity and Aging*, 2nd edn, Rockville MD: Aspen Publishers.

Skinner J.S. (1987). *Exercise Testing and Exercise Prescription for Special Cases. Theoretical Basis and Clinical Application*, Philadelphia: Lea & Febiger.

US Department of Health and Human Services (1986). *Age Words: A Glossary on Health and Aging*, NIH Publication No. 86–1849. Washington DC: USGPO.

Vandervoort A., Hill K., Sandrin M. and Vyse V.M. (1990). Mobility impairment and falling in the elderly. *Physiotherapy Canada*, 42(2): 99–107.

Weston C.F.M., O'Hare J.P., Evans J.M. and Corall R.J.M. (1987). Haemodynamic changes in man during immersion in water at different temperatures. *Clinical Science*, 73: 613–616.

FURTHER READING

Heckheimer E.F. (1989). *Health Promotion of the Elderly in the Community*, Philadelphia, PA: W.B. Saunders.

Ontario Ministry of Health (1993). *A Guide for Community Health Promotion Planning*, Toronto: Queen's Printer.

Appendix

Peter Charles Shelley Campion LDS RCS Eng.

THE CRIBRIFORM PLATE

The cribriform plate is the horizontal component of the ethmoid bone in the central anterior portion of the base of the skull, with a central crest – the crista galli – dividing it into right and left portions. The plate is penetrated by numerous foramina (or holes), through which passes the olfactory nerve. This is the 1st cranial nerve, the nerve of smell arising from the olfactory bulb situated at the anterior part of the base of the brain and which innervates the olfactory mucosa of that region. In addition, there is at least one slit on either side of the crista galli into which dips the dura mater (part of the meninges), the membrane which encloses the brain and the spinal cord. On the nasal side these slits have a covering of very fine nasal olfactory epithelium. Therefore, any infection introduced into the upper reaches of the nasal cavity can involve the nasal mucous membrane and consequently, through the various foramina, the dura mater, the olfactory nerve, the base of the brain and thence to the spinal cord. Not only infections but chemicals, either in solution or gaseous form, can produce unpleasant effects as well as damage to the delicate mucous membrane. Such effects can occur to the tissues in the adult form. In the infant whose tissues are still developing, the trauma is likely to be more devastating.

THE EAR

The ear is divided into three clearly defined compartments – the outer ear (or externa), the middle ear (or media), and the inner ear (or interna). With the exception of the interna, these are connected to the outside.

The outer ear consists of that part of the ear from the auricle, seen on the outside of the skull, to the ear drum (or tympanic membrane). In the neonate and infant, the 'ear hole' (the external auditory meatus) is virtually non-existent and the ear drum itself is on the outside of the skull surrounded by a bony ring known as the tympanic ring. It is hardly necessary in the infant to move the external ear in order to see the ear drum, and infections causing autis externa, chemicals, water pressure or the careless poking of an object into the external auditory meatus can be dangerous and cause damage to delicate tissues. In the adult whose external auditory meatus is well developed with a definite 'S'-shaped curve, protective hairs and wax, the ear drum is far less likely to be damaged. A bubble of air is frequently trapped in the ear before any liquid reaches the ear drum itself. The formation of the adult ear is not complete until the fifth year of life.

The middle ear is a cavity inside the ear drum and consists of three minute bones known as the ossicles. These are activated by the ear drum (tympanic membrane), and multiply the vibrations to the sensors of the inner ear. The cavity of the middle ear is filled with air through the auditory tube (the nasopharynx), which originates at the back of the throat and nose. Any infection of the throat can pass, or be forced up, into the middle ear cavity, which is itself connected with various hollows or air cells in the bone surrounding it, such as the mastoid air cells. Among other vital structures of the middle ear is an exposed portion of the facial nerve. This nerve supplies the muscles of facial expression. Damage or infection to the middle ear can result in conditions such as deafness and facial paralysis.

The inner ear consists of the vestibule, the semi-circular canals and the cochlea – which together form the bony labyrinth – and these are set into the bone of the base of the skull.

This apparatus provides a sense of balance and awareness of position in space. The extremely fine vestibular membrane separates the inner ear from the middle ear. Infections of the middle ear, the surrounding bone and air cells, can involve the inner ear and this may result in otitis interna, causing imbalance, disorientation, distortion or even loss of hearing.

Index

N.B. Page references to figures and tables are italic.

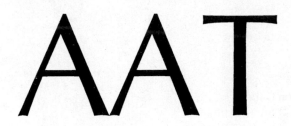

Qualifications and Credit Framework (QCF)
AQ2013
LEVEL 3 DIPLOMA IN ACCOUNTING

WORKBOOK

Spreadsheet Software

2015 Edition

For assessments from September 2015

Third edition June 2015
ISBN 9781 4727 2214 0

Previous edition
ISBN 9781 4727 0948 6

British Library Cataloguing-in-Publication Data
A catalogue record for this book is available from the British
Library

Published by
BPP Learning Media Ltd
BPP House
Aldine Place
London
W12 8AA

www.bpp.com/learningmedia

Printed in the United Kingdom by Ricoh UK Limited
Unit 2
Wells Place
Merstham
RH1 3LG

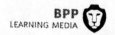

CONTENTS

Chapters and chapter tasks

*Study either Chapters 1 and 2 (Microsoft Office Excel 2007) or
Chapters 3 and 4 (Microsoft Office Excel 2010)*

Spreadsheet practice

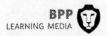

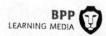

BPP LEARNING MEDIA'S AAT MATERIALS

The AAT's assessments fall within the **Qualifications and Credit Framework** and most papers are assessed by way of an on demand **computer based assessment**. BPP Learning Media has invested heavily to ensure our materials are as relevant as possible for this method of assessment. In particular, our **suite of online resources** ensures that you are prepared for online testing by allowing you to practise numerous online tasks that are similar to the tasks you will encounter in the AAT's assessments.

Resources

The BPP range of resources comprises:

- **Texts**, covering all the knowledge and understanding needed by students, with numerous illustrations of 'how it works', practical examples and tasks for you to use to consolidate your learning. The majority of tasks within the texts have been written in an interactive style that reflects the style of the online tasks we anticipate the AAT will set. When you purchase a Text you are also granted free access to your Text content online.

- **Question Banks**, including additional learning questions plus the AAT's sample assessment(s) and a number of BPP full practice assessments. Full answers to all questions and assessments, prepared by BPP Learning Media Ltd, are included. Our question banks are provided free of charge online.

- **Passcards**, which are handy pocket-sized revision tools designed to fit in a handbag or briefcase to enable you to revise anywhere at anytime. All major points are covered in the Passcards which have been designed to assist you in consolidating knowledge.

- **Workbooks**, which have been designed to cover the units that are assessed by way of computer based project/case study. The workbooks contain many practical tasks to assist in the learning process and also a sample assessment or project to work through.

- **Lecturers' resources**, for units assessed by computer based assessments. These provide a further bank of tasks, answers and full practice assessments for classroom use, available separately only to lecturers whose colleges adopt BPP Learning Media material.

This workbook for Spreadsheet Software has been written specifically to ensure comprehensive yet concise coverage of the AAT's **AQ2013** learning outcomes and assessment criteria.

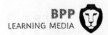

Each chapter contains:

- Clear, step by step explanation of the topic

- Logical progression and linking from one chapter to the next

- Numerous illustrations of 'how it works'

- Interactive tasks within the text of the chapter itself, with answers at the back of the book. The majority of these tasks have been written in the interactive form that students can expect to see in their real assessments

- Test your learning questions of varying complexity, again with answers supplied at the back of the book. The majority of these questions have been written in the interactive form that students can expect to see in their real assessments

The emphasis in all tasks and test questions is on the practical application of the skills acquired.

Supplements

From time to time we may need to publish supplementary materials to one of our titles. This can be for a variety of reasons, from a small change in the AAT unit guidance to new legislation coming into effect between editions.

You should check our supplements page regularly for anything that may affect your learning materials. All supplements are available free of charge on our supplements page on our website at:

www.bpp.com/about-bpp/aboutBPP/StudentInfo#q4

Customer feedback

If you have any comments about this book, please email nisarahmed@bpp.com or write to Nisar Ahmed, AAT Head of Programme, BPP Learning Media Ltd, BPP House, Aldine Place, London W12 8AA.

Any feedback we receive is taken into consideration when we periodically update our materials, including comments on style, depth and coverage of AAT standards.

In addition, although our products pass through strict technical checking and quality control processes, unfortunately errors may occasionally slip through when producing material to tight deadlines.

When we learn of an error in a batch of our printed materials, either from internal review processes or from customers using our materials, we want to make sure customers are made aware of this as soon as possible and the appropriate action is taken to minimise the impact on student learning.

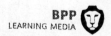

As a result, when we become aware of any such errors we will:

1) Include details of the error and, if necessary, PDF prints of any revised pages under the related subject heading on our 'supplements' page at: www.bpp.com/about-bpp/aboutBPP/StudentInfo#q4

2) Update the source files ahead of any further printing of the materials

3) Investigate the reason for the error and take appropriate action to minimise the risk of reoccurrence.

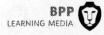

A NOTE ON TERMINOLOGY

The AAT AQ2013 standards and assessments use international terminology based on International Financial Reporting Standards (IFRSs). Although you may be familiar with UK terminology, you need to now know the equivalent international terminology for your assessments.

The following information is taken from an article on the AAT's website and compares IFRS terminology with UK GAAP terminology. It then goes on to describe the impact of IFRS terminology on students studying for each level of the AAT QCF qualification.

Note that since the article containing the information below was published, there have been changes made to some IFRSs. Therefore BPP Learning Media have updated the table and other information below to reflect these changes.

In particular, the primary performance statement under IFRSs which was formerly known as the 'income statement' or the 'statement of comprehensive income' is now called the 'statement of profit or loss' or the 'statement of profit or loss and other comprehensive income'.

What is the impact of IFRS terms on AAT assessments?

The list shown in the table that follows gives the 'translation' between UK GAAP and IFRS.

UK GAAP	IFRS
Final accounts	Financial statements
Trading and profit and loss account	**Statement of profit or loss (or statement of profit or loss and other comprehensive income)**
Turnover or Sales	Revenue or Sales Revenue
Sundry income	Other operating income
Interest payable	Finance costs
Sundry expenses	Other operating costs
Operating profit	Profit from operations
Net profit/loss	Profit/Loss for the year/period
Balance sheet	**Statement of financial position**
Fixed assets	Non-current assets
Net book value	Carrying amount
Tangible assets	Property, plant and equipment

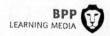

UK GAAP	IFRS
Reducing balance depreciation	Diminishing balance depreciation
Depreciation/Depreciation expense(s)	Depreciation charge(s)
Stocks	Inventories
Trade debtors or Debtors	Trade receivables
Prepayments	Other receivables
Debtors and prepayments	Trade and other receivables
Cash at bank and in hand	Cash and cash equivalents
Trade creditors or Creditors	Trade payables
Accruals	Other payables
Creditors and accruals	Trade and other payables
Long-term liabilities	Non-current liabilities
Capital and reserves	Equity (limited companies)
Profit and loss balance	Retained earnings
Minority interest	Non-controlling interest
Cash flow statement	**Statement of cash flows**

This is certainly not a comprehensive list, which would run to several pages, but it does cover the main terms that you will come across in your studies and assessments. However, you won't need to know all of these in the early stages of your studies – some of the terms will not be used until you reach Level 4. For each level of the AAT qualification, the points to bear in mind are as follows:

Level 2 Certificate in Accounting

The IFRS terms do not impact greatly at this level. Make sure you are familiar with 'receivables' (also referred to as 'trade receivables'), 'payables' (also referred to as 'trade payables'), and 'inventories'. The terms sales ledger and purchases ledger – together with their control accounts – will continue to be used. Sometimes the control accounts might be called 'trade receivables control account' and 'trade payables control account'. The other term to be aware of is 'non-current asset' – this may be used in some assessments.

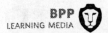

Level 3 Diploma in Accounting

At this level you need to be familiar with the term 'financial statements'. The financial statements comprise a 'statement of profit or loss' (previously known as an income statement), and a 'statement of financial position'. In the statement of profit or loss the term 'revenue' or 'sales revenue' takes the place of 'sales', and 'profit for the year' replaces 'net profit'. Other terms may be used in the statement of financial position – eg 'non-current assets' and 'carrying amount'. However, specialist limited company terms are not required at this level.

Level 4 Diploma in Accounting

At Level 4 a wider range of IFRS terms is needed, and in the case of Financial statements, are already in use – particularly those relating to limited companies. Note especially that a statement of profit or loss becomes a 'statement of profit or loss and other comprehensive income'.

Note: The information above was taken from an AAT article from the 'assessment news' area of the AAT website (www.aat.org.uk). However, it has been adapted by BPP Learning Media for changes in international terminology since the article was published.

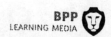

ASSESSMENT STRATEGY

Spreadsheet Software (SPSW) is assessed at Level 3.

The unit may be assessed either using Workplace Evidence (which is locally assessed by a centre) or by completing the Computer Based Assessment which is based on a case study, provided by the AAT but which is also locally assessed by a centre.

The assessment is approximately 2 hours and 30 minutes (plus 15 minutes reading time). The assignment is in one section:

- **Task 1** consists of an assignment asking the learner to design a spreadsheet
- **Task 2** consists of an assignment asking the learner to produce a chart
- **Task 3** consists of an assignment asking the learner to use techniques to calculate data
- **Task 4** consists of an assignment asking the learner to use analysis tools
- **Task 5** contains 5 multiple choice questions

The purpose of the assessment is to allow the learner to demonstrate the skills and knowledge necessary to use spreadsheet software at Level 3.

Competency

The assessment material will normally be provided by the AAT, delivered online and assessed locally. Candidates can provide workplace evidence.

Learners will be required to demonstrate competence in all sections of the assessment.

For the purpose of assessment the competency level for AAT assessment is set at 70 per cent.

The Level descriptor below describes the ability and skills students at this level must successfully demonstrate to achieve competence.

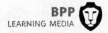

QCF Level descriptor	Summary
	Achievement at Level 3 reflects the ability to identify and use relevant understanding, methods and skills to complete tasks and address problems that, while well defined, have a measure of complexity. It includes taking responsibility for initiating and completing tasks and procedures as well as exercising autonomy and judgement within limited parameters. It also reflects awareness of different perspectives or approaches within an area of study or work.
	Knowledge and understanding
	■ Use factual, procedural and theoretical understanding to complete tasks and address problems that, while well defined, may be complex and non-routine
	■ Interpret and evaluate relevant information and ideas
	■ Be aware of the nature of the area of study or work
	■ Have awareness of different perspectives or approaches within the area of study or work
	Application and action
	■ Address problems that, while well defined, may be complex and non routine
	■ Identify, select and use appropriate skills, methods and procedures
	■ Use appropriate investigation to inform actions
	■ Review how effective methods and actions have been
	Autonomy and accountability
	■ Take responsibility for initiating and completing tasks and procedures, including, where relevant, responsibility for supervising or guiding others
	■ Exercise autonomy and judgement within limited parameters

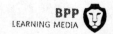

AAT UNIT GUIDE

Spreadsheet Software (SPSW)

Introduction

Please read this document in conjunction with the standards for all relevant units.

This unit is about the learner having the ability to use a software application designed to record data in rows and columns; perform calculations with numerical data and also present the information using charts and graphs.

It fits into the qualification at Level 3, and supports the accounting units, as it enables the learner to use spreadsheets to undertake a range of accounting tasks and produce supporting documentation. Students at Level 3 are required to design a spreadsheet to display data clearly and use a variety of spreadsheet skills in order to complete this unit successfully.

If learners have completed AQ2013 Level 2 they will have gained basic spreadsheet skills in the unit 'Analysing and Presenting Basic Cost and Revenue Information' where they will have learned to enter and edit data. This unit then builds on these skills. If a learner enters directly at Level 3, then they should already have some basic spreadsheet skills to ensure that they can complete this unit successfully.

Learning objectives

The objective of this unit is to equip the learner with a range of spreadsheet skills to enable them to complete both routine and non-routine tasks in the workplace using spreadsheets. It will enable the learner to design and use spreadsheets for a range of accounting purposes using formulae, functions and data analysis tools available on all common spreadsheet software. Learners should be able to display data and information clearly using graphs, tables and charts so it is easily understood by the user(s) of the information.

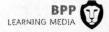

The purpose of the unit

This unit has been designed by e-skills to describe the skills and competencies of an **intermediate** spreadsheet user.

The use of spreadsheet software tools and techniques are defined as 'intermediate' because:

- The range of data entry, manipulation and outputting techniques will be multi-step and at times non-routine or unfamiliar.

- The tools, formulas and functions needed to analyse and interpret the data requires knowledge and understanding (for example, mathematical, logical, statistical or financial).

- The user will take some responsibility for setting up or developing the structure and functionality of the spreadsheet.

Learning outcomes

There are three learning outcomes for this unit – the learner will:

(1) Use a spreadsheet to enter, edit and organise numerical and other data.

(2) Select and use appropriate formulas and data analysis tools and techniques to meet requirements.

(3) Use tools and techniques to present, and format and publish spreadsheet information.

QCF Unit Spreadsheet Software (SPSW)		
Learning Outcome	**Assessment Criteria**	**Covered in Chapters**
Use a spreadsheet to enter, edit and organise numerical and other data	Identify what numerical and other information is needed in the spreadsheet and how it should be structured	**1 & 3**
	Enter and edit numerical and other data accurately	**1 & 3**
	Combine and link data from different sources	**1 & 3**
	Store and retrieve spreadsheet files effectively, in line with local guidelines and conventions where available	**2 & 4**

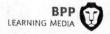

QCF Unit Spreadsheet Software (SPSW)		
Learning Outcome	**Assessment Criteria**	**Covered in Chapters**
Select and use formulas and data analysis tools and techniques to meet requirements	Explain what methods can be used to summarise, analyse and interpret spreadsheet data and when to use them	1 – 4
	Select and use a wide range of appropriate functions and formulas to meet calculation requirements	1 – 4
	Select and use a range of tools and techniques to analyse and interpret data to meet requirements	2 & 4
	Select and use forecasting tools and techniques	2 & 4
Use tools and techniques to present, and format and publish spreadsheet information	Explain how to present and format spreadsheet information effectively to meet needs	1 – 4
	Select and use appropriate tools and techniques to format spreadsheet cells, rows, columns and worksheets effectively	1 – 4
	Select and use appropriate tools and techniques to generate, develop and format charts and graphs	1 – 4
	Select and use appropriate page layout to present, print and publish spreadsheet information	1 & 3
	Explain how to find and sort out any errors in formulas	2 & 4
	Check spreadsheet information meets needs, using IT tools and making corrections as necessary	2 & 4
	Use auditing tools to identify and respond appropriately to any problems with spreadsheets	2 & 4

The following are **examples** of what the learner will be required to be familiar with. However, this is intended only as a guide to the most common areas to be assessed.

- The learner should be familiar with the component parts of a spreadsheet including: workbook, worksheet, column, row, cell, active cell, tab, page and panes/windows and be able to edit and label these.

- The learner should be able to use the following functions – open, save, save as, file name/rename, folder name, rename tab, order worksheets, password protect files, backup and archive information.

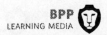

- The learner should be able to use the following functions in editing and entering data across single or multiple cells: insert, delete, justify, input/amend text and numerical data, copy, cut, paste, paste special, clear and find and replace.

- The learner should be able to reorganise data in different formats and link spreadsheets and data including functions such as data sort and filter, V and H look-up and concatenate.

- The learner should be able to use the following functions in analysing and interpreting data: addition, subtraction, multiplication, division, sum, percentages, parentheses, Pivot Table, Pivot Charts, Consolidation, Sort data, Filter Data, Data restriction, Data Validation, Find and replace, Look Up, If, And, Auto sum (count, max, min, sum, average), relative references, absolute references and Date (today, now, day/month/year).

- The learner should be able to lock and hide cells, columns and rows.

- The learner should be able to use the analysis tools within the spreadsheet. This may include, histograms, rank and percentile and moving averages.

- The learner should be able to forecast using trend lines within the spreadsheet.

- The learner should be able to display formulae on the worksheet.

- Learners should be able to title a spreadsheet, insert headers and footers, and tab names.

- They should be able to use the following formatting tools – Currency, date, fixed decimal, 1000 separator, '£', formatting percentages, applying a double underline border to cells, text alignment (including wrap text, shrink to fit, merge cells and orientation), font and font size, cell justification, borders, shading, merge cells, underline, use italics, conditional formatting, page setup (margins, orientation, print area) and be able to print formula.

- Learners should be able to insert and delete columns, rows, cells and to change the row height, column width.

- Learners should be able to hide and unhide cells, columns and rows and protect spreadsheets/cells. They should be able to print with or without gridlines, and have gridlines visible or invisible.

- Learners should be able to produce, title and label all elements and graphs (column, bar, line, pie, scatter, doughnut, bubble) and be able to show different views of these (2D, 3D, clustered, stacked, exploded, combined).

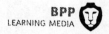

- Learners should know how to use page layouts to present data and scale information for printing purposes.

- Learners should be able to use passwords, both to open and protect documents.

- Learners should be able to check spreadsheets for errors in content and in formulas using the following functions – error checking, trace error and formula auditing.

- Learners should ensure that the information contained within the spreadsheet meets the needs of the recipient.

Delivery guidance

Learners should be able to:

- Design a suitable spreadsheet format using a blank worksheet
- Use existing spreadsheets, and also
- Use spreadsheet templates to meet certain requirements.

Therefore they will need to:

- Identify and select data (numerical and text) to include within a spreadsheet, and to be able to show
- How the spreadsheet should be structured, in terms of both layout and format including appropriate titles and data display formats.

Designing a suitable spreadsheet structure involves:

- Using a blank worksheet to develop a logical structure and format to display prescribed information for specific purpose.
- The designs should ensure that the information is easily understood by the users of that information.

The design and manipulation of data/workbooks covers:

- The use of spreadsheet templates for routine work, and also
- The production of a spreadsheet for a particular reason.

There should be a planned structure to the spreadsheet and the design and layout should be appropriate to the task.

Learners should know and be able to work with all component parts of spreadsheets:

- Cells
- Rows
- Columns
- Tabs

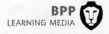

- Pages
- Charts
- Workbooks
- Worksheets and
- Windows

Learners should be able to enter and edit data accurately. This will include both numerical and textual data.

They must be able to:

- Insert data into single and multiple cells
- Clear cells
- Edit cell contents
- Replicate data
- Cut
- Copy
- Paste
- Find and replace
- Add and delete rows and columns
- Use absolute and relative cell references and
- Add data and text to a chart

They should also be able to hide and protect cells, columns and rows and link data.

The learner must be able to store and retrieve spreadsheets – therefore they could be assessed on using:

- Folders (eg create and name) and
- Files, eg
    - Create
    - Name
    - Open
    - Save
    - Save as
    - Print
    - Close
    - Find
    - Share

They should also be able to:

- Use version control
- Import/export files into other documents, and also
- Archive information (backup and restore)

The learner must be able to use font, alignment, styles, page layout, headers and footers to ensure data and information is displayed clearly and meets the specified requirements. Students should be able to proof read information and check formulae to identify and correct errors.

The learner needs to be able to use a wide range of formulae and functions to complete calculations; they should be able to use the design of formulas to meet calculation requirements. These could include mathematical, statistical, financial, conditional, look-up, and logical functions.

They must be able to use a range of techniques to summarise data and then analyse and interpret the results. Assessable summarising tools include:

- Totals and sub-totals
- Sorting of a cell range
- Rank
- Conditional formatting
- Filter rows and columns
- Data restriction
- Tables
- Graphs and charts
- Histograms
- Simple pivot tables and charts

The learner can be assessed on their judgment of when and how to use these methods.

Learners may be assessed on using the tools, formulas and functions (for example, data restrictions, data validation using formula and pivot tables and charts) needed to analyse the information within a spreadsheet.

The learner should then be able to develop the spreadsheets by using forecasting techniques:

- What-if scenarios
- Goal seek, and
- Data tables may be assessed.

The learner needs to be able to use data in different formats and link data in spreadsheets and worksheets using functions such as look-up (V and H), data sort and filter and concatenate.

Spreadsheets should then be prepared for publication or sharing with others. The learner should be able to format spreadsheet contents (cells, rows and columns) to ensure that they meet a competent standard and are easy to read. This may include:

- Height and width and shading for rows and columns and for cells
- Formatting for numbers or text
- Currency
- Percentages
- Number of decimal place
- Dates

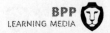

- Font
- Bold, underline and italic
- Alignment
- Text and cell colour
- Shading and borders, and
- Alignment of cell content

Learners must be able to produce the information within the spreadsheet in different formats. They could be assessed on choosing the most appropriate way to display information.

Charts must be correctly labelled (chart title, axis titles, axis scale and include a legend, data label or data table). All chart types may be assessed (2D, 3D, clustered, stacked column, bar, pie, bubble, doughnut, line and scatter graphs and may also include custom types, eg 2 graphs types on 1 axis and pivot table reports).

Learners should be able to change the chart type; move and resize a chart and annotate the chart as needed.

To present print and publish information the learner must ensure that spreadsheet is displayed in the best possible way and adjust the page set up or scale to fit, if necessary, for printing. This includes choosing:

- The font size
- The orientation (portrait or landscape)
- Margins
- Header and footer
- Page breaks
- Page numbering and
- Including a date/time stamp

Learners will need to check the spreadsheets for any errors. This should include:

- Accuracy of numbers and any text
- Accuracy of results
- Correcting errors in formulas
- Checking the layout and format validity
- Using formulae to determine valid entries for cells, the validity, relevance and accuracy of analysis and the interpretation of calculations and results.

Errors, once identified, must be rectified and the learner's ability to do this can be assessed. The learner should be able to:

- Use the help facility
- Sort out errors in formulas (use audit formulas to check for errors)
- Identify and correct errors in circular references, calculations and results.

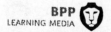

They should also be able to validate data and locate and remove invalid data.

Learners will be assessed on the most common tasks used in the workplace. No accounts specific knowledge is required. Where accounts specific calculations are required, guidance will be provided as to how to calculate these figures. This will ensure that whatever the learner's prior accounting experience/knowledge they will be able to calculate figures, as they will be provided with the necessary information to perform the spreadsheet tasks.

SPREADSHEET SOFTWARE

Do students have to use Microsoft Excel to complete this unit?

No. Students **do not** have to use Microsoft Excel (Excel) in their AAT Spreadsheet Software assessment.

The AAT recognise that a variety of productivity software packages are available and can be used. The only stipulation the AAT make is that the package used must be capable of performing the procedures outlined in the learning outcomes and assessment criteria.

Do students need access to Excel software to use this book?

Students that don't have Excel software may still pick up some useful information from this book.

However, those students with access to Excel will find it easier to work through the practical exercises than users of other accounting software packages.

Why does this Workbook refer to Excel 2007 and Excel 2010?

To explain and demonstrate the skills required in this Unit, it is necessary to provide practical examples and exercises. This requires the use of spreadsheet software.

This book provides examples taken from Excel 2007 and Excel 2010. Microsoft releases new versions of its software every few years, each time hoping to offer technical and user improvements. The basic functions are often the same.

Students should **study either Chapters 1 and 2 (covering Excel 2007) or Chapters 3 and 4 (covering Excel 2010).**

What version do I need?

The illustrations in this book are taken from Excel 2010 and 2007.

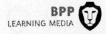

Microsoft released Excel 2010 in June 2010. This newer version of Excel is very similar to Excel 2007 and you can use this book if you are using Excel 2007. However, you may notice some differences in the way that Excel 2010 operates in certain sections.

How do I buy Excel software?

Colleges

If this book is used by students in a college environment, the college will need either Excel 2007 or Excel 2010 installed on student computers.

Microsoft make Excel available to educational institutions at very reasonable rates. Colleges wanting to purchase Excel should **contact Microsoft**. In the UK, the number is 0870 60 70 800.

Individual students

Students are eligible to purchase Microsoft Excel at a discounted price. Visit Amazon's website and search for 'Microsoft Excel student edition'.

Are Excel data files available for use with this book?

Yes. Excel data files are included, either to provide a starting set of data or to show the results of an exercise. You will be given instructions for locating the relevant spreadsheet when you need it.

The spreadsheets referred to in this Workbook are available for download – type **www.bpp.com/aatspreadsheets** into your browser and follow the instructions provided.

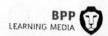

chapter 1:
INTRODUCTION TO SPREADSHEETS (EXCEL 2007)

chapter coverage 📖

This chapter and the next introduce spreadsheets, using Excel 2007. Chapters 3 and 4 cover the same material using Excel 2010. You should study and work through *either* Chapters 1 and 2 *or* Chapters 3 and 4, depending on the Excel software you have.

Spreadsheets have become indispensible tools for the presentation and analysis of accounting data.

This chapter covers:

- ✍ Introduction
- ✍ Basic skills
- ✍ Spreadsheet construction
- ✍ Formulae with conditions
- ✍ Charts and graphs
- ✍ Printing

INTRODUCTION

The vast majority of people who work in an accounting environment are required to use spreadsheets to perform their duties. This fact is reflected in the AAT Standards, which require candidates to be able to produce clear, well-presented spreadsheets, that utilise appropriate spreadsheet functions and formulae.

Uses of spreadsheets

Spreadsheets can be used for a wide range of tasks. Some common applications of spreadsheets are:

- Management accounts
- Cash flow analysis and forecasting
- Reconciliations
- Revenue analysis and comparison
- Cost analysis and comparison
- Budgets and forecasts

Spreadsheet software also provides basic database capabilities which allow simple records to be recorded, sorted and searched.

BASIC SKILLS

In this section we revise some **basic spreadsheet skills**.

The Ribbon

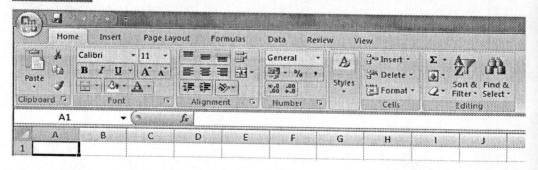

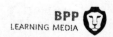

The Office button

The Office button is the circular, multi-coloured icon at the extreme top left of the spreadsheet. It is also a menu button and provides access to some important options.

Office button

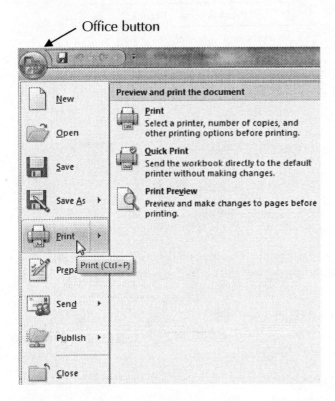

Workbooks and worksheets

At the bottom left of the spreadsheet window you will see tabs which are known as **Worksheets**:

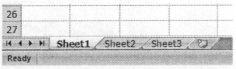

When **New** is selected from the Office button menu, a new **workbook** is created. The workbook consists of one or more **worksheets**. Think of worksheets as **pages** that make up the workbook. By default, a new Excel workbook starts out with three worksheets, although this can be changed (see later).

Worksheets can provide a convenient way of organising information. For example, consider a business consisting of three branches. Worksheets 2 – 4

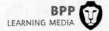

could hold budget information separately for each branch. When entering formulae into cells it is possible to refer to cells in other worksheets within the workbook so it would then be possible for Worksheet 1 to show the totals of the budget information for the whole business. Effectively, a 'three dimensional' structure can be set up. We look at this in more detail later.

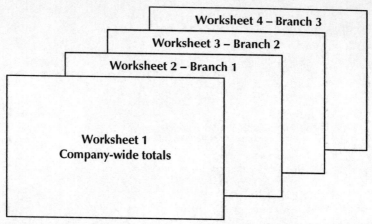

Opening an existing workbook

You can open an existing workbook file by using the menu commands **Office button>Open** and then navigating to the location of the file and double clicking on it.

If you open more than one workbook, each will open in a new window. To swap between open workbooks, click on the **Office button** and choose the workbook you want from the Recent documents list.

Closing a workbook

There are two ways to close a spreadsheet file:

> (1)   Click the **Office button** and choose **Close** at the very bottom.
>
> (2)   Click on either the **'x'** in the top right hand corner of the window or the one just below it.
>
> 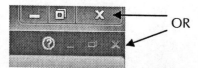 OR
>
> In both cases, if you have made any changes to the spreadsheet you will be asked if you want to save them. Choose **Yes** to save any changes (this will overwrite the existing file), **No** to close the file without saving any changes, or **Cancel** to return to the spreadsheet.

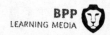

Cell contents

The contents of any cell can be one of the following:

(a) **Text**. A text cell usually contains **words**. Numbers that do not represent numeric values for calculation purposes (eg a Part Number) may be entered in a way that tells Excel to treat the cell contents as text. To do this, enter an apostrophe before the number eg '451.

(b) **Values**. A value is a **number** that can be used in a calculation.

(c) **Formulae**. A formula **refers to other cells** in the spreadsheet, and performs some type of computation with them. For example, if cell C1 contains the formula =A1 – B1, cell C1 will display the result of the calculation subtracting the contents of cell B1 from the contents of cell A1. In Excel, a formula always begins with an equals sign: =. This alerts the program that what follows is a formula and not text or a value. There is a wide range of formulae and functions available.

Formulas and the formula bar

Open the workbook called ExcelExample1. This is one of the files available for download from www.bpp.com/aatspreadsheets. You can open a file by using the menu commands:

Office button>Open

then navigating to and double clicking on the file called ExcelExample1.

Note. Throughout this book we want spreadsheets to recalculate every time a figure is changed. This is the normal or default setting, so it is likely your spreadsheets already do this. But, if they don't, then:

(1) Click the **Microsoft Office Button**, click **Excel Options**, and then click the **Formulas** category.

(2) To recalculate all dependent formulas every time you make a change to a value, formula, or name, in the **Calculation options** section, under **Workbook Calculation**, click **Automatic**. This is the default calculation setting.

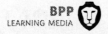

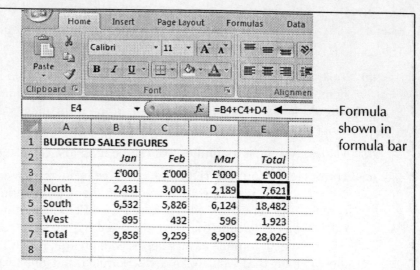

You should see the worksheet illustrated above. Click on cell E4.

Look at the formula bar.

Note. If the formula bar is not visible, choose the **View** tab and check the **Formula Bar** box.

Note the important difference between:

(1)   What is shown in cell E4: 7,621

(2)   What is actually in cell E4: this is shown in the formula bar and it tells us that cell E4 is the result of adding together the contents of cells B4, C4 and D4

The formula bar allows you to see and edit the contents of the active cell. The bar also shows, on the left side, the cell address of the active cell (E4 in the example above).

Select different cells to be the active cell by using the up/down/right/left arrows on your keyboard or by clicking directly on the cell you want to be active. Look at what is in the cell and what is shown in the formula bar.

The **F5** key is useful for moving around within large spreadsheets. If you press the function key **F5**, a **Go To** dialogue box will allow you to specify the cell address you would like to move to. Try this out.

Also experiment by holding down Ctrl and pressing each of the direction arrow keys in turn to see where you end up. Try using the **Page Up** and **Page Down** keys and also try **Home** and **End** and Ctrl + these keys. Try **Tab** and **Shift + Tab**, too. These are all useful shortcuts for moving quickly from one place to another in a large spreadsheet.

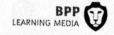

Examples of spreadsheet formulae

Formulae in Microsoft Excel follow a specific syntax. All Excel formulae start with the equals sign =, followed by the elements to be calculated (the operands) and the calculation operators (such as +, -, /, *). Each operand can be a:

- Value that does not change (a constant value, such as the VAT rate)

- Cell or range reference to a range of cells

- Name (a named cell, such as 'VAT')

- Worksheet function (such as 'AVERAGE', which will work out the average value of defined values)

Formulae can be used to perform a variety of calculations. Here are some examples:

(a) =C4*5. This formula **multiplies** the value in C4 by 5. The result will appear in the cell holding the formula.

(b) =C4*B10. This **multiplies** the value in C4 by the value in B10.

(c) =C4/E5. This **divides** the value in C4 by the value in E5. * means multiply and / means divide by.

(d) =C4*B10 – D1. This **multiplies** the value in C4 by that in B10 and then subtracts the value in D1 from the result. Note that generally Excel will perform multiplication and division before addition or subtraction. If in any doubt, use brackets (parentheses): =(C4*B10) – D1.

(e) =C4*120%. This **adds** 20% to the value in C4. It could be used to calculate a price including 20% VAT.

(f) =(C4+C5+C6)/3. Note that the **brackets** mean Excel would perform the addition first. Without the brackets, Excel would first divide the value in C6 by 3 and then add the result to the total of the values in C4 and C5.

(g) = 2^2 gives you 2 **to the power** of 2, in other words 2 squared. Likewise = 2^3 gives you 2 cubed and so on.

(h) = 4^(1/2) gives you the **square root** of 4. Likewise 27^(1/3) gives you the cube root of 27 and so on.

Displaying spreadsheet formulae

It is sometimes useful to see all formulae held in your spreadsheet to enable you to see how the spreadsheet works. There are two ways of making Excel **display the formulae** held in a spreadsheet.

(a) You can 'toggle' between the two types of display by pressing **Ctrl +`** (the latter is the key above the Tab key). Press **Ctrl +`** again to go back to the previous display.

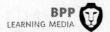

(b)　You can also click on **Formulas>Show Formulas** in the Ribbon.

The formulae for the spreadsheet we viewed earlier are shown below.

	A	B	C	D	E
1	BUDGETED S				
2		Jan	Feb	Mar	Total
3		£'000	£'000	£'000	£'000
4	North	2431	3001	2189	=B4+C4+D4
5	South	6532	5826	6124	=B5+C5+D5
6	West	895	432	596	=B6+C6+D6
7	Total	=B4+B5+B6	=C4+C5+C6	=D4+D5+D6	=E4+E5+E6

The importance of formulae

Look carefully at the example above and note which cells have formulae in them. It is important to realise that:

- If a cell contains a value, such as sales for North in January, then that data is entered as a number.

- If a cell shows the result of a calculation based on values in other cells, such as the total sales for January, then that cell contains a formula.

This is vital, because now if North's January sales were changed to, say, 2,500, the total would be automatically updated to show 9,927. Also the total for North would change to 7,690.

> Try that out by clicking on cell B4 to make it active, then typing 2,500, followed by the Enter key. You should see both the totals change.
>
> Now re-enter the original figure of 2,432 into cell B4.

Similarly, if a number is used more than once, for example a tax rate, it will be much better if the number is input to one cell only. Any other calculations making use of that value should refer to that cell. That way, if the tax rate changes, you only have to change it in one place in the spreadsheet (where it was originally entered) and any calculations making use of it will automatically change.

Your first function

In the example above, totals were calculated using a formula such as:

=+B4+C4+D4

That is fine provided there are not too many items to be included in the total. Imagine, the difficulty if you had to find the total of 52 weeks for a year. Adding up rows or columns is made much easier by using the SUM function. Instead of the formula above, we could place the following calculation in cell E4:

= SUM(B4:D4)

This produces the sum of all the cells in the range B4 to D4. Now it is much easier to add up a very long row of figures (for example, SUM(F5:T5)) or a very long column of figures (for example, SUM(B10:B60)).

There are three ways in which the SUM function can be entered. One way is simply to type =SUM(B4:D4) when E4 is the active cell. However, there is a more visual and perhaps more accurate way.

Make E4 the active cell by moving the cursor to it using the arrow keys or by clicking on it.

Type =Sum(

Click on cell B4

Type a colon :

Click on cell D4

Close the bracket by typing)

Press the Enter key

Another way is to use the AutoSum button, which we cover later.

Editing cell contents

Cell D5 of ExcelExample1 currently contains the value 6,124. If you wish to change the value in that cell from 6,124 to 6,154 there are four options (you have already used the first method).

(a) Activate cell D5, **type** 6,154 and press **Enter**.

To undo this and try the next option press **Ctrl + Z**; this will always undo what you have just done (a very useful shortcut).

(b) **Double-click** in cell D5. The cell will keep its thick outline but you will now be able to see a vertical line flashing in the cell. You can move this line by using the direction arrow keys or the Home and the End keys. Move it to just after the 2, press the **backspace** key on the keyboard and then type 5. Then press **Enter**. (Alternatively, move the vertical line to just in front of the 2, press the **Delete** key on the keyboard, then type 5, followed by the **Enter** key).

When you have tried this press **Ctrl + Z** to undo it.

(c) **Click once** before the number 6,124 in the formula bar. Again, you will get the vertical line which can be moved back and forth to allow editing as in (b) above.

(d) Activate cell D4 and press **F2** at the top of your keyboard. The vertical line cursor will be flashing in cell D4 at the end of the figures entered there and this can be used to edit the cell contents, as above.

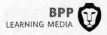

Deleting cell contents

There are a number of ways to delete the contents of a cell:

(a) Make the cell the active cell and press the **Delete** button. The contents of the cell will disappear.

(b) Go to the **Editing** section on the **Home** tab of the Ribbon. Click on the **Clear** button and various options appear. Click **Clear Contents**. You can also achieve this by **right clicking** the cell and choosing **Clear contents**.

Any **cell formatting** (for example, cell colour or border) will not be removed when using either of these methods. To remove formatting click on the **Clear** button on the **Home** tab and select **Clear Formats**. If you want to remove the formatting *and* the contents, click **Clear All**.

Ranges of cells

A range of cells can occupy a single column or row or can be a rectangle of cells. The extent of a range is defined by the rectangle's top left cell reference and the bottom right cell reference. If the range is within a single row or column, it is defined by the references of the start and end cells.

Defining a range is very useful as you can then manipulate many cells at once rather than having to go to each one individually.

The following shows that a rectangular range of cells has been selected from C4 to D6. The range consists of three rows and two columns.

	A	B	C	D	E	F
1	BUDGETED SALES FIGURES					
2		Jan	Feb	Mar	Total	
3		£'000	£'000	£'000	£'000	
4	North	2,431	3,001	2,189	7,621	
5	South	6,532	5,826	6,124	18,482	
6	West	895	432	596	1,923	
7	Total	9,858	9,259	8,909	28,026	
8						
9						

There are several ways of selecting ranges. Try the following:

(1) Click on cell C4, but hold the mouse button down. Drag the cursor down and to the right until the required range has been selected. Then release the mouse button. Now press the **Delete** key. All the cells in this range are cleared of their contents. Reverse this by **Ctrl+Z** and deselect the range by clicking on any single cell.

(2) Click on cell C4 (release the mouse button). Hold down the **Shift** key and press the **down** and **right hand arrows** until the correct range is highlighted.

Deselect the range by clicking on any single cell.

(3) Click on cell C4 (release the mouse button). Hold down the **Shift** key and click on cell D6.

Deselect the range by clicking on any single cell.

Sometimes you may want to select an entire row or column:

(4) Say you wanted to select row 3, perhaps to change all the occurrences of £'000 to a bold font. Position your cursor over the figure 3 defining row 3 and click. All of row 3 is selected. Clicking on the **B** in the font group on the **Home** tab will make the entire row bold:

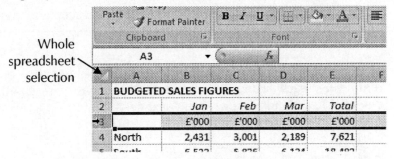

Whole spreadsheet selection

Sometimes you may want to select every cell in the worksheet, perhaps to put everything into a different font:

(5) Click on the triangle shape at the extreme top left of the cells (indicated above). Alternatively you can select the active cells using **Ctrl + A**.

Filling a range of cells

There are a number of labour-saving shortcuts which allow you to quickly fill ranges of cells with headings (such as £'000, or month names) and with patterns of numbers. You can keep the ExcelExercise1 spreadsheet open throughout the following activities and simply open a new spreadsheet on which to experiment.

(1) Create a new spreadsheet (**Office button>New>Create**).

(2) Make cell B3 active and type Jan (or January) into it.

(3) Position the cursor at the bottom right of cell B3 (you will see a black + when you are at the right spot – this is often referred to as the **fill handle**).

(4) Hold down the mouse button and drag the cursor rightwards, until it is under row G. Release the mouse button.

The month names will automatically fill across.

(5) Using the same technique, fill B4 to G4 with £.

(6) Type 'Region' into cell 3A.

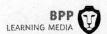

(7) Type the figure 1 into cell A5 and 2 into cell A6. Select the range A5–A6 and obtain the black cross at the bottom right of cell A6. Hold down the mouse key and drag the cursor down to row 10. Release the mouse button.

The figures 1–6 will automatically fill down column A.

Note. If 1 and 3 had been entered into A5 and C6, then 1, 3, 5, 7, 9, 11 would automatically appear. This does **not** work if just the figure 1 is entered into A5.

The AutoSum button Σ

We will explain how to use the AutoSum button by way of a simple example.

(1) Clear your worksheet (**Select all>Delete**).

(2) Enter the following figures in cells A1:B5. (**Hint.** Instead of pressing return after each figure, you can press the down or right arrow to enter the figure and to move to the next cell.)

	A	B
1	400	582
2	250	478
3	359	264
4	476	16
5	97	125

(3) Make cell B6 the active cell and select the Formulas group from the Ribbon. Click the drop-down arrow next to the **Σ AutoSum** button and select **Σ Sum**. The formula =SUM(B1:B5) will appear in the cell. Above cell B6 you will see a flashing dotted line around cells B1:B5. Accept the suggested formula by hitting Enter. 1,465 should appear in B6. Alternatively, you can simply click on the large **Σ** symbol itself, or click on the **Σ AutoSum** button in the **Editing** part of **Home** on the ribbon (see later).

(4) Next, make cell A6 the active cell and repeat the operation for that column. The number 1,582 should appear in cell A6.

(5) Now delete the two totals.

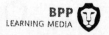

Copying and pasting formulae

You have already seen that formulae are extremely important in spreadsheet construction. In Excel it is very easy to define a formula once and then apply it to a wide range of cells. As it is applied to different cells the cell references in the formula are automatically updated. Say, that in the above example, you wanted to multiply together each row of figures in columns A and B and to display the answer in the equivalent rows of column C.

(1) Make C1 the active cell.

(2) Type =, then click on cell A1, then type * and click on cell B1.

(3) Press **Enter**

The formula =A1*B1 should be shown in the formula bar, and the amount 232,800 should be shown in C1.

(4) Make C1 the active cell and obtain the black + by positioning the cursor at the bottom right of that cell.

(5) Hold down the mouse button and drag the cursor down to row 5.

(6) Release the mouse button.

Look at the formulae in column C. You will see that the cell references change as you move down the column, updating as you move from row to row.

	C3	▼		f_x	=A3*B3
	A	B	C	D	
1	400	582	232800		
2	250	478	119500		
3	359	264	94776		
4	476	16	7616		
5	97	125	12125		

It is also possible to copy whole blocks of cells, with formulae being updated in a logical way.

> (1) Make A1 the active cell and select the range A1:C5, for example, by dragging the cursor down and rightwards.
>
> (2) Press **Ctrl+C** (the standard Windows Copy command) or click on the **Copy** symbol in the **Home** section of the ribbon.
>
>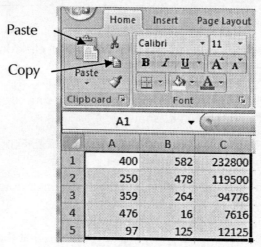
>
> (3) Make E7 the active cell and press **Ctrl+V** or click on the paste button. E7 will become the top right cell of the copied rectangle and will hold 400.
>
> (4) Now, look at the formulae shown in cell G7. It will show =E7*F7. So all cell references in the formulae have been updated relative to one another. This type of copying is called **relative copying**.
>
> (5) **Delete** the range E7:G7.

Paste special

Sometimes you don't want to copy formulae and you only want to copy the displayed values. This can be done using **Paste special**.

> Open the spreadsheet called Paste special example from the files available for download at www.bpp.com/aatspreadsheets.
>
> You will see a simple inventory-type application listing quantities, prices and values. The values are obtained by formulae multiplying together prices and quantities. Say that you just want to copy the values of cells D3:D8, without the underlying formulae.

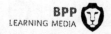

(1) Select the range D3:D8.

(2) Press **Ctrl+C** or the copy icon in the **Clipboard** part of **Home** on the Ribbon.

(3) **Right-click** on cell C12 to make it active, and choose **Paste Special** from the list.

(4) Check the **Values** radio button.

(5) Click **OK**.

The list of figures will be pasted, but if you look in the formula bar, you will see that they are just figures; there are no formulae there.

Note. If you change a quantity or price in the original table, the figures you have just pasted will not change; they have become pure numbers and do not link back to their source.

Inserting and deleting columns and rows

Often you will need to insert or delete whole rows or columns in spreadsheets. This can easily be done and sometimes formulae are correctly updated – but they should always be checked. For this exercise we will go back to using the ExcelExample1 spreadsheet.

Close the spreadsheet you have recently been working on and go back to (using the tabs across the bottom of the screen) or reopen the spreadsheet ExcelExample1.

Let us assume that we have a new region, East and that we want this to be in a row lying between North and South.

(1) Select row 5, by clicking on the 5, then click the right mouse button ('right click') and select **Insert**. You will see rows 5, 6 and 7 move down.

(2) Make B8 the active cell and you will see that the formula in the formula bar is =B4+B6+B7. If we were to put the figures for East into row 5 then those would **not** be correctly included in the total, though B5 has been updated to B6 etc.

(3) Reverse the last step (**Ctrl+Z**).

(4) Now, in cell B7 insert =SUM(B4:B6).

(5) Copy B7 across columns C7 to E7 (black cross and drag across).

(6) Check the formulae that are in cells C7 to E7 to ensure they have all been updated.

(7) Insert a whole row above row 5 (select row 5>right click>**Insert**).

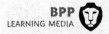

(8) Inspect the formulae in row 8, the new total row.

The formulae in the total row will now be showing =SUM(B4:B7), =SUM(C4:C7), etc. In this case the new row will be included in the total. Effectively, the range over which the totals are calculated has been 'stretched'. Depending how your copy of Excel is set up, you may notice little green triangles in row 8. If so, place your cursor on one and press the exclamation symbol. The triangles are warning that you have included empty cells in your total – not a problem here, but it might have been in some cases. Don't worry if the triangles aren't showing.

(9) Finally delete row 5. Select the whole row by clicking on the 5, then right click and choose **Delete** from the menu.

The cells below Row 5 will move up and the SUM formulae are again updated.

New columns can also be added. Say that we now wanted to include April in the results.

(1) Replace the current formula in E4 with =SUM(B4:D4).

(2) Copy the formula in E4 down through columns 5, 6 and 7. Check that the correct formulae are in cells E4–E7.

(3) Select column E, by clicking on the E, then click the right mouse button ('right click') and select **Insert**. You will see column E move to the right.

(4) Inspect the formulae now in Column F, the new total column.

You will see that the formula in F7 still says = SUM(B7:D7). It has **not been updated** for the extra column.

So, if an extra row or column is inserted in the middle of a range, the formulae is updated because the new row or column probably (but not always) becomes part of the range that has to be added up.

However, if the extra row or column is added at the end of a range (or the start) the formula will not be updated to include that. That's reasonably logical as new items at the very start or end have a greater chance of being headings or something not part of the range to be included in a calculation.

So:

**Whenever columns or rows are added or deleted,
check that formulae affected remain correct.**

Changing column width and height

You may occasionally find that a cell is not wide enough to display its contents. When this occurs, the cell displays a series of hashes ######. There are several ways to deal with this problem:

16

- Column widths can be adjusted by positioning the mouse pointer at the head of the column, directly over the little line dividing two columns. The mouse **pointer** will change to a **cross** with a double-headed arrow through it. Hold down the left mouse button and, by moving your mouse, stretch or shrink the column until it is the right width. Alternatively, you can double click when the double-headed arrow appears and the column will automatically adjust to the optimum width.

- Highlight the columns you want to adjust and choose **Home>Cells>Format>Column Width** from the menu and set the width manually. Alternatively, you can right click the highlighted column(s) and choose **Column width** from the menu.

- Highlight the columns you want to adjust and choose **Home>Format>Autofit Column Width** from the menu and set the width to fit the contents.

Setting column heights works similarly.

Dates

You can insert the current date into a cell by **Ctrl+ ;** (semicolon)

You can insert the current time by **Ctrl+Shift + ;** .

You can insert date and time by first inserting the date, release Ctrl, press space, insert the time. The date can be formatted by going to **Home>Number>Date** and choosing the format required.

Once a date is entered it is easy to produce a sequence of dates.

In a new worksheet, insert the date 1/1/2011 in cell A1.

(1) Format so as to show 01 January 2011.

(2) In A2, insert the date 8/1/2011 and format it to appear as 08 January 2011.

(3) Select cells A1 and A2.

(4) Position the cursor on the bottom right of cell A2 (a black + will appear).

(5) Hold down the mouse button and drag the mouse down to A12.

The cells should fill with dates seven days apart.

(If you see ###### in a cell it means that column A is too narrow, so widen it as explained above.)

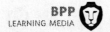

Naming cells

It can be difficult to always have to refer to a cell co-ordinate, eg C12. Cell C12 might contain the VAT rate and it would be more natural (and less error prone) to refer to a name like 'VAT'.

> (1) Open the worksheet called Name example.
>
> (2) Make cell B3 the active one and right click on it.
>
> (3) Select **Name a range**.
>
> (4) Accept the offered name, 'VAT' that Excel has picked up from the neighbouring cell.
>
> (5) Highlight the range D4:D7, right click **Name a range** and accept the offered 'Net'.
>
> (6) In E4 enter =Net*(1 + VAT).
>
> (7) Copy E4 into E5:E7.
>
> You will see the formula bar refers to names. This makes understanding a spreadsheet much easier.

A list of names can be seen using the **Formulas** section of the Ribbon and clicking on **Name Manager**.

Keyboard shortcuts

Here are a few tips to quickly improve the **appearance** of your spreadsheets and speed up your work, using only the keyboard. These are all alternatives to clicking the relevant button in the **Home** section of the Ribbon.

To do any of the following to a cell or range of cells, first **select** the cell or cells and then:

(a) Press **Ctrl + B** to make the cell contents **bold**.

(b) Press **Ctrl + I** to make the cell contents *italic*.

(c) Press **Ctrl + U** to <u>underline</u> the cell contents.

(d) Press **Ctrl + C** to **Copy** the contents of the cells.

(e) Move the cursor and press **Ctrl + V** to **paste** the cell you just copied into the new active cell or cells.

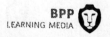

SPREADSHEET CONSTRUCTION

All spreadsheets need to be planned and then constructed carefully. More complex spreadsheet models should include some documentation that explains how the spreadsheet is set-up and how to use it.

There can be a feeling that, because the spreadsheet carries out calculations automatically, results will be reliable. However, there can easily be errors in formulae, errors of principle and errors in assumptions. All too often, spreadsheets offer a reliable and quick way to produce nonsense.

Furthermore, it is rare for only one person to have to use or adapt a spreadsheet and proper documentation is important if other people are to be able to make efficient use of it.

The following should be kept in separate identifiable areas of the spreadsheet:

(1) An inputs and assumptions section containing the variables (eg the amount of a loan and the interest rate, planned mark-ups, assumptions about growth rates).

(2) A calculations section containing formulae.

(3) The results section, showing the outcome of the calculations.

Sometimes it is convenient to combine (2) and (3).

It is also important to:

(1) Document data sources. For example, where did the assumed growth rate come from? If you don't know that, how will you ever test the validity of that data and any results arising from it.

(2) Explain calculation methods. This is particularly important if calculations are complex or have to be done in a specified way.

(3) Explain the variables used in functions. Some functions require several input variables (arguments) and may not be familiar to other users.

(4) Set out the spreadsheet clearly, using underlinings, colour, bold text etc to assist users.

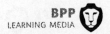

Example: constructing a costing spreadsheet

You want to set up a spreadsheet to record the time you and your colleagues spend on an assignment, and to cost it using your group's internal chargeout rates which are as follows:

Divisional chief accountant	£72.50
Assistant accountant	£38.00
Accounting technician (you)	£21.45
Secretary	£17.30

The spreadsheet needs to show the hours spent and costs per person, by week, for a three-week assignment. The time spent each week is shown below:

	Week 3	Week 2	Week 1
Divisional chief accountant	6 hrs 45 mins	4 hrs 30 mins	–
Assistant accountant	35 hrs	40 hrs	20 hrs
You	37 hrs 30 mins	40 hrs	32 hrs
Secretary	37 hrs 15 mins	32 hrs 15 mins	15 hrs

Setting up the assumptions area

As we will be referring to the chargeout rates for each week's costs, set these up in a separate area of the spreadsheet.

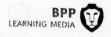

Headings and layout

Next we will enter the various **headings** required.

You want your spreadsheet to look like this:

	A	B	C	D	E	F	G
1	**Internal chargeout rates**						
2	Divisional chief accountant	£72.50					
3	Assistant accountant	£38.00					
4	Accounting technician	£21.45					
5	Secretary	£17.30					
6							
7	**Costs**	*Week 1*	*Week 2*	*Week 3*	**Total**		
8	Divisional chief accountant						
9	Assistant accountant						
10	Accounting technician						
11	Secretary						
12	**Total**						
13							
14	**Hours**	*Week 1*	*Week 2*	*Week 3*	**Total**		
15	Divisional chief accountant						
16	Assistant accountant						
17	Accounting technician						
18	Secretary						
19	**Total**						

(B1 cell reference shown, Sheet1 / Sheet2 / Sheet3 tabs)

Note the following points.

(a) Column A is wider to allow longer items of text to be entered. Depending on how your copy of Excel is set up, this might happen automatically or you may have to drag the line between the A and B columns to the right.

(b) We have used a **simple style for headings**. Headings tell users what data relates to and what the spreadsheet 'does'. We have made some words **bold**.

(c) **Numbers** should be **right aligned** in cells. This usually happens automatically when you enter a number into a cell.

(d) We have left **spaces** in certain rows (after blocks of related items) to make the spreadsheet **easier to use and read**.

(e) Totals have been highlighted by a single line above and a double line below. This can be done by highlighting the relevant cells then going to the **Styles** group in the **Home** section of the Ribbon, clicking on the drop-down arrow and choosing the style you want, in this case '**Totals**'.

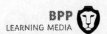

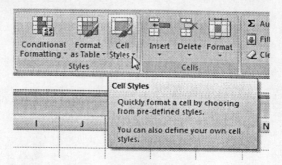

Alternatively, highlight the relevant cells, go to the **Font** area of the **Home** section and click on the drop-down arrow to access the list of **borders** available:

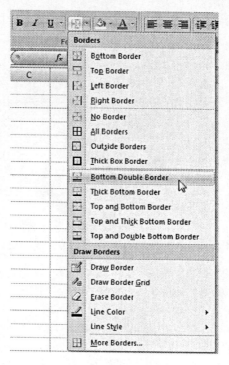

Entering data

Enter the time data in cells B15 to D18. Make sure you enter it correctly – the data is given to you in the order week 3 to week 1 but you would prefer it to be in the order week 1 to week 3. You will need to convert the time to decimal numbers.

	Hours	Week 1	Week 2	Week 3	Total
14	Hours	Week 1	Week 2	Week 3	Total
15	Divisional chief accountant	0	4.5	6.75	
16	Assistant accountant	20	40	35	
17	Accounting technician	32	40	37.5	
18	Secretary	15	32.25	37.25	
19	Total				(Ctrl) ▼
20					
21					
22					
23					
24					

Inserting formulae

The next step is to enter the **formulae** required. For example, in cell B19 you want the total hours for Week 1. In cell B8 you want the total cost of time spent. You could enter this formula as =B15*B2, but you need to make sure that as you copy the formula across for Weeks 2 and 3 you still refer to the chargeout rate in B2.

The quick way to insert a series of formulae is to type in the initial one and then to copy across a row or down a column. You may remember that cell references are cleverly updated as you move along the row or column. This was called **relative copying**. However, that will get us into trouble here. If cell B8 contains the formula =B15*B2 and that is copied one cell to the right, into column D, the formula will become =C15*C2.

The C15 reference is correct because we are progressing along the row, one month at a time, but the C2 reference is incorrect. The location of the chargeout rate does not move: it is **absolute**. To prevent a cell reference being updated during the copying process put a '$' sign in front of the row and/or column reference.

A reference like $A1 will mean that column A is always referred to as you copy across the spreadsheet. If you were to copy down, the references would be updated to A2, A3, A4, etc.

A reference such as A$1 will mean that row 1 is always referred to as you copy down the spreadsheet. If you were to copy across, the references would be updated to B1, C1, D1, etc.

A reference like $A$1 will mean that cell A1 is always referred to no matter what copying of the formula is carried out.

The **function key F4** adds dollar signs to the cell reference, cycling through one, two or zero dollar signs. Press the **F4** key as you are entering the cell address.

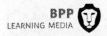

You should end up with the following figures:

	B8	▼	f_x =B15*$B$2			
	A	B	C	D	E	F	G
1	**Internal chargeout rates**					
2	Divisional chief accountant	£72.50				
3	Assistant accountant	£38.00				
4	Accounting technician	£21.45				
5	Secretary	£17.30				
6						
7	**Costs**	*Week 1*	*Week 2*	*Week 3*	*Total*	
8	Divisional chief accountant	0	326.25	489.375		
9	Assistant accountant	760	1520	1330		
10	Accounting technician	686.4	858	804.375		
11	Secretary	259.5	557.925	644.425		
12	**Total**					
13						
14	**Hours**	*Week 1*	*Week 2*	*Week 3*	*Total*	
15	Divisional chief accountant	0	4.5	6.75		
16	Assistant accountant	20	40	35		
17	Accounting technician	32	40	37.5		
18	Secretary	15	32.25	37.25		
19	**Total**					
20						
21						
22						
23						

Note that the formula in B8 refers to cell B15 (Week 1 hours) but to cell $B$2 – the absolute address of the chargeout rate.

The sales figure are untidy: some have comma separators between the thousands, some have one decimal place, some two. To tidy this up we will use the **Number** section of the Ribbon to format these numbers as **Currency**.

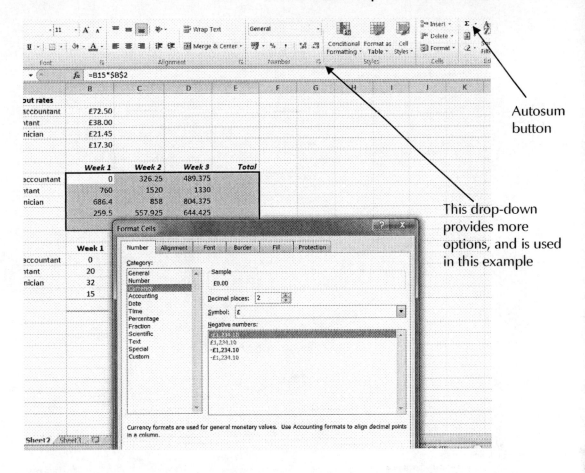

Autosum button

This drop-down provides more options, and is used in this example

---

(1) Select the range of cells B8:E12.

(2) Click in the small arrow just right of the word '**Number**' to open the **Format Cells** window.

(3) Select **Currency**, make sure the **Decimal places** reads 2 and that the £ symbol is showing.

You should see that all the figures in your spreadsheet are now in the same format.

(4) In cell E8, enter a formula to total the hours. This is easiest if you use the Autosum button.

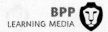

The spreadsheet should now be like this:

	B8	▼		*fx*	=B15*$B$2	
	A	B	C	D	E	F
1	**Internal chargeout rates**					
2	Divisional chief accountant	£72.50				
3	Assistant accountant	£38.00				
4	Accounting technician	£21.45				
5	Secretary	£17.30				
6						
7	**Costs**	*Week 1*	*Week 2*	*Week 3*	*Total*	
8	Divisional chief accountant	£0.00	£326.25	£489.38	£815.63	
9	Assistant accountant	£760.00	£1,520.00	£1,330.00	£3,610.00	
10	Accounting technician	£686.40	£858.00	£804.38	£2,348.78	
11	Secretary	£259.50	£557.93	£644.43	£1,461.85	
12	**Total**	**£1,705.90**	**£3,262.18**	**£3,268.18**	**£8,236.25**	
13						
14	**Hours**	*Week 1*	*Week 2*	*Week 3*	*Total*	
15	Divisional chief accountant	0	4.5	6.75	11.25	
16	Assistant accountant	20	40	35	95	
17	Accounting technician	32	40	37.5	109.5	
18	Secretary	15	32.25	37.25	84.5	
19	**Total**	**67**	**116.75**	**116.5**	**300.25**	
20						
21						
22						

And the formulae behind the cell contents should be:

	A	B	C	D	E
6					
7	Costs	Week 1	Week 2	Week 3	Total
8	Divisional chief accountant	=B15*$B$2	=C15*$B$2	=D15*$B$2	=SUM(B8:D8)
9	Assistant accountant	=B16*$B$3	=C16*$B$3	=D16*$B$3	=SUM(B9:D9)
10	Accounting technician	=B17*$B$4	=C17*$B$4	=D17*$B$4	=SUM(B10:D10)
11	Secretary	=B18*$B$5	=C18*$B$5	=D18*$B$5	=SUM(B11:D11)
12	Total	=SUM(B8:B11)	=SUM(C8:C11)	=SUM(D8:D11)	=SUM(E8:E11)
13					
14	Hours	Week 1	Week 2	Week 3	Total
15	Divisional chief accountant	0	4.5	6.75	=SUM(B15:D15)
16	Assistant accountant	20	40	35	=SUM(B16:D16)
17	Accounting technician	32	40	37.5	=SUM(B17:D17)
18	Secretary	15	32.25	37.25	=SUM(B18:D18)
19	Total	=SUM(B15:B18)	=SUM(C15:C18)	=SUM(D15:D18)	=SUM(E15:E18)
20					
21					
22					

However, after designing the spreadsheet, you find out that the Divisional Chief Accountant has worked for 6 hours in week 4. He also wants you to add in to your calculations the cost of using two laptop computers which were charged out at £100 per week each, for the first 3 weeks. You have also found out that the secretarial chargeout rate was increased by 10% in week 3. You now need to amend the spreadsheet to reflect these changes.

(1)   Insert a column between columns D and E.

(2)   Label E7 and E14 as Week 4.

(3)   Enter the 6 hours in cell E15.

(4)   Enter a formula in cell E8 to calculate the cost of these hours.

(5)   Insert a row between rows 11 and 12.

(6)   Enter Laptops in cells A6 and A12.

(7)   In cell A22, enter Laptops and enter the number of laptops used each week.

(8)   In cell B6 enter the cost of each laptop per week.

(9)   Use a formula in cells B12 to D12 to calculate the cost of the laptops.

(10) Insert two rows between row 6 and 7.

(11) In cell B7, enter the percentage increase in the secretary's chargeout rate. Format this cell as percentage. Amend the formula in cell D13 accordingly.

(12) You may have noticed that the total cost has not altered.   This is because we have inserted rows and columns which were outside the range of the original formula used to calculate the totals. Amend your formulas accordingly.

Tidy the spreadsheet up

The presentation is reasonable as we have taken care of it as we have developed the spreadsheet. This is good practice. You can now apply different formatting techniques – change font colour or cell colour, for example. Save the spreadsheet as 'Costing exercise-finished'.

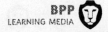

The spreadsheet should now look like this:

	A	B	C	D	E	F
	F15		f_x	=SUM(F10:F14)		
1	**Internal chargeout rates**					
2	Divisional chief accountar	£72.50				
3	Assistant accountant	£38.00				
4	Accounting technician	£21.45				
5	Secretary	£17.30				
6	Laptop cost	£100.00				
7	Chargeout rate	10%				
8						
9	**Costs**	*Week 1*	*Week 2*	*Week 3*	*Week 4*	*Total*
10	Divisional chief accountar	£0.00	£326.25	£489.38	£435.00	£1,250.63
11	Assistant accountant	£760.00	£1,520.00	£1,330.00	£0.00	£3,610.00
12	Accounting technician	£686.40	£858.00	£804.38	£0.00	£2,348.78
13	Secretary	£259.50	£557.93	£708.87	£0.00	£1,526.29
14	Laptops	£200.00	£200.00	£200.00		£600.00
15	Total	£1,905.90	£3,462.18	£3,532.62	£435.00	£9,335.69
16						
17	**Hours**	Week 1	Week 2	Week 3	Week 4	Total
18	Divisional chief accountant		4.5	6.75	6	17.25
19	Assistant accountant	20	40	35		95
20	Accounting technician	32	40	37.5		109.5
21	Secretary	15	32.25	37.25		84.5
22	Total	67	116.75	116.5	6	306.25
23						
24	Laptops	2	2	2		

And the formulas should look like this:

	A	B	C	D	E	F
	F15	▾	ƒₓ =SUM(F10:F14)			
1	Internal chargeout rates					
2	Divisional chief accountant	72.5				
3	Assistant accountant	33				
4	Accounting technician	21.45				
5	Secretary	17.3				
6	Laptop cost	100				
7	Chargeout rate	0.1				
8						
9	Costs		Week 1	Week 2	Week 3	Week 4	Total
10	Divisional chief accountant	=B18*$B$2	=C18*$B$2	=D18*$B$2	=E18*$B$2	=SUM(B10:E10)
11	Assistant accountant	=B19*$B$3	=C19*$B$3	=D19*$B$3	=E19*$B$3	=SUM(B11:E11)
12	Accounting technician	=B20*$B$4	=C20*$B$4	=D20*$B$4	=E20*$B$2	=SUM(B12:E12)
13	Secretary	=B21*$B$5	=C21*$B$5	=D21*($B$5+($B$5*$B$7))	=E21*$B$2	=SUM(B13:E13)
14	Laptops	=B24*$B$6	=C24*$B$6	=D24*$B$6		=SUM(B14:E14)
15	Total	=SUM(B10:B14)	=SUM(C10:C14)	=SUM(D10:D14)	=SUM(E10:E14)	=SUM(F10:F14)
16						
17	Hours		Week 1	Week 2	Week 3	Week 4	Total
18	Divisional chief accountant		4.5	6.75	6	=SUM(B18:E18)
19	Assistant accountant	20	40	35		=SUM(B19:D19)
20	Accounting technician	32	40	37.5		=SUM(B20:D20)
21	Secretary	15	32.25	37.25		=SUM(B21:D21)
22	Total	=SUM(B18:B21)	=SUM(C18:C21)	=SUM(D18:D21)	=SUM(E18:E21)	=SUM(B22:E22)
23						
24	Laptops	2	2	2		

Example: commission calculations

Four telesales staff each earn a basic salary of £14,000 pa. They also earn a commission of 2% of sales. The following spreadsheet has been created to process their commission and total earnings. Give an appropriate formula for each of the following cells.

    (a)   Cell D4
    (b)   Cell E6
    (c)   Cell D9
    (d)   Cell E9

	A	B	C	D	E
1	Sales team salaries and commissions - 200X				
2	Name	Sales	Salary	Commission	Total earnings
3		£	£	£	£
4	Northington	284,000	14,000	5,680	19,680
5	Souther	193,000	14,000	3,860	17,860
6	Weston	12,000	14,000	240	14,240
7	Easterman	152,000	14,000	3,040	17,040
8					
9	Total	641,000	56,000	12,820	68,820
10					
11					
12	Variables				
13	Basic Salary	14,000			
14	Commission rate	0.02			
15					

Solution

Possible formulae are:

(a) =B4*$B$14

(b) =C6+D6

(c) =SUM(D4:D7)

(d) There are a number of possibilities here, depending on whether you set the cell as the total of the earnings of each salesman (cells E4 to E7): =SUM(E4:E7) or as the total of the different elements of remuneration (cells C9 and D9): =SUM(C9:D9). Even better, would be a formula that checked that both calculations gave the same answer. A suitable formula for this purpose would be:

=IF(SUM(E4:E7)=SUM(C9:D9),SUM(E4:E7),"ERROR")

We explain this formula after the next example, don't worry about it at the moment!

Example: actual sales compared with budget sales

A business often compares its results against budgets or targets. It is useful to express differences or **variations as a percentage of the original budget**, for example sales may be 10% higher than predicted.

Continuing the telesales example, a spreadsheet could be set up as follows showing differences between actual sales and target sales, and expressing the difference as a percentage of target sales.

	A	B	C	D	E
1	Sales team comparison of actual against budget sales				
2	Name	Sales (Budget)	Sales (Actual)	Difference	% of budget
3		£	£	£	£
4	Northington	275,000	284,000	9,000	3.27
5	Souther	200,000	193,000	(7,000)	(3.50)
6	Weston	10,000	12,000	2,000	20.00
7	Easterman	153,000	152,000	(1,000)	(0.65)
8					
9	Total	638,000	641,000	3,000	0.47
10					

Give a suitable formula for each of the following cells.

(a) Cell D4

(b) Cell E6

(c) Cell E9

Try this for yourself, before looking at the solution.

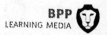

Solution

(a)   =C4 − B4

(b)   =(D6/B6)*100

(c)   =(D9/B9)*100. Note that in (c) you **cannot simply add up the individual percentage differences**, as the percentages are based on different quantities.

FORMULAE WITH CONDITIONS

Suppose the employing company in the above example awards a bonus to people who exceed their target by more than £1,000. The spreadsheet could work out who is entitled to the bonus.

To do this we would enter the appropriate formula in cells F4 to F7. For salesperson Easterman, we would enter the following in cell F7:

=IF(D4>1000,"BONUS"," ")

We will now explain this **IF** function.

IF statements follow the following structure (or 'syntax').

=IF(logical_test, value_if_true, value_if_false)

The logical_test is any value or expression that can be evaluated to Yes or No. For example, D4>1000 is a logical expression; if the value in cell D4 is over 1,000, the expression evaluates to Yes. Otherwise, the expression evaluates to No.

Value_if_true is the value that is returned if the answer to the logical_test is Yes. For example, if the answer to D4>1000 is Yes, and the value_if_true is the text string "BONUS", then the cell containing the IF function will display the text "BONUS".

Value_if_false is the value that is returned if the answer to the logical_test is No. For example, if the value_if_false is two sets of quote marks "" this means display a blank cell if the answer to the logical test is No. So in our example, if D4 is not over 1,000, then the cell containing the IF function will display a blank cell.

Note the following symbols which can be used in formulae with conditions:

   <   less than

   <=   less than or equal to

   =   equal to

   >=   greater than or equal to

   >   greater than

   <>   not equal to

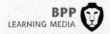
BPP LEARNING MEDIA

Care is required to ensure **brackets** and **commas** are entered in the right places. If, when you try out this kind of formula, you get an error message, it may well be a simple mistake, such as leaving a comma out.

Using the IF function

A company offers a discount of 5% to customers who order more than £10,000 worth of goods. A spreadsheet showing what customers will pay may look like:

	C8				fx	=IF(B8>$C$3, B8*$C$4,0)	
	A	B	C	D	E	F	
1	**Sales discount**						
2							
3	Discount hurdle		10,000				
4	Discount rate		5%				
5							
6	**Customer**	**Sales**	**Discount**	**Net price**			
7		£	£	£			
8	John	12,000	600	11,400			
9	Margaret	9,000	0	9,000			
10	William	8,000	0	8,000			
11	Julie	20,000	1000	19,000			
12							
13							
14							
15							

The formula in cell C8 is as shown: =**IF**(B8>$C$3, B8*$C$4, 0). This means, if the value in B8 is greater than £10,000 multiply it by the contents of C4, ie 5%, otherwise the discount will be zero. Cell D8 will calculate the amount net of discount, using the formula: =B8−C8. The same conditional formula with the cell references changed will be found in cells C9, C10 and C11.

Here is another example for you to try.

Open the spreadsheet called Exam Results (one of the spreadsheets downloaded from www.bpp.com/aatspreadsheets).

There are ten candidates listed together with their marks.

The pass mark has been set at 50%.

See if you can complete column C rows 6–15 so that it shows PASS if the candidate scores 50 or above, and FAIL if the candidate scores less than 50.

Once it's set up and working correctly, change the pass mark in cell B3 to 60 and ensure that the PASS/FAIL indications reflect the change.

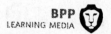

The formulae you need will be based on the one for cell C6.

| | C6 | ▼ | | f_x | =IF(B6>=$B$3, "PASS","FAIL") |

Book3

	A	B	C	D	E	F
1	**Exam results**					
2						
3	Pass mark	50				
4						
5	Candidate	Mark	Pass/fail			
6	Alf	51	PASS			
7	Beth	56	PASS			
8	Charles	82	PASS			
9	David	42	FAIL			
10	Edwina	68	PASS			
11	Frances	36	FAIL			
12	Gary	75	PASS			
13	Hugh	53	PASS			
14	Iris	72	PASS			
15	John	34	FAIL			

Conditional formatting

In addition to the condition determining whether PASS or FAIL appear, you can also conditionally format cell contents – for example, by altering the colour of a cell to highlight problems. This can be done by accessing the **Conditional Formatting** option in the **Styles** section of the **Home** tab of the Ribbon.

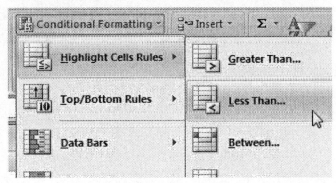

The marks which are less than the value in B3 have been highlighted by making the cell background red and the text white, as illustrated below:

	A	B	C
1	**Exam results**		
2			
3	Pass mark	50	
4			
5	Candidate	Mark	Pass/fail
6	Alf	51	PASS
7	Beth	56	PASS
8	Charles	82	PASS
9	David	42	FAIL
10	Edwina	68	PASS
11	Frances	36	FAIL
12	Gary	75	PASS
13	Hugh	53	PASS
14	Iris	72	PASS
15	John	34	FAIL

To produce the above result:

> Change the pass mark back to 50% if it is still at 60%.
>
> Highlight the numbers in column B.
>
> Click **Conditional formatting>Highlight cell rules>Less than**. You will see there are two white entry boxes.
>
> Click on cell B3. This will be entered automatically into the first box.
>
> Then click on the down arrow next to the second entry box. Click on **Custom format>Fill** and choose the red box. This changes the colour of the cell.
>
> Then click on **Font** and click the down arrow next to 'Automatic', under **Colour** and choose the white box.
>
> Click **OK**.

You can also use Conditional formatting to highlight the top three results for example:

	A	B	C	D
1	**Exam results**			
2				
3	Pass mark	50		
4				
5	**Candidate**	**Mark**	**Pass/fail**	
6	Alf	51	PASS	
7	Beth	56	PASS	
8	Charles	82	PASS	
9	David	42	FAIL	
10	Edwina	68	PASS	
11	Frances	36	FAIL	
12	Gary	75	PASS	
13	Hugh	53	PASS	
14	Iris	72	PASS	
15	John	34	FAIL	
16				
17				
18				
19				
20				

To produce the above result:

> Highlight the numbers in column B.
>
> Click **Conditional formatting>Top/Bottom rules>Top 10 items.**
>
> In the first entry box, change the number from 10 to 3.
>
> In the second entry box, click on **Custom format>Fill** and choose the green box. This changes the colour of the cell.
>
> Then click on **Font** and click the down arrow next to 'Automatic', under **Colour** and choose the white box.
>
> Click **OK.**

Ranking data

The RANK function, one of Excel's statistical functions, ranks the size of a number compared to other numbers in a list a data.

The syntax for the RANK function is:

= RANK (Number, Ref, Order)

Number – the cell reference of the number to be ranked.

Ref – the range of cells to use in ranking the Number.

Order – determines whether the Number is ranked in ascending or descending order. 0 for descending order and 1 for ascending order.

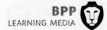

The names in the Exam Results spreadsheet are in alphabetical order. Say you want to keep them in that order but you want to see who came first, second, third etc. You can use RANK to give that information.

	D6			f_x =RANK(B6,$B$6:$B$15,0)			
	A	B	C	D	E	F	G
1	Exam results						
2							
3	Pass mark	50					
4							
5	Candidate	Mark	Pass/fail	Rank			
6	Alf	51	PASS	7			
7	Beth	56	PASS	5			
8	Charles	63	PASS	1			
9	David	42	FAIL	8			
10	Edwina	68	PASS	4			
11	Frances	36	FAIL	9			
12	Gary	73	PASS	2			
13	Hugh	53	PASS	6			
14	Iris	72	PASS	3			
15	John	34	FAIL	10			
16							

To produce the above result:

> Enter Rank in cell D5.
>
> In cell D6, type =RANK(B6,$B$6:$B$15,0). This means that B6 will be ranked within the range B6:B15 in descending order.
>
> Copy the formula to cells B7 to B15.

CHARTS AND GRAPHS

Charts and graphs are useful and powerful ways of communicating trends and relative sizes of numerical data. Excel makes the production of charts relatively easy through the use of the chart wizard.

We will use the Sales discount spreadsheet (one of the spreadsheets downloaded from www.bpp.com/aatspreadsheets) to generate a number of different charts.

	A	B	C	D
1	Sales discount			
2				
3	Discount hurdle		10,000	
4	Discount rate		5%	
5				
6	Customer	Sales	Discount	Net price
7		£	£	£
8	John	12,000	600	11,400
9	Margaret	9,000	0	9,000
10	William	8,000	0	8,000
11	Julie	20,000	1000	19,000

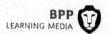

First, we will generate a simple pie chart showing the total sales figure, before discounts.

A simple pie chart

(1) Open the Sales discount spreadsheet.

(2) Place your cursor on the word 'Customer', hold down the mouse button and drag the cursor downwards until you have selected the four names and four sales figures.

(3) Select the **Insert** section from the Ribbon, then **Pie/3-D pie**.

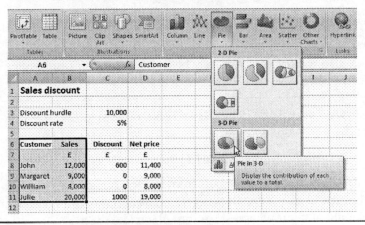

This will generate a pie chart that looks like this:

Sales £

You will see that it already has a title, 'Sales £'. To make any changes to this, double click the area where the title appears, then enter additional text or delete text you do not want. Below we have added 'for 20X6' and brackets around the pound sign.

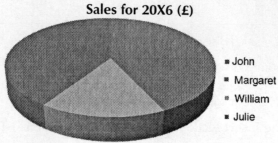

Changing the chart type

If you decide that a different chart may be more suitable for presenting your data you can easily change the chart type.

(1) Click on your chart. The **Chart Tools** options should become available at the top of the window.

(2) Click **Design>Change Chart Type**.

(3) From here, pick some charts from the following chart types to see what they produce: **Bar**, **Bubble**, **Doughnut** and **Line**. For example the doughnut chart will produce something like this:

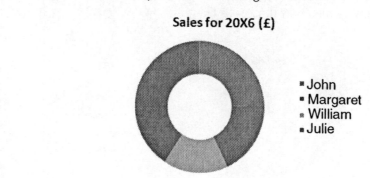

Bar charts

A pie chart is good for showing relative sizes of elements making up a total. However, sometimes you may want to be able to compare how two series of data are moving: sales and gross profit for example. In this case, bar charts (or line charts) are more suitable. Excel makes a distinction between bar charts that show vertical bars and those that show horizontal bars. **When the data is shown** *vertically* Excel refers to the chart as a *'column'* chart whereas if the data is shown *horizontally* it is a *'bar'* chart.

We are going to create a column chart showing the Sales and Net Price figure from the data on the Sales Discount spreadsheet.

(1) Delete your chart by clicking on its outer most frame and pressing the **Delete** key.

(2) Place the cursor on the word 'Customer' and drag the cursor down until all four names have been selected.

(3) Hold down the Ctrl button and select B6:B11. Still holding the Ctrl button down, select D6:D11.

(4) Release the mouse button and Ctrl key.

(5) On the Ribbon, choose **Insert>Column>2D Column**.

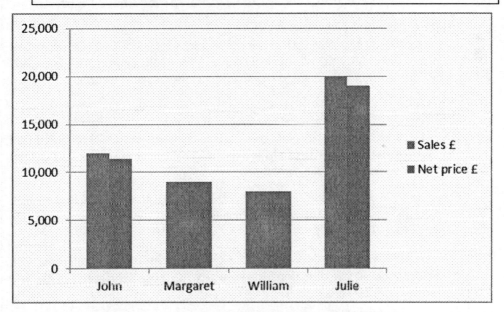

This time there is no automatic chart title so we will need to add one.

Click on the chart. At the top of the window you will see **Chart Tools** appear:

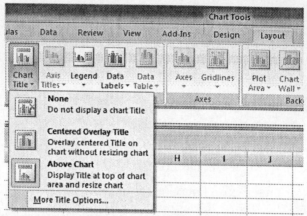

From the **Layout** section, choose **Labels>Chart Title>Above Chart**.

Type in "Sales and Net Prices for 20X6 (£)".

To the right of the chart you will see a description for each column. This is called a Legend. You can move the legend by clicking on the **Legend** button.

You should also label the horizontal axis and the vertical axis.

(1) To label the horizontal axis, click **Layout>Axis Titles>Primary Horizontal Axis>Title below axis** (make sure you are clicked on the chart to see the **Chart Tools** tabs).

(2) The words 'Axis Title' appear at the bottom of the chart. Click on this, then press **Ctrl + A** to select all the words and type in your axis title, in this case 'Customer'.

(3) To label the other axis, this time choose **Primary Vertical Axis**. You have a choice of directions for your text. Choose **Horizontal Title** and type a pound sign.

Note that if you are typing words for the vertical axis title the best option is usually **Rotated Title**. Try experimenting with that now.

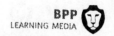

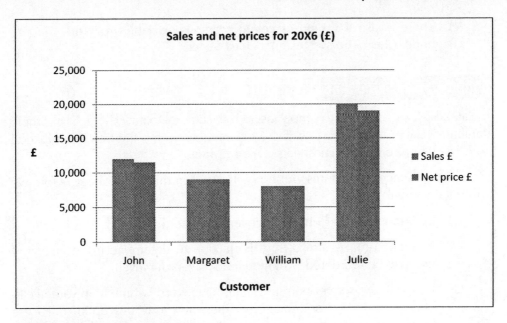

Formatting existing charts

Even after your chart is 'finished' you can change it in a variety of ways.

(a) You can **resize it** simply by selecting it and dragging out one of its corners.

(b) You can change the scale by dragging out the top, base or sides. To do so, hover your cursor over the four dots in the middle of the relevant top, base or side until your cursor turns into a **double ended arrow**. Click and it will turn into a large cross, then drag with the mouse button still held down.

(c) You can change **each element** by **clicking** on it then selecting from the options available on the various **Chart tools** tabs.

(d) You can also select any item of **text** and alter the wording, size or font, or change the **colours** used using the buttons on the **Font** section of the Home part of the ribbon. For example, practice increasing and decreasing the size of the font by clicking on the text you wish to change, then experimenting with the two different sized capital A buttons:

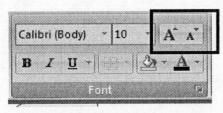

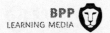

(e) There is also a variety of colour schemes available from the Ribbon, under **Chart Tools > Design > Chart Styles**.

Simple data manipulation

A database can be viewed simply as a collection of data. There is a simple 'database' related to inventory, called Stockman Ltd within the files downloaded from www.bpp.com/aatspreadsheets. **Open it now**.

There are a number of features worth pointing out in this spreadsheet before we start data manipulation.

(1) Each row from 4–15 holds an inventory record.

(2) Column G makes use of the **IF** function to determine if the inventory needs to be reordered (when quantity < reorder level).

(3) In row 2, the spreadsheet uses automatic word wrap within some cells. This can improve presentation if there are long descriptions. To use word wrap, select the cells you want it to apply to then click the **Wrap Text** icon in the **Alignment** section of the **Home** tab. The height of the cells needs to be increased to accommodate more than one line of text. To do this, select the whole row then double click on the line between the row numbers 2 and 3, or instead, select **AutoFit Row Height** as shown below.

The data is currently arranged in part number order.

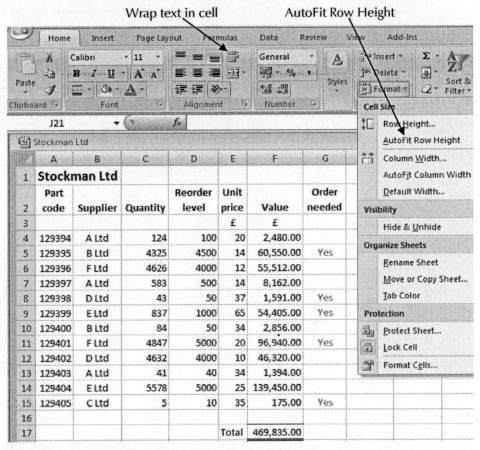

The horizontal rows are records: one record for each inventory type. The vertical columns are attributes (qualities) relating to each record.

Sorting the data

Let's say that we want to sort the data into descending value order.

(1) Select the data range A4:G15.

(2) At the right-hand side of the **Home** section of the Ribbon (and in the **Data** section of the Ribbon) you will see the **Sort & Filter** drop-down menu.

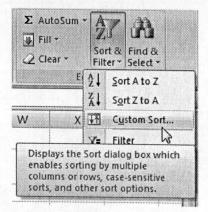

(3) Choose **Custom Sort**.

(4) Sort by Column F, largest to smallest.

(5) Click **OK**.

You will see that the data has been sorted by value.

If you now **Sort by** Supplier (**Order A–Z**) you will have the data arranged by supplier, and within that by value.

PRINTING

Printing spreadsheets

The print options for your spreadsheet may be accessed by selecting **Office button** and **Print>Print**, or pressing **Ctrl + P**. Printing large spreadsheets without checking the print and layout settings will often result in printouts spread messily over several pages.

It is a good idea to at least opt for **Print Preview** to see what your printout will look like before printing.

A better option is to control what prints more precisely. This can be done from the **Page Layout** section of the Ribbon.

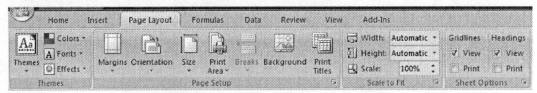

This allows you to, for example, print out selected areas only, include/exclude grid-lines and the column and row headings, alter the orientation of the page and so on.

Open the spreadsheet we saw earlier called Costing Exercise – Finished.

Assume that we only want to print out the Costs without the table at the top showing the assumptions. We want to show the gridlines but not the A, B, C... or 1, 2, 3... that head up columns and rows.

(1) Select the range A9:F24.

(2) Choose **Page Layout>Print Area>Set Print Area** from the Ribbon.

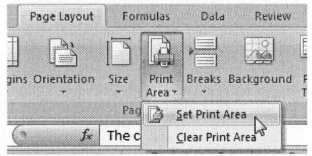

(3) Check the **Print Gridlines** box in **Page Layout>Sheet** options.

(4) Choose **Office Button>Print>Print Preview**.

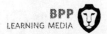

At this point you can check for obvious layout and formatting errors.

Spelling

Before you print, it is wise to check your work for spelling mistakes. To do this click the **Review** tab and select **Spelling**. If you have made any spelling errors Excel will offer alternative **Suggestions** which you can accept by clicking **Change** or ignore by clicking **Ignore** (**Once** or **All**).

If the word is in fact correct (for example, terminology that Excel does not recognise) you can add it to Excel's dictionary by clicking **Add to Dictionary**.

Preparing your spreadsheet for printing: Page set-up

The **Page Setup** area of the **Page Layout** tab on the Ribbon also allows you to specify certain other details that affect how your spreadsheet looks when it prints out.

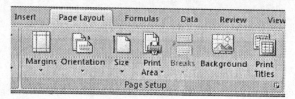

From here you can set the size of the **Margins** (the white spaces that print around the spreadsheet) and choose whether to print the spreadsheet in landscape **Orientation** (ie wider than tall) rather than the default portrait **Orientation** (taller than wide).

If you want to make sure that your spreadsheet will print onto one page, you can choose to Fit 1 page wide by 1 page tall. This can be done by accessing the **Page Setup** options, by clicking on the little arrow in the bottom right corner of the section on the ribbon.

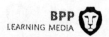

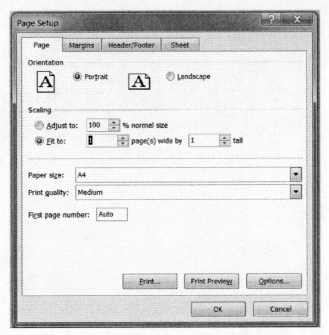

Imagine you are printing out a spreadsheet that will cover several pages. It is important that certain information is present on each page. For example:

- The spreadsheet title
- The page number and total pages
- The author
- The row and column headings

This can be done by accessing the **Page Setup** options, in the way outlined above, or by clicking on the **Print Titles** icon.

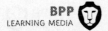

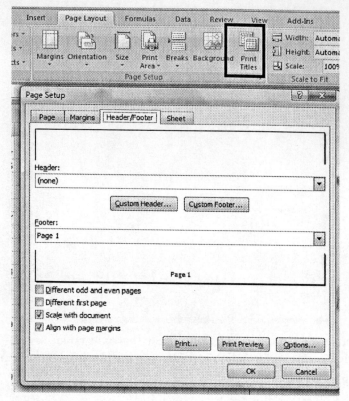

Headers appear at the top of each page. For example, a custom header could be:

Author   Budget for 2012   Date printed

Footers appear at the bottom of each page, for example:

Page   File name

The **Sheet** tab allows you to specify the rows and columns to be repeated on each page. For example, you might want to repeat the months across the top of each page and the type of income down the left of each page.

> We have provided a demonstration spreadsheet in the downloaded files, Print practice. Open it and try the following:
>
> Insert a **Header**: Author name, Title (Budget 2012) Date printed
>
> Insert a **Footer**: Page number, File name
>
> Click **Page setup** (or **Print Titles**)>Header/Footer> **Custom Header** and **Custom Footer**.
>
> Ensure that the headings in column A are repeated on the second page.

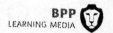

Use this spreadsheet to experiment with page breaks (**Breaks**) and the other remaining options in the **Page Setup** area.

Printing formulae

Occasionally, perhaps for documentation or checking, you might want the spreadsheet formulae to be printed out instead of the calculated results of the formula. To do this:

> (1) Display the formulae on the screen by pressing **Ctrl + `**.
>
> (2) Set the area you want to be printed: **Page Layout > Print Area > Set Area**
>
> (3) Check what the printout will look like **Office button > Print > Print preview**
>
> (4) Adjust as necessary and print out when happy with the display

Printing charts

Charts can be printed either with or without the data on the worksheet.

To print only the chart simply click on it and then press **Ctrl + P**. As always it is wise to **Print Preview** first.

If you also want to print the worksheet data, click away from the chart into any cell. Use **Print Preview** to make sure that the chart is the right size and is in the right position. Then press **Ctrl + P**.

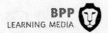

CHAPTER OVERVIEW

- A **spreadsheet** is basically an electronic piece of paper divided into **rows** and **columns**. The intersection of a row and a column is known as a **cell**.

- Essential basic **skills** include how to **move around** within a spreadsheet, how to **enter** and **edit** data, how to **fill** cells, how to **insert** and **delete** columns and rows and how to improve the basic **layout** and **appearance** of a spreadsheet.

- **Relative** cell references (eg B3) change when you copy formulae to other locations or move data from one place to another. **Absolute** cell references (eg $B$3) stay the same.

- A wide range of **formulae** and functions are available within Excel. We looked at the use of conditional formulae that use an **IF** statement.

- A spreadsheet should be given a **title** which clearly defines its purpose. The contents of rows and columns should also be clearly **labelled**. **Formatting** should be used to make the data in the spreadsheet easy to read and interpret.

- **Numbers** can be **formatted** in several ways, for instance with commas, as percentages, as currency or with a certain number of decimal places.

- Excel includes the facility to produce a range of charts and graphs. The **Chart Wizard** provides a tool to simplify the process of chart construction.

- Excel offers data handling including **sorting and ranking**.

- Spreadsheets can be used in a variety of accounting contexts. You should practise using spreadsheets, **hands-on experience** is the key to spreadsheet proficiency.

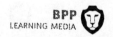

TEST YOUR LEARNING

Test 1

List three types of cell contents.

Test 2

What do the F5 and F2 keys do in Excel?

Test 3

What technique can you use to insert a logical series of data such as 1, 2 .... 10, or Jan, Feb, March etc?

Test 4

How do you display formulae instead of the results of formulae in a spreadsheet?

Test 5

List five possible changes that may improve the appearance of a spreadsheet.

Test 6

What is the syntax (pattern) of an IF function in Excel?

Test 7

The following spreadsheet shows sales of two products, the Ego and the Id, for the period July to September.

	A	B	C	D	E
1	Sigmund Ltd				
2	Sales analysis - quarter 3, 2010				
3		July	August	September	Total
4	Ego	3,000	4,000	2,000	9,000
5	Id	2,000	1,500	4,000	7,500
6	Total	5,000	5,500	6,000	16,500

Devise a suitable formula for each of the following cells.

    (a)   Cell B6

    (b)   Cell E5

    (c)   Cell E6

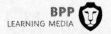

Test 8

The following spreadsheet shows sales, exclusive of VAT, the VAT amounts and the VAT inclusive amounts. The old VAT rate of 17.5% has been used and needs to be updated to the new 20% rate. It is important that this can easily be changed without needing to change any of the formulae in the spreadsheet.

	A	B	C	D
1	Taxable Supplies Ltd		Vat rate	0.175
2				
3		January	February	March
4	Product A	5,000	4,000	3,000
5	Product B	2,000	1,500	4,000
6	Product C	7,000	5,700	4,000
7	Product D	2,000	3,000	1,000
8	Product E	1,000	2,400	6,000
9	Total net	17,000	16,600	18,000
10	VAT	2,975	2,905	3,150
11	Total gross	19,975	19,505	21,150

Suggest suitable formulae for cells:

    (a)   B9

    (b)   C10

    (c)   D11

chapter 2:
MORE ADVANCED SPREADSHEET TECHNIQUES (EXCEL 2007)

---
chapter coverage 📖

In this chapter we explore some of the more advanced aspects of spreadsheets using Excel 2007.

This chapter covers:

✍ Controls, security and sharing

✍ Data manipulation

✍ Three dimensional (multi-sheet) spreadsheets

✍ Changes in assumptions (what-if? analysis)

✍ Statistical function

✍ Combination charts

✍ Error detection and correction

CONTROLS, SECURITY AND SHARING

Back-ups, passwords and cell protection

There are facilities available in spreadsheet packages which can be used as controls – to prevent unauthorised or accidental amendment or deletion of all or part of a spreadsheet. There are also facilities available for hiding data, and for preventing (or alerting) users about incorrect data.

Saving files and backing up

(a) **Save.** When working on a spreadsheet, save your file regularly, as often as every ten minutes, using **Office button>Save** or pressing **Ctrl + S**. This will prevent too much work being lost in the event of a system crash.

Save files in the appropriate **folder** so that they are easy to locate. If you need to save the file to a new folder, choose the '**New folder**' option after clicking **Office button>Save**. Where this option is located depends on the operating system you are using. For example, in Windows 7, you simply click the **New folder** button (see below).

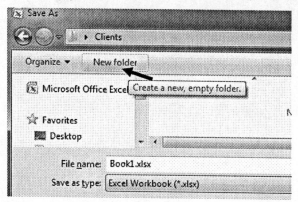

Give the folder a suitable name (for example, the name of the client you are working on or following your employer's standard naming practice).

(b) **Save as.** A simple **save** overwrites the existing file. If you use **Save as** then you can give the file a different name, preserving previous versions. For example Save as 'Budget Edition 1', 'Budget Edition 2', 'Budget Edition 3'. This is much safer than simply relying on the most recent version – which might be beyond fixing!

(c) **Back-ups.** Because data and the computers or storage devices on which it is stored can easily be lost or destroyed, it is vital to take regular copies or back-ups. If the data is lost, the back-up copy can be used to **restore** the data up to the time the back-up was taken. Spreadsheet files should be included in standard backup procedures, for example the daily back-up routine.

The back-ups could be held on a separate external hard drive, or perhaps a USB memory stick, and should stored away from the original data, in case there is a fire or other disaster at the organisation's premises. Alternatively the back-ups can be saved to a network location. Some back-ups are now stored on the Internet.

(d) **AutoRecover.** Excel has a built-in feature that saves copies of all open Excel files at a fixed time interval. The files can be restored if Excel closes unexpectedly, such as during a power failure.

Turn on the AutoRecover feature by clicking **Office button>Excel Options>Save**.

The default time between saves is every 10 minutes. To change this, click the **Save AutoRecover info every** check box and enter any number of minutes between 1 and 120.

In the **AutoRecover file location** box, you can type the path and the folder name of the location in which you want to keep the AutoRecover files.

Protection

(a) **Cell protection/cell locking.** This prevents the user from inadvertently changing cells that should not be changed. There are two ways of specifying which cells should be protected.

(i) All cells are locked except those specifically unlocked.

This method is useful when you want most cells to be locked. When protection is implemented, all cells are locked unless they have previously been excluded from the protection process. You will also see here a similar mechanism for hiding data.

> (1) Once again, open the spreadsheet Costing Exercise–Finished.
>
> (2) Highlight the range B2:B5. This contains some of the assumptions on which the costing exercise is based and this is the only range of cells that we want to be unlocked and available for alteration.
>
> (3) In the **Home** section of the Ribbon, click on the small arrow beside **Fonts** and then choose **Protection**.

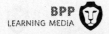

55

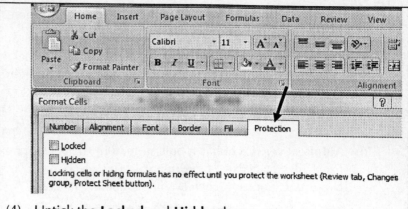

(4) Untick the **Locked** and **Hidden** boxes.

(5) Click on **OK**.

(6) Now go to the **Review** group on the **Ribbon**.

(7) Click on **Protect Sheet**.

(8) Don't enter a password when prompted, simply click **OK**.

Now investigate what you can change on the spreadsheet. You should find that only cells B2:B5 can be changed. If you try to change anything else a message comes up telling you that the cell is protected.

Click on **Unprotected Sheet** to make every cell accessible to change again.

(ii) Most are unlocked, except those specified as being locked.

This method is useful if only a few cells have to be locked.

(1) Open the spreadsheet Sales discount.

(2) Assume that we want to lock only the 10,000 in cell C3 and the 5% figure in cell C4.

(3) Select the whole spreadsheet and, as we did above, click on the small arrow beside **Fonts**. Then choose **Protection** and untick the **Locked** and **Hidden** boxes. The cells can still be changed if you do not do this step.

(4) Select the range of cells C3:C4.

(5) In the **Home** section of the Ribbon go to the **Cells** group and click on **Format**.

(6) Click on **Lock Cell**.

(7) Click on **Protect Sheet** from the same **Format** menu. The cells remain editable if you do not do this step.

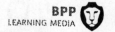

> You are offered the chance to enter a password.
>
> Now you will be prevented from changing just those two cells.

(b) **Passwords**. There are two levels of password.

(i) All access to the spreadsheet can be protected and the spreadsheet encrypted. This can be done by:

> (1) **Office button>Prepare>Encrypt Document**.
>
> (2) You are then asked to enter and verify a password. Heed the warning: if you forget the password, there's no likelihood of recovery of the spreadsheet.
>
> (3) To remove the password protection use:
> **Office button>Prepare>Encrypt Document**
>
> (4) Then delete the asterisks in the password box and click OK.

(ii) The spreadsheet can be password protected from amendment but can be seen without a password. This can be done as follows:

> (1) At the bottom of the **Save As** dialogue click **Tools**.
>
> (2) Choose **General Options**.
>
> (3) You can choose here again a Password to open.
>
> (4) In the Password to modify box type a password, then retype it to confirm and click **OK**.
>
> (5) Click **Save**.

Now, if you close the file and re-open it, you will be asked for a password to get full access, or without the password you can open it in read-only mode so that it can be seen but not changed.

Data validation

Sometimes only a specific type or range of data is valid for a certain cell or cells. For example, if inputting hours worked in a week from a time sheet it could be known that no one should have worked more than 60 hours. It is possible to test data as it is input and to either prevent input completely or simply warn that the input value looks odd. This is known as 'data validation' or 'data restriction'.

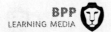

C2		▼		f_x	=A2*B2
	A	B	C	D	
1	Hours	Rate/hr	Pay		
2	10	7	70		

In this simple spreadsheet, C2 holds the only formula; A2 and B2 are cells into which data will be entered, but we want the data to conform to certain rules:

Hours <= 60. If greater than 60, a warning is to be issued.

Rate/hr >=8 and <=20. Data outside that range should be rejected.

(1) Set up a new spreadsheet with the above data and make A2 the active cell. Go to **Data>Data Validation** (in **Data Tools** section).

(2) Under the **Data Validation Settings** tab, **Allow Decimal**, select less than or equal to from the drop-down list and enter 60 as the Maximum.

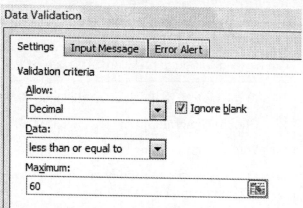

(3) Under the **Input Message** tab enter 'Warning' as the title and 'Hours expected to be less than 60' as the input message.

(4) Under the **Error Alert** tab change the **Style** to Warning, enter 'Attention' as the title and 'Check hours: look too large' as the **Error message**.

(5) Click **OK**.

(6) Now try to enter 70 into A2. You will first see an information message explaining what data is expected, then a warning message and the option to continue.

(7) Now try to set up cell B2 with appropriate messages and to prevent any value outside the range 8–20 from being entered at all.

DATA MANIPULATION

Data manipulation refers to a number of techniques available in Excel for summarising, analysing and presenting data.

Filtering the data

Filtering data allows you to select and display just some of it in the table. This is useful if the table consists of many records but you only wish to view some of them.

Open the Stockman Ltd spreadsheet.

Let's say we just want to find inventory records relating to suppliers B and C.

Select **Filter** from the **Sort & Filter** drop-down menu.

Click on the drop-down arrow that has appeared at the top of the Supplier column.

Deselect (ie click on the box to remove the tick) **Select All**, then select B and C.

Click on **OK**.

Only the records relating to suppliers B and C are visible and these can be manipulated (eg sorted) as an independent subset of the whole table.

Note that the other records are still there and are included in the total value figure. It's simply that they have been hidden for presentation.

You will also see a little funnel symbol at the top of the Supplier column informing that there is filtering in place.

Make all the records visible again by removing the filter:

(1) Drop-down arrow in the Supplier column.
(2) Select **Select All**.
(3) Click on **OK**.
(4) Sort the data back into Part code order if it's not already in that order.

To get rid of the little filter arrows, click on the funnel symbol in the **Sort & Filter** area of the Ribbon to disengage it.

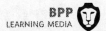

Find and replace

Let's now say that that Supplier A Ltd has been taken over and that its name has changed to Acorn plc.

> (1) Make all the records visible again by removing the filter if you haven't already
>
> (2) Click on the **Find & Select** symbol and select **Find** (or press **Ctrl + F**)
>
> (3) Enter A Ltd in the **Find what**: box
>
> (4) Click on the **Replace** tab and enter Acorn Plc in the **Replace with**: box
>
> (5) Click on **Replace All**
>
> **Note**. You could instead click on **Find & Select > Replace** (or press **Ctrl + H**) as a shortcut.

You should see that all occurrences of A Ltd have been replaced by Acorn plc.

If no range is specified before this step then the whole spreadsheet would be affected. If a range is specified, the search and replace occurs only within that range.

Σ AutoSum

You have already used Σ AutoSum as a way of specifying a range of data to add up. However, the Σ AutoSum drop-down list also contains other useful functions such as:

- **Average**
- **Count numbers**
- **Maximum**
- **Minimum**

Still using the Stockman Ltd spreadsheet:

> (1) Select cells E4..E15
>
> (2) From the **Σ AutoSum** drop-down list (you can find this on both the **Home** and **Formulas** tabs of the Ribbon) select **Max**
>
> You will see 65 appear in cell E16 (just below the last unit price). The formula in that cell is =MAX(E4:E15).
>
> Try some of the other **Σ AutoSum** functions.

The results given by **Σ AutoSum** are always just under a column of data, or immediately to the right of a row of data.

If you want the results to appear in a different cell, you have to type the appropriate formula into that cell. For example, typing =MAX(E4:E15) into cell A20 will show the maximum unit price of the inventory in cell A20.

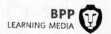

Concatenate

The concatenate function is used to combine two text cells into a single cell.

This is done by using the formula =CONCATENATE(text1, [text 2]…)

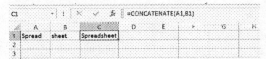

If the formula is used as shown above, the words will be joined together with no space inbetween.

If a space is to be included between the words, this can be achieved by using quotation marks around a single space between the two text references in the formula.

=CONCATENATE(text1, " ",[text 2]…)

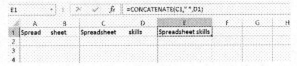

This is particularly useful when joining data such as first name and last name.

Pivot tables

Pivot tables are a very powerful way of analysing data. Look at the following simple example relating to sales by a music company.

	A	B	C
	Pivot table example		
1	Sales data		
2			
3	Customer	Source	Amount spent (£)
4	Bill	CDs	50
5	Chris	Vinyl	10
6	Sandra	Merchandise	30
7	Graham	CDs	45
8	Chris	Merchandise	20
9	Chris	Vinyl	10
10	Chris	CDs	10
11	Caroline	Merchandise	30
12	Graham	Tickets	75
13	Fred	Vinyl	30
14	Bill	CDs	20
15	Graham	CDs	60
16	Chris	Vinyl	10
17	Sandra	Tickets	50
18	Bill	Tickets	26
19	Caroline	Vinyl	24
20			
21		Total	£500

The information has simply been listed and totalled on the spreadsheet. It would be useful to be able to show:

- Sales per customer
- Sales by source

Ideally, we would like to produce a table which displays sales by both source and by customer: this type of table is called a pivot table.

(1) Open the spreadsheet file called Pivot Table Example which contains the above data.

(2) Select the range A4:C19.

(3) On the Ribbon, select **Insert>PivotTable**.

(4) Select the **Existing Worksheet** radio button on the **Create PivotTable** option window.

(5) Enter E4 as the location.

(6) Click **OK**. The PivotTable Field List window opens.

(7) Check Customer, Source, Amount spent (£).

(8) You will see that Customer and Source go by default into Row Labels. The resulting table is quite useful, but not quite what we wanted.

Therefore:

(9) Drag Customer from Row Labels to Column Labels.

The pivot table is now transformed into the two-dimensional table we want.

(10) Tidy it up a little by selecting F5 to L5 and right justifying these names by clicking on the appropriate Home>Alignment button on the Ribbon.

Note the two drop down arrows on the pivot table that allow filtering of the data.

Sum of Amount spent (£)	Column Labels						
Row Labels	Bill	Caroline	Chris	Fred	Graham	Sandra	Grand Total
CDs	70		10		105		185
Merchandise		30	20			30	80
Tickets	26				75	50	151
Vinyl		24	30	30			84
Grand Total	96	54	60	30	180	80	500

If you had difficulty with this, the spreadsheet called 'Pivot Table Result Excel 2007' is available within the downloaded files.

Experiment with different settings. Clicking on the pivot table will bring up the **PivotTable Field List** window again if it has disappeared.

Note that if the original data is altered, the pivot table does *not* change until you right-click on it and select **Refresh** from the list of options.

Pivot charts

The information contained in a pivot table can be visually presented using a pivot chart.

(1) Click on any cell inside the pivot table.

(2) On the insert tab click column and select one of the subtypes. For example, clustered.

Note any changes you make to the pivot table will be immediately reflected in the pivot chart and vice versa.

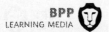

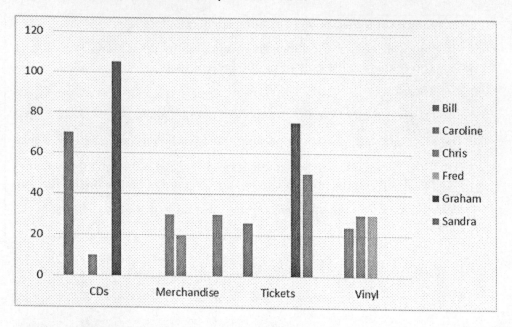

Sharing workbooks

It is possible to share a workbook with colleagues so that the same file can be viewed by more than one person at a time. This can be done in a number of ways.

Send as an attachment

One way to share a spreadsheet with colleagues is to send it as an attachment in an email. If your computer is set up with a mail client such as Microsoft Outlook you can click **Office Button>Send>Email** to quickly send the spreadsheet you are working on as an attachment.

Alternatively, you can first draft the email and attach the spreadsheet using your email program's options and the Windows Explorer menu.

However, if each recipient of the email makes changes to the document, this will lead to the existence of a number of different versions of the same document, and a potential loss of version control. This is not, therefore, a recommended method of sharing spreadsheets.

Save to a shared network server

Another way to make a spreadsheet available to colleagues is to save it in a place on the network server that is also accessible to them. Anyone with access to that particular location will be able to open the file but, if more than one person tries to open the file, only the first person will be able to make changes to it. Anyone else subsequently opening the file will only be able to open a 'Read Only' version of it, so they will be able to view the contents but not make any changes.

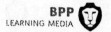

This method prevents loss of version control but is not particularly useful if other people wish to make changes at the same time.

Share workbook method

A more practical method is to use the inbuilt sharing function in Excel. This allows different people to open and make changes to the same document at the same time, and for these changes to be tracked.

Click the **Review** tab on the Ribbon. In the **Changes** section click the **Share Workbook** button. Click the **Editing** tab and select **Allow changes by more than one user at the same time**. From this tab you can also see who has the document open.

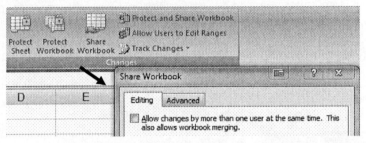

Other settings are available from the **Advanced** tab such as choosing how long to keep the change history for, how frequently to update changes and what to do if users make conflicting changes.

To stop any tracked changes from being lost click **Protect and Share Workbook** and click **Sharing with tracked changes**. This option also allows you to set a password so only those with the password can make changes.

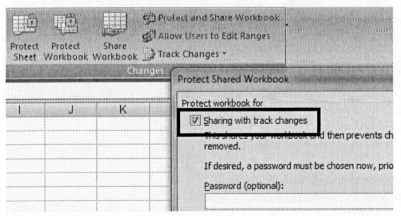

THREE DIMENSIONAL (MULTI-SHEET) SPREADSHEETS

Background

In early spreadsheet packages, a spreadsheet file consisted of a single worksheet. As mentioned earlier, Excel provides the option of multi-sheet spreadsheets, consisting of a series of related sheets.

For example, suppose you were producing a profit forecast for two regions, and a combined forecast for the total of the regions. This situation would be suited to using separate worksheets for each region and another for the total. This approach is sometimes referred to as working in **three dimensions**, as you are able to flip between different sheets stacked in front or behind each other. Cells in one sheet may **refer** to cells in another sheet. So, in our example, the formulae in the cells in the total sheet would refer to the cells in the other sheets.

Excel has a series of 'tabs', one for each worksheet at the bottom of the spreadsheet.

How many worksheets?

Excel can be set up so that it always opens a fresh file with a certain number of worksheets ready and waiting for you. Click on **Office button > Excel Options > Popular**, and set the number **'Include this many sheets'** option to the number you would like each new workbook to contain (sheets may be added or deleted later).

If you subsequently want to insert more sheets you just click on the new sheet tab.

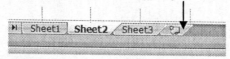

By default sheets are called Sheet 1, Sheet 2 etc. However, these may be changed. To rename a sheet in Excel, right click on its index tab and choose the **Rename** option. You can drag the sheets into different orders by clicking on the tab, holding down the mouse button and dragging a sheet to its new position.

Pasting from one sheet to another

When building a spreadsheet that will contain a number of worksheets with identical structure, users often set up one sheet, then copy that sheet and amend its contents.

To copy a worksheet in Excel, from within the worksheet you wish to copy, select **Home > Cells > Format > Move or Copy Sheet** (or right click the worksheet tab and select **Move or Copy Sheet**) and tick the **Create a copy** box.

BPP
LEARNING MEDIA

A 'Total' sheet would use the same structure, but would contain formulae totalling the individual sheets.

Linking sheets with formulae

Formulae on one sheet may refer to data held on another sheet. The links within such a formula may be established using the following steps.

Step 1   In the cell that you want to refer to a cell from another sheet, type =.

Step 2   Click on the index tab for the sheet containing the cell you want to refer to and select the cell in question.

Step 3   Press **Enter.**

---

(1)   Open the spreadsheet called 3D spreadsheet example.

This consists of three worksheets. The Branch A and Branch B sheets hold simple trading accounts and income statements. There are both numbers and formulae in those sheets. The Company sheet contains only headings, but is set out in the same pattern as the two branch sheets.

We want to combine the Branch figures onto the Company sheet.

(2)   On the Company sheet, make D2 the active cell

(3)   Enter =

(4)   Click on Branch A and click on D2

(5)   Enter +

(6)   Click on Branch B and click on D2

(7)   Press **Enter**

You will see that the formula ='Branch A'!D2+'Branch B'!D2 is now in cell D2 of the Company sheet and that the number displayed is 500,000, the sum of the sales in each branch.

In the Company sheet, copy D2 (**Ctrl+C**) and paste (**Ctrl+V**) to D3, D4, C6, C7, C8, and D9 to complete the income statement.

The company sheet will now look like this:

	A	B	C	D
	3D spreadsheet example [Compatibility Mode]			
1	**Company**		£	£
2	Revenue			500,000
3	Cost of sales			270,000
4	Gross profit			230,000
5	Expenses:			
6	Selling and distribution		70,000	
7	Administration		45,000	
8				115,000
9	Net profit			115,000
10				
11				

This is arithmetically correct, but needs lines to format it correctly.

Use the border facility in **Home>Font** to insert appropriate single and double lines (**borders**) in the cells:

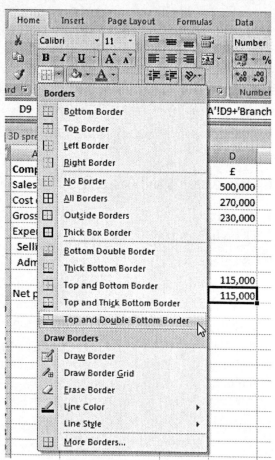

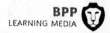

The final consolidated results should look like:

	A	B	C	D
	3D spreadsheet example [Compatibility Mode]			
1	**Company**		£	£
2	Revenue			500,000
3	Cost of sales			270,000
4	Gross profit			230,000
5	Expenses:			
6	Selling and distribution		70,000	
7	Administration		45,000	
8				115,000
9	Net profit			115,000

Note. If you change any figures in Branch A or Branch B, the figures will also change on the Company spreadsheet.

Uses for multi-sheet spreadsheets

There are a wide range of situations suited to the multi-sheet approach. A variety of possible uses follow.

(a) A spreadsheet could use one sheet for variables, a second for calculations, and a third for outputs.

(b) To enable quick and easy **consolidation** of similar sets of data, for example the financial results of two subsidiaries or the budgets of two departments.

(c) To provide different views of the same data. For instance, you could have one sheet of data sorted into product code order and another sorted into product name order.

Formatting data as a table

You can format data within a spreadsheet as a table. This provides you with another way to present and manipulate data.

Creating a table

First we will create a table and then we'll look at what we can do with it.

(1) **Open** the Tables example spreadsheet from the downloaded files. This uses almost the same data as in the previous exercise, so should look familiar to you.

(2) Select the cells that contain the data (A3 to G15).

(3) On the **Home** tab of the Ribbon select **Format as Table** from the **Styles** section.

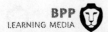

(4) A gallery of styles will appear, so choose one of the formats (any one will do). Check that the correct data for the table is selected in the white box and tick the box **My table has headers**.

(5) Click **OK**.

(6) Your table should now look something like this, depending on which format you chose:

	A	B	C	D	E	F	G
1	Stockman Ltd						
2							
3	Part cod	Supplie	Quantit	Reorder leve	Unit pric	Value	Order neede
4	129394	A Ltd	134	100	20	2,480.00	
5	129395	B Ltd	4325	4500	14	60,550.00	Yes
6	129396	F Ltd	4626	4000	12	55,512.00	
7	129397	A Ltd	583	500	14	8,162.00	
8	129398	D Ltd	43	50	37	1,591.00	Yes
9	129399	E Ltd	837	1000	65	54,405.00	Yes
10	129400	B Ltd	84	50	34	2,856.00	
11	129401	F Ltd	4847	5000	20	96,940.00	Yes
12	129402	D Ltd	4632	4000	10	46,320.00	
13	129403	A Ltd	41	40	34	1,394.00	
14	129404	E Ltd	5578	5000	25	139,450.00	
15	129405	C Ltd	5	10	35	175.00	Yes

You will notice that there are **Sort & Filter** drop down arrows at the top of each column in the header row. This is just one of the benefits of formatting data as a table: automatic **Sort & Filter**.

Other benefits of formatting data as a table

Other benefits include:

(a) **Easy row and column selection**

Move the cursor to the top of the header row of the table and it will change to a thick pointing arrow. When you click, just the data in that column will be selected (and not the empty cells below the data). You can select data rows in a similar way.

The whole table can be selected by hovering near the table's top left corner until the arrow becomes thick and starts pointing towards the bottom right hand corner.

(b) **Visible header row when scrolling**

When you scroll down past the bottom of the table the column letters become the table's column names so long as you have clicked anywhere inside the table before starting scrolling.

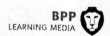

Part code	Supplier	Quantity	Reorder level	Unit price	Value	Order needed
129394	A Ltd	124	100	20	2,480.00	
129395	B Ltd	4325	4500	14	60,550.00	Yes
129396	F Ltd	4626	4000	12	55,512.00	
129397	A Ltd	583	500	14	8,162.00	
129398	D Ltd	43	50	37	1,591.00	Yes
129399	E Ltd	837	1000	65	54,405.00	Yes
129400	B Ltd	84	50	34	2,856.00	
129401	F Ltd	4847	5000	20	96,940.00	Yes
129402	D Ltd	4632	4000	10	46,320.00	
129403	A Ltd	41	40	34	1,394.00	
129404	E Ltd	5578	5000	25	139,450.00	
129405	C Ltd	5	10	35	175.00	Yes

(c) **Automatic table expansion**

Type anything into any of the cells around the table and the table will automatically grow to include your new data. The formatting of the table will automatically adjust (this will also happen if you insert or delete a row or column).

(d) **Automatic formula copying**

If you enter a formula in a cell around the table and click **Enter**, the column will automatically resize to fit the formula, which is automatically copied down to fill the entire column alongside your data.

Changing the design of the table

You can change how the table looks by clicking anywhere in the table and selecting **Design** tab from the **Table Tools** toolbar.

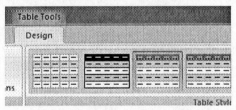

From here there are a number of **Table Style Options** that you can play around with, such as formatting a **First Column** or **Last Column**, adding a **Total Row** and changing the **Table Style**.

You can also choose to give your table a name so that any formula you enter which uses the figures from the table will refer to that table by its name.

So, for example, type 'Parts' into the **Table Name** box:

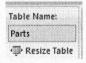

Now any formula entered in the column next to the table will refer to the table by name. Try it!

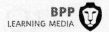

Font		Alignment			Number				Styles			Cells

✓ ƒx =Parts[[#This Row],[Quantity]]*Parts[[#This Row],[Unit price]]

C	D	E	F	G	H	I	J	K	L	M

antit ▼	Reorder leve ▼	Unit pric ▼	Value ▼	Order neede ▼		
		£	£			
124	100	20	2,480.00			
4325	4500	14	60,550.00	Yes	=Parts[[#This Row],[Quantity]]*Parts[[#This Row],[Unit price]]	
4626	4000	12	55,512.00			
583	500	14	8,162.00			
43	50	37	1,591.00	Yes		
837	1000	65	54,405.00	Yes		

Table tools

From the **Design** tab you can also:

- Choose to **Remove Duplicates**, which, as the name suggests, removes duplicate data from the table,

- **Summarize with PivotTable** (see below), and

- Remove the table formatting completely by selecting **Convert to Range**. You may then wish to clear the formatting. You can easily do this by clicking **Clear** on the **Editing** section of the **Home** tab and choosing **Clear formats**.

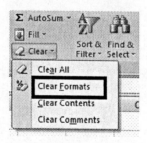

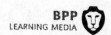

Look-up tables

The Look-up function allows you to find and use data that is held in a table.

VLOOKUP is used for finding data in **v**ertical columns.

HLOOKUP is used for finding data in **h**orizontal rows.

Here is a simple example:

	A	B	C	D	E	F	G	H	I
1	**Salesman Ltd**								
2	Part code	VATcode	Unit price		VAT rate	20.0%			
3			£						
4	129394	1	20.00						
5	129395	1	14.00		Invoice				
6	129396	0	12.00						
7	129397	0	14.00						
8	129398	1	37.00		Part code	Quantity	Unit price	VAT	£
9	129399	0	65.00		129396	10	12.00	0	120.00
10	129400	1	34.00					Net	120.00
11	129401	0	20.00					VAT	0.00
12	129402	1	10.00					Total	120.00
13	129403	0	34.00						
14	129404	0	25.00						
15	129405	1	35.00						
16									
17									

On the left is a price list. If a part has a VAT code of 1, then VAT will be charged at the rate as set in cell F2; if the VAT code is 0, then no VAT is chargeable.

To create this invoice, you would look down the part numbers column until you found 129396. You would then read across to find the unit price and VAT code and, together with the quantity sold, you could create the invoice.

This process has been automated in the spreadsheet Salesman Ltd.

> (1) Open the Spreadsheet called Salesman Ltd.
> (2) Click on cell G9 to reveal the use of the VLOOKUP function.

Cell G9 holds the formula =VLOOKUP(E9,A4:C15,3, FALSE)

This means: look for the value held in cell E9, in the first row of the range A4:C15, and return the value in the third column of the range: it will return the price relating to the part number. FALSE (at the end of the statement) asks it to find an exact match so if a non-existent part code is entered in E9 you will get an error message (**#N/A**).

Similarly, cell H9 holds the formula =VLOOKUP(E9,A4:C15,2) and will return the VAT code relating to the part number.

Cell I11 holds a conditional (IF) function that will calculate VAT if the VAT code is 1 and insert 0 if the VAT code is 0.

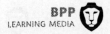

Note that some cells have been formatted to show two decimal places and some to show no decimal places. Cell F2 is formatted as a percentage and, because VAT might need to be changed, VAT is held in only one location with other cells referring to it.

Try out different part codes and quantities in the invoice.

CHANGES IN ASSUMPTIONS (WHAT-IF? ANALYSIS)

We referred earlier to the need to design a spreadsheet so that **changes in assumptions** do **not** require **major changes** to the spreadsheet. In our Costing Exercise workbook we set up two separate areas of the spreadsheet, one for assumptions and opening balances and one for the calculations and results. We could simply change the values in the assumptions cells to see how any changes in assumptions affect the results.

However, if we have more than one value to change, or we want to see the result of a number of different assumption changes we can use one of the three 'What if' functions.

Data tables

A **data table** is a way to see different results by altering an input cell in a formula. You can create one- or two-variable data tables.

Let's try creating a one-variable data table.

---

(1) Open the earlier spreadsheet Mortgage which used the PMT formula.

(2) Enter 1% to 10% in cells E8 to L8 as shown below. You will need to increase the width of cells I8 & J8.

	A	B	C	D	E	F	G	H	I	J	K	L	M	N
1	Assumptions													
2														
3	Annual interest rate		10%											
4	Amount of loan (£)		20,000											
5	Period of loan		20											
6														
7	Calculation of monthly repayments over a reducing balance mortgage lasting (years)													
8					1%	2%	3%	4%	5%	6%	7%	8%	9%	10%
9	Monthly repayment			-£193.00										
10														

(3) Select cells D8 to N9.

(4) **Click Data > What-If Analysis > Data Table.**

(5) Here you want your data table to fill in the values in row 9, based on the results if the value in cell C3 were to change to a different percentage, so choose the **Row input cell** box and enter C3.

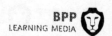

You should get the following results:

	1%	2%	3%	4%	5%	6%	7%	8%	9%	10%
-£193.00	-91.9789	-101.177	-110.92	-121.196	-131.991	-143.286	-155.06	-167.288	-179.945	-193.004

The table would look better if the numbers were formatted in the same way as the first result in cell D9. An easy way to copy a format from one cell to another is to click on the cell whose format you wish to copy then click the **Format Painter** button on the **Clipboard** area of the **Home** tab and then click on the cells you wish to format.

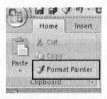

Try it now. Click on cell D9, then click the **Format Painter** button. Now select cells E9:M9. You should see:

	1%	2%	3%	4%	5%	6%	7%	8%	9%	10%
-£193.00	-£91.98	-£101.18	-£110.92	-£121.20	-£131.99	-£143.29	-£155.06	-£167.29	-£179.95	-£193.00

Note. If you double click the **Format Painter** button you can then click any number of cells afterwards to apply that same format. To stop the **Format Painter**, simply click **Esc** (Escape).

Now let's try a two-variable data table using the same workbook. This time we want to see the result if both the interest rate and the number of years of the loan change.

(1) Rename the worksheet you have been working on to 'One variable'. Now select Sheet2 (or insert a new worksheet if necessary) and rename it 'Two variable'. This is the sheet that we will now use.

(2) **Copy** the data on the One variable worksheet (**Ctrl + C**) and paste (**Ctrl + V**) into the new worksheet.

(3) Select cells E8 to N8 and move them up down by one cell (ie to E9 to N9). You can do this by hovering over the selected cells until a cross with four arrow heads appears, then click and drag to cell E9. Alternatively, **Cut** (**Ctrl + X**) and then **Paste** (**Ctrl + V**) to cell E9.

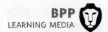

(4) In cells D10 to D14 insert different loan periods. We have used 10, 15, 20, 25 and 30 years as shown below:

-£193.00	1%	2%	3%	4%	5%	6%	7%	8%	9%	10%
10										
15										
20										
25										
30										

(5) Select cells D9 to N14

(6) **Click Data>What-If Analysis>Data Table**

(7) Here you want the data table to fill in the values based on the results if the value in cell C3 were to change to a different percentage (as shown in row 9) and also if the loan period in C5 changes (as shown in column D). So, choose the **Row input cell** box and enter C3 and then select the **Column input cell** box and enter C5.

You should get the following results:

-£193.00	1%	2%	3%	4%	5%	6%	7%	8%	9%	10%
10	-£175.21	-£184.03	-£193.12	-£202.49	-£212.13	-£222.04	-£232.22	-£242.66	-£253.35	-£264.30
15	-£119.70	-£128.70	-£138.12	-£147.94	-£158.16	-£168.77	-£179.77	-£191.13	-£202.85	-£214.92
20	-£91.98	-£101.18	-£110.92	-£121.20	-£131.99	-£143.29	-£155.06	-£167.29	-£179.95	-£193.00
25	-£75.37	-£84.77	-£94.84	-£105.57	-£116.92	-£128.86	-£141.36	-£154.36	-£167.84	-£181.74
30	-£64.33	-£73.92	-£84.32	-£95.48	-£107.36	-£119.91	-£133.06	-£146.75	-£160.92	-£175.51

Format cells E10 to N14 in the same way as cell D9.

Finally practise saving the file as 'Mortgage – Data tables' in a new folder on your computer using **Office button>Save as**. Choose an appropriate name for the folder – it's your choice!

Scenarios

The Scenarios function allows you to change information in cells that affect the final totals of a formula and to prepare instant reports showing the results of all scenarios together.

Using the spreadsheet Costing Exercise – Finished, we will show the result of changing the following assumptions:

(a) The chargeout rate for the Accounting Technician is now £30.00.
(b) The cost of a laptop has increased to £115.00 per week.
(c) The increase in chargeout rate for the secretary has been altered to 8%.

You could simply change the relevant cells in the spreadsheet to reflect these changes in assumptions. However, we are going to use the Scenario Manager function.

BPP
LEARNING MEDIA

(1) Select the **Data** tab and from the **Data Tools** section click **What-If Analysis>Scenario Manager**.

(2) Click **Add** and give the scenario an appropriate name, for example 'Original cash flow'.

(3) Press the tab button or click in the **Changing cells** box and, based on the information we used above, select the cells with the changing data, ignoring the change to the opening bank balance. To select cells that are not next to each other, use the Ctrl button. You should **Ctrl click** on cells B4, B6, B7.

(4) Click **OK**.

(5) You are now asked for **Scenario Values**. This will show the values currently in the cells specified, which are our original figures so click **OK**.

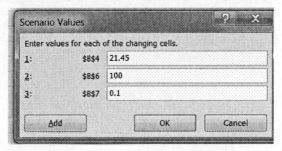

(6) We now need to enter our new values. Click **Add** and type a new **Name** (for example Costing exercise 2). The **Changing Cells** box will already contain the correct cells.

(7) Click **OK**.

(8) In the **Scenario Values** boxes change the values as follows and click **OK**.

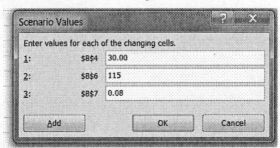

(9) Your second scenario should be highlighted. Now if you click on **Show** the figures in your assumptions table should automatically change and you can view the results.

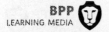

	L22		f_x			
	A	B	C	D	E	F	G
1	**Internal chargeout rates**						
2	Divisional chief accountant	£72.50					
3	Assistant accountant	£38.00					
4	Accounting technician	£30.00					
5	Secretary	£17.30					
6	Laptop cost	£115.00					
7	Chargeout rate	8%					
8							
9	**Costs**	*Week 1*	*Week 2*	*Week 3*	*Week 4*	*Total*	
10	Divisional chief accountant	£0.00	£326.25	£489.38	£435.00	£1,250.63	
11	Assistant accountant	£760.00	£1,520.00	£1,330.00	£0.00	£3,610.00	
12	Accounting technician	£960.00	£1,200.00	£1,125.00	£0.00	£3,285.00	
13	Secretary	£259.50	£557.93	£695.98	£0.00	£1,513.40	
14	Laptops	£230.00	£230.00	£230.00		£690.00	
15	**Total**	**£1,979.50**	**£3,604.18**	**£3,640.35**	**£435.00**	**£10,349.03**	
16							
17	**Hours**	Week 1	Week 2	Week 3	Week 4	Total	
18	Divisional chief accountant		4.5	6.75	6	17.25	
19	Assistant accountant	20	40	35		95	
20	Accounting technician	32	40	37.5		109.5	
21	Secretary	15	32.25	37.25		84.5	
22	**Total**	**67**	**116.75**	**116.5**	**6**	**300.25**	
23							
24	Laptops	2	2	2			
25							
26							
27							

(10) Click back on your original Costing exercise and then click **Show** and the numbers will change back.

Note. You may need to make your screen smaller to view the whole sheet at the same time. You can do this by clicking **View** on the Ribbon, then in the **Zoom** section clicking on **Zoom** and choosing a smaller percentage. 75% should be perfect.

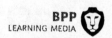

You can also easily and quickly create a report from the scenarios.

	A	B	C	D	E	F
1	**Internal chargeout rates**					
2	Divisional chief accountar	£72.50				
3	Assistant accountant	£38.00				
4	Accounting technician	£30.00				
5	Secretary	£17.30				
6	Laptop cost	£115.00				
7	Chargeout rate	8%				
8						
9	Costs	*Week 1*	*Week 2*	*Week 3*	*Week 4*	*Total*
10	Divisional chief accountar	£0.00	£326.25	£489.38	£435.00	£1,250.63
11	Assistant accountant	£760.00	£1,520.00	£1,330.00	£0.00	£3,610.00
12	Accounting technician	£960.00	£1,200.00	£1,125.00	£0.00	£3,285.00
13	Secretary	£259.50	£557.93	£695.98	£0.00	£1,513.40
14	Laptops	£230.00	£230.00	£230.00		£690.00
15	Total	£2,209.50	£3,834.18	£3,870.35	£435.00	£10,349.03
16						
17	Hours	Week 1	Week 2	Week 3	Week 4	Total
18	Divisional chief accountant		4.5	6.75	6	17.25
19	Assistant accountant	20	40	35		95
20	Accounting technician	32	40	37.5		109.5
21	Secretary	15	32.25	37.25		84.5
22	Total	67	116.75	116.5	6	306.25
23						
24	Laptops	2	2	2		
25						

(1) Click **Data>What-If Analysis>Scenario Manager**.

(2) Click the **Summary** button.

(3) In the **Result cells** box choose the cells to go into the report, ie the ones you want to see the results of. As we are interested in the final cost select cell F315. This creates a separate **Scenario Summary** worksheet. Open the Costing Exercise – What-if spreadsheet if you do not see the following report.

A1				f_x		

	A	B	C	D	E	F	G
1							
2		Scenario Summary					
3				Current Values:	Original costing exercise		Costing exercise 2
5		Changing Cells:					
6		$B$4		£21.45	£21.45		£30.00
7		$B$6		£100.00	£100.00		£115.00
8		$B$7		10%	10%		8%
9		Result Cells:					
10		$F$15		£9,335.69	£9,335.69		£10,349.03
11		Notes: Current Values column represents values of changing cells at					
12		time Scenario Summary Report was created. Changing cells for each					
13		scenario are highlighted in gray.					
14							
15							
16							
17							
18							

Goal seek

What if you already know the result you want from a formula but not the value the formula itself needs to calculate the result? In this case you should use the **Goal Seek** function, which is located in the **Data Tools** section of the **Data** tab on the Ribbon.

Open the original Mortgage spreadsheet from the downloaded files. Let's assume that we have enough income to pay a monthly mortgage payment of £300 and want to know how many years it will take to pay off the mortgage.

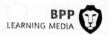

(1) Copy the data on Sheet 1 and paste it to Sheet 2.

(2) Click **Data>What-If Analysis>Goal Seek**.

(3) **Set cell** to D9, as this is the figure we know and enter -300 in the **To value** box (make sure that you enter a negative figure to match the figure already in D9).

(4) Enter C5 in the **By changing cell** box, as this is the figure we are looking for.

(5) Click **OK**.

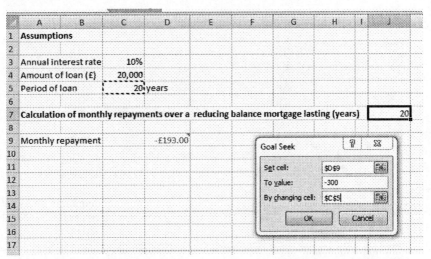

Goal seek will find the solution, 8.14 years, and insert it in cell C5.

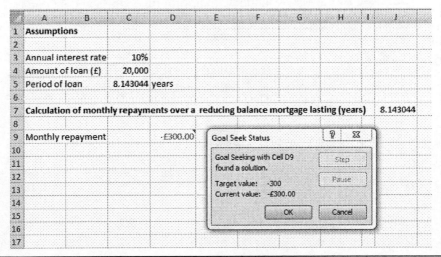

STATISTICAL FUNCTIONS

Linear regression/trends

Excel contains powerful statistical tools for the analysis of information such as how costs vary with production volumes and how sales vary through the year.

Look at the following example of costs and volume:

Month	Volume £	Costs
1	1,000	8,500
2	1,200	9,600
3	1,800	14,000
4	900	7,000
5	2,000	16,000
6	400	5,000

It is clear that at higher production volumes costs are higher, but it would be useful to find a relationship between these variables so that we could predict what costs might be if production were forecast at, say, 1,500 units.

The first investigation we could perform is simply to draw a graph of costs against volume. Volume is the independent variable (it causes the costs) so should run on the horizontal (x) axis.

Open the spreadsheet called Cost_volume and draw a scatter graph showing cost against volume, with appropriate labels and legends.

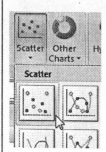

(1)   Select the range B1:C7.

(2)   Using **Insert/Chart** from the Ribbon, choose the top left Scatter graph type).

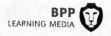

It should look something like the following:

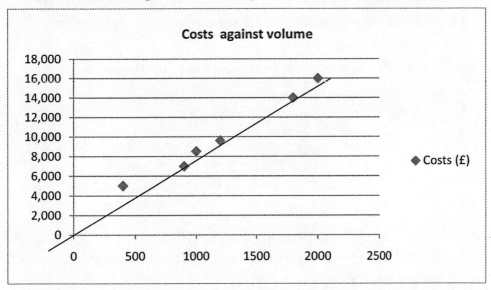

The straight line through the points has been manually drawn here to show that there's clearly a good association between volume and cost because the points do not miss the line by much, but we want to analyse this properly so that we can make a fairly good prediction of costs at output of say 1,500 units.

Lines of the sort above have a general equation of the type:

$$y = mx + b$$

Here **y** = Total costs

x = Volume

m = Variable cost per unit (the slope of the line)

b = The fixed cost (where the line crosses the y axis: the cost even at zero volume)

Excel provides two easy ways of finding the figures we need for predicting values.

Find the trend:

(1) On the same spreadsheet (Cost_volume), enter 1,500 in cell B9.

(2) Now click on cell C9.

(3) From the Ribbon choose **Formulas>More Functions>Statistical**.

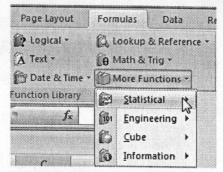

(4) Scroll down the list until you get to **TREND** and choose that.

(5) For **Known_y's** select the range C2:C7.

(6) For **Known_x's** select the range B2:B7.

(These ranges are the raw material which the calculation uses)

For **New_x's**, enter B9, the volume for which we want the costs to be predicted.

The number 12,003 should appear in cell C9. That is the predicted cost for output of 1,500 units – in line with the graph. In practice, we would use 12,000. Altering the value in B9 will produce the corresponding predicted cost.

A second way of analysing this data will allow us to find the variable and fixed costs of the units (**m** and **b** in the equation **y = mx +b**).

(1) To find **m** use the statistical function **LINEST** and assign the **Known_y's** and **Known_x's** as before. You should get the answer 7.01, the variable cost per unit.

(2) To find the intersection, **b**, use the statistical function **INTERCEPT**. You should get the answer 1,486.

Note. These can be used to predict the costs of 1,500 units by saying:

Total costs = 1,486 + 7.01 × 1,500 = 12,001, more or less as before.

The spreadsheet called Cost_volume finished contains the graph, and the three statistical functions just described.

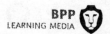

Moving averages

Look at this data

Year	Quarter	Time series	Sales £'000
20X6	1	1	989.0
	2	2	990.0
	3	3	994.0
	4	4	1,015.0
20X7	1	5	1,030.0
	2	6	1,042.5
	3	7	1,036.0
	4	8	1,056.5
20X8	1	9	1,071.0
	2	10	1,083.5
	3	11	1,079.5
	4	12	1,099.5
20X9	1	13	1,115.5
	2	14	1,127.5
	3	15	1,123.5
	4	16	1,135.0
20Y0	1	17	1,140.0

You might be able to see that the data follows a seasonal pattern: for example there always seems to be a dip in Quarter 3 and a peak in Quarter 2. It is more obvious if plotted as a time series of sales against the consecutively numbered quarters.

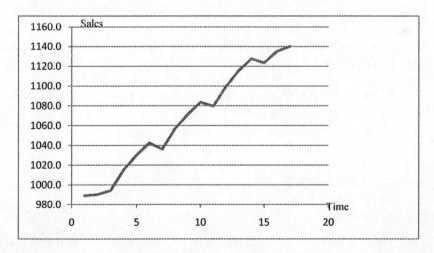

The moving average technique attempts to even out the seasonal variations. Here, because we seem to have data repeating every four readings a four-part

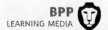

moving average would be appropriate. If you were trading five days a week and wanted to even out the sales, a five-part moving average would be suitable.

The moving average is calculated as follows:

Take the first four figures and average them:

$$\frac{(989.0 + 990.0 + 994.0 + 1,015.0)}{4} = 997.0$$

Then move on one season:

$$\frac{(990.0 + 994.0 + 1,015.0 + 1,030.0)}{4} = 1,007.3$$

and so on, always averaging out all four seasons. Each average will include a high season and a low season.

That's rather tedious to do manually and Excel provides a function to do it automatically. To access this analysis function you must have the Excel Analysis ToolPak installed. If it is installed there will be an **Analysis > Data Analysis** tab in the **Data** section of the Ribbon.

If it is not already installed, you can install it as follows:

(1)   Click the **Microsoft Office Button** , and then click **Excel Options**.

(2)   Click **Add-Ins**, and then from the **Manage** box, select **Excel Add-Ins**.

(3)   Click **Go**.

(4)   In the **Add-Ins available** box, select the **Analysis ToolPak** check box, and then click OK.

Tip. If **Analysis ToolPak** is not listed in the **Add-Ins available** box, click **Browse** to locate it.

If you are prompted that the Analysis ToolPak is not currently installed on your computer, click **Yes** to install it. This may take a little time, so be patient!

---

(1)   Open the spreadsheet called Time series
(2)   Select **Data > Data analysis > Moving average**
(3)   Select D2:D18 as the **Input Range**
(4)   Enter 4 as the **Interval** (a four-part moving average)
(5)   Enter F2 as the **Output Range**
(6)   Check **Chart Output**
(7)   Click on **OK**

Don't worry about the error messages – the first three simply mean that you can't do a four-part average until you have four readings.

Move your cursor onto the moving average figures and move it down, one cell at a time to see how the averages move.

BPP
LEARNING MEDIA

Notice on the graph how the Forecast line (the moving average) is much smoother than the actual figures. This makes predicting future sales much easier.

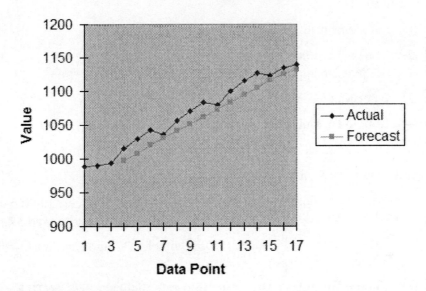

Moving average

Mean, mode and median

These are three measures of what is known as the 'location' of data – they give an indication of whereabouts the data is clustered.

Mean (or arithmetic mean) is the ordinary average (add up the readings and divide by the number of readings).

Mode is the most frequently occurring item. For example, in a shoe shop, the arithmetic mean of shoe sizes is not much use. The shopkeeper is more interested in the most common shoe size.

Median is the value of the middle item if they are arranged in ascending or descending sequence. As well as medians you can have 'quartiles' (upper and lower) dividing the population into top one-quarter, lowest three-quarters (or *vice versa*) and 'deciles' (10:90 splits).

Excel allows all of these measures to be calculated (or identified) easily.

(1) Open the spreadsheet called Student Results.

This lists the exam results of 23 students. They are currently displayed in alphabetical order. Don't worry about the column headed 'Bins' for now.

Enter 'Mean' in cell A28, then make cell B28 active.

(2) Choose **Formulas>Σ AutoSum>Average** and accept the range offered. 58.56 is the arithmetic mean of the marks.

(3) Enter 'Median' in cell A29, then make cell B29 active.

(4) Choose **Formulas>More Functions>Statistical>MEDIAN**.

(5) Enter the range B4:B26 for Number 1.

You should see 57 as the median.

Check this by sorting the data into descending order by score, then counting up to the 12th student, Kate. (She's the middle student and scored 57.)

(6) Enter 'Percentile' in cell A30, 0.75 in cell C30 and then make cell B30 active.

(7) Choose **Formulas>More Functions>Statistical>PERCENTILE**.

(8) Enter the range B4:B26 and C30 as the K value.

The reported value is 68, the figure which divides the top quarter from the bottom three-quarters of students.

(9) Enter 'Mode' in cell A31 then make cell B31 active.

(10) Choose **Formulas>More Functions>Statistical>Mode**.

(11) Enter the range B4:B26.

The reported value is 65 (that occurs more frequently than any other score).

Histograms

A histogram is a graph which shows the frequency with which certain values occur. Usually the values are grouped so that one could produce a histogram showing how many people were 160 – 165cm tall, how many >165 – 170, >170 – 175 and so on.

Excel can produce histogram analyses provided the Analysis ToolPak is installed. Installation was described earlier in the section about time series.

To demonstrate the histogram we will use the Student results spreadsheet again.

BPP
LEARNING MEDIA

(1) Open the Student Results spreadsheet if it is not already open.

You will see that in E5 to E13 is a column called 'Bins'. This describes the groupings that we want our results to be included in, so here we are going up the result in groups (bins) of ten percentage points at a time and the histogram will show how many results are in 0 – 10, 10 – 20, 20 – 30 etc.

(2) Choose **Data>Data Analysis>Histogram**.

(3) Enter the range B4:B26 as the **Input Range**.

(4) Enter E5:E13 as the **Bin Range**.

(5) Choose **New Worksheet Ply** and enter 'Histogram analysis' in the white text box.

(6) Tick **Chart Output**.

(7) Click on **OK**.

The new worksheet will show the data grouped into the 'bins' by frequency and also shows a histogram.

The spreadsheet 'Student Results Finished' shows the finished spreadsheet complete with histogram in the Histogram analysis sheet.

COMBINATION CHARTS

Excel allows you to combine two different charts into one. For example you may wish to compare sales to profits. This is also known as showing two graphs on one axis.

To do this we create a chart from our data as before.

(1) Open the Combination Chart spreadsheet from the downloaded files. This provides data for the number of sales of precious metal in 2009 and 2010. The price at which the precious metal is sold per kilo goes up and down according to the market.

(2) Select the data that will go into your chart (cells A1 to C9).

(3) Click Insert and then choose your chart type. For this example let's choose a **2D clustered column** chart. The chart doesn't really help us to understand the relationship between the two different sets of data.

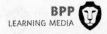

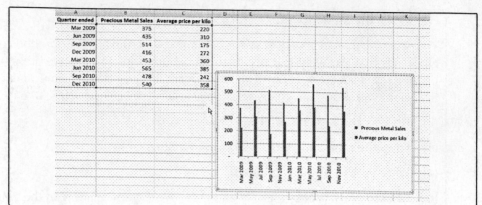

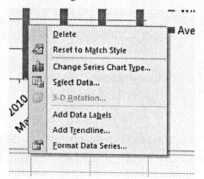

(4) A more visual way of displaying the average price data might be to see it in a line set against the number of sales. So click on any Average price column, right click and select **Change Series Chart Type**.

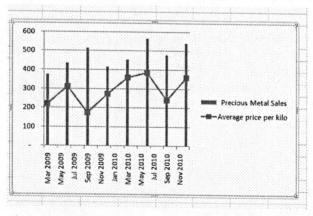

(5) Select **Line with Markers** and click **OK**. The chart will look like this:

(6) The chart still does not make sense as the figures on the left axis are not comparing like with like. So we need to right click again an Average price marker and choose **Format Data Series**.

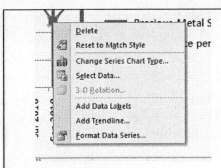

(7) Click **Secondary Axis**.

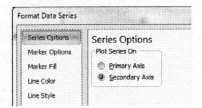

(8) Click **OK**.

(9) Take some time to play with the **Chart Tools**. Give the chart the name 'Precious Metal Sales' and label the axes. The vertical axis on the left should show the 'Number of sales', while the right hand axis should show the 'Price per kilo'.

You should end up with a chart that looks something like:

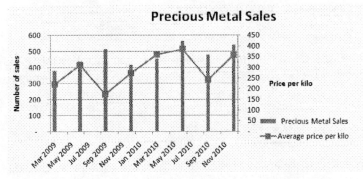

It can clearly be seen that the price per kilo dips in the third quarter of each year, something we could not easily determine without using the combination chart.

ERROR DETECTION AND CORRECTION

It is important to try to detect and correct errors before a spreadsheet is used to make decisions. We've already looked at some ways of trying to prevent wrong input (for example, data validation).

The final part of this chapter covers Excel's built-in help facility, error messages and ways to check that a spreadsheet has been constructed and is being used correctly.

Help

You can use Excel's Help window to quickly find the answer to any questions you may have while using Excel. You can access Help by clicking the **Help** button (the white question mark in the blue circle) in the top right corner of your spreadsheet or by pressing **F1**.

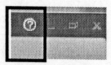

You can either type a search term directly into the white bar, or click on the **book icon** to access a table of help contents.

Or type query here →

Table of contents

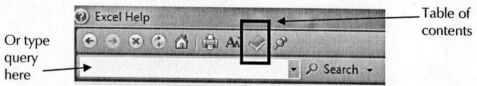

Take some time to explore the results when you type in different search terms. For example, if you found the section on What If analysis challenging, you could type 'What if' into the search bar to receive help on this topic.

Removing circular references

Circular references nearly always mean that there's a mistake in the logic of the spreadsheet. Here's an example:

	A	B
1		
2		£
3	Basic salary	20,000
4	Bonus 10% of total pay	=0.1*B5
5	Total pay	20,000

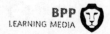

A warning will be displayed by Excel:

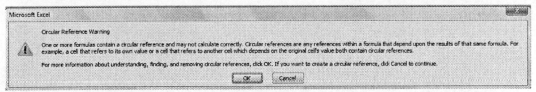

In our example, it is relatively easy to find the cause of the problem, but in a large spreadsheet it can be difficult. Clicking **OK** will provide help and will bring up a help screen referring you to **Formulas>Formula Auditing>Circular References** on the Ribbon.

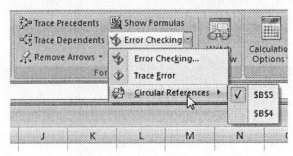

Using trace precedents

Tracing precedents and dependents

As spreadsheets are developed it can become difficult to be sure where figures come from and go to (despite being able to display formulae in all the cells). A useful technique is to make use of the trace precedents and trace dependents options. These are available on the **Formulas** section of the **Ribbon**.

---

(1) Open the Precedent example spreadsheet from the downloaded files and make cell F4 active.

(2) Choose the **Formulas** section of the Ribbon and click on **Trace Precedents** in the **Formula Auditing** group of icons.

You should see:

	A	B	C	D	E	F
1	BUDGETED SALES FIGURES					
2		Jan	Feb	Mar		Total
3		£'000	£'000	£'000		£'000
4	North	2,431	3,001	2,189		7,621
5	South	6,532	5,826	6,124		18,482
6	West	895	432	596		1,923
7	Total	9,858	9,259	8,909		28,026

Now it is very obvious that anything in column E, like April figures will not be included in the total.

(3) Click on **Remove Arrows** in the **Formula Auditing** group.

(4) Make B4 the active cell.

(5) Click on **Trace Dependents**. This will show what cells make use of this cell:

	A	B	C	D	E	F
1	BUDGETED SALES FIGURES					
2		Jan	Feb	Mar		Total
3		£'000	£'000	£'000		£'000
4	North	2,431	3,001	2,189		7,621
5	South	6,532	5,826	6,124		18,482
6	West	895	432	596		1,923
7	Total	9,858	9,259	8,909		28,026

Rounding errors

The ability to display numbers in a variety of formats (eg to no decimal places) can result in a situation whereby totals that are correct may actually look incorrect.

Example: rounding errors

The following example shows how apparent rounding errors can arise.

	A	B	C
1	*Petty cash*		
2	Week ending 31/12/20X6		
3			£
4	Opening balance		231.34
5	Receipts		32.99
6	Payments		-104.67
7	Closing balance		159.66

	A	B	C
1	*Petty cash*		
2	Week ending 31/12/20X6		
3			£
4	Opening balance		231
5	Receipts		33
6	Payments		-105
7	Closing balance		160

Cell C7 contains the formula =SUM(C4:C6). The spreadsheet on the left shows the correct total to two decimal places. The spreadsheet on the right seems to be saying that 231 + 33 – 105 is equal to 160, which is not true, it's 159 (check it). The **reason for the discrepancy** is that both spreadsheets actually contain the values shown in the spreadsheet on the **left**.

However, the spreadsheet on the right has been formatted to display numbers with **no decimal places**. So, individual numbers display as the nearest whole number, although the actual value held by the spreadsheet and used in calculations includes the decimals.

The round function

One solution, that will prevent the appearance of apparent errors, is to use the **ROUND function**. The ROUND function has the following structure: ROUND (value, places). 'Value' is the value to be rounded. 'Places' is the number of places to which the value is to be rounded.

The difference between using the ROUND function and formatting a value to a number of decimal places is that using the ROUND function actually **changes** the **value**, while formatting only changes the **appearance** of the value.

In the example above, the ROUND function could be used as follows. The following formulae could be inserted in cells D4 to D7.

D4 = ROUND(C4,0)
D5 = ROUND(C5,0)
D6 = ROUND(C6,0)
D7 = Round (SUM(D4:D6),0)

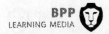
BPP
LEARNING MEDIA

Column C could then be hidden by highlighting the whole column (clicking on the C at the top of the column), then right clicking anywhere on the column and selecting **Hide**. Try this for yourself, hands-on using the Rounding example spreadsheet.

D4			f_x	=ROUND(C4,0)

Book10

	A	B	D	E
1	*Petty cash*			
2	Week ending 31/12/20X6			
3				
4	Opening balance		231	
5	Receipts		33	
6	Payments		-105	
7	Closing balance		159	
8				

Note that using the ROUND function to eliminate decimals results in slightly inaccurate calculation totals (in our example 160 is actually 'more correct' than the 159 obtained using ROUND). For this reason, some people prefer not to use the function, and to make users of the spreadsheet aware that small apparent differences are due to rounding.

Identifying error values

Error checking can be turned on by **Office button>Excel options>Formulas** and checking **Enable background error checking**. There is a list that allows you to decide which errors to be highlighted. If a green triangle appears in a cell, then the cell contains an error.

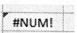

#NUM!

 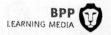

Other information about the nature of the error will also be supplied:

#########	The column is not wide enough to hold the number. Widen the column or choose another format in which to display the number (no green triangle here as it is not a 'real' error – just a presentation problem).
#DIV/0!	Commonly caused by a formula attempting to divide a number by zero (perhaps because the divisor cell is blank).
#VALUE!	Occurs when a mathematical formula refers to a cell containing text, eg if cell A2 contains text the formula =A1+A2+A3 will return #VALUE!. Functions that operate on ranges (eg SUM) will not result in a #VALUE! error as they ignore text values.
#NAME?	The formula contains text that is not a valid cell address, range name or function name. Check the spelling of any functions used (eg by looking through functions under **Formulas > Insert Function**).
#REF!	The formula includes an invalid cell reference, for example a reference to cells that have subsequently been deleted. If you notice the reference immediately after a deletion, use **Ctrl+Z** to reverse the deletion.
#NUM!	This error is caused by invalid numeric values being supplied to a worksheet formula or function. For example, using a negative number with the SQRT (square root) function. To investigate, check the formula and function logic and syntax. The **Formula Auditing** toolbar may help this process (see below).
#N/A	A value is not available to a function or formula, for example omitting a required argument from a spreadsheet function. Again, the **Formula Auditing** toolbar may help the investigation process (see below).

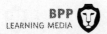

Tracing and correcting errors

If you do see one of the above errors you can trace where it came from by clicking on the cell with the error, then, from the **Formulas** tab of the Ribbon, choose **Formula Auditing** and click the down arrow next to **Error Checking**. Lines will appear pointing to the data that has produced the error.

If you simply click the **Error Checking** button, it will automatically check the current worksheet and alert you to any errors.

Finally, you can click **Evaluate Formula** to be taken step by step through it so that you can identify the error.

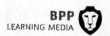

CHAPTER OVERVIEW

- It is important to save and **backup your work regularly**. You can use **Save as** to give various versions of the same document different names.

- It is important to **control the security** of spreadsheets through passwords, locking (protecting) cells against unauthorised or accidental changes, data validation on input.

- Spreadsheet packages permit the user to work with **multiple sheets** that refer to each other. This is sometimes referred to as a three dimensional spreadsheet.

- Excel offers sophisticated data handling including **filtering, pivot tables** and **look-up tables**.

- **Combination charts** allow you to show two sets of data on one axis of your chart.

- Three tools, **Data tables, Scenarios** and **Goal seek**, are available to allow you to explore various results using different sets of values in one or more formulae.

- **Error detection** and prevention is important in spreadsheet design and testing. There are useful facilities available such as tracing precedents and dependents, identification of circular references, and error reports, as well as Excel's built-in help function.

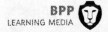

TEST YOUR LEARNING

Test 1

What command is used to save a file under a different name?

Test 2

What part of the Ribbon do you go to set up checking procedures on the input of data?

Test 3

List three possible uses for a multi-sheet (3D) spreadsheet.

Test 4

What does filtering do?

Test 5

What is a trend line?

Test 6

What is the median?

chapter 3:
INTRODUCTION TO SPREADSHEETS (EXCEL 2010)

chapter coverage 📖

This chapter and the next introduce spreadsheets, using Excel 2010. Chapters 1 and 2 cover the same material using Excel 2007. You should study and work through *either* Chapters 1 and 2 *or* Chapters 3 and 4, depending on the Excel software you have.

Spreadsheets have become indispensible tools for the presentation and analysis of accounting data.

This chapter covers:

✍ Introduction

✍ Basic skills

✍ Spreadsheet construction

✍ Formulae with conditions

✍ Charts and graphs

✍ Printing

INTRODUCTION

The vast majority of people who work in an accounting environment are required to use spreadsheets to perform their duties. This fact is reflected in the AAT Standards, which require candidates to be able to produce clear, well-presented spreadsheets, that utilise appropriate spreadsheet functions and formulae.

Uses of spreadsheets

Spreadsheets can be used for a wide range of tasks. Some common applications of spreadsheets are:

- Management accounts
- Cash flow analysis and forecasting
- Reconciliations
- Revenue analysis and comparison
- Cost analysis and comparison
- Budgets and forecasts

Spreadsheet software also provides basic database capabilities which allow simple records to be recorded, sorted and searched.

BASIC SKILLS

In this section we revise some **basic spreadsheet skills**.

The Ribbon

File button

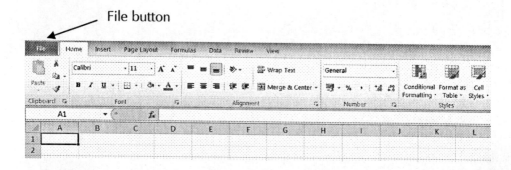

File button

The File button is a menu button and provides access to several options.

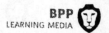

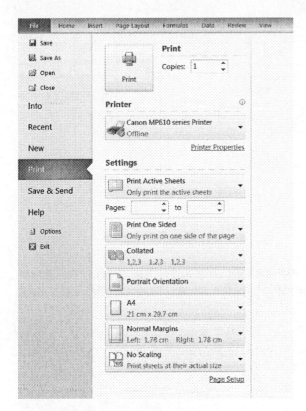

Workbooks and worksheets

At the bottom left of the spreadsheet window you will see tabs which are known as **Worksheets**:

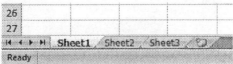

When **New** is selected from the Office button menu, a new **workbook** is created. The workbook consists of one or more **worksheets**. Think of worksheets as **pages** that make up the workbook. By default, a new Excel workbook starts out with three worksheets, although this can be changed (see later).

Worksheets can provide a convenient way of organising information. For example, consider a business consisting of three branches. Worksheets 2 – 4 could hold budget information separately for each branch. When entering formulae into cells it is possible to refer to cells in other worksheets within the workbook so it would then be possible for Worksheet 1 to show the totals of the budget information for the whole business. Effectively, a 'three dimensional' structure can be set up. We look at this in more detail later.

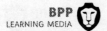

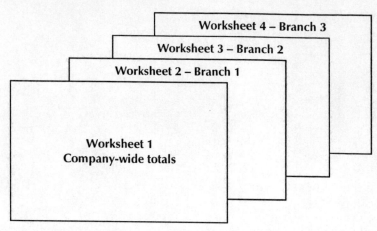

Opening an existing workbook

You can open an existing workbook file by using the menu commands **File button>Open** and then navigating to the location of the file and double clicking on it.

If you open more than one workbook, each will open in a new window. To swap between open workbooks, click on the **File button** and choose the workbook you want from the Recent documents list.

Closing a workbook

There are two ways to close a spreadsheet file:

(1) Click the **File button** and choose **Close** (fourth icon down)

(2) Click on either the **'x'** in the top right hand corner of the window or the one just below it.

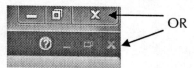

OR

In both cases, if you have made any changes to the spreadsheet you will be asked if you want to save them. Choose **Yes** to save any changes (this will overwrite the existing file), **No** to close the file without saving any changes, or **Cancel** to return to the spreadsheet.

Cell contents

The contents of any cell can be one of the following:

(a) **Text.** A text cell usually contains **words**. Numbers that do not represent numeric values for calculation purposes (eg a Part Number) may be

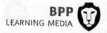

entered in a way that tells Excel to treat the cell contents as text. To do this, enter an apostrophe before the number eg '451.

(b) **Values**. A value is a **number** that can be used in a calculation.

(c) **Formulae**. A formula **refers to other cells** in the spreadsheet, and performs some type of computation with them. For example, if cell C1 contains the formula =A1 – B1, cell C1 will display the result of the calculation subtracting the contents of cell B1 from the contents of cell A1. In Excel, a formula always begins with an equals sign: = . This alerts the program that what follows is a formula and not text or a value. There is a wide range of formulae and functions available.

Formulas and the formula bar

Open the workbook called ExcelExample1. This is one of the files available for download from www.bpp.com/aatspreadsheets. You can open a file by using the menu commands:

File button>Open

then navigating to and double clicking on the file called ExcelExample1.

Note. Throughout this book we want spreadsheets to recalculate every time a figure is changed. This is the normal or default setting, so it is likely your spreadsheets already do this. But, if they don't, then:

(1) Click the **File Button**, click **Excel Options**, and then click the **Formulas** category.

(2) To recalculate all dependent formulas every time you make a change to a value, formula, or name, in the **Calculation options** section, under **Workbook Calculation**, click **Automatic**. This is the default calculation setting.

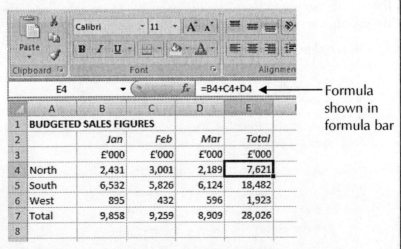

Formula shown in formula bar

You should see the worksheet illustrated above. Click on cell E4.

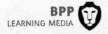

Look at the formula bar.

Note. If the formula bar is not visible, choose the **View** tab and check the **Formula Bar** box.

Note the important difference between:

(1) What is shown in cell E4: 7,621.

(2) What is actually in cell E4: this is shown in the formula bar and it tells us that cell E4 is the result of adding together the contents of cells B4, C4 and D4.

The formula bar allows you to see and edit the contents of the active cell. The bar also shows, on the left side, the cell address of the active cell (E4 in the example above).

Select different cells to be the active cell by using the up/down/right/left arrows on your keyboard or by clicking directly on the cell you want to be active. Look at what is in the cell and what is shown in the formula bar.

The **F5** key is useful for moving around within large spreadsheets. If you press the function key **F5**, a **Go To** dialogue box will allow you to specify the cell address you would like to move to. Try this out.

Also experiment by holding down Ctrl and pressing each of the direction arrow keys in turn to see where you end up. Try using the **Page Up** and **Page Down** keys and also try **Home** and **End** and Ctrl + these keys. Try **Tab** and **Shift + Tab**, too. These are all useful shortcuts for moving quickly from one place to another in a large spreadsheet.

Examples of spreadsheet formulae

Formulae in Microsoft Excel follow a specific syntax. All Excel formulae start with the equals sign =, followed by the elements to be calculated (the operands) and the calculation operators (such as +, -, /, *). Each operand can be a:

- Value that does not change (a constant value, such as the VAT rate).

- Cell or range reference to a range of cells.

- Name (a named cell, such as 'VAT').

- Worksheet function (such as 'AVERAGE', which will work out the average value of defined values).

Formulae can be used to perform a variety of calculations. Here are some examples:

(a) =C4*5. This formula **multiplies** the value in C4 by 5. The result will appear in the cell holding the formula.

(b) =C4*B10. This **multiplies** the value in C4 by the value in B10.

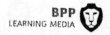

(c) =C4/E5. This **divides** the value in C4 by the value in E5. * means multiply and / means divide by.

(d) =C4*B10 – D1. This **multiplies** the value in C4 by that in B10 and then subtracts the value in D1 from the result. Note that generally Excel will perform multiplication and division before addition or subtraction. If in any doubt, use brackets (parentheses): =(C4*B10) – D1.

(e) =C4*120%. This **adds** 20% to the value in C4. It could be used to calculate a price including 20% VAT.

(f) =(C4+C5+C6)/3. Note that the **brackets** mean Excel would perform the addition first. Without the brackets, Excel would first divide the value in C6 by 3 and then add the result to the total of the values in C4 and C5.

(g) $= 2\wedge2$ gives you 2 **to the power** of 2, in other words 2 squared. Likewise $= 2\wedge3$ gives you 2 cubed and so on.

(h) $= 4\wedge(1/2)$ gives you the **square root** of 4. Likewise $27\wedge(1/3)$ gives you the cube root of 27 and so on.

Displaying spreadsheet formulae

It is sometimes useful to see all formulae held in your spreadsheet to enable you to see how the spreadsheet works. There are two ways of making Excel **display the formulae** held in a spreadsheet.

(a) You can 'toggle' between the two types of display by pressing **Ctrl +`** (the latter is the key above the Tab key). Press **Ctrl +`** again to go back to the previous display.

(b) You can also click on **Formulas>Show Formulas** in the Ribbon.

The formulae for the spreadsheet we viewed earlier are shown below.

	A	B	C	D	E
1	BUDGETED S				
2		Jan	Feb	Mar	Total
3		£'000	£'000	£'000	£'000
4	North	2431	3001	2189	=B4+C4+D4
5	South	6532	5826	6124	=B5+C5+D5
6	West	895	432	596	=B6+C6+D6
7	Total	=B4+B5+B6	=C4+C5+C6	=D4+D5+D6	=E4+E5+E6

The importance of formulae

Look carefully at the example above and note which cells have formulae in them. It is important to realise that:

- If a cell contains a value, such as sales for North in January, then that data is entered as a number.

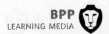

- If a cell shows the result of a calculation based on values in other cells, such as the total sales for January, then that cell contains a formula.

This is vital, because now if North's January sales were changed to, say, 2,500, the total would be automatically updated to show 9,927. Also the total for North would change to 7,690.

Try that out by clicking on cell B4 to make it active, then typing 2,500, followed by the Enter key. You should see both the totals change.

Now re-enter the original figure of 2,432 into cell B4.

Similarly, if a number is used more than once, for example a tax rate, it will be much better if the number is input to one cell only. Any other calculations making use of that value should refer to that cell. That way, if the tax rate changes, you only have to change it in one place in the spreadsheet (where it was originally entered) and any calculations making use of it will automatically change.

Your first function

In the example above, totals were calculated using a formula such as:

=+B4+C4+D4

That is fine provided there are not too many items to be included in the total. Imagine, the difficulty if you had to find the total of 52 weeks for a year. Adding up rows or columns is made much easier by using the SUM function. Instead of the formula above, we could place the following calculation in cell E4:

= SUM(B4:D4)

This produces the sum of all the cells in the range B4 to D4. Now it is much easier to add up a very long row of figures (for example, SUM(F5:T5)) or a very long column of figures (for example, SUM(B10:B60)).

There are three ways in which the SUM function can be entered. One way is simply to type =SUM(B4:D4) when E4 is the active cell. However, there is a more visual and perhaps more accurate way.

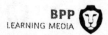

Make E4 the active cell by moving the cursor to it using the arrow keys or by clicking on it.

> Type =Sum(
> Click on cell B4
> Type a colon :
> Click on cell D4
> Close the bracket by typing)
> Press the Enter key

Another way is to use the AutoSum button, which we cover later.

Editing cell contents

Cell D5 of ExcelExample1 currently contains the value 6,124. If you wish to change the value in that cell from 6,124 to 6,154 there are four options (you have already used the first method).

(a) Activate cell D5, **type** 6,154 and press **Enter**.

To undo this and try the next option press **Ctrl + Z**; this will always undo what you have just done (a very useful shortcut).

(b) **Double-click** in cell D5. The cell will keep its thick outline but you will now be able to see a vertical line flashing in the cell. You can move this line by using the direction arrow keys or the Home and the End keys. Move it to just after the 2, press the **backspace** key on the keyboard and then type 5. Then press **Enter**. (Alternatively, move the vertical line to just in front of the 2, press the **Delete** key on the keyboard, then type 5, followed by the **Enter** key).

When you have tried this press **Ctrl + Z** to undo it.

(c) **Click once** before the number 6,124 in the formula bar. Again, you will get the vertical line which can be moved back and forth to allow editing as in (b) above.

(d) Activate cell D4 and press **F2** at the top of your keyboard. The vertical line cursor will be flashing in cell D4 at the end of the figures entered there and this can be used to edit the cell contents, as above.

Deleting cell contents

There are a number of ways to delete the contents of a cell:

(a) Make the cell the active cell and press the **Delete** button. The contents of the cell will disappear.

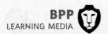

(b) Go to the **Editing** section on the **Home** tab of the Ribbon. Click on the **Clear** button and various options appear. Click **Clear Contents**. You can also achieve this by **right clicking** the cell and choosing **Clear contents**.

Any **cell formatting** (for example, cell colour or border) will not be removed when using either of these methods. To remove formatting click on the **Clear** button on the **Home** tab and select **Clear Formats**. If you want to remove the formatting *and* the contents, click **Clear All**.

Ranges of cells

A range of cells can occupy a single column or row or can be a rectangle of cells. The extent of a range is defined by the rectangle's top left cell reference and the bottom right cell reference. If the range is within a single row or column, it is defined by the references of the start and end cells.

Defining a range is very useful as you can then manipulate many cells at once rather than having to go to each one individually.

The following shows that a rectangular range of cells has been selected from C4 to D6. The range consists of three rows and two columns.

	A	B	C	D	E	F
1	BUDGETED SALES FIGURES					
2		Jan	Feb	Mar	Total	
3		£'000	£'000	£'000	£'000	
4	North	2,431	3,001	2,189	7,621	
5	South	6,532	5,826	6,124	18,482	
6	West	895	432	596	1,923	
7	Total	9,858	9,259	8,909	28,026	
8						
9						

There are several ways of selecting ranges. Try the following:

(1) Click on cell C4, but hold the mouse button down. Drag the cursor down and to the right until the required range has been selected. Then release the mouse button. Now press the **Delete** key. All the cells in this range are cleared of their contents. Reverse this by **Ctrl+Z** and deselect the range by clicking on any single cell.

(2) Click on cell C4 (release the mouse button). Hold down the **Shift** key and press the **down** and **right hand arrows** until the correct range is highlighted.

Deselect the range by clicking on any single cell.

(3) Click on cell C4 (release the mouse button). Hold down the **Shift** key and click on cell D6.

Deselect the range by clicking on any single cell.

Sometimes you may want to select an entire row or column:

(4) Say you wanted to select row 3, perhaps to change all the occurrences of £'000 to a bold font. Position your cursor over the figure 3 defining row 3 and click. All of row 3 is selected. Clicking on the **B** in the font group on the **Home** tab will make the entire row bold:

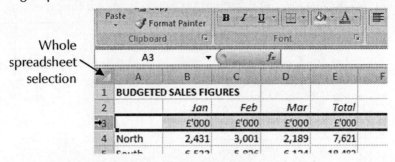

Whole spreadsheet selection

Sometimes you may want to select every cell in the worksheet, perhaps to put everything into a different font:

(5) Click on the triangle shape at the extreme top left of the cells (indicated above). Alternatively you can select the active cells using **Ctrl + A.**

Filling a range of cells

There are a number of labour-saving shortcuts which allow you to quickly fill ranges of cells with headings (such as £'000, or month names) and with patterns of numbers. You can keep the ExcelExercise1 spreadsheet open throughout the following activities and simply open a new spreadsheet on which to experiment.

(1) Create a new spreadsheet (**File button>New. Select Blank workbook.**)

(2) Make cell B3 active and type Jan (or January) into it.

(3) Position the cursor at the bottom right of cell B3 (you will see a black + when you are at the right spot – this is often referred to as the **fill handle**).

(4) Hold down the mouse button and drag the cursor rightwards, until it is under row G. Release the mouse button.

The month names will automatically fill across.

(5) Using the same technique, fill B4 to G4 with £.

(6) Type 'Region' into cell 3A.

(7) Type the figure 1 into cell A5 and 2 into cell A6. Select the range A5–A6 and obtain the black cross at the bottom right of cell A6. Hold down the mouse key and drag the cursor down to row 10. Release the mouse button.

The figures 1–6 will automatically fill down column A.

> **Note.** If 1 and 3 had been entered into A5 and C6, then 1, 3, 5, 7, 9, 11 would automatically appear. This does **not** work if just the figure 1 is entered into A5.

The AutoSum button Σ

We will explain how to use the AutoSum button by way of a simple example.

(1) Clear your worksheet (**Select all > Delete**).

(2) Enter the following figures in cells A1:B5. (**Hint.** Instead of pressing return after each figure, you can press the down or right arrow to enter the figure and to move to the next cell.)

	A	B
1	400	582
2	250	478
3	359	264
4	476	16
5	97	125

(3) Make cell B6 the active cell and select the Formulas group from the Ribbon. Click the drop-down arrow next to the **Σ AutoSum** button and select **Σ Sum**. The formula =SUM(B1:B5) will appear in the cell. Above cell B6 you will see a flashing dotted line around cells B1:B5. Accept the suggested formula by hitting Enter. 1,465 should appear in B6. Alternatively, you can simply click on the large **Σ** symbol itself, or click on the **Σ AutoSum** button in the **Editing** part of **Home** on the ribbon (see later).

(4) Next, make cell A6 the active cell and repeat the operation for that column. The number 1,582 should appear in cell A6.

(5) Now delete the two totals.

Copying and pasting formulae

You have already seen that formulae are extremely important in spreadsheet construction. In Excel it is very easy to define a formula once and then apply it to a wide range of cells. As it is applied to different cells the cell references in the formula are automatically updated. Say, that in the above example, you wanted to multiply together each row of figures in columns A and B and to display the answer in the equivalent rows of column C.

(1)   Make C1 the active cell.

(2)   Type =, then click on cell A1, then type * and click on cell B1.

(3)   Press **Enter**.

The formula =A1*B1 should be shown in the formula bar, and the amount 232,800 should be shown in C1.

(4)   Make C1 the active cell and obtain the black + by positioning the cursor at the bottom right of that cell.

(5)   Hold down the mouse button and drag the cursor down to row 5.

(6)   Release the mouse button.

Look at the formulae in column C. You will see that the cell references change as you move down the column, updating as you move from row to row.

C3			f_x	=A3*B3
	A	B	C	D
1	400	582	232800	
2	250	478	119500	
3	359	264	94776	
4	476	16	7616	
5	97	125	12125	

It is also possible to copy whole blocks of cells, with formulae being updated in a logical way.

(1) Make A1 the active cell and select the range A1:C5, for example, by dragging the cursor down and rightwards.

(2) Press **Ctrl+C** (the standard Windows Copy command) or click on the **Copy** symbol in the **Home** section of the ribbon.

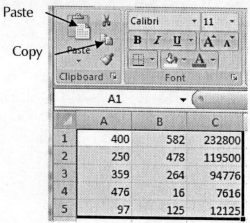

(3) Make E7 the active cell and press **Ctrl+V** or click on the paste button. E7 will become the top right cell of the copied rectangle and will hold 400.

(4) Now, look at the formulae shown in cell G7. It will show =E7*F7. So all cell references in the formulae have been updated relative to one another. This type of copying is called **relative copying**.

(5) **Delete** the range E7:G7.

Paste special

Sometimes you don't want to copy formulae and you only want to copy the displayed values. This can be done using **Paste special**.

Open the spreadsheet called Paste special example from the files available for download at www.bpp.com/aatspreadsheets.

You will see a simple inventory-type application listing quantities, prices and values. The values are obtained by formulae multiplying together prices and quantities. Say that you just want to copy the values of cells D3:D8, without the underlying formulae.

(1) Select the range D3:D8.

(2) Press **Ctrl+C** or the copy icon in the **Clipboard** part of **Home** on the Ribbon.

(3) **Right-click** on cell C12 to make it active, and choose **Paste Special** from the list.

(4) Check the **Values** radio button.

(5) Click **OK**.

The list of figures will be pasted, but if you look in the formula bar, you will see that they are just figures; there are no formulae there.

Note. If you change a quantity or price in the original table, the figures you have just pasted will not change; they have become pure numbers and do not link back to their source.

Inserting and deleting columns and rows

Often you will need to insert or delete whole rows or columns in spreadsheets. This can easily be done and sometimes formulae are correctly updated – but they should always be checked. For this exercise we will go back to using the ExcelExample1 spreadsheet.

Close the spreadsheet you have recently been working on and go back to (using the tabs across the bottom of the screen) or reopen the spreadsheet ExcelExample1.

Let us assume that we have a new region, East and that we want this to be in a row lying between North and South.

(1) Select row 5, by clicking on the 5, then click the right mouse button ('right click') and select **Insert**. You will see rows 5, 6 and 7 move down.

(2) Make B8 the active cell and you will see that the formula in the formula bar is =B4+B6+B7. If we were to put the figures for East into row 5 then those would **not** be correctly included in the total, though B5 has been updated to B6 etc.

(3) Reverse the last step (**Ctrl+Z**).

(4) Now, in cell B7 insert =SUM(B4:B6).

(5) Copy B7 across columns C7 to E7 (black cross and drag across).

(6) Check the formulae that are in cells C7 to E7 to ensure they have all been updated.

(7) Insert a whole row above row 5 (select row 5>right click>**Insert**).

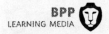

(8) Inspect the formulae in row 8, the new total row.

The formulae in the total row will now be showing =SUM(B4:B7), =SUM(C4:C7), etc. In this case the new row will be included in the total. Effectively, the range over which the totals are calculated has been 'stretched'. Depending how your copy of Excel is set up, you may notice little green triangles in row 8. If so, place your cursor on one and press the exclamation symbol. The triangles are warning that you have included empty cells in your total – not a problem here, but it might have been in some cases. Don't worry if the triangles aren't showing.

(9) Finally delete row 5. Select the whole row by clicking on the 5, then right click and choose **Delete** from the menu.

The cells below Row 5 will move up and the SUM formulae are again updated.

New columns can also be added. Say that we now wanted to include April in the results.

(1) Replace the current formula in E4 with =SUM(B4:D4).

(2) Copy the formula in E4 down through columns 5, 6 and 7. Check that the correct formulae are in cells E4–E7.

(3) Select column E, by clicking on the E, then click the right mouse button ('right click') and select **Insert**. You will see column E move to the right.

(4) Inspect the formulae now in Column F, the new total column.

You will see that the formula in F7 still says = SUM(B7:D7). It has **not been updated** for the extra column.

So, if an extra row or column is inserted in the middle of a range, the formulae is updated because the new row or column probably (but not always) becomes part of the range that has to be added up.

However, if the extra row or column is added at the end of a range (or the start) the formula will not be updated to include that. That's reasonably logical as new items at the very start or end have a greater chance of being headings or something not part of the range to be included in a calculation.

So:

**Whenever columns or rows are added or deleted,
check that formulae affected remain correct.**

Changing column width and height

You may occasionally find that a cell is not wide enough to display its contents. When this occurs, the cell displays a series of hashes ######. There are several ways to deal with this problem:

- Column widths can be adjusted by positioning the mouse pointer at the head of the column, directly over the little line dividing two columns. The mouse **pointer** will change to a **cross** with a double-headed arrow through it. Hold down the left mouse button and, by moving your mouse, stretch or shrink the column until it is the right width. Alternatively, you can double click when the double-headed arrow appears and the column will automatically adjust to the optimum width.

- Highlight the columns you want to adjust and choose **Home>Cells>Format>Column Width** from the menu and set the width manually. Alternatively, you can right click the highlighted column(s) and choose **Column width** from the menu.

- Highlight the columns you want to adjust and choose **Home>Format>Autofit Column Width** from the menu and set the width to fit the contents.

Setting column heights works similarly.

Dates

You can insert the current date into a cell by **Ctrl+ ;** (semicolon)

You can insert the current time by **Ctrl+Shift + ;**.

You can insert date and time by first inserting the date, release Ctrl, press space, insert the time. The date can be formatted by going to **Home>Number>Date** and choosing the format required.

Once a date is entered it is easy to produce a sequence of dates.

In a new worksheet, insert the date 1/1/2011 in cell A1.

(1) Format so as to show 01 January 2011.

(2) In A2, insert the date 8/1/2011 and format it to appear as 08 January 2011.

(3) Select cells A1 and A2.

(4) Position the cursor on the bottom right of cell A2 (a black + will appear).

(5) Hold down the mouse button and drag the mouse down to A12.

The cells should fill with dates seven days apart.

(If you see ###### in a cell it means that column A is too narrow, so widen it as explained above.)

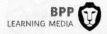

Naming cells

It can be difficult to always have to refer to a cell co-ordinate, eg C12. Cell C12 might contain the VAT rate and it would be more natural (and less error prone) to refer to a name like 'VAT'.

> (1) Open the worksheet called Name example.
>
> (2) Make cell B3 the active one and right click on it.
>
> (3) Select **Name a range**.
>
> (4) Accept the offered name, 'VAT' that Excel has picked up from the neighbouring cell.
>
> (5) Highlight the range D4:D7, right click **Name a range** and accept the offered 'Net'.
>
> (6) In E4 enter =Net*(1 + VAT).
>
> (7) Copy E4 into E5:E7.
>
> You will see the formula bar refers to names. This makes understanding a spreadsheet much easier.

A list of names can be seen using the **Formulas** section of the Ribbon and clicking on **Name Manager**.

Keyboard shortcuts

Here are a few tips to quickly improve the **appearance** of your spreadsheets and speed up your work, using only the keyboard. These are all alternatives to clicking the relevant button in the **Home** section of the Ribbon.

To do any of the following to a cell or range of cells, first **select** the cell or cells and then:

(a) Press **Ctrl + B** to make the cell contents **bold**.

(b) Press **Ctrl + I** to make the cell contents *italic*.

(c) Press **Ctrl + U** to underline the cell contents.

(d) Press **Ctrl + C** to **Copy** the contents of the cells.

(e) Move the cursor and press **Ctrl + V** to **paste** the cell you just copied into the new active cell or cells.

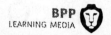

SPREADSHEET CONSTRUCTION

All spreadsheets need to be planned and then constructed carefully. More complex spreadsheet models should include some documentation that explains how the spreadsheet is set-up and how to use it.

There can be a feeling that, because the spreadsheet carries out calculations automatically, results will be reliable. However, there can easily be errors in formulae, errors of principle and errors in assumptions. All too often, spreadsheets offer a reliable and quick way to produce nonsense.

Furthermore, it is rare for only one person to have to use or adapt a spreadsheet and proper documentation is important if other people are to be able to make efficient use of it.

The following should be kept in separate identifiable areas of the spreadsheet:

(1) An inputs and assumptions section containing the variables (eg the amount of a loan and the interest rate, planned mark-ups, assumptions about growth rates).

(2) A calculations section containing formulae.

(3) The results section, showing the outcome of the calculations.

Sometimes it is convenient to combine (2) and (3).

It is also important to:

(1) Document data sources. For example, where did the assumed growth rate come from? If you don't know that, how will you ever test the validity of that data and any results arising from it.

(2) Explain calculation methods. This is particularly important if calculations are complex or have to be done in a specified way.

(3) Explain the variables used in functions. Some functions require several input variables (arguments) and may not be familiar to other users.

(4) Set out the spreadsheet clearly, using underlinings, colour, bold text etc to assist users.

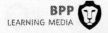

Example: constructing a costing spreadsheet

You want to set up a spreadsheet to record the time you and your colleagues spend on an assignment, and to cost it using your group's internal chargeout rates which are as follows:

Divisional chief accountant	£72.50
Assistant accountant	£38.00
Accounting technician (you)	£21.45
Secretary	£17.30

The spreadsheet needs to show the hours spent and costs per person, by week, for a three-week assignment. The time spent each week is shown below:

	Week 3	Week 2	Week 1
Divisional chief accountant	6 hrs 45 mins	4 hrs 30 mins	–
Assistant accountant	35 hrs	40 hrs	20 hrs
You	37 hrs 30 mins	40 hrs	32 hrs
Secretary	37 hrs 15 mins	32 hrs 15 mins	15 hrs

Setting up the assumptions area

As we will be referring to the chargeout rates for each week's costs, set these up in a separate area of the spreadsheet.

Headings and layout

Next we will enter the various **headings** required.

You want your spreadsheet to look like this:

	A	B	C	D	E	F	G
1	**Internal chargeout rates**						
2	Divisional chief accountant	£72.50					
3	Assistant accountant	£38.00					
4	Accounting technician	£21.45					
5	Secretary	£17.30					
6							
7	**Costs**	*Week 1*	*Week 2*	*Week 3*	*Total*		
8	Divisional chief accountant						
9	Assistant accountant						
10	Accounting technician						
11	Secretary						
12	**Total**						
13							
14	**Hours**	*Week 1*	*Week 2*	*Week 3*	*Total*		
15	Divisional chief accountant						
16	Assistant accountant						
17	Accounting technician						
18	Secretary						
19	**Total**						

Note the following points.

(a) Column A is wider to allow longer items of text to be entered. Depending on how your copy of Excel is set up, this might happen automatically or you may have to drag the line between the A and B columns to the right.

(b) We have used a **simple style for headings**. Headings tell users what data relates to and what the spreadsheet 'does'. We have made some words **bold**.

(c) **Numbers** should be **right aligned** in cells. This usually happens automatically when you enter a number into a cell.

(d) We have left **spaces** in certain rows (after blocks of related items) to make the spreadsheet **easier to use and read**.

(e) Totals have been highlighted by a single line above and a double line below. This can be done by highlighting the relevant cells then going to the **Styles** group in the **Home** section of the Ribbon, clicking on the drop-down arrow and choosing the style you want, in this case '**Totals**'.

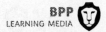

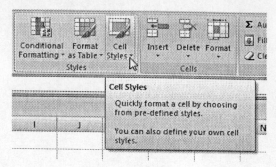

Alternatively, highlight the relevant cells, go to the **Font** area of the **Home** section and click on the drop-down arrow to access the list of **borders** available:

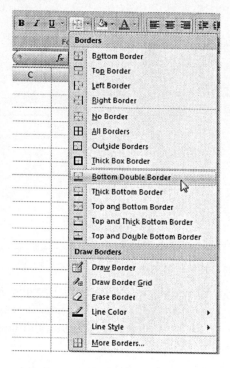

Entering data

Enter the time data in cells B15 to D18. Make sure you enter it correctly – the data is given to you in the order week 3 to week 1 but you would prefer it to be in the order week 1 to week 3. You will need to convert the time to decimal numbers.

		Week 1	Week 2	Week 3	Total
13					
14	Hours	Week 1	Week 2	Week 3	Total
15	Divisional chief accountant	0	4.5	6.75	
16	Assistant accountant	20	40	35	
17	Accounting technician	32	40	37.5	
18	Secretary	15	32.25	37.25	
19	Total				{Ctrl} ▼
20					
21					
22					
23					
24					

Inserting formulae

The next step is to enter the **formulae** required. For example, in cell B19 you want the total hours for Week 1. In cell B8 you want the total cost of time spent. You could enter this formula as =B15*B2, but you need to make sure that as you copy the formula across for Weeks 2 and 3 you still refer to the chargeout rate in B2.

The quick way to insert a series of formulae is to type in the initial one and then to copy across a row or down a column. You may remember that cell references are cleverly updated as you move along the row or column. This was called **relative copying**. However, that will get us into trouble here. If cell B8 contains the formula =B15*B2 and that is copied one cell to the right, into column D, the formula will become =C15*C2.

The C15 reference is correct because we are progressing along the row, one month at a time, but the C2 reference is incorrect. The location of the chargeout rate does not move: it is **absolute**. To prevent a cell reference being updated during the copying process put a '$' sign in front of the row and/or column reference.

A reference like $A1 will mean that column A is always referred to as you copy across the spreadsheet. If you were to copy down, the references would be updated to A2, A3, A4, etc.

A reference such as A$1 will mean that row 1 is always referred to as you copy down the spreadsheet. If you were to copy across, the references would be updated to B1, C1, D1, etc.

A reference like $A$1 will mean that cell A1 is always referred to no matter what copying of the formula is carried out.

The **function key F4** adds dollar signs to the cell reference, cycling through one, two or zero dollar signs. Press the **F4** key as you are entering the cell address.

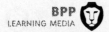

You should end up with the following figures:

B8		fx	=B15*$B$2			
A	B	C	D	E	F	G
1 Internal chargeout rates						
2 Divisional chief accountant	£72.50					
3 Assistant accountant	£38.00					
4 Accounting technician	£21.45					
5 Secretary	£17.30					
6						
7 Costs	Week 1	Week 2	Week 3	Total		
8 Divisional chief accountant	0	326.25	489.375			
9 Assistant accountant	760	1520	1330			
10 Accounting technician	686.4	858	804.375			
11 Secretary	259.5	557.925	644.425			
12 Total						
13						
14 Hours	Week 1	Week 2	Week 3	Total		
15 Divisional chief accountant	0	4.5	6.75			
16 Assistant accountant	20	40	35			
17 Accounting technician	32	40	37.5			
18 Secretary	15	32.25	37.25			
19 Total						
20						
21						
22						
23						

Note that the formula in B8 refers to cell B15 (Week 1 hours) but to cell $B$2 – the absolute address of the chargeout rate.

The sales figure are untidy: some have comma separators between the thousands, some have one decimal place, some two. To tidy this up we will use the **Number** section of the Ribbon to format these numbers as **Currency**.

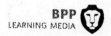

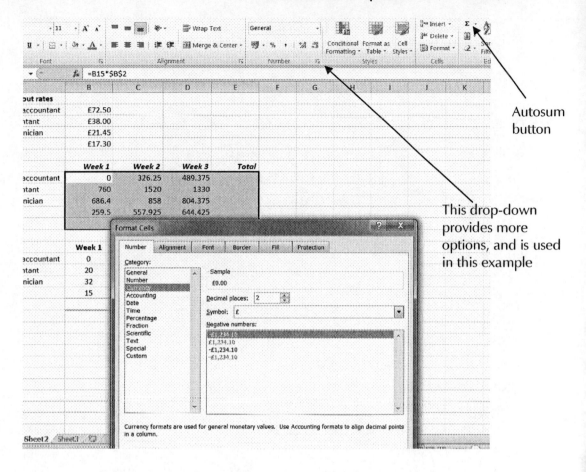

Autosum button

This drop-down provides more options, and is used in this example

---

(1) Select the range of cells B8:E12.

(2) Click in the small arrow just right of the word '**Number**' to open the **Format Cells** window.

(3) Select **Currency**, make sure the **Decimal places** reads 2 and that the £ symbol is showing.

You should see that all the figures in your spreadsheet are now in the same format.

(4) In cell E8, enter a formula to total the hours. This is easiest if you use the Autosum button.

The spreadsheet should now be like this:

	B8	▾	f_x =B15*$B$2		
	A	B	C	D	E	F
1	**Internal chargeout rates**				
2	Divisional chief accountant	£72.50			
3	Assistant accountant	£38.00			
4	Accounting technician	£21.45			
5	Secretary	£17.30			
6					
7	**Costs**	*Week 1*	*Week 2*	*Week 3*	*Total*
8	Divisional chief accountant	£0.00	£326.25	£489.38	£815.63
9	Assistant accountant	£760.00	£1,520.00	£1,330.00	£3,610.00
10	Accounting technician	£686.40	£858.00	£804.38	£2,348.78
11	Secretary	£259.50	£557.93	£644.43	£1,461.85
12	**Total**	**£1,705.90**	**£3,262.18**	**£3,268.18**	**£8,236.25**
13					
14	**Hours**	*Week 1*	*Week 2*	*Week 3*	*Total*
15	Divisional chief accountant	0	4.5	6.75	11.25
16	Assistant accountant	20	40	35	95
17	Accounting technician	32	40	37.5	109.5
18	Secretary	15	32.25	37.25	84.5
19	**Total**	**67**	**116.75**	**116.5**	**300.25**
20					
21					
22					

And the formulae behind the cell contents should be:

	A	B	C	D	E
6					
7	**Costs**		*Week 1*	*Week 2*	*Week 3*	*Total*
8	Divisional chief accountant	=B15*$B$2	=C15*$B$2	=D15*$B$2	=SUM(B8:D8)
9	Assistant accountant	=B16*$B$3	=C16*$B$3	=D16*$B$3	=SUM(B9:D9)
10	Accounting technician	=B17*$B$4	=C17*$B$4	=D17*$B$4	=SUM(B10:D10)
11	Secretary	=B18*$B$5	=C18*$B$5	=D18*$B$5	=SUM(B11:D11)
12	**Total**	=SUM(B8:B11)	=SUM(C8:C11)	=SUM(D8:D11)	=SUM(E8:E11)
13					
14	**Hours**		*Week 1*	*Week 2*	*Week 3*	*Total*
15	Divisional chief accountant	0	4.5	6.75	=SUM(B15:D15)
16	Assistant accountant	20	40	35	=SUM(B16:D16)
17	Accounting technician	32	40	37.5	=SUM(B17:D17)
18	Secretary	15	32.25	37.25	=SUM(B18:D18)
19	**Total**	=SUM(B15:B18)	=SUM(C15:C18)	=SUM(D15:D18)	=SUM(E15:E18)
20					
21					
22					

However, after designing the spreadsheet, you find out that the Divisional Chief Accountant has worked for 6 hours in week 4. He also wants you to add in to your calculations the costs of using two laptop computers which were charged out at £100 per week each, for the first 3 weeks. You have also found out that the secretarial chargeout rate was increased by 10% in week 3. You now need to amend the spreadsheet to reflect these changes.

(1) Insert a column between columns D and E.

(2) Label E7 and E14 as Week 4.

(3) Enter the 6 hours in cell E15.

(4) Enter a formula in cell E8 to calculate the cost of these hours.

(5) Insert a row between rows 11 and 12.

(6) Enter Laptops in cells A6 and A12.

(7) In cell A22, enter Laptops and enter the number of laptops used each week.

(8) In cell B6 enter the cost of each laptop per week.

(9) Use a formula in cells B12 to D12 to calculate the cost of the laptops.

(10) Insert two rows between row 6 and 7.

(11) In cell B7, enter the percentage increase in the secretary's chargeout rate. Format this cell as persentage. Amend the formula in cell D13 accordingly.

(12) You may have noticed that the total cost has not altered. This is because we have inserted rows and columns which were outside the range of the original formula used to calculate the totals. Amend your formulas accordingly.

Tidy the spreadsheet up

The presentation is reasonable as we have taken care of it as we have developed the spreadsheet. This is good practice. You can now apply different formatting techniques – change font colour or cell colour, for example. Save the spreadsheet as Costing Exercise-finished.

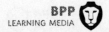

The spreadsheet should now look like this:

	A	B	C	D	E	F	G
	F15			f_x	=SUM(F10:F14)		
1	**Internal chargeout rates**						
2	Divisional chief accountant	£72.50					
3	Assistant accountant	£38.00					
4	Accounting technician	£21.45					
5	Secretary	£17.30					
6	Laptop cost	£100.00					
7	Chargeout rate	10%					
8							
9	**Costs**	*Week 1*	*Week 2*	*Week 3*	*Week 4*	*Total*	
10	Divisional chief accountant	£0.00	£326.25	£489.38	£435.00	£1,250.63	
11	Assistant accountant	£760.00	£1,520.00	£1,330.00	£0.00	£3,610.00	
12	Accounting technician	£686.40	£858.00	£804.38	£0.00	£2,348.78	
13	Secretary	£259.50	£557.93	£708.87	£0.00	£1,526.29	
14	Laptops	£200.00	£200.00	£200.00		£600.00	
15	**Total**	**£1,705.90**	**£3,262.18**	**£3,332.62**	**£435.00**	**£9,335.69**	
16							
17	**Hours**	Week 1	Week 2	Week 3	Week 4	Total	
18	Divisional chief accountant		4.5	6.75	6	17.25	
19	Assistant accountant	20	40	35		95	
20	Accounting technician	32	40	37.5		109.5	
21	Secretary	15	32.25	37.25		84.5	
22	Total	**67**	**116.75**	**116.5**	**6**	**300.25**	
23							
24	Laptops	2	2	2			
25							
26							
27							

And the formulas should look like this:

	F15	▾	fx	=SUM(F10:F14)	

	A	B	C	D	E	F
1	**Internal chargeout rates**					
2	Divisional chief accountant	72.5				
3	Assistant accountant	38				
4	Accounting technician	21.45				
5	Secretary	17.3				
6	Laptop cost	100				
7	Chargeout rate	0.1				
8						
9	**Costs**	*Week 1*	*Week 2*	*Week 3*	*Week 4*	*Total*
10	Divisional chief accountant	=B18*$B$2	=C18*$B$2	=D18*$B$2	=E18*$B$2	=SUM(B10:E10)
11	Assistant accountant	=B19*$B$3	=C19*$B$3	=D19*$B$3	=E19*$B$2	=SUM(B11:E11)
12	Accounting technician	=B20*$B$4	=C20*$B$4	=D20*$B$4	=E20*$B$2	=SUM(B12:E12)
13	Secretary	=B21*$B$5	=C21*$B$5	=D21*($B$5+($B$5*$	=E21*$B$2	=SUM(B13:E13)
14	Laptops	=B24*$B$6	=C24*$B$6	=D24*$B$6		=SUM(B14:E14)
15	**Total**	=SUM(B10:B13)	=SUM(C10:C13)	=SUM(D10:D13)	=SUM(E10:E13)	=SUM(F10:F14)
16						
17	**Hours**	Week 1	Week 2	Week 3	Week 4	Total
18	Divisional chief accountant		4.5	6.75	6	=SUM(B18:E18)
19	Assistant accountant	20	40	35		=SUM(B19:D19)
20	Accounting technician	32	40	37.5		=SUM(B20:D20)
21	Secretary	15	32.25	37.25		=SUM(B21:D21)
22	Total	=SUM(B18:B21)	=SUM(C18:C21)	=SUM(D18:D21)	=SUM(E18:E21)	=SUM(B22:D22)
23						
24	Laptops	2	2	2		
25						
26						
27						
28						

Example: commission calculations

Four telesales staff each earn a basic salary of £14,000 pa. They also earn a commission of 2% of sales. The following spreadsheet has been created to process their commission and total earnings. Give an appropriate formula for each of the following cells.

    (a)   Cell D4

    (b)   Cell E6

    (c)   Cell D9

    (d)   Cell E9

	A	B	C	D	E
1	Sales team salaries and commissions - 200X				
2	Name	Sales	Salary	Commission	Total earnings
3		£	£	£	£
4	Northington	284,000	14,000	5,680	19,680
5	Souther	193,000	14,000	3,860	17,860
6	Weston	12,000	14,000	240	14,240
7	Easterman	152,000	14,000	3,040	17,040
8					
9	Total	641,000	56,000	12,820	68,820
10					
11					
12	Variables				
13	Basic Salary	14,000			
14	Commission rate	0.02			
15					

Solution

Possible formulae are:

(a) =B4*$B$14

(b) =C6+D6

(c) =SUM(D4:D7)

(d) There are a number of possibilities here, depending on whether you set the cell as the total of the earnings of each salesman (cells E4 to E7): =SUM(E4:E7) or as the total of the different elements of remuneration (cells C9 and D9): =SUM(C9:D9). Even better, would be a formula that checked that both calculations gave the same answer. A suitable formula for this purpose would be:

=IF(SUM(E4:E7)=SUM(C9:D9),SUM(E4:E7),"ERROR")

We explain this formula after the next example, don't worry about it at the moment!

Example: actual sales compared with budget sales

A business often compares its results against budgets or targets. It is useful to express differences or **variations as a percentage of the original budget**, for example sales may be 10% higher than predicted.

Continuing the telesales example, a spreadsheet could be set up as follows showing differences between actual sales and target sales, and expressing the difference as a percentage of target sales.

130

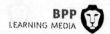

	A	B	C	D	E
1	Sales team comparison of actual against budget sales				
2	Name	Sales (Budget)	Sales (Actual)	Difference	% of budget
3		£	£	£	£
4	Northington	275,000	284,000	9,000	3.27
5	Souther	200,000	193,000	(7,000)	(3.50)
6	Weston	10,000	12,000	2,000	20.00
7	Easterman	153,000	152,000	(1,000)	(0.65)
8					
9	Total	638,000	641,000	3,000	0.47
10					

Give a suitable formula for each of the following cells.

(a) Cell D4

(b) Cell E6

(c) Cell E9

Try this for yourself, before looking at the solution.

Solution

(a) =C4 – B4

(b) =(D6/B6)*100

(c) =(D9/B9)*100. Note that in (c) you **cannot simply add up the individual percentage differences**, as the percentages are based on different quantities

FORMULAE WITH CONDITIONS

Suppose the employing company in the above example awards a bonus to people who exceed their target by more than £1,000. The spreadsheet could work out who is entitled to the bonus.

To do this we would enter the appropriate formula in cells F4 to F7. For salesperson Easterman, we would enter the following in cell F7:

=IF(D4>1000,"BONUS"," ")

We will now explain this **IF** function.

IF statements follow the following structure (or 'syntax').

=**IF(logical_test, value_if_true, value_if_false)**

The logical_test is any value or expression that can be evaluated to Yes or No. For example, D4>1000 is a logical expression; if the value in cell D4 is over 1,000, the expression evaluates to Yes. Otherwise, the expression evaluates to No.

Value_if_true is the value that is returned if the answer to the logical_test is Yes. For example, if the answer to D4>1000 is Yes, and the value_if_true is the text string "BONUS", then the cell containing the IF function will display the text "BONUS".

Value_if_false is the value that is returned if the answer to the logical_test is No. For example, if the value_if_false is two sets of quote marks "" this means display a blank cell if the answer to the logical test is No. So in our example, if D4 is not over 1,000, then the cell containing the IF function will display a blank cell.

Note the following symbols which can be used in formulae with conditions:

<	less than
<=	less than or equal to
=	equal to
>=	greater than or equal to
>	greater than
<>	not equal to

Care is required to ensure **brackets** and **commas** are entered in the right places. If, when you try out this kind of formula, you get an error message, it may well be a simple mistake, such as leaving a comma out.

Using the IF function

A company offers a discount of 5% to customers who order more than £10,000 worth of goods. A spreadsheet showing what customers will pay may look like:

	C8			f_x	=IF(B8>$C$3, B8*$C$4,0)	
	A	B	C	D	E	F
1	Sales discount					
2						
3	Discount hurdle		10,000			
4	Discount rate		5%			
5						
6	Customer	Sales	Discount	Net price		
7		£	£	£		
8	John	12,000	600	11,400		
9	Margaret	9,000	0	9,000		
10	William	8,000	0	8,000		
11	Julie	20,000	1000	19,000		
12						
13						
14						
15						

The formula in cell C8 is as shown: =**IF**(B8>$C$3, B8*$C$4, 0). This means, if the value in B8 is greater than £10,000 multiply it by the contents of C4, ie 5%, otherwise the discount will be zero. Cell D8 will calculate the amount net of

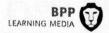

discount, using the formula: =B8–C8. The same conditional formula with the cell references changed will be found in cells C9, C10 and C11.

Here is another example for you to try.

Open the spreadsheet called Exam Results (one of the spreadsheets downloaded from www.bpp.com/aatspreadsheets).

There are ten candidates listed together with their marks.

The pass mark has been set at 50%.

See if you can complete column C rows 6 – 15 so that it shows PASS if the candidate scores 50 or above, and FAIL if the candidate scores less than 50.

Once it's set up and working correctly, change the pass mark in cell B3 to 60 and ensure that the PASS/FAIL indications reflect the change.

The formulae you need will be based on the one for cell C6.

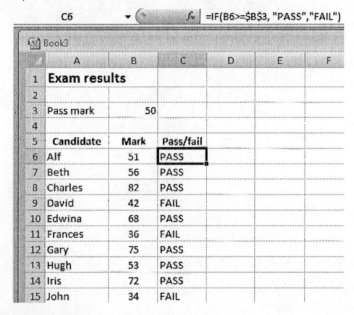

Conditional formatting

In addition to the condition determining whether PASS or FAIL appear, you can also conditionally format cell contents – for example, by altering the colour of a cell to highlight problems. This can be done by accessing the **Conditional Formatting** option in the **Styles** section of the **Home** tab of the Ribbon.

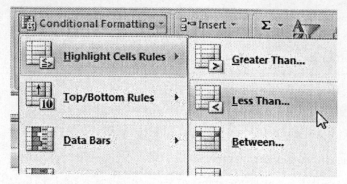

The marks which are less than the value in B3 have been highlighted by making the cell background red and the text white, as illustrated below:

	A	B	C
1	**Exam results**		
2			
3	Pass mark	50	
4			
5	**Candidate**	**Mark**	**Pass/fail**
6	Alf	51	PASS
7	Beth	56	PASS
8	Charles	82	PASS
9	David	42	FAIL
10	Edwina	68	PASS
11	Frances	36	FAIL
12	Gary	75	PASS
13	Hugh	53	PASS
14	Iris	72	PASS
15	John	34	FAIL

To produce the above result:

> Change the pass mark back to 50% if it is still at 60%.
>
> Highlight the numbers in column B.
>
> Click **Conditional formatting>Highlight cell rules>Less than**. You will see there are two white entry boxes.
>
> Click on cell B3. This will be entered automatically into the first box.
>
> Then click on the down arrow next to the second entry box. Click on **Custom format>Fill** and choose the red box. This changes the colour of the cell.
>
> Then click on **Font** and click the down arrow next to 'Automatic', under **Colour** and choose the white box.
>
> Click **OK**.

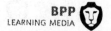

You can also use Conditional formatting to highlight the top three results for example:

	A	B	C	D
1	**Exam results**			
2				
3	Pass mark	50		
4				
5	**Candidate**	**Mark**	**Pass/fail**	
6	Alf	51	PASS	
7	Beth	56	PASS	
8	Charles	82	PASS	
9	David	42	FAIL	
10	Edwina	68	PASS	
11	Frances	36	FAIL	
12	Gary	75	PASS	
13	Hugh	53	PASS	
14	Iris	72	PASS	
15	John	34	FAIL	
16				
17				
18				
19				
20				

To produce the above result:

> Highlight the numbers in column B.
>
> Click **Conditional formatting > Top/Bottom rules > Top 10 items.**
>
> In the first entry box, change the number from 10 to 3.
>
> In the second entry box, click on **Custom format > Fill** and choose the green box. This changes the colour of the cell.
>
> Then click on **Font** and click the down arrow next to 'Automatic', under **Colour** and choose the white box.
>
> Click **OK.**

Ranking data

The RANK function, one of Excel's statistical functions, ranks the size of a number compared to other numbers in a list a data.

The syntax for the RANK function is:

= **RANK (Number, Ref, Order)**

Number – the cell reference of the number to be ranked.

Ref – the range of cells to use in ranking the Number.

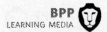

Order – determines whether the Number is ranked in ascending or descending order. 0 for descending order and 1 for ascending order.

The names in the Exam Results spreadsheet are in alphabetical order. Say you want to keep them in that order but you want to see who came first, second, third etc. You can use RANK to give that information.

	D6			f_x	=RANK(B6,$B$6:$B$15,0)		
	A	B	C	D	E	F	G
1	Exam results						
2							
3	Pass mark	50					
4							
5	Candidate	Mark	Pass/fail	Rank			
6	Alf	51	PASS	7			
7	Beth	56	PASS	5			
8	Charles	82	PASS	1			
9	David	42	FAIL	8			
10	Edwina	68	PASS	4			
11	Frances	36	FAIL	9			
12	Gary	75	PASS	2			
13	Hugh	53	PASS	6			
14	Iris	72	PASS	3			
15	John	34	FAIL	10			
16							

To produce the above result:

> Enter Rank in cell D5.
>
> In cell D6, type =RANK(B6,$B$6:$B$15,0). This means that B6 will be ranked within the range B6:B15 in descending order.
>
> Copy the formula to cells B7 to B15.

CHARTS AND GRAPHS

Charts and graphs are useful and powerful ways of communicating trends and relative sizes of numerical data. Excel makes the production of charts relatively easy through the use of the chart wizard.

We will use the Sales discount spreadsheet (one of the spreadsheets downloaded from www.bpp.com/aatspreadsheets) to generate a number of different charts.

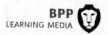

	A	B	C	D
1	**Sales discount**			
2				
3	Discount hurdle		10,000	
4	Discount rate		5%	
5				
6	**Customer**	**Sales**	**Discount**	**Net price**
7		£	£	£
8	John	12,000	600	11,400
9	Margaret	9,000	0	9,000
10	William	8,000	0	8,000
11	Julie	20,000	1000	19,000

First, we will generate a simple pie chart showing the total sales figure, before discounts.

A simple pie chart

(1) Open the Sales discount spreadsheet.

(2) Place your cursor on the word 'Customer', hold down the mouse button and drag the cursor downwards until you have selected the four names and four sales figures.

(3) Select the **Insert** section from the Ribbon, then **Pie/3-D pie**.

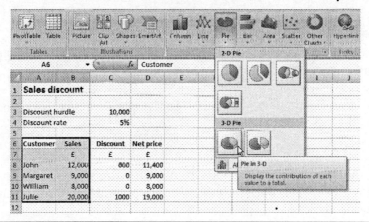

This will generate a pie chart that looks like this:

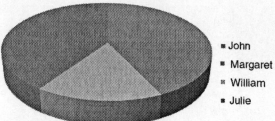

You will see that it already has a title, 'Sales £'. To make any changes to this, double click the area where the title appears, then enter additional text or delete text you do not want. Below we have added 'for 20X6' and brackets around the pound sign.

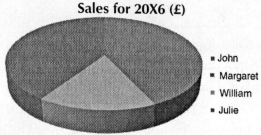

Changing the chart type

If you decide that a different chart may be more suitable for presenting your data you can easily change the chart type.

> (1) Click on your chart. The **Chart Tools** options should become available at the top of the window.
>
> (2) Click **Design>Change Chart Type**.
>
> (3) From here, pick some charts from the following chart types to see what they produce: **Bar**, **Bubble**, **Doughnut** and **Line**. For example the doughnut chart will produce something like this:

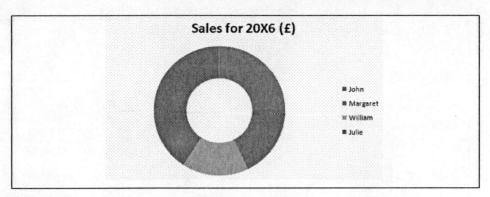

Bar charts

A pie chart is good for showing relative sizes of elements making up a total. However, sometimes you may want to be able to compare how two series of data are moving: sales and gross profit for example. In this case, bar charts (or line charts) are more suitable. Excel makes a distinction between bar charts that show vertical bars and those that show horizontal bars. **When the data is shown *vertically* Excel refers to the chart as a *'column'* chart whereas if the data is shown *horizontally* it is a *'bar'* chart.**

We are going to create a column chart showing the Sales and Net Price figure from the data on the Sales Discount spreadsheet.

(1) Delete your chart by clicking on its outer most frame and pressing the **Delete** key.

(2) Place the cursor on the word 'Customer' and drag the cursor down until all four names have been selected.

(3) Hold down the Ctrl button and select B6:B11. Still holding the Ctrl button down, select D6:D11.

(4) Release the mouse button and Ctrl key.

(5) On the Ribbon, choose **Insert>Column>2D Column**.

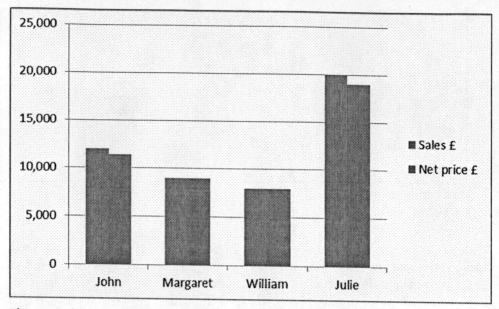

This time there is no automatic chart title so we will need to add one.

Click on the chart. At the top of the window you will see **Chart Tools** appear:

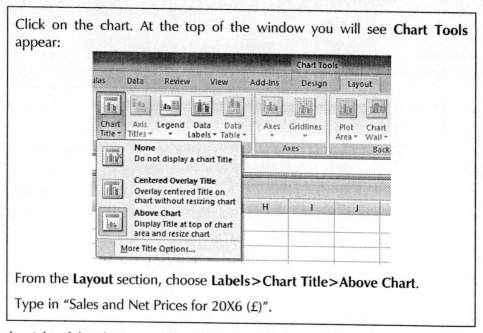

From the **Layout** section, choose **Labels>Chart Title>Above Chart**.

Type in "Sales and Net Prices for 20X6 (£)".

To the right of the chart you will see a description for each column. This is called a Legend. You can move the legend by clicking on the **Legend** button.

You should also label the horizontal axis and the vertical axis.

(1) To label the horizontal axis, click **Layout>Axis Titles>Primary Horizontal Axis>Title below axis** (make sure you are clicked on the chart to see the **Chart Tools** tabs).

(2) The words 'Axis Title' appear at the bottom of the chart. Click on this, then press **Ctrl + A** to select all the words and type in your axis title, in this case 'Customer'.

(3) To label the other axis, this time choose **Primary Vertical Axis**. You have a choice of directions for your text. Choose **Horizontal Title** and type a pound sign.

Note that if you are typing words for the vertical axis title the best option is usually **Rotated Title**. Try experimenting with that now.

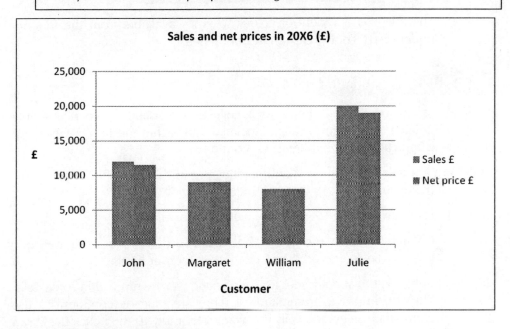

Formatting existing charts

Even after your chart is 'finished' you can change it in a variety of ways.

(a) You can **resize it** simply by selecting it and dragging out one of its corners.

(b) You can change the scale by dragging out the top, base or sides. To do so, hover your cursor over the four dots in the middle of the relevant top, base or side until your cursor turns into a **double ended arrow**. Click and it will turn into a large cross, then drag with the mouse button still held down.

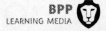

(c) You can change **each element** by **clicking** on it then selecting from the options available on the various **Chart tools** tabs.

(d) You can also select any item of **text** and alter the wording, size or font, or change the **colours** used using the buttons on the **Font** section of the Home part of the ribbon. For example, practice increasing and decreasing the size of the font by clicking on the text you wish to change, then experimenting with the two different sized capital A buttons:

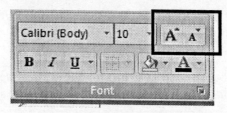

(e) There is also a variety of colour schemes available from the Ribbon, under **Chart Tools > Design > Chart Styles**.

Simple data manipulation

A database can be viewed simply as a collection of data. There is a simple 'database' related to inventory, called Stockman Ltd within the files downloaded from www.bpp.com/aatspreadsheets. **Open it now.**

There are a number of features worth pointing out in this spreadsheet before we start data manipulation.

(1) Each row from 4–15 holds an inventory record.

(2) Column G makes use of the **IF** function to determine if the inventory needs to be reordered (when quantity < reorder level).

(3) In row 2, the spreadsheet uses automatic word wrap within some cells. This can improve presentation if there are long descriptions. To use word wrap, select the cells you want it to apply to then click the **Wrap Text** icon in the **Alignment** section of the **Home** tab. The height of the cells needs to be increased to accommodate more than one line of text. To do this, select the whole row then double click on the line between the row numbers 2 and 3, or instead, select **AutoFit Row Height** as shown below.

The data is currently arranged in part number order.

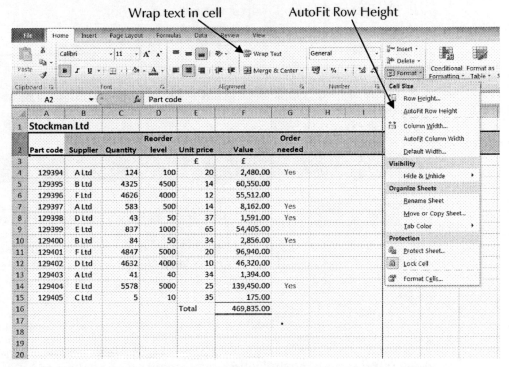

The horizontal rows are records: one record for each inventory type. The vertical columns are attributes (qualities) relating to each record.

Sorting the data

Let's say that we want to sort the data into descending value order.

(1) Select the data range A4:G15.

(2) At the right-hand side of the **Home** section of the Ribbon (and in the **Data** section of the Ribbon) you will see the **Sort & Filter** drop-down menu.

> (3) Choose **Custom Sort**.
>
> (4) Sort by Column F, largest to smallest.
>
> (5) Click **OK**.

You will see that the data has been sorted by value.

If you now **Sort by** Supplier (**Order A – Z**) you will have the data arranged by supplier, and within that by value.

PRINTING

Printing spreadsheets

The print options for your spreadsheet may be accessed by selecting **File button** and **Print**, or pressing **Ctrl + P**. Printing large spreadsheets without checking the print and layout settings will often result in printouts spread messily over several pages.

It is a good idea to at least opt for **Print Preview** to see what your printout will look like before printing.

A better option is to control what prints more precisely. This can be done from the **Page Layout** section of the Ribbon.

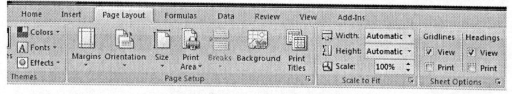

This allows you to, for example, print out selected areas only, include/exclude grid-lines and the column and row headings, alter the orientation of the page and so on.

> Open the spreadsheet we saw earlier called Costing Exercise – Finished.
>
> Assume that we only want to print out the cash flow without the table at the top showing the assumptions. We want to show the gridlines but not the A, B, C... or 1, 2, 3... that head up columns and rows.
>
> (1) Select the range A9:F24.
>
> (2) Choose **Page Layout>Print Area>Set Print Area** from the Ribbon.

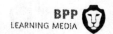

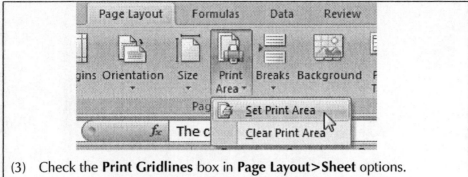

(3)   Check the **Print Gridlines** box in **Page Layout>Sheet** options.

(4)   Choose **Office Button>Print>Print Preview**.

At this point you can check for obvious layout and formatting errors.

Spelling

Before you print, it is wise to check your work for spelling mistakes. To do this click the **Review** tab and select **Spelling**. If you have made any spelling errors Excel will offer alternative **Suggestions** which you can accept by clicking **Change** or ignore by clicking **Ignore** (**Once** or **All**).

If the word is in fact correct (for example, terminology that Excel does not recognise) you can add it to Excel's dictionary by clicking **Add to Dictionary**.

Preparing your spreadsheet for printing: Page set-up

The **Page Setup** area of the **Page Layout** tab on the Ribbon also allows you to specify certain other details that affect how your spreadsheet looks when it prints out.

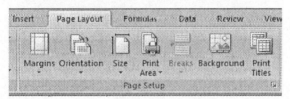

From here you can set the size of the **Margins** (the white spaces that print around the spreadsheet) and choose whether to print the spreadsheet in landscape **Orientation** (ie wider than tall) rather than the default portrait **Orientation** (taller than wide).

If you want to make sure that your spreadsheet will print onto one page, you can choose to Fit 1 page wide by 1 page tall. This can be done by accessing the **Page Setup** options, by clicking on the little arrow in the bottom right corner of the section on the ribbon.

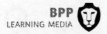

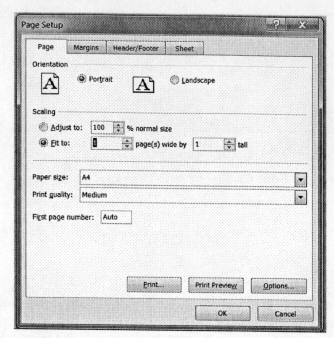

Imagine you are printing out a spreadsheet that will cover several pages. It is important that certain information is present on each page. For example:

- The spreadsheet title
- The page number and total pages
- The author
- The row and column headings

This can be done by accessing the **Page Setup** options, in the way outlined above, or by clicking on the **Print Titles** icon.

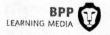

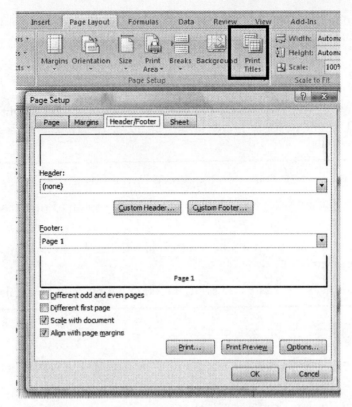

Headers appear at the top of each page. For example, a custom header could be:

Author   Budget for 2013   Date printed

Footers appear at the bottom of each page, for example:

Page   File name

The **Sheet** tab allows you to specify the rows and columns to be repeated on each page. For example, you might want to repeat the months across the top of each page and the type of income down the left of each page.

We have provided a demonstration spreadsheet in the downloaded files, Print practice. Open it and try the following:

    Insert a **Header**: Author name, Title (Budget 2013) Date printed

    Insert a **Footer**: Page number, File name

Click **Page setup (or Print Titles)>Header/Footer> Custom Header** and **Custom Footer**.

Ensure that the headings in column A are repeated on the second page.

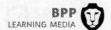

Use this spreadsheet to experiment with page breaks (**Breaks**) and the other remaining options in the **Page Setup** area.

Printing formulae

Occasionally, perhaps for documentation or checking, you might want the spreadsheet formulae to be printed out instead of the calculated results of the formula. To do this:

> (1)   Display the formulae on the screen by pressing **Ctrl + `** .
>
> (2)   Set the area you want to be printed: **Page Layout > Print Area > Set Area**
>
> (3)   Check what the printout will look like **Office button > Print > Print preview**
>
> (4)   Adjust as necessary and print out when happy with the display

Printing charts

Charts can be printed either with or without the data on the worksheet.

To print only the chart simply click on it and then press **Ctrl + P**. As always it is wise to **Print Preview** first.

If you also want to print the worksheet data, click away from the chart into any cell. Use **Print Preview** to make sure that the chart is the right size and is in the right position. Then press **Ctrl + P**.

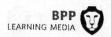

CHAPTER OVERVIEW

- A **spreadsheet** is basically an electronic piece of paper divided into **rows** and **columns**. The intersection of a row and a column is known as a **cell**.

- Essential basic **skills** include how to **move around** within a spreadsheet, how to **enter** and **edit** data, how to **fill** cells, how to **insert** and **delete** columns and rows and how to improve the basic **layout** and **appearance** of a spreadsheet.

- **Relative** cell references (eg B3) change when you copy formulae to other locations or move data from one place to another. **Absolute** cell references (eg $B$3) stay the same.

- A wide range of **formulae** and functions are available within Excel. We looked at the use of conditional formulae that use an **IF** statement.

- A spreadsheet should be given a **title** which clearly defines its purpose. The contents of rows and columns should also be clearly **labelled**. **Formatting** should be used to make the data in the spreadsheet easy to read and interpret.

- **Numbers** can be **formatted** in several ways, for instance with commas, as percentages, as currency or with a certain number of decimal places.

- Excel includes the facility to produce a range of charts and graphs. The **Chart Wizard** provides a tool to simplify the process of chart construction.

- Excel offers data handling including **sorting and ranking**.

- Spreadsheets can be used in a variety of accounting contexts. You should practise using spreadsheets, **hands-on experience** is the key to spreadsheet proficiency.

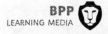

TEST YOUR LEARNING

Test 1

List three types of cell contents.

Test 2

What do the F5 and F2 keys do in Excel?

Test 3

What technique can you use to insert a logical series of data such as 1, 2 ....
10, or Jan, Feb, March etc?

Test 4

How do you display formulae instead of the results of formulae in a
spreadsheet?

Test 5

List five possible changes that may improve the appearance of a spreadsheet.

Test 6

What is the syntax (pattern) of an IF function in Excel?

Test 7

The following spreadsheet shows sales of two products, the Ego and the Id,
for the period July to September.

	A	B	C	D	E
1	Sigmund Ltd				
2	Sales analysis - quarter 3, 2010				
3		July	August	September	Total
4	Ego	3,000	4,000	2,000	9,000
5	Id	2,000	1,500	4,000	7,500
6	Total	5,000	5,500	6,000	16,500

Devise a suitable formula for each of the following cells.

(a) Cell B6
(b) Cell E5
(c) Cell E6

Test 8

The following spreadsheet shows sales, exclusive of VAT, the VAT amounts and the VAT inclusive amounts. The old VAT rate of 17.5% has been used and needs to be updated to the new 20% rate. It is important that this can easily be changed without needing to change any of the formulae in the spreadsheet.

	A	B	C	D
1	Taxable Supplies Ltd		Vat rate	0.175
2				
3		January	February	March
4	Product A	5,000	4,000	3,000
5	Product B	2,000	1,500	4,000
6	Product C	7,000	5,700	4,000
7	Product D	2,000	3,000	1,000
8	Product E	1,000	2,400	6,000
9	Total net	17,000	16,600	18,000
10	VAT	2,975	2,905	3,150
11	Total gross	19,975	19,505	21,150

Suggest suitable formulae for cells:

    (a)   B9

    (b)   C10

    (c)   D11

chapter 4:
MORE ADVANCED SPREADSHEET TECHNIQUES (EXCEL 2010)

---

chapter coverage 📖

In this chapter we explore some of the more advanced aspects of spreadsheets using Excel 2010.

This chapter covers:

- ✍ Controls, security and sharing
- ✍ Data manipulation
- ✍ Three dimensional (multi-sheet) spreadsheets
- ✍ Changes in assumptions (what-if? analysis)
- ✍ Statistical functions
- ✍ Combination charts
- ✍ Error detection and correction

CONTROLS, SECURITY AND SHARING

Back-ups, passwords and cell protection

There are facilities available in spreadsheet packages which can be used as controls – to prevent unauthorised or accidental amendment or deletion of all or part of a spreadsheet. There are also facilities available for hiding data, and for preventing (or alerting) users about incorrect data.

Saving files and backing up

(a) **Save.** When working on a spreadsheet, save your file regularly, as often as every ten minutes, using **File button>Save** or pressing **Ctrl + S**. This will prevent too much work being lost in the event of a system crash.

Save files in the appropriate **folder** so that they are easy to locate. If you need to save the file to a new folder, choose the **'New folder'** option after clicking **File button>Save**. Where this option is located depends on the operating system you are using. For example, in Windows 7, you simply click the **New folder** button (see below).

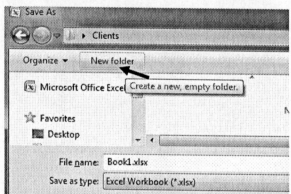

Give the folder a suitable name (for example, the name of the client you are working on or following your employer's standard naming practice).

(b) **Save as.** A simple **save** overwrites the existing file. If you use **Save as** then you can give the file a different name, preserving previous versions. For example Save as 'Budget Edition 1', 'Budget Edition 2', 'Budget Edition 3'. This is much safer than simply relying on the most recent version – which might be beyond fixing!

(c) **Back-ups.** Because data and the computers or storage devices on which it is stored can easily be lost or destroyed, it is vital to take regular copies or back-ups. If the data is lost, the back-up copy can be used to **restore** the data up to the time the back-up was taken. Spreadsheet files should be included in standard backup procedures, for example the daily back-up routine.

The back-ups could be held on a separate external hard drive, or perhaps a USB memory stick, and should stored away from the original data, in case there is a fire or other disaster at the organisation's premises. Alternatively the back-ups can be saved to a network location. Some back-ups are now stored on the Internet.

(d) **AutoRecover**. Excel has a built-in feature that saves copies of all open Excel files at a fixed time interval. The files can be restored if Excel closes unexpectedly, such as during a power failure.

Turn on the AutoRecover feature by clicking **File button>Excel Options>Save**.

The default time between saves is every 10 minutes. To change this, click the **Save AutoRecover info every** check box and enter any number of minutes between 1 and 120.

In the **AutoRecover file location** box, you can type the path and the folder name of the location in which you want to keep the AutoRecover files.

Protection

(a) **Cell protection/cell locking**. This prevents the user from inadvertently changing cells that should not be changed. There are two ways of specifying which cells should be protected.

(i) All cells are locked except those specifically unlocked.

This method is useful when you want most cells to be locked. When protection is implemented, all cells are locked unless they have previously been excluded from the protection process. You will also see here a similar mechanism for hiding data.

---

(1) Open the spreadsheet Costing Exercise–Finished.

(2) Highlight the range B2:B5. This contains some of the assumptions on which the cash flow forecast is based and this is the only range of cells that we want to be unlocked and available for alteration.

(3) In the **Home** section of the Ribbon, click on the small arrow beside **Fonts** and then choose **Protection**.

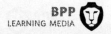

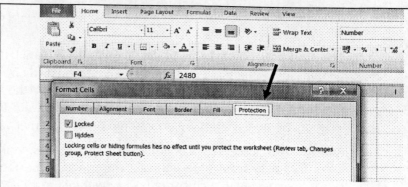

(4) Untick the **Locked** and **Hidden** boxes.

(5) Click on **OK**.

(6) Now go to the **Review** group on the **Ribbon**.

(7) Click on **Protect Sheet**.

(8) Don't enter a password when prompted, simply click **OK**.

Now investigate what you can change on the spreadsheet. You should find that only cells B2:B5 can be changed. If you try to change anything else a message comes up telling you that the cell is protected.

Click on **Unprotect Sheet** to make every cell accessible to change again.

(ii) Most are unlocked, except those specified as being locked.

This method is useful if only a few cells have to be locked.

(1) Open the spreadsheet Sales discount.

(2) Assume that we want to lock only the 10,000 in cell C3 and the 5% figure in cell C4.

(3) Select the whole spreadsheet and, as we did above, click on the small arrow beside **Fonts**. Then choose **Protection** and untick the **Locked** and **Hidden** boxes. The cells can still be changed if you do not do this step.

(4) Select the range of cells C3:C4.

(5) In the **Home** section of the Ribbon go to the **Cells** group and click on **Format**.

(6) Click on **Lock Cell**.

(7) Click on **Protect Sheet** from the same **Format** menu. The cells remain editable if you do not do this step.

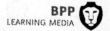

> You are offered the chance to enter a password.
>
> Now you will be prevented from changing just those two cells.

(b) **Passwords**. There are two levels of password.

   (i) All access to the spreadsheet can be protected and the spreadsheet encrypted. This can be done by:

   > (1) **File button > Info > Protect Workbook > Encrypt with Password.**
   >
   > (2) You are then asked to enter and verify a password. Heed the warning: if you forget the password, there's no likelihood of recovery of the spreadsheet.
   >
   > (3) To remove the password protection use:
   > **File button > Info > Protect Workbook > Encrypt with Password**
   >
   > (4) Then delete the asterisks in the password box and click OK.

   (ii) The spreadsheet can be password protected from amendment but can be seen without a password. This can be done as follows:

   > (1) At the bottom of the **Save As** dialogue click **Tools**.
   >
   > (2) Choose **General Options**.
   >
   > (3) You can choose here again a Password to open.
   >
   > (4) In the Password to modify box type a password, then retype it to confirm and click **OK**.
   >
   > (5) Click **Save**.

   Now, if you close the file and re-open it, you will be asked for a password to get full access, or without the password you can open it in read-only mode so that it can be seen but not changed.

Data validation

Sometimes only a specific type or range of data is valid for a certain cell or cells. For example, if inputting hours worked in a week from a time sheet it could be known that no one should have worked more than 60 hours. It is possible to test data as it is input and to either prevent input completely or simply warn that the input value looks odd. This is known as 'data validation' or 'data restriction'.

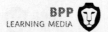

C2			f_x	=A2*B2
A	B	C	D	
1	Hours	Rate/hr	Pay	
2	10	7	70	

In this simple spreadsheet, C2 holds the only formula; A2 and B2 are cells into which data will be entered, but we want the data to conform to certain rules:

Hours <= 60. If greater than 60, a warning is to be issued.

Rate/hr >=8 and <=20. Data outside that range should be rejected.

(1) Set up a new spreadsheet with the above data and make A2 the active cell. Go to **Data>Data Validation** (in **Data Tools** section).

(2) Under the **Data Validation Settings** tab, **Allow Decimal**, select less than or equal to from the drop-down list and enter 60 as the Maximum.

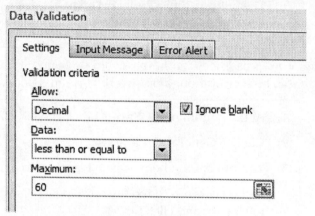

(3) Under the **Input Message** tab enter 'Warning' as the title and 'Hours expected to be less than 60' as the input message.

(4) Under the **Error Alert** tab change the **Style** to Warning, enter 'Attention' as the title and 'Check hours: look too large' as the **Error message**.

(5) Click **OK**.

(6) Now try to enter 70 into A2. You will first see an information message explaining what data is expected, then a warning message and the option to continue.

(7) Now try to set up cell B2 with appropriate messages and to prevent any value outside the range 8–20 from being entered at all.

DATA MANIPULATION

Data manipulation refers to a number of techniques available in Excel for summarising, analysing and presenting data.

Filtering the data

Filtering data allows you to select and display just some of it in the table. This is useful if the table consists of many records but you only wish to view some of them.

> Open the Stockman Ltd spreadsheet.
>
> Let's say we just want to find inventory records relating to suppliers B and C.
>
> Select **Filter** from the **Sort & Filter** drop-down menu.
>
> Click on the drop-down arrow that has appeared at the top of the Supplier column.
>
> Deselect (ie click on the box to remove the tick) **Select All**, then select B and C.
>
> Click on **OK**.

Only the records relating to suppliers B and C are visible and these can be manipulated (eg sorted) as an independent subset of the whole table.

Note that the other records are still there and are included in the total value figure. It's simply that they have been hidden for presentation.

You will also see a little funnel symbol at the top of the Supplier column informing that there is filtering in place.

> Make all the records visible again by removing the filter:
>
> (1)   Drop-down arrow in the Supplier column.
> (2)   Select **Select All**.
> (3)   Click on **OK**.
> (4)   Sort the data back into Part code order if it's not already in that order.
>
> To get rid of the little filter arrows, click on the funnel symbol in the **Sort & Filter** area of the Ribbon to disengage it.

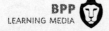

Find and replace

Let's now say that that Supplier A Ltd has been taken over and that its name has changed to Acorn plc.

> (1) Make all the records visible again by removing the filter if you haven't already
>
> (2) Click on the **Find & Select** symbol and select **Find** (or press **Ctrl + F**)
>
> (3) Enter A Ltd in the **Find what:** box
>
> (4) Click on the **Replace** tab and enter Acorn Plc in the **Replace with:** box
>
> (5) Click on **Replace All**
>
> **Note.** You could instead click on **Find & Select>Replace** (or press **Ctrl + H**) as a shortcut.

You should see that all occurrences of A Ltd have been replaced by Acorn plc.

If no range is specified before this step then the whole spreadsheet would be affected. If a range is specified, the search and replace occurs only within that range.

Σ AutoSum

You have already used Σ AutoSum as a way of specifying a range of data to add up. However, the Σ AutoSum drop-down list also contains other useful functions such as:

- **Average**
- **Count numbers**
- **Maximum**
- **Minimum**

Still using the Stockman Ltd spreadsheet:

> (1) Select cells E4..E15
>
> (2) From the **Σ AutoSum** drop-down list (you can find this on both the **Home** and **Formulas** tabs of the Ribbon) select **Max**
>
> You will see 65 appear in cell E16 (just below the last unit price). The formula in that cell is =MAX(E4:E15).
>
> Try some of the other **Σ AutoSum** functions.

The results given by **Σ AutoSum** are always just under a column of data, or immediately to the right of a row of data.

If you want the results to appear in a different cell, you have to type the appropriate formula into that cell. For example, typing =MAX(E4:E15) into cell A20 will show the maximum unit price of the inventory in cell A20.

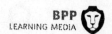

Concatenate

The concatenate function is used to combine two text cells into a single cell.

This is done by using the formula =CONCATENATE(text1, [text 2]…)

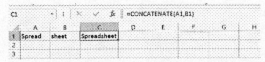

If the formula is used as shown above, the words will be joined together with no space inbetween.

If a space is to be included between the words, this can be achieved by using quotation marks around a single space between the two text references in the formula.

=CONCATENATE(text1, " ",[text 2]…)

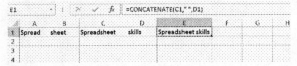

This is particularly useful when joining data such as first name and last name.

Pivot tables

Pivot tables are a very powerful way of analysing data. Look at the following simple example relating to sales by a music company.

	A	B	C
			Pivot table example
1	Sales data		
2			
3	Customer	Source	Amount spent (£)
4	Bill	CDs	50
5	Chris	Vinyl	10
6	Sandra	Merchandise	30
7	Graham	CDs	45
8	Chris	Merchandise	20
9	Chris	Vinyl	10
10	Chris	CDs	10
11	Caroline	Merchandise	30
12	Graham	Tickets	75
13	Fred	Vinyl	30
14	Bill	CDs	20
15	Graham	CDs	60
16	Chris	Vinyl	10
17	Sandra	Tickets	50
18	Bill	Tickets	26
19	Caroline	Vinyl	24
20			
21		Total	£500

The information has simply been listed and totalled on the spreadsheet. It would be useful to be able to show:

- Sales per customer
- Sales by source

Ideally, we would like to produce a table which displays sales by both source and by customer: this type of table is called a pivot table.

(1) Open the spreadsheet file called Pivot Table Example which contains the above data.

(2) Select the range A4:C19.

(3) On the Ribbon, select **Insert>PivotTable**.

(4) Select the **Existing Worksheet** radio button on the **Create PivotTable** option window.

(5) Enter E4 as the location.

(6) Click **OK**. The PivotTable Field List window opens.

(7) Check Customer, Source, Amount spent (£).

(8) You will see that Customer and Source go by default into Row Labels. The resulting table is quite useful, but not quite what we wanted.

Therefore:

(9) Drag Customer from Row Labels to Column Labels.

The pivot table is now transformed into the two-dimensional table we want.

(10) Tidy it up a little by selecting F5 to L5 and right justifying these names by clicking on the appropriate Home>Alignment button on the Ribbon.

Note the two drop down arrows on the pivot table that allow filtering of the data.

Sum of Amount spent (£)	Column Labels						
Row Labels	Bill	Caroline	Chris	Fred	Graham	Sandra	Grand Total
CDs	70		10		105		185
Merchandise		30	20			30	80
Tickets	26				75	50	151
Vinyl		24	30	30			84
Grand Total	96	54	60	30	180	80	500

If you had difficulty with this, the spreadsheet called 'Pivot Table Result Excel 2010' is available within the downloaded files.

Experiment with different settings. Clicking on the pivot table will bring up the **PivotTable Field List** window again if it has disappeared.

Note that if the original data is altered, the pivot table does *not* change until you right-click on it and select **Refresh** from the list of options.

Pivot charts

The information contained in a pivot table can be visually presented using a pivot chart.

(1) Click on any cell inside the pivot table.

(2) On the insert tab click Pivot chart and select one of the graph types. For example, clustered column

Note any changes you make to the pivot table will be immediately reflected in the pivot chart and vice versa.

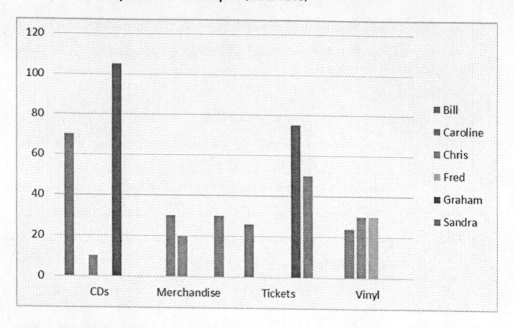

Sharing workbooks

It is possible to share a workbook with colleagues so that the same file can be viewed by more than one person at a time. This can be done in a number of ways.

Send as an attachment

One way to share a spreadsheet with colleagues is to send it as an attachment in an email. If your computer is set up with a mail client such as Microsoft Outlook you can click **File Button>Save & Send>Send Using Email** to quickly send the spreadsheet you are working on as an attachment.

Alternatively, you can first draft the email and attach the spreadsheet using your email program's options and the Windows Explorer menu.

However, if each recipient of the email makes changes to the document, this will lead to the existence of a number of different versions of the same document, and a potential loss of version control. This is not, therefore, a recommended method of sharing spreadsheets.

Save to a shared network server

Another way to make a spreadsheet available to colleagues is to save it in a place on the network server that is also accessible to them. Anyone with access to that particular location will be able to open the file but, if more than one person tries to open the file, only the first person will be able to make changes to it. Anyone else subsequently opening the file will only be able to open a 'Read Only' version of it, so they will be able to view the contents but not make any changes.

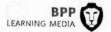

This method prevents loss of version control but is not particularly useful if other people wish to make changes at the same time.

Share workbook method

A more practical method is to use the inbuilt sharing function in Excel. This allows different people to open and make changes to the same document at the same time, and for these changes to be tracked.

Click the **Review** tab on the Ribbon. In the **Changes** section click the **Share Workbook** button. Click the **Editing** tab and select **Allow changes by more than one user at the same time**. From this tab you can also see who has the document open.

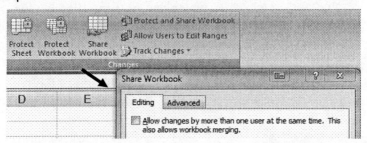

Other settings are available from the **Advanced** tab such as choosing how long to keep the change history for, how frequently to update changes and what to do if users make conflicting changes.

To stop any tracked changes from being lost click **Protect and Share Workbook** and click **Sharing with tracked changes**. This option also allows you to set a password so only those with the password can make changes.

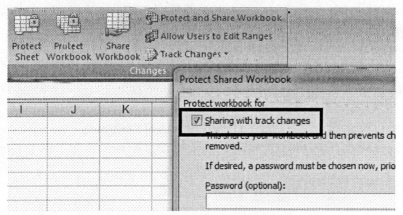

THREE DIMENSIONAL (MULTI-SHEET) SPREADSHEETS

Background

In early spreadsheet packages, a spreadsheet file consisted of a single worksheet. As mentioned earlier, Excel provides the option of multi-sheet spreadsheets, consisting of a series of related sheets.

For example, suppose you were producing a profit forecast for two regions, and a combined forecast for the total of the regions. This situation would be suited to using separate worksheets for each region and another for the total. This approach is sometimes referred to as working in **three dimensions**, as you are able to flip between different sheets stacked in front or behind each other. Cells in one sheet may **refer** to cells in another sheet. So, in our example, the formulae in the cells in the total sheet would refer to the cells in the other sheets.

Excel has a series of 'tabs', one for each worksheet at the bottom of the spreadsheet.

How many worksheets?

Excel can be set up so that it always opens a fresh file with a certain number of worksheets ready and waiting for you. Click on **Office button > Excel Options > Popular**, and set the number **'Include this many sheets'** option to the number you would like each new workbook to contain (sheets may be added or deleted later).

If you subsequently want to insert more sheets you just click on the new sheet tab.

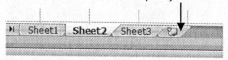

By default sheets are called Sheet 1, Sheet 2 etc. However, these may be changed. To rename a sheet in Excel, right click on its index tab and choose the **Rename** option. You can drag the sheets into different orders by clicking on the tab, holding down the mouse button and dragging a sheet to its new position.

Pasting from one sheet to another

When building a spreadsheet that will contain a number of worksheets with identical structure, users often set up one sheet, then copy that sheet and amend its contents.

To copy a worksheet in Excel, from within the worksheet you wish to copy, select **Home > Cells > Format > Move or Copy Sheet** (or right click the worksheet tab and select **Move or Copy Sheet**) and tick the **Create a copy** box.

A 'Total' sheet would use the same structure, but would contain formulae totalling the individual sheets.

Linking sheets with formulae

Formulae on one sheet may refer to data held on another sheet. The links within such a formula may be established using the following steps.

Step 1   In the cell that you want to refer to a cell from another sheet, type =.

Step 2   Click on the index tab for the sheet containing the cell you want to refer to and select the cell in question.

Step 3   Press **Enter**.

---

(1)   Open the spreadsheet called 3D spreadsheet example.

This consists of three worksheets. The Branch A and Branch B sheets hold simple trading accounts and income statements. There are both numbers and formulae in those sheets. The Company sheet contains only headings, but is set out in the same pattern as the two branch sheets.

We want to combine the Branch figures onto the Company sheet.

(2)   On the Company sheet, make D2 the active cell.

(3)   Enter =

(4)   Click on Branch A and click on D2.

(5)   Enter +

(6)   Click on Branch B and click on D2.

(7)   Press **Enter**.

You will see that the formula ='Branch A'!D2+'Branch B'!D2 is now in cell D2 of the Company sheet and that the number displayed is 500,000, the sum of the sales in each branch.

In the Company sheet, copy D2 (**Ctrl+C**) and paste (**Ctrl+V**) to D3, D4, C6, C7, C8, and D9 to complete the income statement.

The company sheet will now look like this:

	A	B	C	D
	3D spreadsheet example [Compatibility Mode]			
1	**Company**		£	£
2	Revenue			500,000
3	Cost of sales			270,000
4	Gross profit			230,000
5	Expenses:			
6	Selling and distribution		70,000	
7	Administration		45,000	
8				115,000
9	Net profit			115,000
10				
11				

This is arithmetically correct, but needs lines to format it correctly.

Use the border facility in **Home>Font** to insert appropriate single and double lines (**borders**) in the cells:

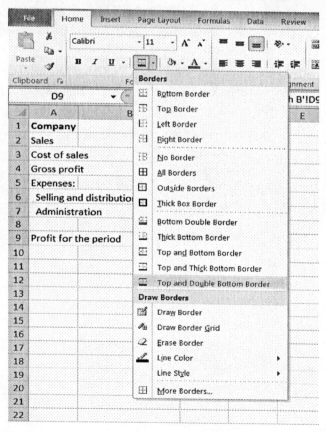

The final consolidated results should look like:

	A	B	C	D
	3D spreadsheet example [Compatibility Mode]			
1	**Company**		£	£
2	Revenue			500,000
3	Cost of sales			270,000
4	Gross profit			230,000
5	Expenses:			
6	Selling and distribution		70,000	
7	Administration		45,000	
8				115,000
9	Net profit			115,000

Note that if you change any figures in Branch A or Branch B, the figures will also change on the Company spreadsheet.

Uses for multi-sheet spreadsheets

There are a wide range of situations suited to the multi-sheet approach. A variety of possible uses follow.

(a) A spreadsheet could use one sheet for variables, a second for calculations, and a third for outputs.

(b) To enable quick and easy **consolidation** of similar sets of data, for example the financial results of two subsidiaries or the budgets of two departments.

(c) To provide different views of the same data. For instance, you could have one sheet of data sorted into product code order and another sorted into product name order.

Formatting data as a table

You can format data within a spreadsheet as a table. This provides you with another way to present and manipulate data.

Creating a table

First we will create a table and then we'll look at what we can do with it.

(1) **Open** the Tables example spreadsheet from the downloaded files. This uses almost the same data as in the previous exercise, so should look familiar to you.

(2) Select the cells that contain the data (A3 to G15).

(3) On the **Home** tab of the Ribbon select **Format as Table** from the **Styles** section.

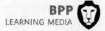

(4)   A gallery of styles will appear, so choose one of the formats (any one will do). Check that the correct data for the table is selected in the white box and tick the box **My table has headers**.

(5)   Click **OK**.

(6)   Your table should now look something like this, depending on which format you chose:

	A	B	C	D	E	F	G
1	Stockman Ltd						
2							
3	Part code	Supplier	Quantity	Reorder level	Unit price	Value	Order needed
4	129394	A Ltd	124	100	20	2,480.00	
5	129395	B Ltd	4325	4500	14	50,550.00	Yes
6	129396	F Ltd	4525	4000	12	55,512.00	
7	129397	A Ltd	583	500	14	8,162.00	
8	129398	D Ltd	41	50	37	1,591.00	Yes
9	129399	E Ltd	837	1000	65	54,405.00	Yes
10	129400	B Ltd	84	50	34	2,856.00	
11	129401	F Ltd	4847	5000	20	96,940.00	Yes
12	129402	D Ltd	4532	4000	10	46,320.00	
13	129403	A Ltd	41	40	34	1,394.00	
14	129404	E Ltd	5578	5000	25	139,450.00	
15	129405	C Ltd	5	10	35	175.00	Yes

You will notice that there are **Sort & Filter** drop down arrows at the top of each column in the header row. This is just one of the benefits of formatting data as a table: automatic **Sort & Filter**.

Other benefits of formatting data as a table

Other benefits include:

(a)   **Easy row and column selection**

Move the cursor to the top of the header row of the table and it will change to a thick pointing arrow. When you click, just the data in that column will be selected (and not the empty cells below the data). You can select data rows in a similar way.

The whole table can be selected by hovering near the table's top left corner until the arrow becomes thick and starts pointing towards the bottom right hand corner.

(b)   **Visible header row when scrolling**

When you scroll down past the bottom of the table the column letters become the table's column names so long as you have clicked anywhere inside the table before starting scrolling.

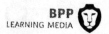

Part code	Supplier	Quantity	Reorder level	Unit price	Value	Order needed
4	129394	A Ltd	124	100	20	2,480.00	
5	129395	B Ltd	4325	4500	14	60,550.00	Yes
6	129396	F Ltd	4626	4000	12	55,512.00	
7	129397	A Ltd	583	500	14	8,162.00	
8	129398	D Ltd	43	50	37	1,591.00	Yes
9	129399	E Ltd	837	1000	65	54,405.00	Yes
10	129400	B Ltd	84	50	34	2,856.00	
11	129401	F Ltd	4847	5000	20	96,940.00	Yes
12	129402	D Ltd	4632	4000	10	46,320.00	
13	129403	A Ltd	41	40	34	1,394.00	
14	129404	E Ltd	5578	5000	25	139,450.00	
15	129405	C Ltd	5	10	35	175.00	Yes
16							

(c) **Automatic table expansion**

Type anything into any of the cells around the table and the table will automatically grow to include your new data. The formatting of the table will automatically adjust (this will also happen if you insert or delete a row or column).

(d) **Automatic formula copying**

If you enter a formula in a cell around the table and click **Enter**, the column will automatically resize to fit the formula, which is automatically copied down to fill the entire column alongside your data.

Changing the design of the table

You can change how the table looks by clicking anywhere in the table and selecting **Design** tab from the **Table Tools** toolbar.

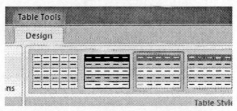

From here there are a number of **Table Style Options** that you can play around with, such as formatting a **First Column** or **Last Column**, adding a **Total Row** and changing the **Table Style**.

You can also choose to give your table a name so that any formula you enter which uses the figures from the table will refer to that table by its name.

So, for example, type 'Parts' into the **Table Name** box:

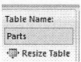

Now any formula entered in the column next to the table will refer to the table by name. Try it!

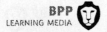

Font		Alignment			Number		Styles		Cells

=Parts[[#This Row],[Quantity]]*Parts[[#This Row],[Unit price]]

C	D	E	F	G	H	I	J	K	L	M

antit	Reorder level	Unit price	Value	Order needed						
		£	£							
124	100	20	2,480.00							
4325	4500	14	60,550.00	Yes	=Parts[[#This Row],[Quantity]]*Parts[[#This Row],[Unit price]]					
4626	4000	12	55,512.00							
583	500	14	8,162.00							
43	50	37	1,591.00	Yes						
837	1000	65	54,405.00	Yes						

Table tools

From the **Design** tab you can also:

- Choose to **Remove Duplicates**, which, as the name suggests, removes duplicate data from the table.

- Remove the table formatting completely by selecting **Convert to Range**. You may then wish to clear the formatting. You can easily do this by clicking **Clear** on the **Editing** section of the **Home** tab and choosing **Clear formats**.

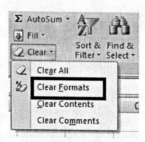

BPP
LEARNING MEDIA

Look-up tables

The Look-up function allows you to find and use data that is held in a table.

VLOOKUP is used for finding data in **v**ertical columns.

HLOOKUP is used for finding data in **h**orizontal rows.

Here is a simple example:

	A	B	C	D	E	F	G	H	I
1	**Salesman Ltd**								
2	**Part code**	**VATcode**	**Unit price**		VAT rate	20.0%			
3			£						
4	129394	1	20.00						
5	129395	1	14.00		**Invoice**				
6	129396	0	12.00						
7	129397	0	14.00						
8	129398	1	37.00		*Part code*	*Quantity*	*Unit price*	*VAT*	£
9	129399	0	65.00		129396	10	12.00	0	120.00
10	129400	1	34.00					Net	120.00
11	129401	0	20.00					VAT	0.00
12	129402	1	10.00					Total	120.00
13	129403	0	34.00						
14	129404	0	25.00						
15	129405	1	35.00						
16									
17									

On the left is a price list. If a part has a VAT code of 1, then VAT will be charged at the rate as set in cell F2; if the VAT code is 0, then no VAT is chargeable.

To create this invoice, you would look down the part numbers column until you found 129396. You would then read across to find the unit price and VAT code and, together with the quantity sold, you could create the invoice.

This process has been automated in the spreadsheet Salesman Ltd.

---

(1) Open the Spreadsheet called Salesman Ltd.
(2) Click on cell G9 to reveal the use of the VLOOKUP function.

Cell G9 holds the formula =VLOOKUP(E9,A4:C15,3, FALSE)

This means: look for the value held in cell E9, in the first row of the range A4:C15, and return the value in the third column of the range: it will return the price relating to the part number. FALSE (at the end of the statement) asks it to find an exact match so if a non-existent part code is entered in E9 you will get an error message (**#N/A**).

Similarly, cell H9 holds the formula =VLOOKUP(E9,A4:C15,2) and will return the VAT code relating to the part number.

Cell I11 holds a conditional (IF) function that will calculate VAT if the VAT code is 1 and insert 0 if the VAT code is 0.

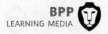

Note that some cells have been formatted to show two decimal places and some to show no decimal places. Cell F2 is formatted as a percentage and, because VAT might need to be changed, VAT is held in only one location with other cells referring to it.

Try out different part codes and quantities in the invoice.

CHANGES IN ASSUMPTIONS (WHAT-IF? ANALYSIS)

We referred earlier to the need to design a spreadsheet so that **changes in assumptions** do **not** require **major changes** to the spreadsheet. In our Costing Exercise workbook we set up two separate areas of the spreadsheet, one for assumptions and opening balances and one for the calculations and results. We could simply change the values in the assumptions cells to see how any changes in assumptions affect the results.

However, if we have more than one value to change, or we want to see the result of a number of different assumption changes we can use one of the three 'What-if' functions.

Data tables

A **data table** is a way to see different results by altering an input cell in a formula. You can create one- or two-variable data tables.

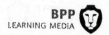

Let's try creating a one-variable data table.

(1) Open the earlier spreadsheet Mortgage which used the PMT formula.

(2) Enter 1% to 10% in cells E8 to L8 as shown below. You will need to increase the width of cells I8 & J8.

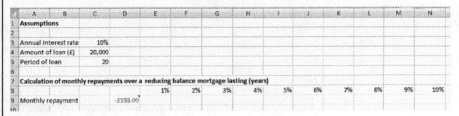

(3) Select cells D8 to N9.

(4) **Click Data>What-If Analysis>Data Table**.

(5) Here you want your data table to fill in the values in row 9, based on the results if the value in cell C3 were to change to a different percentage, so choose the **Row input cell** box and enter C3.

You should get the following results:

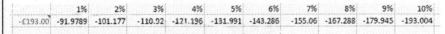

The table would look better if the numbers were formatted in the same way as the first result in cell D9. An easy way to copy a format from one cell to another is to click on the cell whose format you wish to copy then click the **Format Painter** button on the **Clipboard** area of the **Home** tab and then click on the cells you wish to format.

Try it now. Click on cell D9, then click the **Format Painter** button. Now select cells E9:M9. You should see:

	1%	2%	3%	4%	5%	6%	7%	8%	9%	10%
-£193.00	-£91.98	-£101.18	-£110.92	-£121.20	-£131.99	-£143.29	-£155.06	-£167.29	-£179.95	-£193.00

Note. If you double click the **Format Painter** button you can then click any number of cells afterwards to apply that same format. To stop the **Format Painter**, simply click **Esc** (Escape).

Now let's try a two-variable data table using the same workbook. This time we want to see the result if both the interest rate and the number of years of the loan change.

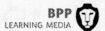

(1) Rename the worksheet you have been working on to 'One variable'. Now select Sheet2 (or insert a new worksheet if necessary) and rename it 'Two variable'. This is the sheet that we will now use.

(2) **Copy** the data on the One variable worksheet (**Ctrl + C**) and paste (**Ctrl + V**) into the new worksheet.

(3) Select cells E8 to N8 and move them up down by one cell (ie to E9 to N9). You can do this by hovering over the selected cells until a cross with four arrow heads appears, then click and drag to cell E9. Alternatively, **Cut (Ctrl + X)** and then **Paste (Ctrl + V)** to cell E9.

(4) In cells D10 to D14 insert different loan periods. We have used 10, 15, 20, 25 and 30 years as shown below:

-£193.00	1%	2%	3%	4%	5%	6%	7%	8%	9%	10%
10										
15										
20										
25										
30										

(5) Select cells D9 to N14.

(6) Click **Data>What-If Analysis>Data Table**.

(7) Here you want the data table to fill in the values based on the results if the value in cell C3 were to change to a different percentage (as shown in row 9) and also if the loan period in C5 changes (as shown in column D). So, choose the **Row input cell** box and enter C3 and then select the **Column input cell** box and enter C5.

You should get the following results:

-£193.00	1%	2%	3%	4%	5%	6%	7%	8%	9%	10%
10	-£175.21	-£184.03	-£193.12	-£202.49	-£212.13	-£222.04	-£232.22	-£242.66	-£253.35	-£264.30
15	-£119.70	-£128.70	-£138.12	-£147.94	-£158.16	-£168.77	-£179.77	-£191.13	-£202.85	-£214.92
20	-£91.98	-£101.18	-£110.92	-£121.20	-£131.99	-£143.29	-£155.06	-£167.29	-£179.95	-£193.00
25	-£75.37	-£84.77	-£94.84	-£105.57	-£116.92	-£128.86	-£141.36	-£154.36	-£167.84	-£181.74
30	-£64.33	-£73.92	-£84.32	-£95.48	-£107.36	-£119.91	-£133.06	-£146.75	-£160.92	-£175.51

Format cells E10 to N14 in the same way as cell D9.

Finally practise saving the file as 'Mortgage – Data tables' in a new folder on your computer using **File button>Save as**. Choose an appropriate name for the folder – it's your choice!

Scenarios

The Scenarios function allows you to change information in cells that affect the final totals of a formula and to prepare instant reports showing the results of all scenarios together.

Using the spreadsheet Costing Exercise – Finished, we will show the result of changing the following assumptions:

(a)   The chargeout rate for the Accounting Technician is now £30.00.
(b)   The cost of a laptop has increased to £115.00 per week.
(c)   The increase in chargeout rate for the secretary has been altered to 8%.

You could simply change the relevant cells in the spreadsheet to reflect these changes in assumptions. However, we are going to use the Scenario Manager function.

---

(1)   Select the **Data** tab and from the **Data Tools** section click **What-If Analysis>Scenario Manager**.

(2)   Click **Add** and give the scenario an appropriate name, for example 'Original costing exercise'.

(3)   Press the tab button or click in the **Changing cells** box and, based on the information we used above, select the cells with the changing data, ignoring the change to the opening bank balance. To select cells that are not next to each other, use the Ctrl button. You should **Ctrl click** on cells B4, B6, B7.

(4)   Click **OK.**

(5)   You are now asked for **Scenario Values**. This will show the values currently in the cells specified, which are our original figures so click **OK.**

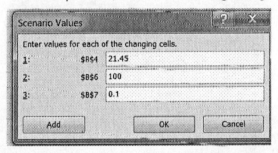

(6)   We now need to enter our new values. Click **Add** and type a new **Name** (for example Costing exercise 2). The **Changing Cells** box will already contain the correct cells.

(7)   Click **OK.**

---

(8) In the **Scenario Values** boxes change the values as follows and click **OK**.

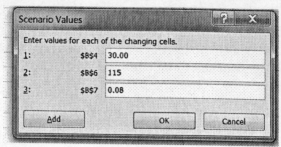

(9) Your second scenario should be highlighted. Now if you click on **Show** the figures in your assumptions table should automatically change and you can view the results.

L22		f_x				
A	B	C	D	E	F	G
1 Internal chargeout rates						
2 Divisional chief accountant	£72.50					
3 Assistant accountant	£38.00					
4 Accounting technician	£30.00					
5 Secretary	£17.30					
6 Laptop cost	£115.00					
7 Chargeout rate	8%					
8						
9 Costs	Week 1	Week 2	Week 3	Week 4	Total	
10 Divisional chief accountant	£0.00	£326.25	£489.38	£435.00	£1,250.63	
11 Assistant accountant	£760.00	£1,520.00	£1,330.00	£0.00	£3,610.00	
12 Accounting technician	£960.00	£1,200.00	£1,125.00	£0.00	£3,285.00	
13 Secretary	£259.50	£557.93	£695.98	£0.00	£1,513.40	
14 Laptops	£230.00	£230.00	£230.00		£690.00	
15 Total	£1,979.50	£3,604.18	£3,640.35	£435.00	£10,349.03	
16						
17 Hours	Week 1	Week 2	Week 3	Week 4	Total	
18 Divisional chief accountant		4.5	6.75	6	17.25	
19 Assistant accountant	20	40	35		95	
20 Accounting technician	32	40	37.5		109.5	
21 Secretary	15	32.25	37.25		84.5	
22 Total	67	116.75	116.5	6	300.25	
23						
24 Laptops	2	2	2			
25						
26						
27						

(10) Click back on your original Costing exercise and then click **Show** and the numbers will change back.

Note. You may need to make your screen smaller to view the whole sheet at the same time. You can do this by clicking **View** on the Ribbon, then in the **Zoom** section clicking on **Zoom** and choosing a smaller percentage. 75% should be perfect.

You can also easily and quickly create a report from the scenarios.

(1) Click **Data>What-If Analysis>Scenario Manager**.

(2) Click the **Summary** button.

(3) In the Result cells box choose the cells to go into the report, ie the ones you want to see the results of. As we are interested in the final cost select cell F15. This creates a separate Scenario Summary worksheet. Open the Costing Exercise – What-if spreadsheet if you do not see the following report.

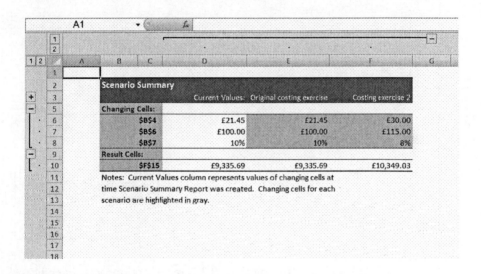

Goal seek

What if you already know the result you want from a formula but not the value the formula itself needs to calculate the result? In this case you should use the **Goal Seek** function, which is located in the **Data Tools** section of the **Data** tab on the Ribbon.

Open the original Mortgage spreadsheet from the downloaded files. Let's assume that we have enough income to pay a monthly mortgage payment of £300 and want to know how many years it will take to pay off the mortgage.

(1) Copy the data on Sheet 1 and paste it to Sheet 2.

(2) Click **Data>What-If Analysis>Goal Seek.**

(3) **Set cell** to D9, as this is the figure we know and enter -300 in the **To value** box (make sure that you enter a negative figure to match the figure already in D9).

(4) Enter C5 in the **By changing cell** box, as this is the figure we are looking for.

(5) Click **OK.**

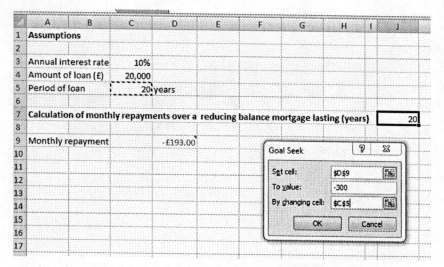

Goal seek will find the solution, 8.14 years, and insert it in cell C5.

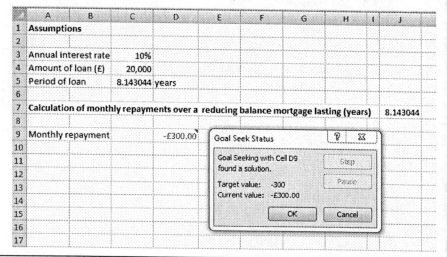

BPP
LEARNING MEDIA

STATISTICAL FUNCTIONS

Linear regression/trends

Excel contains powerful statistical tools for the analysis of information such as how costs vary with production volumes and how sales vary through the year.

Look at the following example of costs and volume:

Month	Volume	Costs
	Units	£
1	1,000	8,500
2	1,200	9,600
3	1,800	14,000
4	900	7,000
5	2,000	16,000
6	400	5,000

It is clear that at higher production volumes costs are higher, but it would be useful to find a relationship between these variables so that we could predict what costs might be if production were forecast at, say, 1,500 units.

The first investigation we could perform is simply to draw a graph of costs against volume. Volume is the independent variable (it causes the costs) so should run on the horizontal (x) axis.

Open the spreadsheet called Cost_volume and draw a scatter graph showing cost against volume, with appropriate labels and legends.

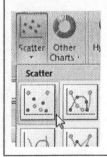

(1) Select the range B1:C7.

(2) Using **Insert/Charts** from the Ribbon, choose the top left Scatter graph type).

It should look something like the following:

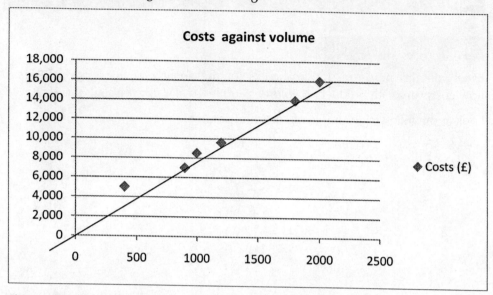

The straight line through the points has been manually drawn here to show that there's clearly a good association between volume and cost because the points do not miss the line by much, but we want to analyse this properly so that we can make a fairly good prediction of costs at output of say 1,500 units.

Lines of the sort above have a general equation of the type:

$$y = mx + b$$

Here **y** = Total costs

    x = Volume

    m = Variable cost per unit (the slope of the line)

    b = The fixed cost (where the line crosses the y axis: the cost even at zero volume)

Excel provides two easy ways of finding the figures we need for predicting values.

Find the trend:

(1)   On the same spreadsheet (Cost_volume), enter 1,500 in cell B9.

(2)   Now click on cell C9.

(3)   From the Ribbon choose **Formulas>More Functions>Statistical**.

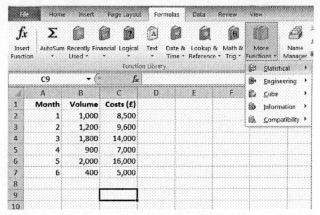

(4)   Scroll down the list until you get to **TREND** and choose that.

(5)   For **Known_y's** select the range C2:C7.

(6)   For **Known_x's** select the range B2:B7.

(These ranges are the raw material which the calculation uses)

For **New_x's**, enter B9, the volume for which we want the costs to be predicted.

The number 12,003 should appear in cell C9. That is the predicted cost for output of 1,500 units – in line with the graph. In practice, we would use 12,000. Altering the value in B9 will produce the corresponding predicted cost.

A second way of analysing this data will allow us to find the variable and fixed costs of the units (**m** and **b** in the equation $y = mx + b$).

(1)   To find **m** use the statistical function **LINEST** and assign the **Known_y's** and **Known_x's** as before. You should get the answer 7.01, the variable cost per unit.

(2)   To find the intersection, **b**, use the statistical function **INTERCEPT**. You should get the answer 1,486.

Note. These can be used to predict the costs of 1,500 units by saying:

Total costs = $1,486 + 7.01 \times 1,500 = 12,001$, more or less as before.

The spreadsheet called Cost_volume finished contains the graph, and the three statistical functions just described.

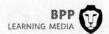

Moving averages

Look at this data

Year	Quarter	Time series	Sales £'000
20X6	1	1	989.0
	2	2	990.0
	3	3	994.0
	4	4	1,015.0
20X7	1	5	1,030.0
	2	6	1,042.5
	3	7	1,036.0
	4	8	1,056.5
20X8	1	9	1,071.0
	2	10	1,083.5
	3	11	1,079.5
	4	12	1,099.5
20X9	1	13	1,115.5
	2	14	1,127.5
	3	15	1,123.5
	4	16	1,135.0
20Y0	1	17	1,140.0

You might be able to see that the data follows a seasonal pattern: for example there always seems to be a dip in Quarter 3 and a peak in Quarter 2. It is more obvious if plotted as a time series of sales against the consecutively numbered quarters.

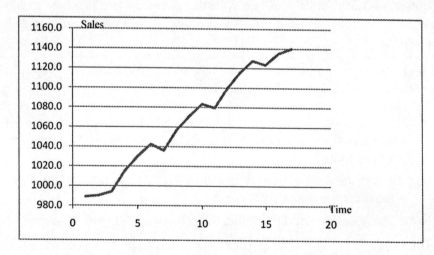

The moving average technique attempts to even out the seasonal variations. Here, because we seem to have data repeating every four readings a four-part

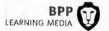

moving average would be appropriate. If you were trading five days a week and wanted to even out the sales, a five-part moving average would be suitable.

The moving average is calculated as follows:

Take the first four figures and average them:

$$\frac{(989.0 + 990.0 + 994.0 + 1,015.0)}{4} = 997.0$$

Then move on one season:

$$\frac{(990.0 + 994.0 + 1,015.0 + 1,030.0)}{4} = 1,007.3$$

and so on, always averaging out all four seasons. Each average will include a high season and a low season.

That's rather tedious to do manually and Excel provides a function to do it automatically. To access this analysis function you must have the Excel Analysis ToolPak installed. If it is installed there will be an **Analysis > Data Analysis** tab in the **Data** section of the Ribbon.

If it is not already installed, you can install it as follows:

(1)   Click the **File Button**, and then click **Excel Options**.

(2)   Click **Add-Ins**, and then from the **Manage** box, select **Excel Add-Ins**.

(3)   Click **Go**.

(4)   In the **Add-Ins available** box, select the **Analysis ToolPak** check box, and then click OK.

Tip. If **Analysis ToolPak** is not listed in the **Add-Ins available** box, click **Browse** to locate it.

If you are prompted that the Analysis ToolPak is not currently installed on your computer, click **Yes** to install it. This may take a little time, so be patient!

---

(1)   Open the spreadsheet called Time series.
(2)   Select **Data > Data analysis > Moving average**.
(3)   Select D2:D18 as the **Input Range**.
(4)   Enter 4 as the **Interval** (a four-part moving average).
(5)   Enter F2 as the **Output Range**.
(6)   Check **Chart Output**.
(7)   Click on **OK**.

Don't worry about the error messages – the first three simply mean that you can't do a four-part average until you have four readings.

Move your cursor onto the moving average figures and move it down, one cell at a time to see how the averages move.

Notice on the graph how the Forecast line (the moving average) is much smoother than the actual figures. This makes predicting future sales much easier.

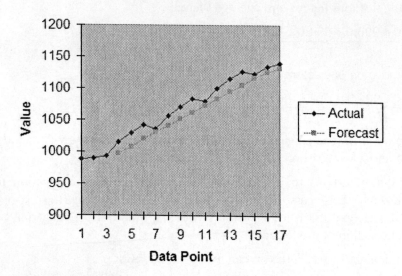

Mean, mode and median

These are three measures of what is known as the 'location' of data – they give an indication of whereabouts the data is clustered.

Mean (or arithmetic mean) is the ordinary average (add up the readings and divide by the number of readings).

Mode is the most frequently occurring item. For example, in a shoe shop, the arithmetic mean of shoe sizes is not much use. The shopkeeper is more interested in the most common shoe size.

Median is the value of the middle item if they are arranged in ascending or descending sequence. As well as medians you can have 'quartiles' (upper and lower) dividing the population into top one-quarter, lowest three-quarters (or *vice versa*) and 'deciles' (10:90 splits).

Excel allows all of these measures to be calculated (or identified) easily.

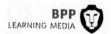

(1) Open the spreadsheet called Student Results.

This lists the exam results of 23 students. They are currently displayed in alphabetical order. Don't worry about the column headed 'Bins' for now.

Enter 'Mean' in cell A28, then make cell B28 active.

(2) Choose **Formulas>Σ AutoSum>Average** and accept the range offered. 58.56 is the arithmetic mean of the marks.

(3) Enter 'Median' in cell A29, then make cell B29 active.

(4) Choose **Formulas>More Functions>Statistical>MEDIAN**.

(5) Enter the range B4:B26 for Number 1.

You should see 57 as the median.

Check this by sorting the data into descending order by score, then counting up to the 12th student, Kate. (She's the middle student and scored 57.)

(6) Enter 'Percentile' in cell A30, 0.75 in cell C30 and then make cell B30 active.

(7) Choose **Formulas>More Functions>Statistical>PERCENTILE.EXC**

(8) Enter the range B4:B26 and C30 as the K value.

The reported value is 68, the figure which divides the top quarter from the bottom three-quarters of students.

(9) Enter 'Mode' in cell A31 then make cell B31 active.

(10) Choose **Formulas>More Functions>Statistical>Mode**.

(11) Enter the range B4:B26.

The reported value is 65 (that occurs more frequently than any other score).

Histograms

A histogram is a graph which shows the frequency with which certain values occur. Usually the values are grouped so that one could produce a histogram showing how many people were 160 – 165cm tall, how many >165 – 170, >170 – 175 and so on.

Excel can produce histogram analyses provided the Analysis ToolPak is installed. Installation was described earlier in the section about time series.

To demonstrate the histogram we will use the Student results spreadsheet again.

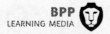

(1) Open the Student Results spreadsheet if it is not already open.

You will see that in E5 to E13 is a column called 'Bins'. This describes the groupings that we want our results to be included in, so here we are going up the result in groups (bins) of ten percentage points at a time and the histogram will show how many results are in 0 – 10, 10 – 20, 20 – 30 etc.

(2) Choose **Data>Data Analysis>Histogram**.

(3) Enter the range B4:B26 as the **Input Range**.

(4) Enter E5:E13 as the **Bin Range**.

(5) Choose **New Worksheet Ply** and enter 'Histogram analysis' in the white text box.

(6) Tick **Chart Output**.

(7) Click on **OK**.

The new worksheet will show the data grouped into the 'bins' by frequency and also shows a histogram.

The spreadsheet 'Student Results Finished' shows the finished spreadsheet complete with histogram in the Histogram analysis sheet.

COMBINATION CHARTS

Excel allows you to combine two different charts into one. For example you may wish to compare sales to profits. This is also known as showing two graphs on one axis.

To do this we create a chart from our data as before.

(1) Open the Combination Chart spreadsheet from the downloaded files. This provides data for the number of sales of precious metal in 2009 and 2010. The price at which the precious metal is sold per kilo goes up and down according to the market.

(2) Select the data that will go into your chart (cells A1 to C9)

(3) Click Insert and then choose your chart type. For this example let's choose a **2D clustered column** chart. The chart doesn't really help us to understand the relationship between the two different sets of data.

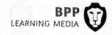

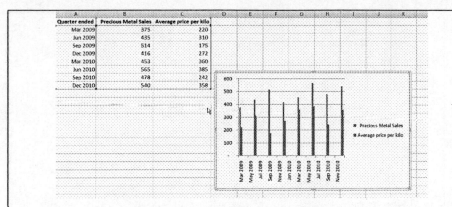

Quarter ended	Precious Metal Sales	Average price per kilo
Mar 2009	375	220
Jun 2009	435	310
Sep 2009	514	175
Dec 2009	416	272
Mar 2010	453	360
Jun 2010	565	385
Sep 2010	478	242
Dec 2010	540	358

(4) A more visual way of displaying the average price data might be to see it in a line set against the number of sales. So click on any Average price column, right click and select **Change Series Chart Type**.

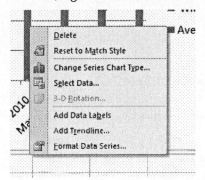

(5) Select **Line with Markers** and click **OK**. The chart will look like this:

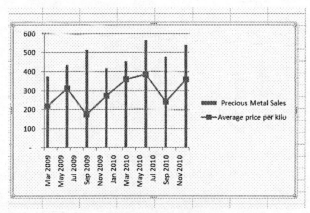

(6) The chart still does not make sense as the figures on the left axis are not comparing like with like. So we need to right click again an Average price marker and choose **Format Data Series**.

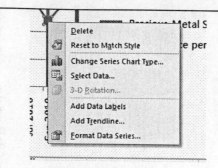

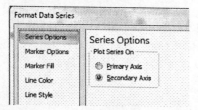

(7) Click **Secondary Axis**.

(8) Click **OK**.

(9) Take some time to play with the **Chart Tools**. Give the chart the name 'Precious Metal Sales' and label the axes. The vertical axis on the left should show the 'Number of sales', while the right hand axis should show the 'Price per kilo'.

You should end up with a chart that looks something like:

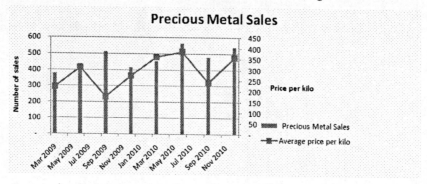

It can clearly be seen that the price per kilo dips in the third quarter of each year, something we could not easily determine without using the combination chart.

ERROR DETECTION AND CORRECTION

It is important to try to detect and correct errors before a spreadsheet is used to make decisions. We've already looked at some ways of trying to prevent wrong input (for example, data validation).

The final part of this chapter covers Excel's built-in help facility, error messages and ways to check that a spreadsheet has been constructed and is being used correctly.

Help

You can use Excel's Help window to quickly find the answer to any questions you may have while using Excel. You can access Help by clicking the **Help** button (the white question mark in the blue circle) in the top right corner of your spreadsheet or by pressing **F1**.

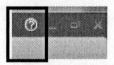

You can either type a search term directly into the white bar, or click on the **book icon** to access a table of help contents.

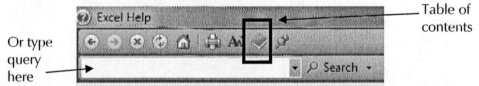

Take some time to explore the results when you type in different search terms. For example, if you found the section on What If analysis challenging, you could type 'What if' into the search bar to receive help on this topic.

Removing circular references

Circular references nearly always mean that there's a mistake in the logic of the spreadsheet. Here's an example:

	A	B
1		
2		£
3	Basic salary	20,000
4	Bonus 10% of total pay	=0.1*B5
5	Total pay	20,000

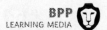

A warning will be displayed by Excel:

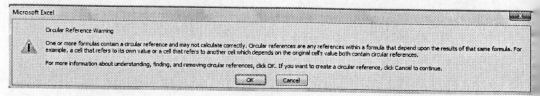

In our example, it is relatively easy to find the cause of the problem, but in a large spreadsheet it can be difficult. Clicking **OK** will provide help and will bring up a help screen referring you to **Formulas>Formula Auditing>Circular References** on the Ribbon.

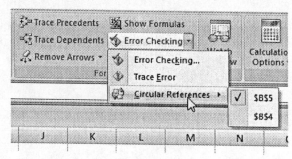

Using trace precedents

Tracing precedents and dependents

As spreadsheets are developed it can become difficult to be sure where figures come from and go to (despite being able to display formulae in all the cells). A useful technique is to make use of the trace precedents and trace dependents options. These are available on the **Formulas** section of the **Ribbon**.

(1) Open the Precedent example spreadsheet from the downloaded files and make cell F4 active.

(2) Choose the **Formulas** section of the Ribbon and click on **Trace Precedents** in the **Formula Auditing** group of icons.

You should see:

	A	B	C	D	E	F
1	BUDGETED SALES FIGURES					
2		Jan	Feb	Mar		Total
3		£'000	£'000	£'000		£'000
4	North	2,431	3,001	2,189		7,621
5	South	6,532	5,826	6,124		18,482
6	West	895	432	596		1,923
7	Total	9,858	9,259	8,909		28,026

Now it is very obvious that anything in column E, like April figures will not be included in the total.

(3) Click on **Remove Arrows** in the **Formula Auditing** group.

(4) Make B4 the active cell.

(5) Click on **Trace Dependents**. This will show what cells make use of this cell:

	A	B	C	D	E	F
1	BUDGETED SALES FIGURES					
2		Jan	Feb	Mar		Total
3		£'000	£'000	£'000		£'000
4	North	2,431	3,001	2,189		7,621
5	South	6,532	5,826	6,124		18,482
6	West	895	432	596		1,923
7	Total	9,858	9,259	8,909		28,026

Rounding errors

The ability to display numbers in a variety of formats (eg to no decimal places) can result in a situation whereby totals that are correct may actually look incorrect.

Example: rounding errors

The following example shows how apparent rounding errors can arise.

	A	B	C
1	*Petty cash*		
2	Week ending 31/12/20X6		
3			£
4	Opening balance		231.34
5	Receipts		32.99
6	Payments		-104.67
7	Closing balance		159.66

	A	B	C
1	*Petty cash*		
2	Week ending 31/12/20X6		
3			£
4	Opening balance		231
5	Receipts		33
6	Payments		-105
7	Closing balance		160

Cell C7 contains the formula =SUM(C4:C6). The spreadsheet on the left shows the correct total to two decimal places. The spreadsheet on the right seems to be saying that 231 + 33 – 105 is equal to 160, which is not true, it's 159 (check it). The **reason for the discrepancy** is that both spreadsheets actually contain the values shown in the spreadsheet on the **left**.

However, the spreadsheet on the right has been formatted to display numbers with **no decimal places**. So, individual numbers display as the nearest whole number, although the actual value held by the spreadsheet and used in calculations includes the decimals.

The round function

One solution, that will prevent the appearance of apparent errors, is to use the **ROUND function**. The ROUND function has the following structure: ROUND (value, places). 'Value' is the value to be rounded. 'Places' is the number of places to which the value is to be rounded.

The difference between using the ROUND function and formatting a value to a number of decimal places is that using the ROUND function actually **changes** the **value**, while formatting only changes the **appearance** of the value.

In the example above, the ROUND function could be used as follows. The following formulae could be inserted in cells D4 to D7.

D4 = ROUND(C4,0)
D5 = ROUND(C5,0)
D6 = ROUND(C6,0)
D7 = Round (SUM(D4:D6),0)

Column C could then be hidden by highlighting the whole column (clicking on the C at the top of the column), then right clicking anywhere on the column and selecting **Hide**. Try this for yourself, hands-on using the Rounding example spreadsheet.

D4			f_x	=ROUND(C4,0)

	A	B	D	E
1	*Petty cash*			
2	Week ending 31/12/20X6			
3				
4	Opening balance		231	
5	Receipts		33	
6	Payments		-105	
7	Closing balance		159	
8				

Note that using the ROUND function to eliminate decimals results in slightly inaccurate calculation totals (in our example 160 is actually 'more correct' than the 159 obtained using ROUND). For this reason, some people prefer not to use the function, and to make users of the spreadsheet aware that small apparent differences are due to rounding.

Identifying error values

Error checking can be turned on by **File button > Excel options > Formulas** and checking **Enable background error checking**. There is a list that allows you to decide which errors to be highlighted. If a green triangle appears in a cell, then the cell contains an error.

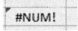

Other information about the nature of the error will also be supplied:

#########	The column is not wide enough to hold the number. Widen the column or choose another format in which to display the number (no green triangle here as it is not a 'real' error – just a presentation problem).
#DIV/0!	Commonly caused by a formula attempting to divide a number by zero (perhaps because the divisor cell is blank).
#VALUE!	Occurs when a mathematical formula refers to a cell containing text, eg if cell A2 contains text the formula =A1+A2+A3 will return #VALUE!. Functions that operate on ranges (eg SUM) will not result in a #VALUE! error as they ignore text values.
#NAME?	The formula contains text that is not a valid cell address, range name or function name. Check the spelling of any functions used (eg by looking through functions under **Formulas > Insert Function**).
#REF!	The formula includes an invalid cell reference, for example a reference to cells that have subsequently been deleted. If you notice the reference immediately after a deletion, use **Ctrl+Z** to reverse the deletion.
#NUM!	This error is caused by invalid numeric values being supplied to a worksheet formula or function. For example, using a negative number with the SQRT (square root) function. To investigate, check the formula and function logic and syntax. The **Formula Auditing** toolbar may help this process (see below).
#N/A	A value is not available to a function or formula, for example omitting a required argument from a spreadsheet function. Again, the **Formula Auditing** toolbar may help the investigation process (see below).

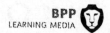

Tracing and correcting errors

If you do see one of the above errors you can trace where it came from by clicking on the cell with the error, then, from the **Formulas** tab of the Ribbon, choose **Formula Auditing** and click the down arrow next to **Error Checking**. Lines will appear pointing to the data that has produced the error.

If you simply click the **Error Checking** button, it will automatically check the current worksheet and alert you to any errors.

Finally, you can click **Evaluate Formula** to be taken step by step through it so that you can identify the error.

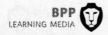

CHAPTER OVERVIEW

- It is important to save and **backup your work regularly**. You can use **Save as** to give various versions of the same document different names.

- It is important to **control the security** of spreadsheets through passwords, locking (protecting) cells against unauthorised or accidental changes, data validation on input.

- Spreadsheet packages permit the user to work with **multiple sheets** that refer to each other. This is sometimes referred to as a three dimensional spreadsheet.

- Excel offers sophisticated data handling including **filtering, pivot tables** and **look-up tables**.

- **Combination charts** allow you to show two sets of data on one axis of your chart.

- Three tools, **Data tables, Scenarios** and **Goal seek**, are available to allow you to explore various results using different sets of values in one or more formulae.

- **Error detection** and prevention is important in spreadsheet design and testing. There are useful facilities available such as tracing precedents and dependents, identification of circular references, and error reports, as well as Excel's built-in help function.

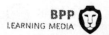

TEST YOUR LEARNING

Test 1

What command is used to save a file under a different name?

Test 2

What part of the Ribbon do you go to set up checking procedures on the input of data?

Test 3

List three possible uses for a multi-sheet (3D) spreadsheet.

Test 4

What does filtering do?

Test 5

What is a trend line?

Test 6

What is the median?

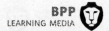

PRACTICE ACTIVITIES

---
chapter coverage 📖

These activities enable you to practise some of the skills and techniques introduced in earlier chapters.

✎ The activities are suitable for both Excel 2007 and Excel 2010.

✎ Each activity requires you to create or open a specified spreadsheet with the suffix Question, eg Activity 1 Question.

✎ No printed answers are provided, but a spreadsheet which solves the problem will have a matching name with suffix Answer, eg Activity 1 Answer.

✎ The opening spreadsheets and answers for each activity are provided in the files available for download from www.bpp.com/aatspreadsheets.

✎ Some activities have no initial spreadsheet. The answer is a spreadsheet with the appropriate activity reference.

✎ The main coverage of each activity is set out below.

Contents

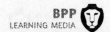

1 ZUMBO

Open the spreadsheet Activity 1 Question.

	A	B	C	D	E
1	Zumbo Enterprises Ltd				
2					
3	Invoice				
4					
5	Date		40608		
6	Account		2141432		
7	Customer		J Jones		
8			21 The Cutting, Anytown AY1 2WR		
9					
10	Product cc	Product description	Quantity	Unit price	Net
11					£
12	1234	2 metre steel bar	10	12.33	123.3
13					0
14					0
15					0
16					0
17	Total net				123.3
18	VAT	0.20			24.66
19	Total Gross				147.96

Layout needs to be improved so that the screen looks more like:

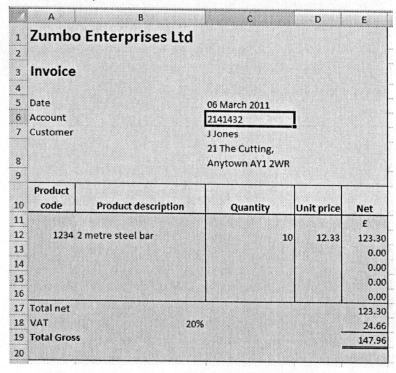

	A	B	C	D	E
1	**Zumbo Enterprises Ltd**				
2					
3	**Invoice**				
4					
5	Date		06 March 2011		
6	Account		2141432		
7	Customer		J Jones		
8			21 The Cutting, Anytown AY1 2WR		
9					
10	Product code	Product description	Quantity	Unit price	Net
11					£
12	1234	2 metre steel bar	10	12.33	123.30
13					0.00
14					0.00
15					0.00
16					0.00
17	Total net				123.30
18	VAT		20%		24.66
19	Total Gross				147.96
20					

Adjust font, borders, alignment, cell colour and number of decimal places to improve presentation.

2 IML

Open the spreadsheet Activity 2 Question.

Activity 2 Question				
	A	B	C	D	E
1	International Magazines Limited: Sales by Region Jan–Jun 2011				
2		Europe	America	Rest of the world	Total
3	Woman's Day	251,208	163,514	105,000	£ 519,722
4	Blue!	202,262	136,290	78,485	£ 417,036
5	Easy Cooking	143,588	86,040	114,900	£ 344,528
6	Sorted!	27,795	6,234	14,769	£ 48,798
7	Total	£624,852	£392,078	£313,154	£1,330,083

You work in the accounts department of International Magazines Limited (IML). IML publish four magazines, which are sold throughout the world. One of the spreadsheets you work on, shown above, analyses sales by magazine and world region.

Follow the instructions below to create several charts using the Chart Wizard.

(i) Select cells **A2:D6** (ensure these are the only cells selected, do not include the totals).

(ii) Use the chart wizard button to insert three charts of that data: 2D clustered column, 2D stacked column and 3D clustered column.

(iii) Enter a suitable title for each graph.

(iv) Adjust their sizes and positions by obtaining the correct pointer shape, holding down the mouse button and dragging.

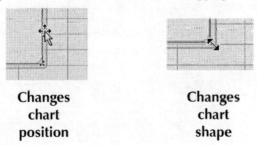

Changes chart position   **Changes chart shape**

3 CASH FLOW EXERCISE

You want to set up a simple six-month cash flow projection in such a way that you can use it to estimate how the **projected cash balance** figures will **change** in total when any **individual item** in the projection is **altered**. You have the following information.

(a) Sales were £45,000 per month in 20X5, falling to £42,000 in January 20X6. Thereafter they are expected to increase by 3% per month (ie February will be 3% higher than January, and so on).

(b) Debts are collected as follows.

   (i) 60% in month following sale
   (ii) 30% in second month after sale
   (iii) 7% in third month after sale
   (iv) 3% remains uncollected

(c) Purchases are equal to cost of sales, set at 65% of sales.

(d) Overheads were £6,000 per month in 20X5, rising by 5% in 20X6.

(e) Opening cash is an overdraft of £7,500.

(f) Dividends: £10,000 final dividend on 20X5 profits payable in May.

(g) Capital purchases: plant costing £18,000 will be ordered in January. 20% is payable with order, 70% on delivery in February and the final 10% in May.

Setting up the assumptions area

These assumptions have been set up in an opening spreadsheet for you.

Open the file Activity 3 – Assumptions. Columns B and G contain the numbers or values making up the assumptions to be used in the cash flow exercise.

	D13	▼	f_x	Payable May				
	A	B	C	D	E	F	G	H
4								
5	Historical monthly sales 2005 (£)	45,000		Purchases = cost of sales.			65%	of sales
6	Projected sales Jan 20X6 (£)	42,000		Monthly overheads 20X5 (£)			6,000	
7	Monthly sales growth (20X6 onwards)	3%		Rise in monthly overheads 20X6			5%	
8	Collection of debts:			Opening cash balance (O/d)			-7,500	
9	Month following sales	60%		Dividends (payable May 20X6, £)			10,000	
10	2nd month following sales	30%		Capital expenditure			18,000	
11	3rd month following sales	7%		Payable January			20%	
12	Uncollected	3%		Payable February			70%	
13				Payable May			10%	
14								
15								

You are required to design a spreadsheet to give a cash flow forecast for six months (January to June).

 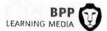

4 DITTORI

Dittori Ltd has a sales ledger package which does not offer an aged receivables option. You have decided to set up a simple spreadsheet to monitor ageing by region. You have been able to export the following information from the sales ledger, as at 31 May 20X6. This data is contained in a spreadsheet – file Activity 4 Question.

Region	Current	1 month	2 month	3 month	4 month	5 month +
Highlands	346.60	567.84	32.17	–	–	54.8
Strathclyde	24,512.05	28,235.50	4,592.50	1,244.80	51.36	942.57
Borders	1,927.77	–	512.88	–	–	–
North West	824.80	14,388.91	2,473.53	–	482.20	79.66
North East	14,377.20	12,850.00		3,771.84	1,244.55	–
Midlands	45,388.27	61,337.88	24,001.02	4,288.31	1,391.27	4,331.11
Wales	14,318.91	5,473.53	21.99	4,881.64	512.27	422.5
East Anglia	157.20	943.68	377.40	1,500.87	15.33	247.66
South West	9,528.73	11,983.39	3,771.89	6,228.77	1,008.21	214.51
South East	68,110.78	83,914.54	29,117.96	24,285.10	14,328.90	5,422.50
France	6,422.80	7,451.47	5,897.55	2,103.70	140.50	3,228.76
Other EU	5,433.88	4,991.90	5,012.70	4,223.80	1,022.43	1,984.29
Rest of World	1,822.70	4,529.67	277.50	3,491.34	–	–

Task

Prepare a spreadsheet which will extend the above analysis to total receivables by region and the percentage of debt in each age category and the percentage by region.

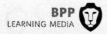

5 PIVOT

Open the file Activity 5 Question. An extract from this spreadsheet is shown below.

	A	B	C	D
1	Issue No	Quantity	Colour	Shape
2	1473	159	Blue	Square
3	1474	84	Yellow	Square
4	1475	120	Green	Triangular
5	1476	125	Blue	Round
6	1477	153	Yellow	Triangular
7	1478	99	Blue	Round
8	1479	137	Blue	Triangular
9	1480	199	Red	Square
10	1481	16	Red	Round
11	1482	158	Green	Square
12	1483	29	Red	Triangular
13	1484	118	Yellow	Square
14	1485	167	Blue	Round
15	1486	177	Red	Triangular
16	1487	168	Green	Square
17	1488	110	Red	Round
18	1489	181	Red	Square
19	1490	168	Blue	Square
20	1491	31	Red	Square
21	1492	86	Green	Triangular
22	1493	160	Green	Triangular
23	1494	120	Red	Square
24	1495	101	Blue	Triangular
25	1496	141	Red	Triangular
26	1497	187	Blue	Triangular
27	1498	62	Green	Square
28	1499	177	Blue	Triangular
29	1500	148	Green	Square
30	1501	175	Red	Triangular
31	1502	131	Red	Square
32	1503	67	Blue	Square
33	1504	18	Blue	Round

The spreadsheet shows the quantity of components of various types that were issued from stores to production during a period. Components come in four colours (blue, red, green and yellow) and three shapes (square, round and triangular).

Task

Use Microsoft Excel's Pivot Table feature to analyse and summarise this data by colour and by shape in a two-dimensional table as shown below:

Sum of quantity	Colour				
Shape	Blue	Green	Red	Yellow	Grand total
Round					
Square					
Triangular					
Grand total					

6 HEIGHT AND WEIGHT

The spreadsheet Activity 6 Question contains data about a number of people's height and weight. Open that spreadsheet. The data is presently in alphabetical order by name of person.

Tasks

Just below the list of data use **statistical functions** to work out:

(a) Mean height and mean weight (175.56, 70.3).

(b) Number of people in the sample (25).

(c) Minimum height and minimum weight (169, 58.2).

(d) Maximum height and maximum weight (182, 84.5).

(e) Mode for height and mode for weight (the most common readings, 175, 67.4).

(f) Median for height and median for weight (the middle reading, 175, 70.1).

(g) Sort the table of data by height and check the mode and median obtained for height.

(h) Sort the table of data by weight and check the mode and median obtained for weight.

(i) Draw a scatter graph of weight (y) against height (x).

(j) Use the Trend function to estimate, to one decimal place, the weight of someone who is 175.5 cm tall (70.2 kg).

(k) Set up a bin range on your spreadsheet with values of 169, 170,....182, and produce a histogram for heights.

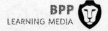

207

7 RETIREMENT

Open the spreadsheet Activity 7 Question.

	A	B
1	Retirement age	65
2		
3	Name	Vic
4	Age	66
5		
6	Years to retirement	Retired
7		
8		
9	Name	Age
10	Annette	38
11	Josephine	43
12	Mike	32
13	Paula	70
14	Vandana	42
15	Omar	34
16	Vic	66
17		

Tasks

In B4 insert a VLOOKUP function which will display the age of the person whose name is typed into cell B3.

In B6 insert the number of years to retirement (with reference to the value in B1). If the person has reached retirement age or is older B6 should state 'Retired'.

8 CHECK DATA

Open the spreadsheet Activity 8 Question.

Tasks

Change the font to Arial, size 10 apart from the title 'Questionnaire Analysis'. Change the headings to Arial size 12, bold and red. Adjust column widths if necessary.

Sort the table into female and male.

You need to use Data Validation to ensure that only people aged between 30 and 50 are to be included.

Show all cells which are outside of the data validation, take a screenshot (Alt + Print Screen) and paste it into a new worksheet named Validation.

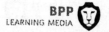

9 ORDER FORM

You will use a LOOKUP function to determine the rate of discount to be used when buying items from a wholesale retailer.

Open the workbook Activity 9 Question.

Tasks

Enter 12 in cell B7.

Enter a HLOOKUP function in cell B9 to return the correct discount rate for the number of items ordered. Format this cell as percentage.

Enter a formula in cell B11 to calculate the value of the order before discount.

Enter a formula in cell E11 to calculate the discount based on the rate shown in cell B9.

Enter a formula in cell B13 to calculate the value of the order after discount.

Now enter a VLOOKUP function in cell B9 to return the correct discount rate for the items ordered.

You should get the same answers as when using the HLOOKUP function.

10 EMPLOYEES

Open the workbook Activity 10 Question.

Tasks

(a) Insert a column between Date of birth and Department and title Age.

Using 31 March 2012 as the date, calculate the age of each employee.

(b) It has been decided to give a £25 bonus to all employees over the age of 40 (ie employees aged 40 and above) who have had fewer than 2 days absence in the year.

Enter Bonus in cell G1.

Use a nested IF function in cell G2, entering 25 in the Value_if_true field and 0 in the Value_if_false field (ie If age is greater than or equal to 40 *and* absence is less than 2, then a bonus is due).

Copy this formula down the Bonus column.

(c) In cell C22 enter Number of employees over 40. Use the COUNTIF function in cell D22 to calculate the number of employees over 40.

In cell C23 enter Average age of employees. Use the AVERAGE function in cell D23 to calculate the average age of employees.

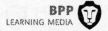

(d) Label cell H1 Retirement year.

In cell H2 use the YEAR function to find the year of birth for each employee and add 66 to it – this will give the year in which the employee can retire.

Copy this formula down the Retirement year column.

(e) Insert a column between First and Date of birth and title it Name.

Use the CONCATENATE function to join together the First name and Surname with a space in between. Hide columns A and B. Hide zeros in columns Absence and Bonus.

AAT AQ2013 SAMPLE ASSESSMENT

Assessment Book

This assignment is in **one** section.

You are required to open or download an existing spreadsheet (from LearnPlus or from a memory stick provided by your assessor) called **Assessment data** for some of these tasks.

All spreadsheets should be titled and contain a footer with your name, date and AAT registration number.

Answers are available for download. Type www.bpp.com/aatspreadsheets into your web browser.

You have two and a half hours (plus 15 minutes reading time) to complete the tasks and a high degree of accuracy is required.

You **MUST** save your work at regular intervals during this assessment to prevent you losing work.

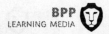

JA Muddlestone is a wholesaler of surplus stock which they resell to small traders, either via the sales team or over the internet on EBid. You are employed as an accounts clerk in the company. The computer system has crashed and the backup will not load due to a technical problem.

The accountant has asked you to collate some figures into a spreadsheet to give an overview of the activity for the last year.

Over the past year the monthly results have been as follows:

Sales

January	£45,360
February	£53,630
March	£89,340
April	£106,209
May	£119,416
June	£104,197

Expenses

January	£17,262
February	£21,837
March	£23,709
April	£31,286
May	£36,899
June	£36,401

Cost of sales

January	£15,626
February	£18,404
March	£22,416
April	£27,435
May	£31,533
June	£32,189

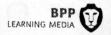

Task 1

Open a new workbook and save this as 'your initial, surname, date (DD.MM.YY)'
For example JSmith12.12.10SHS.

(a) Prepare a spreadsheet showing all the figures for sales, expenses and cost of sales. Formulate cells for January to show gross profit and net profit then copy these formulas into the remaining cells for February to June. Gross profit is sales less cost of sales, and net profit is gross profit less expenses. Use formulae to total each column.

(b) Gross profit margin is calculated as gross profit expressed as a percentage of sales revenue, and net profit margin as net profit expressed as a percentage of sales revenue. Use formula to calculate these figures for each month, and format the result as a percentage rounded to two decimal places.

(c) Title this worksheet as 'J A Muddlestone Monthly Figures for 2013' in Arial 10 Bold font in one merged cell centred over the data. Ensure all columns have appropriate headings in bold, and that all totals are displayed in bold font. Save as worksheet JAM 1.

(d) Copy JAM1 to a new worksheet and display as formula. Save this worksheet as JAM1(F). Print out one legible copy of JAM1 and JAM1(F), ensuring they each fit on to an A4 page.

Task 2

Open the EBid worksheet.

(a) Open a new worksheet and copy into it the information from the EBID worksheet. Give the new worksheet the title 'Ebid History' using font size 16, and centre the title on the page. Format headings to bold and ensure column widths and row heights are suitable. Then use the spellcheck function to check and resolve any errors.

(b) Insert a row between books and collectables, input 'coins' in column 'Auction Type', and '1910 SHILLING' in column 'Item'. Input bids 1 to 12 of £4, £31, £65, £84, £198, £175, £205, £265, £320, £289, £400 and £432, respectively.

(c) Insert two new columns between columns B and C using the column headings 'AVERAGE' and 'MEDIAN'. Use appropriate functions to calculate these for each of the items listed.

(d) Change the format of all numerical cells to currency rounded to the nearest

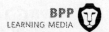

£. Use conditional formatting to change cell content to red for the highest bid for each item on the worksheet.

(e) Produce a line chart to show the bid history of JP computers. Insert the line chart below the bid figures, ensuring it is appropriately labelled and has a suitable title. Save worksheet as E-BID and print, ensuring the data and graph will fit on a sheet of A4 paper.

Task 3

Parkins Motors are a large car dealership, selling a range of luxury cars and accessories.

(a) Open the sales commission data for Parkins Cars – there are two worksheets for this, 'Saleforce results' and 'Parkins % commission rates'.

Copy and paste the data from the Parkins salesforce worksheet into a new worksheet, then use this and the data in the Parkins % commission rates worksheet. Insert formulae to calculate:

- (i) The commission earned by each sales person on each make of car (to two decimal places)

- (ii) The total of sales revenue earned by each sales person

- (iii) The total commissions earned by each sales person

- (iv) The total value of sales revenue for each make of car

- (v) The total value of commission for each make of car

(b) Format the spreadsheet with:

- Titles in bold

- Currency figures to two decimal places

- Column width adjusted as necessary, so that all figures and headings are visible

(c) Sort the spreadsheet alphabetically by family name order. Save the worksheet with the name 'Parkinsalphalist'.

(d) Copy the information from 'Parkinsalphalist' to a new worksheet. On the new worksheet, use a function to calculate the average value of total sales per sales person, clearly identifying this.

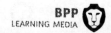

(e) If any salesperson has total sales of more than 20% above the average value for sales made by all the sales force, then a bonus of 0.5% of their individual total sales figure should be given. Head a column 'BONUS', use an 'IF' statement to calculate this bonus, and then total all bonuses to be paid.

(f) Insert a column to the left of all data and head this RANK. Then rank the spreadsheet by total sales value, from the highest to the lowest value. Display the results in ranked descending order of sales value. Save as worksheet with file name 'Parkinsranked'. Print this worksheet.

Task 4

Parkins Motors also sell a range of car accessories. These are sold across the country in showrooms, across the internet and from their own catalogue.

(a) Open the 'accessories' worksheet and copy this data to a new worksheet. Create two pivot tables: one to show the total sales revenue from the different ways the good were sold, and one to show the total sales revenue from each city in column B.

The pivot tables should be displayed to the right of the data provided, one under the other. Save this, naming the worksheet as 'Pivots'. Fill the cells yellow to show the city and the amount with the highest sales revenue, and the type of sale and amount that has the highest sales revenue.

Task 5

Short answer questions

Note. Candidates **must** tick a box to indicate their answer for each Task 5 question.

Example: ☐ Answer 1

☑ Answer 2

☐ Answer 3

I have **clicked** the box beside 'Answer 2' to indicate this is my chosen answer.

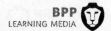

(a) If you wanted to annotate the data in a pie chart, what would you do?

☐ Name the axes.

☐ Use a legend.

☐ Write an explanation next to the chart.

☐ Give the chart a title.

(b) What would you use the PMT function for?

☐ Calculate the interest rate if you know the term and monthly payments of a loan.

☐ Calculate the term when you know the principal and interest rate of a loan.

☐ Calculate the payment if you have the principal, interest rate and term of a loan.

☐ Do a permanent memory transfer of data across workbooks.

(c) What does the error message '#REF!' mean?

☐ You have used a function instead of a formula.

☐ The formula you have entered is invalid.

☐ There is a problem with the cell reference.

☐ You have made an error with a mathematical sign.

(d) You require users to amend figures within a worksheet, but you also wish to prevent people writing in a number of key cells. What would you do?

☐ Hide the cells.

☐ Protect the cells.

☐ Use conditional formatting.

☐ Ask them not to alter anything on the worksheet.

(e) You need to use the Euro sign on a work sheet. What do you do?

☐ You cannot do this as it is not on the keyboard.

☐ Use an E as a recognised abbreviation.

☐ Format the cell as currency, and then select 'Euro'.

☐ Write 'Euro' as a heading to the column.

BPP PRACTICE ASSESSMENT

This assessment is in one section. All spreadsheets should be titled and contain a footer with your name, date and AAT registration number. You are required to open or download an existing spreadsheet (from the internet or from a memory stick provided by your assessor) for some of these tasks.

It is called 'Practice assessment data' and it comprises various worksheets within the workbook.

Answers are available for download. Type www.bpp.com/aatspreadsheets into your web browser.

You have two and a half hours to complete the tasks and a high degree of accuracy is required.

Open a new workbook and save it as PRACTICE ASSESSMENT ONE.

Scenario

Energysparks Ltd is a company which manufactures electrical goods. It operates three separate divisions in the UK: South West, Midlands and Wales. Performance figures for the last three months have just been made available, and you have been asked to provide an analysis of how the three divisions, and the company as a whole, have been performing. You have been supplied with the following data:

Sales:

South West	£399,000
Midlands	£598,650
Wales	£498,500

Cost of sales:

South West	£250,000
Midlands	£375,000
Wales	£375,000

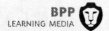

Overheads:

South West	£85,000
Midlands	£150,000
Wales	£100,000

Number of employees:

South West	120
Midlands	135
Wales	130

Total hours available:

South West	55,200
Midlands	63,000
Wales	75,000

Total hours worked:

South West	51,072
Midlands	63,856
Wales	68,040

Units produced and sold:

South West	319,200
Midlands	399,100
Wales	324,000

Task 1

(1.1) Enter the above data into a new worksheet (alter column widths as necessary) and use formulae to calculate the following for each area and as a total for the company (insert columns/rows as necessary):

- Gross profit
- Net profit
- Gross profit margin (gross profit divided by sales)
- Net profit margin (net profit divided by sales)
- Cost per unit (cost of sales divided by units produced)
- Output per worker (units produced divided by number of employees)
- Sales revenue per hour worked (sales divided by total hours worked)
- Labour utilisation rate (total hours worked divided by total hours available)

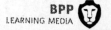

(1.2) The performance indicators gross profit margin, net profit margin and labour utilisation rate should be formatted as a percentage; sales per hour worked and cost per unit should be formatted as currency, and all figures should be expressed to 2 decimal places. Output per worker should be rounded up to the nearest whole number. Ensure the 1000's separator is used where appropriate.

(1.3) Insert the title 'Performance Indicators for Energysparks Ltd' and name the worksheet 'Perf Ind'. The title should be formatted as bold, Arial, font size 12, and should be centred across the page.

(1.4) Format the performance indicators calculated above as bold, italic and coloured blue.

(1.5) Print a copy of the worksheet and also print a copy showing the formulae used.

Task 2

(2.1) Produce a line graph to show the cost per unit and sales revenue per hour worked for each area. This chart should be titled 'Productivity indicators' and saved to a new worksheet; give the worksheet an appropriate name.

Task 3

(3.1) Open the Climates worksheet and copy the data to a new worksheet in the Practice Assessment One workbook.

(3.2) Calculate the average rainfall and average temperature for each City. Format the average rainfall and temperature to 1 decimal place.

(3.3) Label two rows as Minimum temperature and Maximum temperature and calculate the minimum and maximum temperature for each city.

(3.4) Use conditional formatting to highlight any month where the rainfall exceeds 10 cm.

(3.5) Use conditional formatting to highlight the highest temperature for each city.

(3.6) Save the worksheet as Climates and print a copy.

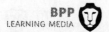

Task 4

(4.1) Open the worksheet Surveys and copy the data to a new worksheet in the Practice Assessment One workbook.

(4.2) Alter the font to Arial, size 12. Adjust column widths if necessary.

(4.3) Sort the table into alphabetical order by Surname. Save the worksheet as Survey Results.

(4.4) Create a PivotTable to show the number of men and women in each town in a new worksheet. Title the pivot table 'Female and male analysis'.

(4.5) Rename the worksheet Pivottown.

(4.6) Go back to the Survey Results worksheet. Use Data Validation to ensure that only people aged between 25 and 60 are to be included, ie born between 1 January 1952 and 31 December 1987. The Error Alert should read 'Persons should be between ages 25 and 60 only'.

(4.7) To test that your validation works, alter the year in the DOB for Robert Best to 1990.

(4.8) Show all cells which are outside of the data validation, take a screenshot (Alt + Print Screen) showing the first page with invalid data circled and paste into a new worksheet named Data Validation.

(4.9) Save your work (the data validation will disappear) and print a copy of the Survey results worksheet, fit to three pages tall.

Task 5

(5.1) Open the worksheet Invoice list and copy the data to a new worksheet in Practice Assessment One.

(5.2) Use a VLOOKUP formula to find the company names from the Customer list worksheet.

(5.3) The current rate of VAT is 20%, although it may change in the future. Use a formula to calculate the VAT amount for each invoice and the total of the invoice; use this formula for all invoices.

(5.4) The company operates a trade discount scheme. If the goods ordered are more than £750, then a discount of 5% is allowed. Insert a column between Amount and VAT and label accordingly. Use an IF statement to calculate any trade discount due.

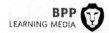

(5.5) If trade discount is taken, then this will affect the amount of VAT, as VAT is calculated on the discounted amount; amend your formula for VAT to take this into account.

(5.6) Format the worksheet so that zero values are not shown.

(5.7) Save this worksheet as Invoices and print a copy.

Task 6

Short answer questions:

(6.1) Which of the following is NOT useful at displaying negative numbers?

☐ Line graph

☐ Pie chart

☐ Column chart

☐ Bar chart

(6.2) The format in a formula '$B$9' is an example of what?

☐ Relative referencing

☐ Conditional formatting

☐ Currency

☐ Absolute referencing

(6.3) What does the error message '#VALUE!' mean?

☐ Value exceeds 1,000,000,000

☐ You are trying to multiply text by a number

☐ You have made an error with a mathematical sign

☐ You have tried to divide by zero

(6.4) What would you use the COUNTIF function for?

☐ Count the number of IF statements in a worksheet

☐ Count the number of cells that contain values

☐ Count the number of cells that meet a given condition

☐ Count the number of cells that are blank

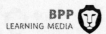

(6.5) You want to enable users to amend the data in a spreadsheet but not the formulas in key cells. What would you do?

☐ Press CTRL and `

☐ Protect and hide the cells

☐ Protect the worksheet

☐ Hide the cells

TEST YOUR LEARNING – ANSWERS

CHAPTER 1 Introduction to spreadsheets (Excel 2007)

1   Text, values or formulae.

2   F5 opens a GoTo dialogue box which is useful for navigating around large spreadsheets. F2 puts the active cell into edit mode.

3   You can use the technique of 'filling' – selecting the first few items of a series and dragging the lower right corner of the selection in the appropriate direction.

4   Select Formulas on the Ribbon then click Show Formulas. Alternatively press Ctrl + `.

5   Removing gridlines, adding shading, adding borders, using different fonts and font sizes, presenting numbers as percentages or currency or to a certain number of decimal places.

6   =IF(logical test, value if true, value if false)

7   (a)   =Sum(B4:B5) or =B4+B5
      (b)   =Sum(B5:D5)
      (c)   =Sum(E4:E5) or =Sum(B6:D6) or best of all to check for errors:
            =IF(SUM(E4:E5)= Sum(B6:D6), Sum(B6:D6),"Error")

8   (a)   =SUM(B4:B8)
      (b)   =C9*D1
      (c)   =D9+D10 or =D9*(1+D1)

CHAPTER 2 More advanced spreadsheet techniques (Excel 2007)

1   Save as

2   Data > Data Validation

3   The construction of a spreadsheet model with separate Input, Calculation and Output sheets. They can help consolidate data from different sources. They can offer different views of the same data.

4   Filtering allows you to see only areas of a table where there are certain values. Other items are filtered from view.

5   The trend line shows how one variable (for example cost) increases as another does (for example volume of production).

6   If data is ranked in ascending or descending order the median is the value of the middle item.

CHAPTER 3 Introduction to spreadsheets (Excel 2010)

1   Text, values or formulae.

2   F5 opens a GoTo dialogue box which is useful for navigating around large spreadsheets. F2 puts the active cell into edit mode.

3   You can use the technique of 'filling' – selecting the first few items of a series and dragging the lower right corner of the selection in the appropriate direction.

4   Select Formulas on the Ribbon then click Show Formulas. Alternatively press Ctrl + `.

5   Removing gridlines, adding shading, adding borders, using different fonts and font sizes, presenting numbers as percentages or currency or to a certain number of decimal places.

6   =IF(logical test, value if true, value if false)

7   (a)   =Sum(B4:B5) or =B4+B5
      (b)   =Sum(B5:D5)
      (c)   =Sum(E4:E5) or =Sum(B6:D6) or best of all to check for errors:
             =IF(SUM(E4:E5)= Sum(B6:D6), Sum(B6:D6),"Error")

8   (a)   =SUM(B4:B8)
      (b)   =C9*D1
      (c)   =D9+D10 or =D9*(1+D1)

CHAPTER 4 More advanced spreadsheet techniques (Excel 2010)

1   Save as

2   Data > Validation

3   The construction of a spreadsheet model with separate Input, Calculation and Output sheets. They can help consolidate data from different sources. They can offer different views of the same data.

4   Filtering allows you to see only areas of a table where there are certain values. Other items are filtered from view.

5   The trend line shows how one variable (for example cost) increases as another does (eg volume of production).

6   If data is ranked in ascending or descending order the median is the value of the middle item.

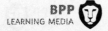

Test your learning – answers

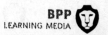

INDEX

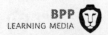